Emerging Trends in the Diagnosis and Intervention of Neurodevelopmental Disorders

Sanjeev Kumar Gupta
All India Institute of Speech and Hearing, India

Srinivasan Venkatesan
All India Institute of Speech and Hearing, India

S.P. Goswami
All India Institute of Speech and Hearing, India

Rajeev Kumar
Indian Institute of Technology Kharagpur, India

A volume in the Advances in Medical Technologies and Clinical Practice (AMTCP) Book Series

IGI Global
DISSEMINATOR OF KNOWLEDGE

Published in the United States of America by
IGI Global
Medical Information Science Reference (an imprint of IGI Global)
701 E. Chocolate Avenue
Hershey PA, USA 17033
Tel: 717-533-8845
Fax: 717-533-8661
E-mail: cust@igi-global.com
Web site: http://www.igi-global.com

Library of Congress Cataloging-in-Publication Data

Names: Gupta, Sanjeev Kumar, 1983- editor. | Venkatesan, S., 1961- editor. | Goswami, S. P. (Satpal P.), 1973- editor. | Kumar, Rajeev (Professor of computer science & engineering), editor.
Title: Emerging trends in the diagnosis and intervention of neurodevelopmental disorders / Sanjeev Kumar Gupta, Srinivasan Venkatesan, S.P. Goswami, and Rajeev Kumar, editors.
Description: Hershey, PA : Medical Information Science Reference, [2019] | Includes bibliographical references.
Identifiers: LCCN 2018011653| ISBN 9781522570042 (hardcover) | ISBN 9781522570059 (ebook)
Subjects: | MESH: Neurodevelopmental Disorders
Classification: LCC RC348 | NLM WM 168 | DDC 616.8/0475--dc23 LC record available at https://lccn.loc.gov/2018011653

This book is published in the IGI Global book series Advances in Medical Technologies and Clinical Practice (AMTCP) (ISSN: 2327-9354; eISSN: 2327-9370)

British Cataloguing in Publication Data
A Cataloguing in Publication record for this book is available from the British Library.

Advances in Medical Technologies and Clinical Practice (AMTCP) Book Series

Srikanta Patnaik
SOA University, India
Priti Das
S.C.B. Medical College, India

ISSN:2327-9354
EISSN:2327-9370

Mission

Medical technological innovation continues to provide avenues of research for faster and safer diagnosis and treatments for patients. Practitioners must stay up to date with these latest advancements to provide the best care for nursing and clinical practices.

The **Advances in Medical Technologies and Clinical Practice (AMTCP) Book Series** brings together the most recent research on the latest technology used in areas of nursing informatics, clinical technology, biomedicine, diagnostic technologies, and more. Researchers, students, and practitioners in this field will benefit from this fundamental coverage on the use of technology in clinical practices.

Coverage

- Patient-Centered Care
- Clinical Nutrition
- Clinical Data Mining
- Medical Imaging
- Biometrics
- Clinical High-Performance Computing
- Biomedical Applications
- Clinical Studies
- Neural Engineering
- Nursing Informatics

IGI Global is currently accepting manuscripts for publication within this series. To submit a proposal for a volume in this series, please contact our Acquisition Editors at Acquisitions@igi-global.com or visit: http://www.igi-global.com/publish/.

The Advances in Medical Technologies and Clinical Practice (AMTCP) Book Series (ISSN 2327-9354) is published by IGI Global, 701 E. Chocolate Avenue, Hershey, PA 17033-1240, USA, www.igi-global.com. This series is composed of titles available for purchase individually; each title is edited to be contextually exclusive from any other title within the series. For pricing and ordering information please visit http://www.igi-global.com/book-series/advances-medical-technologies-clinical-practice/73682. Postmaster: Send all address changes to above address.

Titles in this Series

For a list of additional titles in this series, please visit: www.igi-global.com/book-series

Optimized Genetic Programming Applications Emerging Research and Opportunities
Bahrudin Hrnjica (University of Bihac, Bosnia and Herzegovina) and Ali Danandeh Mehr (Antalya Bilim University, Turkey)
Medical Information Science Reference • ©2019 • 310pp • H/C (ISBN: 9781522560050) • US $225.00 (our price)

Design and Development of Affordable Healthcare Technologies
Arindam Bit (National Institute of Technology Raipur, India)
Medical Information Science Reference • ©2018 • 388pp • H/C (ISBN: 9781522549697) • US $245.00 (our price)

Optimizing Health Literacy for Improved Clinical Practices
Vassilios E. Papalois (Imperial College, UK) and Maria Theodosopoulou (Imperial College, UK)
Medical Information Science Reference • ©2018 • 338pp • H/C (ISBN: 9781522540748) • US $235.00 (our price)

Electrocardiogram Signal Classification and Machine Learning Emerging Research and Opportunities
Sara Moein (Mount Sinai School of Medicine, USA)
Medical Information Science Reference • ©2018 • 196pp • H/C (ISBN: 9781522555803) • US $160.00 (our price)

Research Advancements in Pharmaceutical, Nutritional, and Industrial Enzymology
Shashi Lata Bharati (North Eastern Regional Institute of Science and Technology, India) and Pankaj Kumar Chaurasia (Babasaheb Bhimrao Ambedkar Bihar University, India)
Medical Information Science Reference • ©2018 • 549pp • H/C (ISBN: 9781522552376) • US $255.00 (our price)

Microbial Cultures and Enzymes in Dairy Technology
Şebnem Öztürkoğlu Budak (Ankara University, Turkey) and H. Ceren Akal (Ankara University, Turkey)
Medical Information Science Reference • ©2018 • 413pp • H/C (ISBN: 9781522553632) • US $265.00 (our price)

Multifunctional Nanocarriers for Contemporary Healthcare Applications
Md. Abul Barkat (K.R. Mangalam University, India) Harshita A.B. (K.R. Mangalam University, India) Sarwar Beg (Jubilant Generics, India) and Farhan J. Ahmad (Jamia Hamdard, India)
Medical Information Science Reference • ©2018 • 602pp • H/C (ISBN: 9781522547815) • US $265.00 (our price)

Biomedical Signal and Image Processing in Patient Care
Maheshkumar H. Kolekar (Indian Institute of Technology Patna, India) and Vinod Kumar (Indian Institute of Technology Roorkee, India)
Medical Information Science Reference • ©2018 • 312pp • H/C (ISBN: 9781522528296) • US $265.00 (our price)

IGI Global
DISSEMINATOR OF KNOWLEDGE

701 East Chocolate Avenue, Hershey, PA 17033, USA
Tel: 717-533-8845 x100 • Fax: 717-533-8661
E-Mail: cust@igi-global.com • www.igi-global.com

Editorial Advisory Board

List of Reviewers

Table of Contents

Detailed Table of Contents

in many rare neurodevelopmental disorders, but the pathophysiology of audiological findings are seldom investigated. In this chapter, the authors highlight the possible relationship between underlying cause and the resultant audiological symptoms in some of the rare neurodevelopmental disorders. Further, the research studies on the audiological profiling in such disorders are discussed.

The chapter highlights the feeding and swallowing issues seen in children with neuro-developmental disorders, types, and extent of the problem across different disorders; its relation with the neuro-development of the child; effect on the quality of life of the parents/caregivers along with the child, specifically in the Indian context. It also focuses on the importance of assessment, team approach, and review of available tests for the assessment of feeding and swallowing problems in these children. The chapter is also going to give a few insights into the challenges faced by speech-language pathologists during the assessment of the feeding and swallowing issues in these children in the Indian scenario. The chapter will also include a section on applications of ICF model to feeding and swallowing issues in children with neurodevelopmental disorders.

Pediatric hearing aid fitting has always been a challenge for an audiologist. There are lots of technological advances in the field of hearing aids which are yet to be verified and used in the pediatric population. The chapter focuses on reviewing the recent advancements in hearing aid technology which can benefit children with hearing impairment. It is attempted to determine the application of these technology in pediatric hearing aid fitting. The lack of translational research to provide empirical evidence in this area is highlighted. It is stressed in the chapter that audiologists should use their clinical knowledge and use appropriate verification methods to make appropriate recommendations in pediatric hearing aid fitting.

The chapter attempts at bringing out an overview of linguistic-based deficits in neurodevelopmental disordered (NDD) population. Clinical linguistics as a discipline has provided a different dimension to view each patient as a distinctive case and has brought out the utilization of comprehensive depiction of individual skill patterns and deficits. As the NDDs are heterogeneous in nature, understanding their language deficits using achievement tests might not provide a clear description of these disorders. Hence, controlled experimental investigations using varied methodological designs could help in tapping their common linguistic variations which may augment key professionals to better identify, assess, and rehabilitate these individuals. While appreciating all these factors, the chapter provides first-hand information on some of the neuro-developmental disorders and also the language-based diagnostic markers to identify them.

The current chapter has reviewed the functional and structural brain connectivity in children with autism spectrum disorders (ASD). Neuropathological studies of the cerebral cortex in autism indicate abnormalities of synaptic and columnar structure and of neuronal migration. The MRI morphometry in young children with autism reveals excessive volume of cerebrum or cerebral white matter or increased total brain volume. The absence of such a volume difference in adults suggests that early hyperplasia in autism is followed by a plateau during which brain growth in normal subjects catches up. The developmental course of brain connectivity and the categorization potential of different connectivity process are important topics that are investigated by different studies. Finally, several studies contribute to a better understanding of the links between cellular abnormalities in the autistic cortex (both cerebral and cerebellar) and disturbances in network connectivity.

The high prevalence of autism spectrum disorder (ASD) has provided a spectrum of diagnostic methodologies ranging from screening scales to technological techniques. The technology-based techniques, especially eye trackers, are shifting the traditional subjective approaches to objective, leading to early ASD screening and intervention. The eye gaze deficits marked by eye trackers are the valid biomarkers of ASD, but the trackers are not clinically available. Another reason for non-availability is the limited number of methodologies which can meaningfully analyze gaze data. The assistance of new technologies into eye tracker system explored here can (1) detect gaze patterns and cognitive abilities of individuals at the single platform and (2) analyze eye movements and events automatically using deep learning system rather than manual interpretation of raw data. These types of systems, if implemented, have the potential to assist clinicians for better ASD diagnosis and intervention approaches.

The chapter intends to highlight the use of eye tracker, a tool that tracks eye movements, as a potential tool to aid diagnosis of specific learning disabilities along with psychometric tests. The issue of identifying and assessing children for specific learning disabilities is very difficult and crucial for the psychological, social, and personal wellbeing of the child growing into an adult. A common technique for diagnosing specific learning disabilities is the need of the hour. The eye is considered to be the window to the brain. Any differences in the eye movement can reflect disorders or diseases in the functional areas of cerebral cortex, brain stem, cerebellum, and other areas of the brain. The most important contribution of eye tracking research is it allows examination of different aspects of cognitive performance in moment-to-moment details on very simple tasks and infer the neurobiological basis of cognitive processes. Therefore, the chapter focuses on studies related to use of eye trackers as a futuristic technique in the diagnosis of specific learning disabilities.

Section 2
Neurodevelopmental Disorders: Intervention and Certification

The recent studies show that the children with learning disabilities numbers have been gradually increased in India. Though the main reason for the cause of this disorder is unknown, the authors strongly believe that this neurological disorder is explained as a genetic disorder passed from elder hierarchy to the next generation. With the available resources, the awareness programs are limited to urban areas only on account of using current technology in diagnosing disorders. In developed countries, it is seen that new technologies taking birth every day for the treatment of these disorders. This includes LCD 3D display, Kinect games, computer games (psychotherapeutic) in therapy sessions, etc. These kinds of games make children more attentive towards the intervention bringing new changes in the day-to-day lives of the children. In this chapter, a new algorithm has been highlighted for the intervention of children with dyslexia by using the Android application as a source to increase the level of perception and sound-symbol association of the respective alphabets used and studied.

Recent biological and behavioral studies indicate that several unhealthy alterations in ways of living (i.e., consumption-pattern, leisure activities, sleep routine, postures, breathing, stress-level, and use of high-tech gadgets) may be related with aggravation and augmentation of neurodevelopmental disorders. In this backdrop, it is important to recognize that yoga offers holistic knowledge for correction in lifestyle to not only prevent but also manage and alleviate neurodevelopmental disorders. Unfortunately, clinicians have been relying in their practice rather heavily on intrusive and pharmacological interventions and avoiding the use of sustainable techniques. Therefore, in order to increase awareness and promote its use in clinical settings, present work is ventured on the understanding effectiveness of and challenges in utilizing yogic practices for neurodevelopmental rehabilitation. It also identifies priorities for future research and action to amplify applicability of yogic lifestyle in hospitals, clinics, and other public health centers.

A play is referred to the language of children through which they express and communicate their feelings, thoughts, and behavior in a playful way. Play therapy enables children to gain an understanding of themselves and the world around them and helps them to overcome behavioral, emotional, social, and various other issues through play activities. The chapter majorly focuses on the effectiveness of play therapy in different neurodevelopmental disorders. Recent trends and studies suggested that play therapy is one of the most favored therapeutic approaches used in the children with various neurodevelopmental disorders.

With the emerging fields of medical jurisprudence and forensic medicine, cases of neurodevelopmental disorders in engagement or conflict with law are on the rise. Affected persons as alibi, victims, or perpetrators of crime are dotting as civil or criminal proceedings in contemporary courts. Rehabilitation specialists must be conversant with the medico-legal process, their duties, and responsibilities as subject experts to witness given their role in the certification of these cases. They must be aware of the problems and issues in certification during clinical practice. This chapter outlines the concerns related to estimation, measurement, and disability certification. Case vignettes are used to illustrate sample court proceedings during deposition before the attorney and at the time of cross-examination. Empirical research is reviewed before concluding this narrative with an agenda for future action to move away from traditional medical models toward understanding these disorders from human rights and person-in-environment perspectives.

Foreword

The edited volume of Neuro-Developmental Disorders (NDD) is a most welcome addition to libraries and professionals working in multidisciplinary teams dealing with NDD. Section 1 comprising of 8 chapters deal with multiple disorders coming under the umbrella of NDD such as Developmental Delays (DD), Intellectual Disability (ID), Autism Spectrum Disorder (ASD) and Cerebral Palsy (CP). All the chapters deal with overviews giving incidence and prevalence of the above conditions. The second section covers intervention and certification issues. However, the last and the most important chapter on certification and medico-legal aspect of NDD is a singular contribution that brings accountability and ethics into the foreground of the paraprofessionals who work with NDD population.

Each chapter can be read as a stand-alone chapter as well. Good number case illustrations, compact descriptive tables, extensive references and most importantly operationally defined key terms at the end of each of the chapters; enhance the quality of this contribution. Chapter 1 is a scholarly overview of NDD highlighting its conceptualizations, complex nature with overlapping manifestation of the conditions. It starts with a case study to make it an interesting read. Several case vignettes are interspersed in the text. This is followed by a compact table of 9 causes and correlates of NDD. These cover diet based, sensory, metabolic, neuroanatomy, neurophysiology, prenatal, natal/obstetric chromosomal and environmental causes. Similar compact table is offered for treatments. Various types of disorders and their classifications are discussed. Several theories such as social learning, family systems, synactive and socio-cultural theories, along with biology based theories and evolutionary theories are discussed. These are conventional psychological theories and not specific to NDD. But the Rights-based approach that is specific to NDD is highlighted even in the last chapter. The diagnostic challenge of overlapping syndromes too is described. The chapter also highlights the challenges of care taking patterns, especially in the world dominated by visual media. Though disorders are anchored to biological systems, there are in dynamic interaction with family, school, cultural and global interactive network. This comprehensive overview enables the reader to put together various available pieces in the chapters to follow into the puzzle that is NDD.

Chapter 2 is a review chapter, focusing specially on "rare NDD" which is outside the ambit of the previous chapter. It enhances the incidence and prevalence of hearing deficits in different disorders under NDD. Rare disorders are defined as prevalent one in 1000 to 2000. The review covers 7000 rare disorders out of which 15% have significant hearing loss. But these are caused by the disorders themselves. 8 specific syndromes including musculo skeletal system, endocrine and metabolic systems are discussed. This descriptive account gives very useful information. The chapter is not intended to be meta-analysis.

Feeding and swallowing problems as present in different disorders under NDD are described in Chapter 3. The focus is on assessment. There are four components namely oral, triggering of swallowing reflex, pharyngeal phase and esophageal phase. Table 4 briefly gives a very precise description. Feeding disorders are provided with case illustrations for Cerebral Palsy (CP), Intellectual Disability (ID) and Autism Spectrum Disorders. Some modes of medical and non-medical assessment are specific to disorders, while others are common to all the disorders as summarized in Table 2. Table 3 provides details of body structure, activities, participation, emotional and personal social factors. This highlights the combination of biological, psychological and environmental contributions. One study in the Indian context providing Feeding Handicap Index (FHIC) has 38 items, physical, factional and emotional domains. It has been validated on CP, ADHD and ASD children. Ethical aspects are rightly flagged, and early intervention and creation of public awareness are recommended. Yet the treatment of NDD remains a challenge as it requires a multidisciplinary approach to deal with the client and caregivers.

Chapter 4 is on Application of advanced hearing aid technology in paediatric hearing aid fitting technologies such as Directional microphones, Digital noise reduction algorithms, open fit receivers as against closed ones, Frequency lowering technology and Channel FreeTM hearing aids are described. Most importantly, valuable information provided on their advantages and disadvantages for the younger and older children being at variance with the experience of adult patients. Evidence-based approach to research is recommended, yet it is rendered very difficult to as there are large number of technology aids marketed and upgraded frequently and are very expensive. While the actual use tends to spread very slowly amongst the user population. A word of caution from the authors is that it is better to rely on the feedback on the use of these aids by the children and their parents than relying on the marketing claims.

NDD is viewed from Clinical Linguistic perspective in Chapter 5, developmentally delayed and intellectually disabled are studied based on assessment. An excellent table provides a list of commonly used tools. These consist of tests of Intelligence, SLD and Communication Disorders, ASD, Motor Disorders, ADHD and Sensory Impairments. The aspects affected by these conditions are phonetics, phonology, syntax, morphology, semantics, pragmatics and also mean length of sentence. However, these occur in different combinations in different disorders, especially so, when there is overlap. Language achievement tests do not evaluate dynamic processing in real time.

Chapter 6 is on recent advances and neural connectivity in autism. The focus is on structural and functional connectivity in children with ASD. Multiple findings are quoted implicating various parts of brain, early onset related to the specific brain regions. These are studied through PET, MR1, fMR1, blood flow studies of physiological aspects in a heterogeneous group of NDD. However, in present chapter focus is on ASD.

Chapter 7 deals with eye tracker as an assistive tool to diagnose ASD. This offers a new approach to qualitatively as well as quantitatively monitor eye movements as a diagnostic tool. Seventeen studies are given in detail in the table. These tools are expensive, too complex and require training to administer. There is an additional chapter that is Chapter 8, that deals with eye tracking specifically in SLD but it adds very little to the earlier chapter.

To summarise this section, the eight chapters give descriptive account of NDD, their characteristics, conceptualization, assessment and possible interventions. Both common disorders such as ASD, CP, ADHD and SLD along with some rare disorders that do not fall in their ambit are provided. To conclude, this section does not comprehensively cover the issues to be addressed. But it fills the vacuum in the conceptualization with some useful information. When one has a mix of symptoms, disorders and varied assessment findings, the research outcome compounded. For example, ICD 11 views NDD (under cluster 2) and does not include ADHD under this cluster. Many of the diagnostic categories such as elimination, eating/feeding disorders and selective mutism are in the yet to be assigned to any group.

Developmental learning disorder with impairment in written expression is characterized by significant and persistent difficulties in learning academic skills related to writing, such as spelling accuracy, grammar and punctuation accuracy, and organization and coherence of ideas in writing. The individual's performance in written expression is markedly below what would be expected for chronological age and level of intellectual functioning and results in significant impairment in the individual's academic or occupational functioning. Developmental learning disorder with impairment in written expression is not due to a disorder of intellectual development, sensory impairment (vision or hearing), a neurological or motor disorder, lack of availability of education, lack of proficiency in the language of academic instruction, or psychosocial adversity. Terms such as Dyslexia, academic skills deficit disorder or Specific Learning disability are used interchangeably with term referred above as Developmental Learning disorder.

Nature of learning, language, feeding processes as well as neural connectivity and eye tracking are discussed. The above chapters provide much needed details about phenomenology, assessment and possible aetiology of NDD. This section can act as a spring board for evidence-based research in the Indian context.

Section 2 shares the plight of all 'process and outcome evaluation' in therapeutic interventions. It is hard enough to find evidence-based study through meta-analysis among adults. With children, it is much harder as developmental and socio-cultural contexts play a key role. It will suffice to say NDD group is the most challenging group to provide intervention. This section highlights these issues. Thus, if the chapter titles may appear idiosyncratic and intriguing, it must be condoned. Pet assisted therapy with some proven efficacy, diet related therapy in ASD, a popular yet somewhat biased view of its efficacy, biofeedback backed by research among adults, remains through popular, need to be empirically examined with NDD children. Play is much recommended for children, but evidence-based research is required for NDD group. Finally, much touted Android applications seem to suggest that unless time intensive individually tailored algorithms are developed, it is too early, to judge its effectiveness. It may be said animal-assisted, play and behavioural and other therapies that work with children should be tried for the NDD groups.

More specifically, Chapter 9 focuses on Animal Associated Therapies and demands for more physician participation in practice and research. It is recommended as an adjunct to other therapies. The chapter provides an excellent overview of its use in the health, education and therapy in the treatment of ASD. Fascinating details are offered about the various animals used in very positive results. Cautions are given about personal safety and hygiene. However, evidence-based research is possible only with the cooperation of the treating physician. The chapter highlights the need to educate, motivate and carry out research by multidisciplinary teams deals with NDD. The chapter ends with solutions and recommendations to educate, motivate, research by multidisciplinary teams who use this intervention. However, availability of Pet assisted interventions though desirable for NDD group, experienced therapists are hard to come by across India, though available in very few places like Pune. Their use especially in institutions can be very effective in enhancing quality of life especially for child population.

Chapter 10 is titled "Autism and Diet: An Insight Approach." The focus is on pre and post nature maternal nutrition and nutrition and brain development of the foetus, infant and child along with its effects on cognitive abilities. Roles of various nutrients in the mother and the child are described. Feeding difficulties in ASD is highlighted. There is a chart on Gluten Free Diet – gluten is one of the commonly implicated culprits. Parent education, nutritional supplements and behavioural treatments are recommended.

Chapter 11 deals with Application of Biofeedback (BF) in NDD. BF is a non-invasive technique to electronically monitor normal autonomic bodily functions such as skin conductance, brain waves, heartbeat, respiration, palatograph (tongue and palate) and visual imaging. The feedback given along any of the above channels, enables the subject to gain control over the respective psychological and physiological functions by the subject himself. Though much research is available for adults, the use of BF in NDD is largely unexplored. A suggested model by the author is a five-tier model which described in detail as a possible framework. A review of studies in 7 diagnostic categories is methodically listed out with relevant details. There is strong possibility and promise but it is a long way to go before the efficacy is proven.

Chapter 12 is "Learn Easy: Android Application as a Technological Intervention for Children With Dyslexia." The term Dyslexia being term used by lay persons does not fall under the current classificatory systems. The authors list out multiple computer games. They report that new algorithms were developed for three children and were found to be effective and show 40% to 50% improvement. Generalizability is questionable as we are dealing with a very heterogenous entity. Perhaps each child's own profile of varied academic skill deficits should be used to develop individually tailored algorithm for that particular child.

Chapter 13, "Yogic Care for NDD Rehabilitation: Bringing Life Into Treatment, Management, and Prevention," is an ambitious and a curious title. A reasonable overview of various yogic techniques is given as applicable to adult population. Details of research in yoga, challenges are highlighted in depth for adult population. Specific issues of the above NDD population have received scant attention.

Chapter 14 is on play therapy for NDD. Description of play methods, practitioner's applications to various groups of disorders of children are described. The Axline model of child centred play therapy is described in detail. Theoretically anchored approaches such as psychoanalytic, Structured, Adlerian, parent interaction based therapies are described. The wide range of specific play activities such as toys used for play activities individual feeling/word games are described. However, only two studies are reported on play in the NDD group. Efficacy of play therapy has been supported in other disorders. But it is essential to tailor the play techniques have been supported in other disorders in the context of the salient features of ASD in particular. There are specifically developed play techniques for ASD group but it is hard to access the information or get trained in their use.

Chapter 15 is on certification and medico-legal aspects of neurodevelopmental disorders in India. The last and the most important contribution to the compilation. The theme of certification is the least understood and most essential component in the bread and butter aspects of rehabilitation of NDD especially in the legal context. Majority of the practitioners are unaware of legal complications arising out of their wards symptoms. An extensive list of the legal terms is elaborated at the end of the chapter and is a must read for everyone involved with NDD – both when young and across ages as these present in courts. The chapter attempts to move away from medical model of certification to NDD advocacy/ activism by paraprofessional multidisciplinary team members.

The chapter is an extraordinary documentation of legal scenario elsewhere in the world and focus especially in the Indian context. The approach advocates strongly rights-based approach. This is an important guideline for not only NDD rehabilitation team, but also for mental health teams consisting of clinical psychologists, psychiatric social workers, psychiatric nurses, care takers in institution and homes. The main responsibility rests on them to protect their vulnerable clients within the legal system. List of tools of assessment and clarification criteria are given in detail which can be very useful to any practitioner with multiple disorders (Table 1 and 2). This is followed by seven illustrative case vignettes. The authors' own such cites of 75 cases with legal system at seven levels. These cover marriage, education, health, housing, reimbursement, employment, inheritance, citizenship and political participation. Heinous crimes by minors (legal) illustration examines the dilemma of adult with reliability and validity of certificates as cause or consequence of individual's condition. According to the authors the actual percentage of disability is not as critical as the actual consequence of the impact of impairment. This is the finest discussions on forensic aspects and is highly recommended to the readers.

My compliments to the editor for bringing out this excellent compilation. There may be a good number of excellent and extensive works being carried out in many centres for NDD in India. Unfortunately, by not publishing the practitioners keep the benefits only to a limited population and prevent other practitioners from learning from them. This leads to reinventing the same exercises, which is entirely due to lack of networking among the paraprofessionals. In this context, this book offers many deep insights. It is left to the reader to assimilate what is valuable and reject the spurious claims.

Malavika Kapur
National Institute of Advanced Studies, India

Preface

The initiative to edit and produce this book was inspired by the children with neurodevelopmental disorders (NDDs). Due to the awareness and early identification of the children, more children are being diagnosed with NDDs. NDDs encompass a group of conditions with onset during the developmental period. It includes intellectual disabilities, communication disorders, autism spectrum disorder, attention-deficit/hyperactivity disorder (ADHD), specific learning disorder, and motor disorders. Two or more of these conditions frequently co-occur. These disorders affect language, cognitive, motor, learning, behavioral, and social development with lifelong consequences.

The World Health Organization estimates that 15-20% of children, worldwide, have disabilities; 85% of which are in developing countries (World Health Organization, 2011). As per 2011 Census of India, there are 7,862,921 children with disability in the below 19 year age group, including 1,410,158 visual impairment, 1,594,249 hearing impairment, 683,702 speech disorder, 1,045,656 movement disorder, 595,089 intellectual disability, 678,441 multiple disability, and 1,719,845 other disabilities (Ministry of Home Affairs, Government of India, 2011). Silberberg et al. (2014) conducted a study in India and reported the countrywide results (excluding Tribal data) revealed that from 10% (Hilly areas), 13% (Urban areas), to 18% (Rural areas) of children ages 2-9 yrs were found to have one or more NDDs. The tribal prevalence was 4.96%, perhaps reflecting lower infant and child survival.

Boyle et al. (2011) reported the prevalence of developmental disabilities based on parental responses to survey questions. Approximately 15% of children in the United States aged between 3 to 17 years were affected by NDDs, including ADHD, learning disabilities, intellectual disability, cerebral palsy, autism, seizures, stuttering or stammering, moderate to profound hearing loss, blindness, and other developmental delays, in 2006–2008. Among these conditions, ADHD and learning disabilities had the greatest prevalence. Many children affected by NDDs have more than one of these conditions: for example, about 4% of U.S. children have both ADHD and a learning disability (Pastor & Reuben, 2008). Early screening, identification and assessment can be a valuable tool in determining diagnosis, prognosis, functional abilities and formulating clinical intervention for such population.

Children's brain is plastic at the early age and can be adapted with drill practices and cognitive training programs. The term 'brain plasticity' refers to the capacity of the central nervous system to modify its structure and function. Cioni, Inguaggiato, and Sgandurra (2016) reported that early identification of infants at risk for NDDs is a major prerequisite for intervention programs. This ensures that interventions which aim to positively modify the natural history of these disorders can start in the first weeks or months of life. There is empirical support for the clinical utility of cognitive training in ADHD (Abikoff, 1991), computerized training of working memory in ADHD (Klingberg, Forssberg, & Westerberg, 2002; Klingberg et al., 2005), cognitive training technologies in autism spectrum disorders (Wass & Porayska-

Pomsta, 2014), auditory training in autism (Bettison, 1996), and executive function training in learning disabilities (Gupta & Venkatesan, 2014a; Gupta & Venkatesan, 2014b). The behavioral intervention program is also effective to improve the skill behavior and to reduce the problem behaviors in NDDs.

Early screening, identification, assessment, diagnosis, and rehabilitation of NDDs can help affected children to improve the quality of life and lessen the economic and social burden on the caregiver. Parent or caregiver is the backbone for the treatment. Training of the parent or caregiver and teachers is the need of the hour for the sustainable rehabilitation of children with NDDs. Conducive environment for the children with NDDs is effective not only for the physical wellbeing but also for mental health. A multidisciplinary team can be helpful to deal with most of the aspects of NDDs.

While addressing children with NDDs and their behavior problems, health and rehabilitation professionals should also consider caregiver's physical and psychosocial health, as this may also have an impact on children's well-being (Lach et al., 2009). Craig et al. (2016) suggested that both mothers and fathers of children with different type of NDDs should be supported with interventions and resources to empower them with the knowledge and skills to reduce their stress and to enhance their quality of life.

Emerging Trends in the Diagnosis and Intervention of Neurodevelopmental Disorders can be used as a stepping stone for further research and clinical practice in the field of NDDs. This book offers a range of useful topics from analysis of themes and issues to certification of NDDs for stimulating ideas, debate, and discussion by researchers, academician, and practitioners for the pursuit of sustainable intervention and long-term care of the affected person. This book is organized into two sections and 15 chapters. Section one, which covers chapter one to chapter eight, elaborates on characteristics, issues and assessment of NDDs. Section two, which covers chapter nine to chapter fifteen, focuses on intervention and certification of NDDs. A brief description of each of the chapters is given below.

SECTION 1: NEURODEVELOPMENTAL DISORDERS – CHARACTERISTICS, ISSUES, AND ASSESSMENT

Chapter 1 attempts to highlight the origins, history, classification, theories, nature, types, and misperceptions about NDDs. The fears of making no diagnosis, patient's perspective, evidence-based practice, and static versus dynamic diagnosis, cultural practices, and other related issues in Indian scene are also addressed.

Chapter 2 reports the possible relationship between underlying cause and the resultant audiological symptoms in some of the rare NDDs. Further, the research studies on the audiological profiling in such disorders are discussed.

Chapter 3 highlights the feeding and swallowing issues in children with NDDs. It focuses on the types, extent of the problem across different disorders, its relation with the neurodevelopment of the child, effect on the quality of life of the parents/caregivers along with the child, specifically in the Indian context. The chapter also covers the importance of assessment, team approach, and review of available tests for the assessment of feeding and swallowing problems in these children.

Chapter 4 reviews the recent advancements in the hearing aid technology which can benefit children with hearing impairment. The author attempts to determine the application of advanced technologies in pediatric hearing aid fitting. The lack of translational research to provide empirical evidence in this area is highlighted. It is suggested that audiologists should use their clinical acumen and use appropriate verification methods to make appropriate recommendations in pediatric hearing aid fitting.

Chapter 5 attempts at bringing out an overview of linguistic-based deficits in NDDs. Clinical Linguistics as a discipline has provided a different dimension to view each patient as a distinctive case and has brought out the utilization of comprehensive depiction of individual skill patterns and deficits. The current chapter provides first-hand information on some of the NDDs and also the language based diagnostic markers to identify them.

Chapter 6 reviews the functional and structural brain connectivity in children with autism spectrum disorder (ASD). The chapter reports neuroanatomical defects in ASD, that occur during the early stages of brain development such as hypoplasia at specific areas as well as excessive cerebral growth lead to abnormalities in the development of functional systems of autism.

Chapter 7 covers the technology-based techniques, especially eye trackers for ASD screening and intervention. The chapter reports the assistance of new technologies into eye tracker system and explores the potential to assist clinicians for better ASD diagnosis and intervention approaches.

Chapter 8 intends to highlight the use of eye tracker as a potential tool to aid diagnosis of specific learning disabilities along with psychometric tests. The chapter focuses on eye tracking system, eye tracking paradigms, data analysis & coding, and studies related to use of eye trackers as a futuristic technique in the diagnosis of specific learning disabilities.

SECTION 2: NEURODEVELOPMENTAL DISORDERS – INTERVENTION AND CERTIFICATION

Chapter 9 reports animal-assisted therapy may be an effective alternative method for treating ASD. The chapter also discusses the necessity for physician participation, the reasons for the lack of clinician participation in such research, and recommendations for encouraging physician and policymaker participation in specifically targeted research studies for ASD.

Chapter 10 evaluates the role and effectiveness of diet in children with ASD. The children with ASD may be sensitive to the taste, smell, colour and texture of foods. Therefore chapter highlights various issues pertaining to ASD such as the impact of maternal nutrition, nutritional deficiencies and GFCF diet in ASD.

Chapter 11 covers the application of biofeedback as a therapeutic module for the children with NDDs. This chapter outlines the meaning, nature, types, protocols, procedure, practices, challenges, benefits, future research directions and limitations in the use of biofeedback for the population of NDDs.

Chapter 12 highlights the importance of LearnEasy-Android application in the treatment of children with dyslexia. The chapter highlights a new algorithm for the intervention of children with dyslexia by using the Android application as a source to increase the level of perception and sound-symbol association of the respective alphabets used and studied.

Chapter 13 presents yoga as a therapeutic approach and reports that yoga offers holistic knowledge for correction in lifestyle to not only prevent but also manage and alleviate NDDs. In order to increase awareness and promote the use of yoga in clinical settings, the present chapter is ventured on the understanding effectiveness of and challenges in utilizing yogic practices for neurodevelopmental rehabilitation.

Chapter 14 reports the definition of play and play therapy and also highlights the effectiveness of play therapy in various NDDs. Play therapy is one of the most favored therapeutic approaches used in the children with various NDDs.

Chapter 15 outlines the concerns related to estimation, measurement and disability certification. The rehabilitation or medical professionals must be aware of the problems and issues in certification during clinical practice. The authors have given the case vignettes to illustrate sample court proceedings during deposition before the attorney and at the time of cross-examination. The authors also advocate the human rights and person-in-environment model rather than traditional medical model.

In conclusion, this book is intended to throw light upon various perspectives of NDDs. As a comprehensive collection of current research findings, this publication provides researchers, practitioners, academicians, health care professionals, and policymakers a complete understanding of NDDs issues, challenges, certification and their rehabilitation.

Sanjeev Kumar Gupta
All India Institute of Speech and Hearing, India

Srinivasan Venkatesan
All India Institute of Speech and Hearing, India

S. P. Goswami
All India Institute of Speech and Hearing, India

Rajeev Kumar
Indian Institute of Technology Kharagpur, India

REFERENCES

Abikoff, H. (1991). Cognitive training in ADHD children: Less to it than meets the eye. *Journal of Learning Disabilities*, *24*(4), 205–209. doi:10.1177/002221949102400404 PMID:1875155

Bettison, S. (1996). The long-term effects of auditory training on children with autism. *Journal of Autism and Developmental Disorders*, *26*(3), 361–374. doi:10.1007/BF02172480 PMID:8792266

Boyle, C. A., Boulet, S., Schieve, L. A., Cohen, R. A., Blumberg, S. J., Yeargin-Allsopp, M., ... Kogan, M. D. (2011). Trends in the prevalence of developmental disabilities in US children, 1997–2008. *Pediatrics*, *127*(6), 1034–1042. doi:10.1542/peds.2010-2989 PMID:21606152

Cioni, G., Inguaggiato, E., & Sgandurra, G. (2016). Early intervention in neurodevelopmental disorders: Underlying neural mechanisms. *Developmental Medicine and Child Neurology*, *58*(S4), 61–66. doi:10.1111/dmcn.13050 PMID:27027609

Craig, F., Operto, F. F., De Giacomo, A., Margari, L., Frolli, A., Conson, M., ... Margari, F. (2016). Parenting stress among parents of children with neurodevelopmental disorders. *Psychiatry Research*, *242*, 121–129. doi:10.1016/j.psychres.2016.05.016 PMID:27280521

Gupta, S. K., & Venkatesan, S. (2014a). Reappraisal of research on executive function training in children with learning disabilities. *International Journal of Psychology and Psychiatry*, *2*(1), 7–18. doi:10.5958/j.2320-6233.2.1.002

Gupta, S. K., & Venkatesan, S. (2014b). Efficacy of training program on executive functions in children with learning disability. *Guru Journal of Behavioral and Social Sciences, 2*(2), 283-291. Retrieved from http://gjbss.org/wp-content/uploads/2014/03/gjbss_Vol2_Issue2_Paper1.pdf

Klingberg, T., Fernell, E., Olesen, P. J., Johnson, M., Gustafsson, P., Dahlström, K., ... Westerberg, H. (2005). Computerized training of working memory in children with ADHD-A randomized, controlled trial. *Journal of the American Academy of Child and Adolescent Psychiatry, 44*(2), 177–186. doi:10.1097/00004583-200502000-00010 PMID:15689731

Klingberg, T., Forssberg, H., & Westerberg, H. (2002). Training of working memory in children with ADHD. *Journal of Clinical and Experimental Neuropsychology, 24*(6), 781–791. doi:10.1076/jcen.24.6.781.8395 PMID:12424652

Lach, L. M., Kohen, D. E., Garner, R. E., Brehaut, J. C., Miller, A. R., Klassen, A. F., & Rosenbaum, P. L. (2009). The health and psychosocial functioning of caregivers of children with neurodevelopmental disorders. *Disability and Rehabilitation, 31*(8), 607–618. doi:10.1080/09638280802242163 PMID:19360498

Ministry of Home Affairs, Government of India. (2011). *Census of India, 2011*. Retrieved from: http://censusindia.gov.in/ 2011-common/censusdataonline.html

Pastor, P. N., & Reuben, C. A. (2008). Diagnosed attention deficit hyperactivity disorder and learning disability: United States, 2004-2006. *Vital and Health Statistics. Series 10, Data from the National Health Survey*, (237): 1–14. PMID:18998276

Silberberg, D., Arora, N., Bhutani, V., Durkin, M., Gulati, S., Nair, M., & Pinto-Martin, J. (2014). Neuro-developmental disorders in India-From epidemiology to public policy (I10-1.006). *Neurology, 82*(10Supplement), I10–I11.

Wass, S. V., & Porayska-Pomsta, K. (2014). The uses of cognitive training technologies in the treatment of autism spectrum disorders. *Autism, 18*(8), 851–871. doi:10.1177/1362361313499827 PMID:24129912

World Health Organization. (2011). *World Report on Disability 2011*. Retrieved from: http://www.unicef.org/protection/ World_report_on_disability_eng.pdf

Acknowledgment

First and foremost, we would like to thank all the authors for their research contributions and scientific knowledge, which they have meticulously put in a consolidated manner in the form of a chapter.

Secondly, we wish to graciously thank and acknowledge the active involvement of the editorial advisory board members and reviewers for the improvement of the quality, coherence, content, organisation and presentation of the chapters. Some of the authors also served as reviewers. We highly admire their dual role.

Editing a book is a challenging academic work and required mutual support from the authors, reviewers and many more for the quality of content and timely completion of the book project. Therefore, we would like to thank everyone who has helped us directly or indirectly. We look forward to collaborating with them on another exciting and interesting project.

We are also thankful to Dr. S. R. Savithri, Director, All India Institute of Speech and Hearing, Mysuru for providing the support and encouraging us to work relentlessly for the benefit of the individual with disabilities and their caregivers.

Finally, we thank the IGI Global team, Hershey, PA, for their wonderful eEditorial Discovery online platform, which makes the editorial task easy and fast.

Sanjeev Kumar Gupta
All India Institute of Speech and Hearing, India

Srinivasan Venkatesan
All India Institute of Speech and Hearing, India

S. P. Goswami
All India Institute of Speech and Hearing, India

Rajeev Kumar
Indian Institute of Technology Kharagpur, India

Section 1

Neurodevelopmental Disorders:

Characteristics, Issues, and Assessment

Chapter 1
Analysis of Themes and Issues in Neurodevelopmental Disorders

Srinivasan Venkatesan
All India Institute of Speech and Hearing, India

ABSTRACT

The study of neurodevelopmental disorders is beset with many issues and pitfalls. If its types are attempted to be explained at the molar developmental, environmental, and behavioral level, there is another explanation at the molecular brain or genetic level. The clinician can stumble into an error at any level while addressing these conditions. The origins and history of the neurodevelopmental model are followed in this chapter by sections on classification, theories, nature, types, and misperceptions. A lifespan approach, use of clinical reasoning, and decision making to sift critical signals from considerable noise during diagnosis are cautioned. The fears of making no diagnosis, patient's perspective, evidence-based practice, and static versus dynamic diagnosis, cultural practices, and other related issues in Indian scene are addressed. Ongoing and unexplored areas like use of animal models, delay versus difference approach, and contemporary parenting practices are explained with a status report on available treatments and engagements to be undertaken in future.

INTRODUCTION

The typical story is about a single child born to a highly paid career-driven professional couple in their mid-thirties. They are married from the different language and cultural backgrounds. There is often a short stint abroad during the first two years of their child's life with a huge mismatch between their native languages or culture to the foreign one. Often friendless in the foreign soil, save their weekend partying companions of Indian origin, they would have employed a babysitter to look after the child during the day. The toddler is kept engaged by the babysitter for feeding, dressing, watching television, or fiddling the latest versions of electronic gadgets. Opportunities for peer play outside their apartment are restricted if not absent. Either there is fear of infection or there are no similar aged kids from the

DOI: 10.4018/978-1-5225-7004-2.ch001

same ethnic background. Armed with this baggage of skewed and under-stimulated early childhood history, the child is back to India on a vacation only to discover his same-aged cousins are toilet trained, speaking fluently, or about to leave for a preschool. The grandparents, often belonging to a language different from the child's mother, struggle to communicate with their grandchild given the different accent and poor English.

Shocked and surprised by the developmental lag in their child, the parents rush to seek a series of consultations. The professionals, on their part, consulting from their closed air-conditioned chambers instruct the parent to set the child free for that momentary observation. When left free, the ever hand-held child rushes around in excitement of the new environment. He does not respond to the doctor's call for restraint much to the chagrin and felt shame or insult by the parents. Meanwhile, the doctor has already decided on the diagnosis for the child as 'autism' or 'attention deficit hyperactivity disorder'. He prescribes medicines with tips on restricted diet, vitamin supplements, scans, EEG investigations, and yoga. Meanwhile, discussions begin at home to retain the child with grandparents in India while the working parents get back abroad with a promise to relocate at least one of them by resigning their job. The grandparents are left to begin the second journey of care giving the grandson. Having lost touch with such skills over the decades, a local helper is recruited. The child develops behavior issues which are perforce yielded, handled inconsistently, and attributed to his primary condition. The local preschools give admission to the toddler only to soon realise that he is lacking in social, play, communication and motor activities although 'gifted' in handling gadgetry. Thereafter, the tussle for rejection by the school and the plea for retention by the guardians begin.

The neurodevelopment framework is based on a synthesis of research from neuroscience, molecular or developmental genetics, neuroimaging, cognitive psychology, child and adolescent development, and related fields concerned about brain functions. It is to do with how these functions affect behavior and even their illness, disease, or disorder manifestations. Rapid advances in these disciplines over the last 2-3 decades have influenced the conceptualization of neurodevelopmental disorders (NDD). With a characteristic developmental perspective, the signs and symptoms of NDD are sought to be understood within the context of the brain growth trajectory. It uses the phenomena like gene mutations, unfolding genetic architecture, myelination, the influence of environment on genes (called epigenetics), and DNA methylation as core concerns to explain the molecular basis of NDD. This model posits that the illness is the end stage of the abnormal neurodevelopmental process that began years before the onset of the illness. For example, developmental insults as early as the first trimester can lead to the activation of pathologic neural circuits during adolescence leading to the emergence of positive or negative symptoms as schizophrenia (Fatemi & Folsom, 2009). Beginning from embryonic mal-development, there is assumed cortical mal-development with insults hitting during two critical time points once at early brain development and once again during adolescence (Keshavan, 1999).

ETIOLOGY

Given below is a short list of causes attributed to NDD:

- Evidence from brain pathology (enlargement of cerebro-vascular system, changes in gray and white matters and abnormal laminar organization);

- Genetics (changes in the normal expression of proteins that are involved in the early migration of neurons and glia, cell proliferation, axonal outgrowth, synaptogenesis, and apoptosis);
- Environmental factors (obstetric complications, births due to prenatal viral or bacterial infections);
- Gene-environmental interactions (candidate genes are regulated by hypoxia, micro-deletions and micro-duplications or over-representation of pathogen-related genes;
- Multiple markers of congenital abnormalities, such as agenesis of corpus callosum, stenosis of Sylvian aqueduct, the presence of low set ears, epicanthic folds, and wide spaces between first and second toes are suggestive of first trimester anomalies;
- Abnormal dermatoglyphics is indicating a second-trimester event, and;
- The presence of pre-morbid soft neurological signs in children who develop later NDD is all characteristic features frequently noted in the literature.

In an extensive profile of commonly reported birth factors from available case records of a clinical population of nearly 1500 cases with NDD, it was found that attempted abortion, use of teratogenic drugs, maternal ill health and hypertension were among the prenatal factors, absent birth cry, unsupervised delivery at home, absent birth cry, and low birth weight were among natal factors, and convulsions following high-grade fever was listed under postnatal factors (Venkatesan & Rao, 1996).

Further, prenatal exposure to rubella or influenza in the first trimester, the presence of maternal antibodies has been all identified as potential environmental risk factors (Arndt, Stodgell, & Rodier, 2005). Brain gene expressions are also implicated as biological markers in deciphering the molecular mechanisms for the genesis of certain forms of NDD. It may not be that the genes and/or environment act alone. Their interactions combined with obstetric complications maybe increasing the risk for these disorders. NDD is predominantly understood as genetic in origin. It has been thought as falling under many groups. The first includes a large number of individually rare syndromes with genetic causes. The second group is idiopathic cases with no known cause. Critics of this model claim that it does not fully account for a number of features in most NDD, including the long gap between neurodevelopmental insult and the development of symptoms. Another viewpoint is that different forms of NDD (such as autism, schizophrenia, and bipolar disorder probably share the same genetic overlap (Carrol & Owen, 2009).

By default, one must expect or search for aetiology of NDD in isolation or as a relatively curious admixture of genetic, intrauterine, prenatal or natal exposure to toxins, inborn errors of metabolism, infections or other obstetric complications, poor maternal health, and environmental factors that aggravate the propensity or predilections to develop these conditions (Kelleher & Corvin, 2015). Complex human phenotypes of NDD range from autism, ADHD, to schizophrenia, bipolar disorder, OCD, addictions, as well as anxiety are shown to have multiple risk factors, wide differences in individual vulnerability and resilience to early insults or exposure which leave an impression of the causes as probably being multi-factorial in nature (De Felice, Ricceri, Venerosi, Chiarotti, & Calamandrei, 2015). Based on their hypothesized genetic etiology, NDD are divided into four sub-groups. Those based on: (a) abnormal number of chromosomes (Down's syndrome with a trisomy of a chromosome); (b) chromosomal micro-deletions in certain regions (William's Beuren Syndrome; (c) single gene affected conditions (Fragile X Syndrome), and; (d) complex aetiologies (autism and schizophrenia). Questions remain whether the shared genetic basis of NDD really does exist and if so, can they be objectively and reliably mapped at all (Jensen & Girirajan, 2017). Wherein genetic mutations and polymorphisms are involved, do they occur in a single gene or a cluster of genes (Batool & Arooj, 2016)?

Inheritance of one NDD also confers an increased risk for other similar disorders in the same family. For example, monozygotic twins are reported to have higher concordance rates for ADHD and SLD than for autism. Relatives of schizophrenia are reported as more likely to develop bipolar disorder, depression, or anxiety as compared to the general population. Models to explain the immune etiology of NDD have included direct cause-effect relationship to the endocrine system and gastrointestinal tract (Bilbo & Schwartz, 2012). The molecular landscape has become more complex with the discovery of a micro RNA-small sequence of approximately 22 nucleotides from non-coding RNA (Khansari & Sperlagh, 2012). Similarly, mitochondrial dysfunctions and NDD is found to be statistically correlated although no disease provoking mechanism has been demonstrated (Marazziti, Baroni, Picchetti, Landi, Silvestri, Vatteroni, & Dell'Osso, 2012). Meanwhile, studies on fatty-acid metabolism, especially omega-3 deficits, are noted in NDD (McNamara & Strawn, 2013). Another inhibitory/excitatory imbalance model attempts to explain the social and cognitive deficits in NDD (Rubenstein & Merzenich, 2003). A link between hypothalamic-pituitary-adrenal hormonal effects to the symptoms of these disorders is proposed (Romano, Cosentino, Laviola, & De Filippis, 2016). Microbiome refers to a community of microorganisms such as bacteria, fungi, and viruses that inhabit a particular environment, especially within the human body. Emerging evidence suggests that the gut microbiota plays a role in shaping cognitive networks encompassing emotional and social domains in NDD (Kelly, Minuto, Cryan, Clarke, & Dinan, 2017; Tognini, 2017). Several other epigenetic pathways are being implicated to NDD, such as, anomalies in synaptogenesis (formation of synapses between neurons), myelination (a sheath covering nerve cell that serves as electrical insulation), DNA methylation (a mechanism which controls gene expression), etc.

Going through all of these, searches for 'biomarkers' as a measured characteristic which may be used as an indicator of some biological state or condition, are being initiated. For example, the recent discovery of MRI biomarker in the form of excess fluid surrounding the brain in toddlers who are siblings of a patient with autism (Shen, Nordahi, Young, Wotton-Gorges, Lee, Liston, Harrington, Ozonoff, & Amarai, 2013) has led to a program on early intervention. Attempts are on to establish genetic markers through linkage analysis at the individual as well as population levels. However, till date, biomarkers have not been shown to be a reliable and valid measure of the aetiological processes in NDD. Association studies on candidate genes and genome-wide linkage analyses have identified many susceptibility chromosomal regions and genes, but considerable efforts to replicate association have been surprisingly often disappointing (Martens & van Loo, 2007). While the search for neurobiological and genetic causes in NDD is on, proponents of the environmental basis for these conditions are not far behind. The notion of intra-uterine environment and the susceptibility of the growing fetus, especially the brain and nervous system, to toxic chemicals in the first trimester of pregnancy (such as thalidomide, misoprostol, and valproic acid) is well recorded (Landrigan, Lambertini, & Birnbaum, 2012). Exposure to insecticides, flame retardants, lead, ethyl alcohol, mercury, or several other chemicals causing developmental neurotoxicity is reiterated (Landrigan, 2010). A summary list of causes and correlates of NDD, although not claimed to be exhaustive, is given in Table 1.

In sum, moving from genes to neurobiology in NDD is not a smooth flow. No single risk factor explains NDD. Both inherited and non-inherited factors contribute and their effects are independent. These conditions are familial and heritable. Even as the arena to understand the causative elements in NDD is still unclear, treatment approaches are equally diverse, multiple, ad hoc, tentative, lacking in specificity, and not necessarily always evidence-based (Homberg, Kyzar, Stewart, Nguyen, Poudel, Echevarria... & Pittman, 2016; Hu, Chahrour, & Walsh, 2014). Genetic contributions to disorder do not necessarily mean that medications are the treatment of choice (Thapar, Cooper, Eyre, & Langley, 2013).

Table1. Summary List of Causes and Correlates of NDD

Category of Cause	Examples
Diet-Based	Alpha Protein Deficit, Diet Disturbances, Enzyme Dysfunction, Food Additives, Food Allergies, GFCF, Leaky Gut, Nutritional Deficiency, Poor Nutrition, Low Levels of Fatty Acids, Protein Energy Malnutrition or Marasmus, Kwashiorkor, vitamin and mineral deficiency (Zinc, Magnesium and Vitamin B6), Oxidative Stress, etc.
Sensory	Auditory, Gustatory, Hypersensitivity, Hyposensitivity, Excitatory, Inhibitory, Olfactory, Tactile, Vestibular, Visual, pain and hearing sensitivity most affected by autism, sensory dysregulation is reported in ADHD, etc.
Metabolic	Maternal antibodies and cytokines, untreated phenylketonuria, disorders of cholesterol and tetrahydrobiopterin metabolism, etc.
Neuroanatomy/ Neurophysiology	Amygdala Neurons, Missing brain protein, Poor Bone Morphogenetic Proteins (BMP) Signalling, CNS Malformations, mitochondrial aberrations, disrupted fetal immunity, higher gray matter than white matter volumes observed in autism, smaller brainstem volume and cortical surface area seen in Prader-Willi Syndrome, abnormalities in the development of astrocytes, etc.
Prenatal	Maternal use of tobacco, drugs and alcohol, exposure to teratogenic pesticides (endosulfan), Vitamin and Folic Acid Deficiency, ultrasound, x-ray or ionized radiation, Exposure to Polychlorinated biphenyls used as cooling agents in fridges, Arsenic, Mercury or Lead Poisoning, Syphilis/HIV/Viral Infection, Maternal Chronic Illness, Rubella, Toxoplasmosis, Preeclampsia, Placental Insufficiency, maternal antibodies crossing the placenta, etc.
Natal/Obstetric	Difficult Labour, Anoxia, Hypoxia, Absent Birth Cry, Prematurity, Preterm, Post Term, Low Birth Weight, Birth Trauma/Injury, Neoplasm, MMR Vaccine, Infectious Diseases like Meningitis or Encephalitis, Rh Incompatibility, Gestational diabetes, breech, Paternal & Maternal Ageing, etc.
Chromosomal	Abnormalities by way of extra or deficient in number, micro-deletion of chromosomes, pre-synaptic dysfunction, synapse disconnection, etc.
Environmental	Accidents, physical trauma, closed head injuries, crushing injury, poor parenting, emotional trauma, Excess Hygiene, deprivation or poor stimulation, refrigerated mother, excess preoccupation with gadgetry, poor sleep habits or hygiene, familial, Environmental Toxicants like plastic-derived chemicals, persistent organic pollutants, heavy metals, etc.

ORIGINS AND HISTORY

The notion of early insults to development of the brain or central nervous system unfolding as the individual develops or grows is ancient. Although the neurodevelopmental models were pioneered to explain schizophrenia (Kochunov & Hong, 2014; Gupta & Kulhara, 2010), thereafter, it has been used to explain many neuropsychiatric conditions including anorexia nervosa (Connan, Campbell, Katzman, Lightman, & Treasure, 2003), Angel man Syndrome (Micheletti, Palestra, Martelli, Accorsi, Alli, Glordano, Trebeschi, & Fazzi, 2016; Li & Qiu, 2014; Summers, 2012), Prader-Willi Syndrome, Backwith-Wiedemann Syndrome, Fragile X Syndrome, Rett syndrome, Rubinstein-Taybi Syndrome, Williams Syndrome (Chailangkarn, Trujillo, Freitas, Hrvoj-Mihic, Herai, Diana, ... & Stefanacci, 2016), alcoholism, psychoses (Read, Fosse, Moskowitz, & Perry, 2014), obsessive compulsive disorder (OCD; Ivarsson, Weidle, Skarphedinsson, & Valderhaug, 2017; Rosenberg & Keshavan, 1998), and bipolar disorder (O' Shea & McInnis, 2016), substance use (Fishbein, Rose, Darcey, Belcher, & VanMeter, 2016).

The neurodevelopmental *m*odel owes its origins to the Scottish psychiatrist Thomas Clouston, who coined the term 'developmental psychosis' in 1873 when he pointed to the frequency of a family history *a*nd minor physical abnormalities in a group of insane patients. Emile Kraepelin later named it 'signs of degeneracy' in schizophrenia and called the mental illness as a form of dementia. From this perspective, it came to be viewed as adult-onset NDD marked by the progressive decline of brain functioning.

However, in the 1980s, there was a renewed interest in the role of obstetric complications and seasonal influences as the neurodevelopmental basis for schizophrenia. Based on this model, assessment, case formulation, labeling, and therapeutic interventions are all advocated by physical, occupational and speech therapists (Solomon, Hessl, Chiu, Olsen, & Hendren, 2009; Couriel, Bisse, Miller, Thomas, & Clarke, 1993). Historically, the physiology, pharmacology, and treatment targets of these disorders were conceptualized in terms of neurons, neurotransmitter levels, and synaptic receptors.

The neurodevelopmental hypothesis was proposed in the United States (Weinbeger, 1987) and in the United Kingdom (Lewis & Murray, 1987). Later, neuropathological reports of abnormalities in the hippocampus in affected brains or disrupted neuronal migration were invoked to lend support to this model. Other ideas like prenatal exposure to influenza were also attributed. It has been always difficult to prove a causal link for these observations in individual patients. Despite these setbacks, this hypothesis marched on fuelled by cohort studies which showed subtle developmental delays, solitariness, and intellectual deficits in pre-schizophrenic children. A part of the success of this approach can be attributed to its elasticity. It exists in several forms at some point to the effect of pre and peri-natal hazards on early brain development, others attribute it to deviations in brain maturation in adolescence (Keshavan, 1999). As a whole, there is a wide range of developmental points when causative 'lesions' might arise. Moreover, some of these conditions dubbed as NDD are not degenerative in the sense of their being marked by gliosis, a proliferation of glial cells in the affected areas of the brain.

Much effort has been devoted to the study of biological markers by way of mapping pattern of brain electrophysiology, fMRI, or cognitive performance. Termed as 'endophenotypes' they are measurable parameters they are sometimes termed as intermediate phenotypes because they are thought to be on the pathway between genes and the clinical phenotype. The study of intermediate phenotypes has also not yielded many positive results. Whole genome scanning or the studying a single gene candidate in an individual has given genetic researchers a fresh avenue. The attempt is to compare the genetic profile of normal controls and a group of people with the disease condition. Comparison of large-scale samples is expected to lead to the identification of susceptibility genes.

The move away from the use of typical antipsychotics, such as chlorpromazine and haloperidol since the development of new antipsychotics like clozapine, risperidone and olanzapine have renewed interest in dopamine. These new agents initially marketed as superior to the earlier drugs for controlling certain positive symptoms failed miserably in ameliorating negative symptoms and for cognitive impairment. Other social-psychological movements during those times like deinstitutionalization and works on optimum expressed emotions, use of cognitive behavior therapies have all moderated the excessive enthusiasm on neurodevelopmental issues. These developments have changed definitions, diagnosis, and dimensions on taxonomy and classification of the diseases or disorders (Herwegen, Riby, & Farran, 2015). Thus, the Diagnostic & Statistical Manual (DSM) criteria used in the United States, and the guidelines for International Classification of Diseases (ICD), followed by signatory nations of the World Health Organization (WHO) have since then undergone drastic changes. Perhaps the frustration with the inconsistencies and changeability of NDD, it has led to the contemporary viewpoint that these conditions may exist as different symptoms occurring in differing degrees in different people. Clinicians are busy prescribing medicines for individual cases whereas the researchers are recruiting subjects from various diagnostic categories and normal controls. There is growing concern and consensus that all the conditions under NDD should be integrated and subsumed under a single entity as developmental delay or difference but complimented by ratings on different dimensions like positive/skill behaviors and negative/problem behaviors. As it stands today, the story of NDD is still evolving. It is not a closed one.

Technological advances have often held the key to define NDD. Rather than questioning the basic premise or validity of the model itself, the debate is on early versus late developmental lesions. So central has become the model that the entire classificatory systems have been revised to fit into them. Epidemiology has become more than a mere head-counting exercise. It is used as the basis for a new genetics. A newfound optimism has erupted on how molecular genetics holds the key for many answers they were looking for through population genetics. To put things in perspective and explain the origins of the neurodevelopmental notions, one may have to take refuge under the 'terroir model' of neurodevelopment (Figure 1). The gene-environment interaction is understood as five layered model with the surface representing the personal expression and symptoms we see as phenotypes of the underlying unseen core that represents the genes of that person held as genotype. Interventions targeted at level four might include behavioral interventions such as applied behavior analysis, physiotherapy, occupational therapy, speech and language therapy and cognitive behavior therapy. Level three targeted interventions include pharmacotherapy while interventions targeting level two might be a biomedical approach like methylation through methylcobalamin or folinic acid; a nutraceutical approach such an omega 3 fatty acids, or high dose micronutrients, or antioxidants targeting oxidative stress, inflammation, or immune function. A level one intervention could be gene modification. None of these interventions targets solely one level (Hagerman & Hendren, 2014; p. 5; Riva, Bellugi, & Denckla, 2005).

The conditions which are now deemed as falling under the category of NDD was earlier explained or understood based on overt symptoms. Later, they were explained on the basis of presumed underlying causes. While these shifting trends from molar to molecular is appreciated, one must wait and see the trends that are likely to emerge in terms of nomenclature, labeling, taxonomy, assessment, intervention for these conditions in future. It will also have ideological, political, economic and social overtures. Admittedly, there is still very less known about the molecular basis of these disorders.

Figure 1. Terroir model (Source: Hagerman & Hendren, 2014; p. 5)

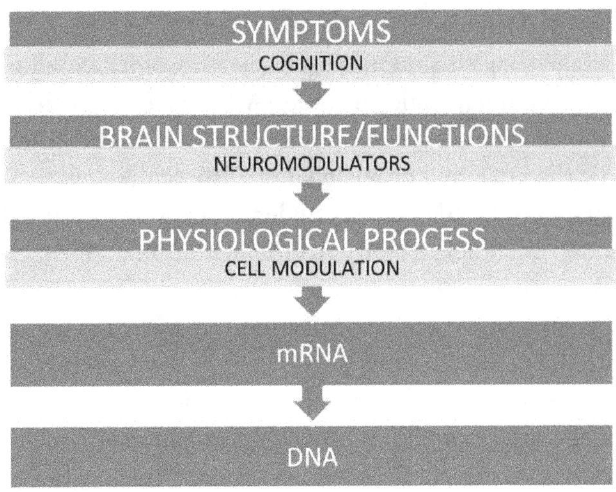

TYPES AND OFFICIAL CLASSIFICATION

There is no single agreed upon list of NDD. In the current psychiatric nosology, NDD is classified on the basis of observable behavioral, phenomenological, and/or morphological features. Even though the identification of molecular substrates for these conditions has long been underway there is little success in listing their biomarkers. In short, the accumulating data suggest, perhaps not surprisingly in retrospect, that genetic risks do not conform to the boundaries defined in the current, categorical diagnostic nosology (State & Levitt, 2011). Questions are raised whether biologically based disorders can be identified or classified based on behaviourally defined criteria for diagnosis and treatment. The specific behaviors included in the diagnostic frameworks may be able to tell individual differences. To conclude that such behaviors constitute abnormality might be largely based on arbitrary decisions strongly influenced by cultural values and expectations (Norbury & Sparks, 2013). It is recommended that an etiology based diagnosis and classification of NDD would be more appropriate. Wilska and Kaski (2001) explored the possibility of aetiological classification based on timing and type of injury to the central nervous system (CNS). They divided them as genetic causes, CNS malformations and multiple malformation syndromes of unknown origin, external prenatal factors, perinatally acquired disorders (−1 to +4 weeks from delivery); post-natal acquired disorders, and untraceable or unclassified causes.

The two major diagnostic classification systems for mental and behaviour disorders used across the world are the DSM published by American Psychiatric Association and ICD issued by WHO. Until the publication of DSM-III (APA, 1980) and DSM-IV (APA, 1994) and DSM-IV-TR (APA, 2000), there is no mention of the term NDD. However, many of the clinical conditions listed under its 'Axis I: Disorders usually first diagnosed in infancy, childhood, or adolescence' have since then been renamed as 'neurodevelopmental disorders' and along with its list of diagnostic categories first appear in the DSM-5 (APA, 2013). The multiaxial system of diagnosis is now abandoned in DSM-5. These disorders:

typically manifest early in development, often before the child enters grade school, and are characterized by developmental deficits that produce impairments of personal, social, academic, or occupational functioning. (APA, 2013, p. 31)

The official list under DSM-5 includes: intellectual disability (intellectual developmental disorder), global developmental delay, language disorder, speech sound disorder, childhood onset fluency disorder (stuttering), social (pragmatic) communication disorder, ASD, ADHD, specific learning disability (SLD), developmental coordination disorder, stereotypic movement disorder, Tourette's disorder, persistent (chronic) motor or vocal tic disorder, and provisional tic disorder. A new section titled as 'neurodevelopmental disorders' was first introduced officially under the DSM, 5th Edition by replacing its earlier 4th Edition wherein the old label 'Disorders usually first diagnosed in infancy, childhood, or adolescence' was used. The DSM-5 classification includes two new categories of brain dysfunction: NDD with onset in developmental period and major neurocognitive disorders (e.g. Alzheimer's disease) with onset in later life (Harris, 2014). It emphasizes clinical formulation whereby the diagnostician can specify association with a known genetic condition by name as well as mention the clinical significance of the disorder by stating the thresholds of a person's distress or impairment in relation to ones daily life.

ICD-10 describes a distinct axis of NDD as a group of conditions with three main criteria: onset in infancy or childhood, impairments related to central nervous system maturation; and expressed steadily without remissions or relapse (WHO, 2008). The Chapter V, Mental and Behavioural Disorders of International Statistical Classification of Diseases and Related Health Problems, 10th Revision (ICD-10; WHO, 1993) makes no distinct mention of the term 'NDD' except one stray observation that 'children also develop HIV-associated NDD characterised by development delay, hypertonia, microcephaly, and basal ganglia calcification' (WHO, 1993; p. 54). However, a list of conditions close to what may be presumed as NDD is available in this classification, such as, a developmental disorder of scholastic skills, autistic disorder, Rett's syndrome, childhood disintegrative disorder, Asperger's Syndrome, Pervasive Developmental Disorder. With Working Groups moving towards the ICD-11 to be published shortly, the indications are that there will be a change in name, definition, and framework for several NDD in consonance with DSM-5 (Salvador-Carulla, Bertelli, & Martinez-Leal, 2018; Doemberg & Hollander, 2016; Carulla, Reed, Vaez-Azizi, Cooper, Leal, Bertelli, ... & Girimaji, 2011). With the advent of rights-based person-in-environment approach, the contemporary ICF-CY (WHO, 2007) is also up-in-arms against the symptom-oriented medical models of ICD and DSM. In the absence of biomarkers, diagnostic criteria for what is presumed as NDD will continue to depend on the phenomenology of surface features of behavior (Mahdi, Viljoen, Yee, Selb, Singhal, Almodayfer, ... & Bölte, 2017; Bölte, Schipper, Robison, Wong, Selb, Singhal ... & Zwaigenbaum, 2014).

A key element in the diagnostic decision making for NDD continues to be based on molar observations or reporting of overt signs and symptoms (Baird, 2013). This is in spite of the continuing notions of NDD being founded upon the assumed brain-behavior molecular inter-relationships (Gabriele, Tobon, D'Agostino, & Testa, 2018). The persistent question is, whether there is a common genetic etiology that explains the high degree of co-morbidity among these disorders? These apparent contradictions have prompted questions like: Are we searching for a needle in a haystack? Are we searching for a needle in different haystacks? Or are we searching for the same needles in different haystacks?

With another growing differentiation between congenital neurodevelopmental and neuropsychiatric disorders, with significant aetiological heterogeneity between these two conditions, are there candidate genes that are commonly shared to represent an interconnected molecular system (Cristino, Williams, Hawi, An, Bellgrove, Schwartz, da F Costa, & Claudianos, 2014)? If this is so, by implication for their treatment, is it possible to reverse certain molecular, electrophysiological and behavioral deficits associated with these disorders in adults by genetic or pharmacological manipulations (Castren, Elgersma, Maffel, & Hagerman, 2012)? Unfortunately, the answers to these questions are only more questions. Are we getting somewhere there? It is not that we have actually got there. The diagnosis of NDD is fraught with several problems, issues, and challenges. Clinicians need a clear understanding of 'developmental standards' expected of same age peers before viewing a client's behavior in that background and context. Understanding the nature, type or extent of non-verbal communication social and play is critical in the evaluation or diagnosis of NDD (McNeil, 2017). The recent advances in gene discovery in the area of NDDs have to lead to a re-conceptualization of diagnostic boundaries of many psychiatric conditions. Since they continue to be based on overt or observable behavioral symptoms, it throws the question whether there is need to develop an alternative, more biologically relevant nosology (Kim & State, 2014)?

A differential diagnosis is a systematic method of diagnosis used to identify the presence of a disorder where multiple alternatives may be possible. Children with NDDs represent a very heterogeneous population, which suggests that having a common diagnosis does not always imply the same presentation of symptoms or the same response to treatment efforts. Therefore, differential diagnosis is imperative as similar behavioral manifestations may exist across disorders and similar behaviors may manifest differently within a disorder. By understanding the commonalities and differences within NDDs, one can appropriately differentiate among them and implement the most effective interventions to address the unique needs of the child.

A variety of theories are postulated to explain NDD. The ***theory of mind*** seeks to explain a related set of intellectual abilities that enable us to understand how others have beliefs, desires, plans, hopes, information and intentions like our own although different from us. It involves joint attention, complex perceptual recognition like face and gaze processing, language, composite executive functions, such as tracking intentions, goals and moral reasoning, emotion processing like recognition, empathy and imitation. The maturation of several brain systems combined with parenting, social relations, training and education shape these behaviors which are characteristically affected in NDD (Korkmaz, 2011). Others have proposed a ***compensation-based theory*** of NDD which views that the human brain has the ability to rely on alternative neural routes when there is brain damage. Focal brain damage during pre/perinatal period may be compensated for by early reallocation of function to intact brain regions. There can be shallow compensation as in developing good social skills by a student with a learning disability, or deep compensation as mastery in non-academic activities. It could also be a matter of genuinely delayed neural maturation (Livingston & Happe, 2017). ***Social learning theory*** has been proposed as a framework for recreational therapy intervention in children with NDD (Johnson, 2017). By doing so, the higher incidence of obesity, emotional and mental health issues, and behavior problems are seen in these persons as a consequence of which intervention is needed. Other theories on abnormal neurodevelopment have posited prenatal and perinatal alterations. A ***family systems theory*** attempts to explain NDD in the socio-cultural context (Helps, 2016; Goepfert, Mule, von Hahn, Visco, & Siegel, 2015). ***Biology-based theories*** try to understand or explain NDD based on factors like epigenetics, neurodevelopment, and plasticity alone although such unidirectional searches have not gained success. Going by the observations that persons with NDD are 'doubly vulnerable' owing to their impaired cognition, communication, mobility or limited social interactions, and are prone to suffer from systemic social, economic and political discriminations that prevent access to better opportunities, ***rights-based theories*** argue for improvements in their quality of life (Racine, Caron, & Stanton-Jean, 2018). ***Evolutionary theories*** based on Darwinism ask the question as to why NDD was not eliminated by natural selection (Ploeger & Galis, 2011). Another ***synactive theory*** of development is proposed by Heildelise Als, American neuropsychologist as a keyword to NDD (Maltese, 2017). It identifies an interactive and hierarchical process including five subsystems: (1) neuro-vegetative or autoimmune system; (2) motor system; (3) behavior system; (4) attention-to-interaction system, and; (5) self-regulation system. Attempts are on to apply ***Vygotsky's Socio-cultural Learning Theory*** and its concept of Zone of Proximal Development (ZPD) to understand NDD (Yan-bin, 2009).

DIAGNOSTIC CHALLENGES

Diagnostic decision making is not an all or none phenomenon. There are various types, levels and shades of it. It progresses in discrete interconnected stages beginning data mining, a decision tree, diagnostic routing through provisional to the final diagnosis, wading through differential diagnosis, labeling, and classification until the eventual communication of the condition is made to the affected individual and/or their family. The culminating point of this entire progression is eventual understanding and acceptance of the nomenclature before proceeding to intervention or treatment planning and programming. Diagnostic success leads to therapeutic success. There are pitfalls at every stage of this rather elaborate scientific process of arriving at a diagnosis. The clinician can stumble into diagnostic error or pseudo-diagnosis. It must take into account considerations like misperceptions about diagnosis, lifespan approach, use of clinical reasoning and decision making to sift critical signals from considerable noise while attempting a diagnosis, the fears of making no diagnosis, patient's perspective on diagnosis, evidence-based diagnosis, static versus dynamic diagnosis, cultural practices in diagnosis, and others. Some key problems and issues related to diagnostic decision making especially with relevance to NDD in the country is given below.

(i) Overlapping Boundaries

A frequently encountered issue by practicing clinicians in the context of diagnosis is the overlapping boundaries between conditions that are deemed as NDD. The most common confusions happen between Intellectual Developmental Disorder (IDD), ASD and Schizophrenia Spectrum Disorders (SSD). Owing to their similarities in clinical presentation, a failure to invest time or effort by the diagnostician, poor reporting by informants, a hurried clinic based observation, or such other factors can contribute to diagnostic errors (Bertelli, Merli, Bradley, Keller, Varrucciu, Furia, & Panocchia, 2015). Clinical experience shows that there is incongruence or lack of agreement not only between parents describing the behavioral assets and deficits in a given child but also, between parent reports and professional observations of the same child. The tendency for misdiagnosis is greatest between childhood psychoses and those with globalized developmental delays (Dossetor, 2007). Wherein persistent biological disturbances related to sleep and appetite is present, it may be taken as a discriminatory feature towards a diagnosis of psychoses more than autism. However, these complaints need to be authenticated by a proper record of sleep diaries, family sleep practices, and daytime activity level of the child. Faulty sleeping or feeding practices, when probed in detail, often emerge for a simple correction rather than a prescription of drugs for the same. Moreover, the relatively lower levels of diurnal physical activities in most children with NDD may predispose them to have decreased nocturnal sleep or even lowered appetite which cannot be construed as biological disturbances.

(ii) Diagnostic Conundrum

The scenario of diagnosis for NDD in India poses some unique issues and problems. There is a growing popularity of child psychiatry clinical conditions like autism, attention deficit hyperactivity disorder (ADHD) and SLD. Take the instance of diagnostic overshadowing, wherein a clinician or caregiver tends to attribute each and every behavior of the child after a brief observation within the four walls of a clinic as a reflection of their primary condition. A problem behavior in a child with IDD, for example, may be interpreted as due to that condition than owing to caregiver mismanagement (Jones, Howard, & Thornicroft, 2008; Reiss & Szyszko, 1983; Reiss, Levitan, & Szyszko, 1982).

While there has been a significant rise by almost four times in the quantum of publications on SLD in India from the base years <=1990s to the present (Venkatesan, 2017a), it is noted that there is no uniformity in the nomenclature, definition, and/or inclusion/exclusion criteria as adopted by the various researchers. This makes it futile to attempt a meta-analysis or any meaningful comparison between these research papers. A similar conclusion was made in another related but different study on concept analysis of SLD across 30 online or offline research articles as published by authors of Indian origin across 26 indexed national and international journals in 2014-15 (Venkatesan, 2016). More than half of the reviewed publications gave no operational definition of SLD. They did not explain its meaning, or enunciate its features. Moreover, a comparative analysis of the similarities and differences between 23 official definitions of learning disabilities derived from various sources showed a plurality with little agreement on what qualities characterize the condition (Venkatesan, 2017b). Given these diagnostic confusions on what is what is not SLD Indian context (Venkatesan, 2012) and given the demonstration that its presenting complaints vary with age/stage at which they are seen (Venkatesan, 2007), a culture-specific lifespan-based model on diagnostic decision tree has been proposed (Venkatesan, 2017c). The decision tree-based approach to identification and diagnosis of SLD offers a dynamic mapping background for prospective practitioners by invoking a longitudinal lifespan perspective on changing presenting complaints, its causes, characteristics and consequences in given instances of such affected students.

The preceding discourse on diagnostic confusions and challenges with regard to SLD is equally true for autism. Till date, there is no official India-specific estimate on the prevalence of autism. Despite the growing popularity of the term and added to this, there is rampant ignorance about this condition both in parents and professionals. A study on netizen searches in a virtual group covering nearly 3500 email transactions showed that the participating parents reported greatest concerns regarding therapy, treatment and management techniques (49.39%; Rank 1) for their wards identified as autism. This was followed by other concerns, such as, on or about their behavior problems (43.31%; Rank 4), consulting (42.61%; Rank 5); peer approval (35.62%; Rank 6), causes (31.69%; Rank 7), diagnostic clarifications (31.64%; Rank 8) and least regarding issues on advocacy (17.49%; Rank 15) (Venkatesan & Purusotham, 2008).

Probably the more disturbing trend in contemporary Indian society is the growing awareness as well as predilection among many neo-literate, elite and net savvy parents to browse the net to arrive at self-diagnosis of their children. Twin working affluent parents who have well provided for their infants and toddlers but left them under-stimulated without same age peer interactions is increasingly becoming the order of the day. For any given 24-hour cycle, apart from an 8-9 hour sleeping engagement, and another 2-3 hour feeding activity, toddlers are reported to be left alone, or with electronic gadgets. The amount of adult-child interactions per day overshoots child-child interactions. The 4 to 5 year old has never had an occasion or opportunity to observe, play with or mentor younger than their age children. In a related study, it was shown that children with IDD spent 9.61% of the time in a day 'watching television' and only 4.12% of the time 'playing with peers'. A sub-sample analysis in the same study of children with autism showed that they spent 21.23% time 'watching television' and 14.62% of a day 'playing alone' (Venkatesan, 2004a). It is also shown that leisure activities and community exposure of persons with NDD are characteristically low which is further aggravated by their lack of needed skills for social interaction and self-determination (Venkatesan & Yashodharakumar, 2016).

If under-stimulation is an anathema to many affected children with NDD, the phenomenon of over-stimulation is equally prevalent in few sections of parenting. Affluence and rabid materialistic consumerism in the neo-rich or neo-elite urban parents among the young wealthy couples have led to the loss of caregiving skills. As applied to infants, toddlers, preschoolers and young children, the result in the pampered child syndrome. There is this phenomenon of ***latchkey kid*** who is in an empty home most of the time during a day either because the twin parents are working or ever busy, or that the child is left to the care of grandparents or a paid babysitter. On their part, the end caregivers leave the child with e-gadgets using which s/he becomes overly proficient at the cost of uncultivated speech or social skills. Parenting kids on a fast track by over scheduling or compressing all activities within their short span. Children are expected to or made to act and behave like adults. By doing so, the pressure is on the kids to even lose out their childhood. Children are not pets and should not be treated as such. Many times, the child's academic presentations mistaken as competencies are either caregiver prompted, facilitated or induced in the form of parroted speech without really comprehending their meaning.

CASE VIGNETTE #1

Rishi, aged 4 years, single child, was reported to have extraordinary skills in browsing the net, downloading pictures of swanky cars, and pointing at them correctly when named by the parent. He was with I-pod, laptops, television, music, babbling to imaginary persons on phone, picture reading or simply staring at a spot on the wall. Since he was born pre-term and had a few bouts of breath-holding spells during the first two years (which the parents misunderstood as fits) they were extra careful not to deny or deprive anything. He was not exposed to children of his age group for fear of an infection or that they would take away his toys, ignore or bully him. Most of the time in a given day, the boy had 'adult-child' interaction only with parents. There was no opportunity for 'child-child' interactions or the child as an older companion to another younger one. Closer observation of the parent-child interactions also showed that most of 'special' skills exhibited by the child were unwittingly prompted or cued by the caregivers. During the clinical interview, the child recited days in a week, months in the year, names of ten wild and domestic animals, the great oceans, continents, gave out spellings out of a prepared list of 5-7 letter words in English, and rote counted numbers 1-1000. However, he could not meaningfully count and give away even less than five objects and did not spell even three letter words outside the list. Even the questions on the list were to be asked in the same order as given there if one wanted the correct answers. Further, it was seen that the child sat continually for more than fifteen minutes if one were to go through the drill in the same order. Whenever a different order of presentation was used or a more difficult question was asked, the child started flapping hands, made peculiar sounds, repeatedly turned the eye-gaze away from the task, or eventually threw a tantrum.

There has been a consistently growing argument that problem behaviors in children with NDD are a symptomatic expression of a cry for help. The presenting complaints are disguised forms of communication by the affected child. Children overly stressed or expected to perform beyond their levels resort to either internalizing or externalizing forms of conduct disturbances. Internalizing problem behaviors are typically directed towards oneself (as in anxiety, fears, or self-harm), just as externalizing ones have an outer trajectory (as in harming others, throwing things, damaging property or telling lies). Consequences or events following the problem behavior are shown to mediate or aggravate their occurrence. Going by this rationale, consequence mapping is suggested as a solution for their remediation (Venkatesan, 2017d). Even as the parents are unable to differentiate between skill and problem behaviors, the prevalence of multiple, ambiguous, inconsistent, self-contradictory ad hoc and arbitrary consequences for given problem behaviors is reported to explain the behavioral issues in these children. Parents are frequent culprits of using incomplete, ineffective, and inadequate discipline strategies which spill over to appear as causative when they are contributory, sustaining or maintaining factors rather than a part of the inherent symptoms of NDD.

Addressing the key issues and problems related to pseudo-diagnosis of children as cases of autism, a detailed individualized re-evaluation covering manifold processes and techniques was undertaken (Venkatesan, 2015a). The study highlighted about 65 critical clinical aspects contributing to diagnostic errors in relation to children suspected of autism. The major sources of error emanated from the case history, informant reporting, the absence of observation-based assessment, poor developmental history, etc.

Extension of the concept of NDD has resulted in an exaggerated preoccupation to look for telltale signs and symptoms even in as young as babies suspected of autism. Probably to intimidate, the net is full of notes, writings, or warnings on this theme. Lists are given to identify potential 'autism in babies' as early as six months! The commonly listed signs are: lack of smiling by six months, infrequent imitation of sounds, smiles, laughter and facial expressions by nine months, delay in babbling and cooing by twelve months, unresponsive to name or sounds of familiar voice by 6-12 months, poor eye contact when being smiled at or during feed times, infrequently seeking attention, lack of pointing or gesturing by 9-10 months age, repetitive behaviours, delayed motor development have all been touted as early baby signs of autism. To cap it all, there is also a baby autism checklist. Another list adds signs like visual or auditory tracking, absence of waving bye, or noises to gain attention, disinterest in what's going on around them, not connecting with friends, peers or others, not playing 'pretend' games, speaking in abnormal tone of voice, with odd pitch or rhythm, responding to question by repeating than answering it, not comprehending simple directions, statements or questions, or taking literal meaning without understanding the underlying irony, humour and sarcasm, being sensitive or reacting unusually to smells, sights, textures, and sounds, following rigid routines, not being ready to adapt to changes, preoccupation with narrow range of interests or topics, unusual attachments to objects, hand flapping, rocking, spinning, etc. Regression of any kind is announced as a serious warning sign of autism. Any loss of speech, babbling, gestures, or social skills should be taken very seriously, as regression is a major red flag for autism. Such over enthusiastic searches can do more harm than help for children who are more different than they are disabled.

(iii) Animal Behavior and NDD

In recent years, a new line of thought is being propagated. Do animals perceive, think or behave in the same manner as people with autism? Taking a cue from Mary Temple Grandin, an American Professor of Animal Science at Colorado State University, it is postulated that non-human animals typically behave like humans with autism. Animals do not have verbal language. They store memories as pictures, sounds or other sensory impressions. They lack word-based memories (Vallortigara, Snyder, Kaplan, Bateson, Clayton, & Rogers, 2008; Temple & Johnson, 2005). Animal models have been invoked to understand ADHD (Russell, 2007; Russell, Sagvolden, & Johansen, 2005) and OCD (Alonso, Lopez-Sola, Real, Segalas, & Menchon, 20-15). These models generally fall into three classes: repetitive behavior associated with targeted insults to the CNS; repetitive behavior induced by pharmacological agents; and such behavior associated with restricted environments and experience. Animals like deer mice and dogs are known to exhibit repetitive and restrictive behaviors like compulsive grooming or imitative vocalization of songbirds by social learning associated with environmental restriction due to their confinement (Crawley, 2012; Lewis, Tanimura, Lee, & Bodfish, 2007). Zoochosis (a portmanteau of the words 'zoo' and 'psychosis') is a new term that is being used to refer to a range of psychological problems exhibited by animals confined in zoos or other places of long-term captivity. Behavior symptoms may include bar biting, continual tongue licking, neck twisting, rocking, vomiting, coprophagia, rocking, swaying, over-grooming and/or self-mutilation are observed. Animal studies have shown that dogs, goldfish, monkeys, and sheep can recognize other fellow animals as well as human faces from photographic portraits. Goats and horses have the capacity to communicate with other people by gazing at them when facing a problem that they cannot solve alone. Trained bumblebees are able to discriminate between ten different colored artificial flowers five of them containing sugar water and five of them containing bitter quinine. Goldfish can not only listen to music but they can also distinct from one composer to another. Cows are not stupid. They have excellent problem-solving skills that involve the use of logic. Once they master how to solve a problem, they celebrate by jumping, wagging their tails and running happily (Pearson, 1962).

Stimming of self-stimulatory behaviors occurs due to under-stimulation or overstimulation. Stimming can be visual (such as seeing fans or flipping through books), auditory (listening to the same music or sounds), tactile (teeth grinding, self scratching or nail biting), verbal (using the same words or noises), taste and smell (licking or sniffing repeatedly), vestibular and proprioceptive (spinning or rocking). Many of these types of self-stimulation behaviors are not entirely different from what is seen in domesticated pets (Cheng, 2003; 1992; Sadowski & Dembinski, 1973; Meyerson, Wilkins, & Sawyer, 1969). From the foregoing, it is implied that use of animal-assisted interventions could help affected persons with NDD. It is shown that social behaviors increase in children with autism in the presence of animals as compared to toys (O'Haire, McKenzie, Beck, & Slaughter 2013). A case-controlled study on horse riding intervention for children with autism has shown a significant reduction in severity of symptoms between the pre- to post-test conditions (Harris & Williams, 2017). Similarly, the calming, socializing, motivating and cognitive effects of animal-assisted interventions are being increasingly explored even for benefit of children with ADHD (Busch, Tucha, Talarovicova, Fuermaier, Lewis-Evans, & Tucha, 2016).

(iv) Are They All Only Developmental Differences or Lags?

While the reliability and validity of the diagnostic category of NDD are under attack, there is a proposal that the excesses and/or deficits in the behaviors of these children may be simply developmental differences-more or less, albeit in different areas or domains. For example, one child may show greater delays in a receptive speech just as another may have an overly laggard expressive speech. Yet another may be deficient in play-social behaviors, while it may be to do with motor coordination affected for the next child. Of course, there are or can be children who are laggard in all areas simultaneously.

CASE VIGNETTE #2

Mahanidhi, aged 3 ½ years, the single child, was brought with complaints of harms self, flaps hands, poor eye contact, and refuses to eat. The child was born in India but was soon moved to Dubai where the father worked. In the foreign country, the whole day, the mother-child spent their time staying indoors, watching television, listening to rhymes, and playing on the iPod. It was only when they visited home in last summer the parents realized that their boy was laggard. Other same age cousins were speaking in sentences, played with one another or were toilet trained, attended preschool, and remained away from their parents most of the time during the day. The contrast in their child's behavior prompted them to seek professional consultation resulting in their understanding of their child's condition as 'autism'. Following this, they browsed the net and found that their ward showed most of the symptoms they read there. On their own, they decided to stop giving milk, wheat, and colored soft drinks to the child.

Developmental history showed delayed milestones. Parents were found to be grossly unaware of the expected ages for the specific sensory, motor, self-care, speech, social, and play milestones. They were continuing to maintain the boy in diapers, disallowed the boy from playing outside with water or in the sand. He was kept away from other same-aged peers for fear of infection. The mother maintained a rigid schedule of feeds and timing for the toilet and daily ablutions. In consultation with specialists, the child was put on Piracetam-a brain tonic, a drug not approved by the US Food and Drug Administration for any medical use.

The child showed 2-word utterances of noun-plus-verb forms. He never used other forms of speech. He followed repetitive situation mediated commands used by the parents often associated with gestures. He sands a few nursery rhymes, rote recited 1-10, A-Z, pointed to the same set of animals, vegetables, fruits and vehicles that was shown to him from a picture book. He hesitated to climb the ladder, could not slide, play on a see-saw, sits or stand and swing. He lacked meaningful counting, could not differentiate big-small, boy-girl, darkness-light, or left-right. His favorite past time was to be with toy vehicles and pretend their sounds. He would throw a tantrum when stopped from doing what he wanted to do. The parents gave into his wishes before his tempers worsened.

The absence of structured, systematic and sequence paced opportunities, over-indulgent parenting, the language-culture mismatch between parent-child, within or outside the family, or alternatively, over-packed exposure is the common concomitant seen in the case histories of these children. In a related study, parents of children with IDD were guided on a regular basis to undertake a home-based training program for skill enhancement with supporting verbal and written guidelines, simple and pragmatic record keeping procedures, specific toys or teaching aids to be used, behavioural or reward techniques to be followed along with bibliotherapeutic materials to be used for a program covering six months. Results showed maximum gains in 'pre-academic skills' (Venkatesan, 2004b). A typical shortcoming in contemporary parents is their abject unawareness about the developmental sequences of behaviors in children. This leads to inaccurate target setting on what to teach their children with NDD. It is shown that parent estimates of their children's developmental ages including intelligence and emotions are suspect as they tend to either over-estimate or under-estimate (Chandler, Howlin, Simonoff, Kennedy, & Baird, 2016; Karstad, Kvello, Wichstrom, & Berg-Nielsen, 2014; Glascoe & Sandler, 1995). Wherein this developmental perspective is appreciated, the clinician is likely to condone many regressed but developmentally age appropriate play behaviors as shown by their aimless running, pushing chair, banging objects and/or excitement in new places or with new faces.

(v) Parenting

To start with, the discovery of their child as NDD is an emotionally shattering experience for many mothers. In most cases, the battle begins for seeking permission from their spouse and other family elders on whether they should go for a professional consultation. After exhausting all well-meaning but failed advice of the family seniors, gurus, and magical-religious dispensations, they have to then shop for medicines or other palliatives. It is shown that parents go through a long-drawn itinerary of shopping for professional help which is influenced by the gender, severity, age, diagnostic condition of the child as well as allied demographic variables (Venkatesan, 2007). It is reported that parents made at least 3-4 non-professional consultations with a minimum of the one-year time lag between each of them before meeting a rehabilitation expert. The older children with NDD are not taken as frequently for consultations as the younger ones below 24 months. The study highlighted the need and importance of restricting the superfluous doctor-shopping sprees in parents of these children. Among the well identified or reported barriers in optimizing home training programs for parents of children with NDD, are frequent ill health in the child, inadequate supports from spouse or neighbours, demands of childcare from other unaffected siblings, shortage of reading materials on child care, or a defeatist attitude that there is no felt return on investment for all their efforts or expenditure of energies (Venkatesan, 2009).

The burden of implementing home-based training programs for children with IDD is recognized as difficulties in transportation, managing problem behaviors, adjusting to other demands of daily living, and understanding the technical jargon of the service providers (Venkatesan & Das, 1994). Other related issues like parenting by proxy through grandparents, elder siblings, extended family members, paid maids or others adds to the behavioral issues in many such children (Bonis, 2016). Hyper-parenting with an over-scheduled lifestyle seeks to create only successful children. Enrichment activities or an overdose of it and overzealous rearing patterns typically end in passing the latent anxiety in the parents to the child. It is common for mothers to attempt to showcase that their so-called 'autistic' or 'developmentally delayed' child is indeed capable of some of the other 'special' things. One mother felt that her child was gifted in identifying the flags of several countries. Another informed that 5-year girl could spell even 7-9 letter words by typing on a word processor or by picking the right strip among several such alternatives placed before her. However, upon closer observation, it was seen that this ability in the child was over-practiced and restricted to only the given word list. Burnout as a combination of fatigue, shame, guilt anger, frustration, and body ailments has been reported from nurture-overload in mothers of children with autism thereby calling for periodic rest, recuperation, relaxation, and recreation as counter coping strategy (Varghese & Venkatesan, 2013).

CASE VIGNETTE #3

Mala, aged 5 ½ years, single child, with no exposure to peers or schooling, twin working parents was reared by grandparents. One parent was a weekend visitor. The other would stopover once in a month. The grandparents provided for feeding and daily care. They left the child to watch television or listen to nursery rhymes the whole day. He was still in diapers and not toilet trained. The mother was worried why her child had poor eye contact, never missed her, did not go out to play with other children, was ill-prepared to join the school, and refusal to eat. His speech was restricted to using 2-3 word utterances which were often the repetitions of what the only four caregivers in the child's life made use in front of him. When denied or upset in the routines, the child would shout, throw things, fall on the floor, bite or push others and cry continually. To avoid such events, they seldom changed the routine. Whenever the child's problem behaviors went across the board, they would take him out, explain or advice to behave well, scold, shout back, carry or show affection, give him an edible, give the mobile game, put on television, tickle him to laughter and so on. Behavior assessment showed a developmental age level performance of around 2 years with little or no exposure to most of the tasks listed therein. A cursory check of parent estimations of the age of expected behaviors for various activities was far beyond or below the normative list. For example, they thought that children get toilet trained only after six, dress/undress shorts after three, or that they drink from cup or glass after four. Either want of time, fear of infection, or lack of cooperation from the child was given as reasons disallowing the child from peer play, taking him to public places, allowing him to care for himself.

Problem behavior management forms the other side of home-based skill training programs for children with NDD. The consumer demand for professional help to identify or manage problem behaviors is reported as the second most sought-after service by parents, teachers and/or caregivers of these children (Peshawaria, Venkatesan, & Menon, 1990; Peshawaria, Venkatesan, Mohapatra, & Menon, 1990; Peshawaria, Venkatesan, & Menon, 1988). While there are well-established problem behavior assessment tools, training programs, manuals, and modules available for use by stakeholders in the country

(Venkatesan, 2015b; 2004c; Peshawaria & Venkatesan, 1992a; 1992b), among the reported barriers in optimizing problem behavior interventions for children with NDD are, disagreements among caregivers in prioritizing problem behaviours, perception that such intervention programs are laborious and time-consuming, or that there are minimal or absent supports from the spouse or their family and/or that they expect instantaneous solutions (Venkatesan, 2017e). A great barrier to optimizing the limited potentials of children with NDD is the typically high expectations of parents followed by unrealistic goal setting for their skill training. By using a need-based 'W' question matrix, data elicitation on different aspects of goal setting, including what objectives are set, who plans them, when, where, or how they are earmarked for the children it was a found that the onus of training fell entirely upon the mothers. The teaching objectives were overly skewed toward activities involving pre-academic, academic and communication skills. Low priority was accorded to teaching self-help, social-play, safety, prevocational, and life skills (Venkatesan, 2015c; 2015d). There was an imposed agenda-setting, over-expectancy error and demand over-load resulting in the child's achievement deficit which was perceived as pendency, non-compliance or failed habilitation. The study showed implications for more realistic goal setting, program planning and for optimum benefits for these children (Venkatesan, Yashodharakumar, Gupta, & Vasudha, 2015).

A significant contribution in this area has been the development and validation of an 'Activity Checklist for Preschool Children with Developmental Disabilities' (ACPC-DD; Venkatesan, 2004b) and its add-on titled as 'Toy Kit for Kids with Developmental Disabilities: User Manual' (Venkatesan, 2004d). The 3-tier 'Toy Kits' have been exclusively designed, assembled, developed and standardized for children with developmental disabilities between 0-2 years (infant level), 2-4 years (toddler level) and 4-6 years (preschool level). A utility analysis of the assembled toy kits based on ratings of consumer judgments has received favourable feedback for some of its high ends features like having a 'supporting manual', 'reinforcement value', 'entertainment attraction', 'education worth', while being fair on lower end values related to minimum cost (Venkatesan, 2012). Despite positive reviews on the 'toy kits' (Venkatesan, 2012; Karande, 2011; Srivastava, 2011), one is unsure whether the children are indeed being given play materials.

Toys are integral ingredients in the lives of children. They enable and empower them. In a related study, a toy index based on identified parameters as reported by parent respondent was developed as a contemporary benchmark for targeted children with and without developmental disabilities. Results showed an overall impoverished mean toy index of 8.60 against standard comparison group. Boys than girls showed greater ownership and parents spend more money on toys for them as also children from urban than those from rural areas (Venkatesan & Yashodharakumar, 2017a; Venkatesan, 2014). These findings are backed by another observation that parents view their children are unable to make choices on the procurement of toys or that they require guidance for their routine use. They also shared apprehensions that toys are unaffordable, or dispensable luxuries. Dispensing of toys to children with NDD is also deemed as unsafe or risky (Venkatesan & Yashodharakumar, 2017b).

Play activities and behaviors of children with IDD are repeatedly reported to be a passive observer of others (Khoshali & Venkatesan, 2007). Their play behaviors are reported as characterised by poor eye-to-eye contact with peers, lack of understanding of the rules or their breach during the game, the absence of skills to share one's belongings or respect the ownership of others, poor or nil waiting for skills, and inability to observe safety rules or precautions (Venkatesan, 2000). The consequence of all this is self-indulgence, autistic or solitary play. Many of them are keen to observe other children at play which indicates their seeking for sociability or gregariousness. However, this tendency is quickly extinguished following their repeated exclusion or rejection by peers. Some of these rejected children are observed to imitate their peer play after a gap of time which is interpreted as delayed echolalia or echopraxia. With regard to toy or pet play, these children show an initial curiosity but need tutoring to enable their actual unassisted, creative or functional use. The bottom line is that there is no instance of any child with or without NDD which is reported as 'never plays' (Venkatesan & Ravindran, 2012).

TREATMENT

Although the etiology of NDD is largely unknown, and since an interactive interplay of genetic and environmental factors are thought to be involved, many interventions have cropped up although most of them are hyped by the online and offline media. Sadly, most of them are not supported by empirical research. They are classified as based on nutritional supplements, bio-medical therapies, diet controls, sensory stimulation, educational-behavioral interventions, gadgetry-or-computer assisted or instrument mediated therapies, use of drugs or medicines, or adoption of alternative systems of medicine. A list of intervention strategies, although not backed by evidence-based double-blind case-controlled studies, is listed in Table 2.

Animal studies on mouse models of NDD have been used to suggest that it is possible to reverse certain molecular, electrophysiological and behavioral deficits associated with these conditions by using certain genetic or pharmacological manipulations. Even though translation from animal experimentation to clinical practice is challenging, it is suggested that critical period-like plasticity can be reactivated by environmental manipulations or pharmacotherapy for the treatment of these conditions (Castren, Elgersma, Maffel, & Hagerman, 2012).

Ideally and typically, a behavior assessment and case formulation in the form of a theoretically based explanation leading to a treatment plan is often the precursor to interventions in NDD. The formulation typically describes the underlying neurodevelopmental processes from the genetic core to the surface symptoms in a way that it leads to biomedical and psychosocial interventions. These interventions can improve environmental interactions, enhance developmental progression, reverse neurobiological dysfunction, prevent kindling and sensitization, protect through high-risk periods, and promote or create healthy neurodevelopment (Hendren, Goldani, & Hagerman, 2014; p. 1). Many times, multi-sensory environment manipulation or stimulation as part of early social enrichment program has proved to be beneficial in reversing brain dysfunction or retarding the slowing down process in NDD. The need or value of psycho-education to optimise the effects of home training in children with NDD requires the greatest emphasis. The future awaits answers for questions related to aging in NDD (Hagerman, Ligsay, & Goldberg, 2016). Related questions are: what are the long-term outcomes of these conditions? Can there be autism or ADHD in the elderly? Other upcoming areas for research include: preclinical models, experimental therapeutics, early identification and intervention, psychiatric co-morbidities, ecological assessment, neuro-technologies, parental/caregiver quality of life, diagnostic considerations not being in compartmentalized boxes but along overlapping dimensional lines, or considering diagnostic decision making in NDD itself as 'work in progress'.

Table 2. Summary List of Treatments for NDD

Category of Therapy	Examples
Nutrition-Diet Based	Almond, Aloe Vera Juice, Brown Barley, Brown Rice, Calcium, Carbohydrate Diet, Cod Liver Oil, Essential Fatty Acids, Feingold's Diet, Feldenkrais Therapy, Fish Oil, Gerson Diet (Fruit & Vegetable Juice), Gluten and Casein Free Diet, Multivitamin Therapy, No Phenol Diet, Omega-3, Ornish Diet (Low fat vegetarian foods), Probiotic Foods, Fatty Acids, Rice Milk, Ketogenic Diet, Zeolite Therapy, etc
Bio-Medical	Candida Albicans, Antibiotic Treatment, Chelation, DAN Doctors, DMG, DMPS Therapy, Detoxification, Fertility Treatment, Live Cell Therapy, Maggot Debridement Therapy, MDT/Larva Therapy, Gene Therapy, Stem Cell Therapy, Exome Sequencing, Genetic Restorations or Manipulations, Genetic Counselling, etc.
Education-Behavior Based	Alternate Communication Methods (Sign Language, Picture Exchange Communication System, Signalling, Makaton, Physiotherapy, Occupational Therapy, The Bobath Concept, Applied Behavior Analysis, Cognitive Behavior Therapy, Conductive Education, Floor Time Intervention, Discrete Trial Training (DTT), Early Intensive Behavior Intervention (EIBI), Face Talk, Facilitated Communication, Family Therapy, Family Focussed Early Language Program, the Son-Rise Program®, Com DEALL, Social Stories, Sensory Integration Therapy (SIT), Treatment and Education of Autistic and Related Communication Handicapped Children (TEACCH), Parent Training (Incredible Years Program, Early Bird Program, Hypnotherapy, Home Schooling/Teaching, Mindfulness Training, Portage Program, Prompt Therapy, Relationship Development Intervention (RDI), Social Skills Training, Verbal Behavior Intervention, etc
Sensory	Animal Assisted Therapy, Aroma Therapy, Arts-Based Therapy, Auditory Integration Therapy, Brushing Therapy, Cranio-sacral Therapy, Dance Therapy, Deep Pressure Therapy, Deep Sound Therapy, Drum Therapy, Group Touching, Holding Therapy, Hydrotherapy, Laughter Therapy, Movement Therapy, Music Therapy, Phototherapy, Rolfing, Swimming, Therapeutic Massage, etc
Alternative Systems of Medicine	Acupuncture, Acupressure, Ayurveda, Biosys or Magnet Therapy, Brain Gym, Chinese Medicine or Quigong, Homeopathy, Osteopathy, Chiropractic Treatment, Dr. Oswal's G Therapy, Faith Healing, Feng Sui, Hair Analysis and Treatment Protocol, Gemmology, Herbal Medicine, Reflexology, Aroma Therapy, Massage Therapy, Love Therapy, Meditation, Miracle Therapy, Nature Cure, Naturopathy, Neuro-Linguistic Programming, Numerology, Nameology, Pranic Healing, Reiki, Siddha, Spiritual Medicine, Tibetan Medicine, Unani, Yoga, etc
Medication/Drug	Antidepressants, Antiepileptic, Antipsychotic, Benzodiazepines, Melatonin, Psychostimulants, Adderal, Benedryl, Botox Injection, Carbamazepine, Cucrumin, Pemoline, Encepabol, Learnol Plus, Olanzepine, Mentat Tonic, Nystatin, Phenol Injectin, Piracetam, Prozac, Quetipine, Resperidl, Ritalin, Secretin, Senetin, Straterra, etc.
Instrument-Based	Advanced Biomechanical Rehabilitation, Electrical Stimulation, Foot Nerve Therapy, Light Sound Therapy, Neurofeedback/Biofeedback, Video Therapy, Pay Attention High Tech Armband, etc
Computer Assisted	ACTIVATE ™, C8 Sciences, Fit Brains Software, My Brain Solutions, Brain Beat Interactive Metronome, Atentiv EEG-based brain-to-computer interface, Mind Sparke Video Game, Myndlift Mobile NF App, Brain Train Computerized Cognitive Training System, Play Attention, Secret Agent Society is computer enabled social/emotional skills training program, Mental Imagery Therapy for Autism (MITA), etc.

CONCLUSION

In sum, the field of NDD is not a straight walk. It needs to work hard to first justify its nomenclature based on the edifice of the molecular premise to explain brain-genetics-environment-behavior tetrad that it is supposed to be built upon. Its current reliance on outward behavioral symptoms with the yet-to-be-proven one-to-one biological basis for each type of NDD has raised debate and suspicion. Further, their interaction effects, either singly or multiply, has posted a great challenge as highlighted by the proverbial search for a needle in the haystack or a white cat in a snowstorm. Nonetheless, this is no excuse to escape or abandon this search in the individual as well as groups of cases. However, caution is needed against misinterpreting every passing sign or symptom in such cases as pathognomonic of NDD.

REFERENCES

Alonso, P., Lopez-Sola, C., Real, E., Segalas, C., & Menchon, J. M. (2015). Animal models of obsessive-compulsive disorder: Utility and limitations. *Neuropsychiatric Disease and Treatment*, *11*, 1939–1955. doi:10.2147/NDT.S62785 PMID:26346234

American Psychiatric Association. (1980). *Diagnostic and Statistical Manual of Mental Disorders* (3rd ed.). Washington, DC: Author.

American Psychiatric Association. (1994). *Diagnostic and Statistical Manual of Mental Disorders* (4th ed.). Washington, DC: Author.

American Psychiatric Association. (2000). *Diagnostic and Statistical Manual of Mental Disorders-IV-TR*. Washington, DC: Author.

American Psychiatric Association. (2013). *Diagnostic and Statistical Manual of Mental Disorders* (5th ed.). Arlington, VA: Author.

Arndt, T. L., Stodgell, C. J., & Rodier, P. M. (2005). The teratology of autism. *The International Journal of Neuroscience*, *23*, 189–199. PMID:15749245

Baird, G. (2013). Editorial: Classification of diseases and the neurodevelopmental disorders: The challenges for DSM-5 and ICD-11. *Developmental Medicine and Child Neurology*, *55*(3), 200–201. doi:10.1111/dmcn.12087 PMID:23398148

Batool, A., & Arooj, M. (2016). Complex neurodevelopmental disorders and their genetic aetiologies. *International Journal of Scientific & Technology Research*, *5*(9), 57–67.

Bertelli, M. O., Merli, M. P., Bradley, E., Keller, R., Varrucciu, N., Furia, C. D., & Panocchia, N. (2015). The diagnostic boundary between autism spectrum disorder, intellectual developmental disorder, and schizophrenia spectrum disorders. *Advances in Mental Health and Intellectual Disabilities*, *9*(5), 243–264. doi:10.1108/AMHID-05-2015-0024

Bilbo, S. D., & Schwartz, J. M. (2012). The immune system and developmental programming of brain and behavior. *Frontiers in Neuroendocrinology*, *33*(3), 267–286. doi:10.1016/j.yfrne.2012.08.006 PMID:22982535

Bölte, S., Schipper, E., Robison, J. E., Wong, V. C., Selb, M., Singhal, N., ... Zwaigenbaum, L. (2014). Classification of functioning and impairment: The development of ICF core sets for autism spectrum disorder. *Autism Research*, *7*(1), 167–172. doi:10.1002/aur.1335 PMID:24124074

Bonis, S. (2016). Stress and parents of children with autism: A review of the literature. *Issues in Mental Health Nursing*, *37*(3), 153–163. doi:10.3109/01612840.2015.1116030 PMID:27028741

Busch, C., Tucha, L., Talarovicova, A., Fuermaier, A. B. M., Lewis-Evans, B., & Tucha, O. (2016). Animal-assisted interventions for children with attention-deficit/hyperactivity disorder: A theoretical review and consideration of future research directions. *Psychological Reports*, *118*(1), 292–331. doi:10.1177/0033294115626633 PMID:29693527

Carroll, L. S., & Owen, M. J. (2009). Genetic overlap between autism, schizophrenia and bipolar disorder. *Genome Medicine*, *1*(102), 1–7. PMID:19886976

Carulla, L. S., Reed, G. M., Vaez-Azizi, L. M., Cooper, S. A., Leal, R., Bertelli, M., ... Girimaji, S. C. (2011). Intellectual developmental disorders: Towards a new name, definition and framework for "mental retardation/intellectual disability" in ICD-11. *World Psychiatry; Official Journal of the World Psychiatric Association (WPA)*, *10*(3), 175–180. doi:10.1002/j.2051-5545.2011.tb00045.x PMID:21991267

Castren, E., Elgersma, Y., Maffel, L., & Hagerman, R. (2012). Treatment of neurodevelopmental disorders in adulthood. *The Journal of Neuroscience*, *32*(41), 14074–14079. doi:10.1523/JNEUROSCI.3287-12.2012 PMID:23055475

Chailangkarn, T., Trujillo, C. A., Freitas, B. C., Hrvoj-Mihic, B., Herai, R. H., Diana, X. Y., ... Stefanacci, L. (2016). A human neurodevelopmental model for Williams syndrome. *Nature*, *536*(7616), 338–343. doi:10.1038/nature19067 PMID:27509850

Chandler, S., Howlin, P., Simonoff, E., Kennedy, J., & Baird, G. (2016). Comparison of the parental estimate of developmental age with measured IQ in children with neurodevelopmental disorders. *Child: Care, Health and Development*, *42*(4), 486–493. doi:10.1111/cch.12346 PMID:27126521

Cheng, M. F. (1992). For whom does the female dove coo? A case for the role of vocal self-stimulation. *Animal Behaviour*, *43*(6), 1035–1044. doi:10.1016/S0003-3472(06)80016-3

Cheng, M. F. (2003). Vocal self-stimulation: From the ring dove story to emotion-based vocal communication. *Advances in the Study of Behavior*, *33*, 309–353. doi:10.1016/S0065-3454(03)33007-4

Connan, F., Campbell, I. C., Katzman, M., Lightman, S. L., & Treasure, J. (2003). A neurodevelopmental model for anorexia nervosa. *Physiology & Behavior*, *79*(1), 13–24. doi:10.1016/S0031-9384(03)00101-X PMID:12818706

Couriel, J. M., Bisse, R., Miller, R., Thomas, A., & Clarke, M. (1993). Assessment of feeding problems in neurodevelopmental handicap: A team approach. *Archives of Disease in Childhood*, *69*(5), 609–613. doi:10.1136/adc.69.5.609 PMID:7504911

Crawley, J. N. (2012). Translational animal models of autism and neurodevelopmental disorders. *Dialogues in Clinical Neuroscience*, *14*(3), 293–305. PMID:23226954

Cristino, A. S., Williams, S. M., Hawi, Z., An, J.-Y., Bellgrove, M. A., Schwartz, C. E., ... Claudianos, C. (2014). Neurodevelopmental and neuropsychiatric disorders represent an interconnected molecular system. *Molecular Psychiatry*, *19*(3), 297–301. doi:10.1038/mp.2013.16 PMID:23439483

De Felice, A., Ricceri, L., Venerosi, A., Chiarotti, F., & Calamandrei, G. (2015). Multifactorial origin of neurodevelopmental disorders: Approaches to understanding complex aetiologies. *Toxics*, *3*(1), 89–129. doi:10.3390/toxics3010089 PMID:29056653

Doemberg, E., & Hollander, E. (2016). Neurodevelopmental disorders (ASD and ADHD): DSM-5, ICD-10, and ICD-11. *CNS Spectrums*, *21*(4), 295–299. doi:10.1017/S1092852916000262 PMID:27364515

Dossetor, D. R. (2007). 'All that glitters is not gold': Misdiagnosis of psychosis in pervasive developmental disorders-A case series. *Clinical Child Psychology and Psychiatry, 12*(4), 537–548. doi:10.1177/1359104507078476 PMID:18095536

Fatemi, S. H., & Folsom, T. D. (2009). The neurodevelopmental hypothesis of schizophrenia revisited. *Schizophrenia Bulletin, 35*(1), 528–548. doi:10.1093chbulbn187 PMID:19223657

Fishbein, D. H., Rose, E. J., Darcey, V. L., Belcher, A. M., & VanMeter, J. W. (2016). Neurodevelopmental precursors and consequences of substance use during adolescence: Promises and pitfalls of longitudinal neuroimaging strategies. *Frontiers in Human Neuroscience, 10*, 296. doi:10.3389/fnhum.2016.00296 PMID:27445743

Gabriele, M., Tobon, L., D'Agostino, G., & Testa, G. (2018). The chromatin basis of neurodevelopmental disorders: Rethinking dysfunction along the molecular and temporal axes. *Progress in Neuro-psychopharmacology and Biological Psychiatry, S0278-5846*(17), 30538-30539. doi:10.1016/j.pnpbp.2017.12.013

Glascoe, F. P., & Sandler, H. (1995). Value of parents' estimate of children's developmental ages. *The Journal of Pediatrics, 127*(5), 831–835. doi:10.1016/S0022-3476(95)70184-2 PMID:7472847

Goepfert, E., Mule, C., von Hahn, E., Visco, Z., & Siegel, M. (2015). Family systems interventions for families of children with autism spectrum disorder. *Child and Adolescent Psychiatric Clinics of North America, 24*(3), 571–583. doi:10.1016/j.chc.2015.02.009 PMID:26092740

Gupta, S., & Kulhara, P. (2010). What is schizophrenia: A neurodevelopmental or neurodegenerative disorder or a combination of both? A critical analysis. *Indian Journal of Psychiatry, 52*(1), 21-27. doi: 14.4103/0019-6645.68891

Hagerman, R. J., & Hendren, R. L. (2014). *Treatment of neurodevelopmental disorders: Targeting neurobiological mechanisms*. Oxford, UK: Oxford University Press. doi:10.1093/med/9780199937806.001.0001

Hagerman, R. J., Ligsay, A., & Goldberg, J. (2016). Aging with neurodevelopmental disorders: On-call assessment and future directions. In *On-Call Geriatric Psychiatry: Handbook of Principles and Practice* (pp. 341–351). New York: Springer International Publishing; doi:10.1007/978-3-319-30346-8_26

Harris, A., & Williams, J. M. (2017). The impact of a horse riding intervention on the social functioning of children with autism spectrum disorder. *International Journal of Environmental Research and Public Health, 14*(4), E776. doi:10.3390/ijerph14070776 PMID:28708075

Harris, J. C. (2014). A new classification of neurodevelopmental disorders in DSM-5. *Current Opinion in Psychiatry, 27*(2), 95–97. doi:10.1097/YCO.0000000000000042 PMID:24441422

Helps, S. (2016). Systemic psychotherapy with families where someone has an autism spectrum condition. *NeuroRehabilitation, 38*(3), 223–230. doi:10.3233/NRE-161314 PMID:27030899

Hendren, R. L., Goldani, A., & Hagerman, R. J. (2014). Overview of neurodevelopmental processes and the assessment of patients with neurodevelopmental disorders. In R. J. Hagerman & R. L. Hendren (Eds.), *Treatment of neurodevelopmental disorders: Targeting neurobiological mechanisms*. Oxford, UK: Oxford University Press. doi:10.1093/med/9780199937806.003.0001

Herwegen, J. V., Riby, D., & Farran, E. K. (2015). Neurodevelopmental disorders: Definitions and issues. In J. V. Herwegen & D. Riby (Eds.), *Neurodevelopmental disorders: Research challenges and solutions* (pp. 3–19). New York: Psychology Press.

Homberg, J. R., Kyzar, E. J., Stewart, A. M., Nguyen, M., Poudel, M. K., Echevarria, D. J., ... Pittman, J. (2016). Improving treatment of neurodevelopmental disorders: Recommendations based on preclinical studies. *Expert Opinion on Drug Discovery*, *11*(1), 11–25. doi:10.1517/17460441.2016.1115834 PMID:26558752

Hu, W. F., Chahrour, M. H., & Walsh, C. A. (2014). The diverse genetic landscape of neurodevelopmental disorders. *Annual Review of Genomics and Human Genetics*, *15*(1), 195–213. doi:10.1146/annurev-genom-090413-025600 PMID:25184530

Ivarsson, T., Weidle, B., Skarphedinsson, G., & Valderhaug, R. (2017). Neurobiological and neurodevelopmental perspectives on OCD and their clinical implications. In J. S. Abramowitz, D. McKay, & E. A. Storch (Eds.), *The Wiley Handbook of Obsessive Compulsive Disorders*. Chichester, UK: John Wiley & Sons; doi:10.1002/9781118890233.ch15

Jensen, M., & Girirajan, S. (2017). Mapping a shared genetic basis for neurodevelopmental disorders. *Genome Medicine*, *9*(1), 109. doi:10.118613073-017-0503-4 PMID:29241461

Johnson, J. (2017). Social learning theory as a framework for recreational therapy intervention in children with neurodevelopmental disorders. *Illuminare: A Student Journal in Recreation, Parks, and Tourism Studies, 15*(1).

Jones, S., Howard, L., & Thornicroft, G. (2008). Diagnostic overshadowing: Worse physical health care for people with mental illness. *Acta Psychiatrica Scandinavica*, *118*(3), 169–171. doi:10.1111/j.1600-0447.2008.01211.x PMID:18699951

Karande, S. (2011). Book Review: Toy kit for kids with developmental disabilities: User manual. Indian Paediatrics, 48(10), 830.

Karstad, S. B., Kvello, O., Wichstrom, L., & Berg-Nielsen, T. S. (2014). What do parents know about their children's comprehension of emotions? The accuracy of parental estimates in a community sample of pre-schoolers. *Child: Care, Health and Development*, *40*(3), 346–353. doi:10.1111/cch.12071 PMID:23601022

Kelleher, E., & Corvin, A. (2015). Overlapping aetiology of neurodevelopmental disorders. In K. J. Mitchell (Ed.), *The genetics of neurodevelopmental disorders*. Hoboken, NJ: John Wiley & Sons. Mitchell. doi:10.1002/9781118524947.ch2

Kelly, J. R., Minuto, C., Cryan, J. F., Clarke, G., & Dinan, T. G. (2017). Cross talk: The microbiota and neurodevelopmental disorders. *Frontiers in Neuroscience*, *15*(11), 490. doi:10.3389/fnins.2017.00490 PMID:28966571

Keshavan, M. S. (1999). Development, disease, and degeneration in schizophrenia: A unitary pathophysiological model. *Journal of Psychiatric Research*, *33*(6), 513–521. doi:10.1016/S0022-3956(99)00033-3 PMID:10628528

Khansari, P. S., & Sperlagh, B. (2012). Inflammation in neurological and psychiatric diseases. *Inflammopharmacology, 20*(3), 103–107. doi:10.100710787-012-0124-x PMID:22361843

Khoshali, A. K., & Venkatesan, S. (2007). Play behaviors of children with mental retardation. *Psychological Studies, 52*(1), 90–94.

Kim, Y. S., & State, M. W. (2014). Recent challenges to the psychiatric diagnostic nosology: A focus on the genetics and genomics of neurodevelopmental disorders. *International Journal of Epidemiology, 43*(2), 465–475. doi:10.1093/ije/dyu037 PMID:24618187

Kochunov, P., & Hong, L. E. (2014). Neurodevelopmental and neurodegenerative models of schizophrenia: White matter at the center stage. *Schizophrenia Bulletin, 40*(4), 721–728. doi:10.1093chbulbu070 PMID:24870447

Korkmaz, B. (2011). Theory of mind and neurodevelopmental disorders of childhood. *Pediatric Research, 69*(5 Part 2), 101R–108R. doi:10.1203/PDR.0b013e318212c177 PMID:21289541

Landrigan, P. J. (2010). What causes autism? Exploring the environmental contribution. *Current Opinion in Pediatrics, 22*(2), 219–225. doi:10.1097/MOP.0b013e328336eb9a PMID:20087185

Landrigan, P. J., Lambertini, L., & Birnbaum, L. S. (2012). A research strategy to discover the environmental causes of autism and neurodevelopmental disorders. *Environmental Health Perspectives, 120*(7), a258–a260. doi:10.1289/ehp.1104285 PMID:22543002

Lewis, M. H., Tanimura, Y., Lee, L. W., & Bodfish, J. W. (2007). Animal models of restricted repetitive behavior autism. *Behavioural Brain Research, 176*(1), 66–74. doi:10.1016/j.bbr.2006.08.023 PMID:16997392

Lewis, S. W., & Murray, R. M. (1987). Is schizophrenia a neurodevelopmental disorder? *British Medical Journal (Clinical Research Ed.), 296*, 681–682. PMID:3117295

Li, G., & Qiu, S. (2014). Neurodevelopmental underpinnings of Angelman Syndrome. *Journal of Bioanalysis & Biomedicine, 6*(6), 52–56. doi:10.4172/1948-593X.1000111 PMID:26491538

Livingston, L. A., & Happe, F. (2017). Conceptualizing compensation in neurodevelopmental disorders: Reflections from autism spectrum disorders. *Neuroscience and Biobehavioral Reviews, 80*, 729–742. doi:10.1016/j.neubiorev.2017.06.005 PMID:28642070

Mahdi, S., Viljoen, M., Yee, T., Selb, M., Singhal, N., Almodayfer, O., ... Bölte, S. (2017). An international qualitative study of functioning in autism spectrum disorder using the World Health Organization international classification of functioning, disability and health framework. *Autism Research, 11*(3), 463–475. doi:10.1002/aur.1905 PMID:29226604

Maltese, A., Gallai, B., Marotta, R., Lavano, F., Lavano, S. M., Tript, G., & Romano, P., D'Oro, & Salerno, M. (2017). The syntactive theory of development: The keyword for neurodevelopmental disorders. *Acta Medica Mediterranea, 33*, 1257. doi:10.19193/0393-6384_2017_2S_194

Marazziti, D., Baroni, S., Picchetti, M., Landi, P., Silvestri, S., Vatteroni, E., & Catena Dell'Osso, M. (2012). Psychiatric disorders and mitochondrial dysfunctions. *European Review for Medical and Pharmacological Sciences, 16*(2), 270–275. PMID:22428481

Martens, G. J. M., & van Loo, K. M. J. (2007). Genetic and environmental factors in complex neurodevelopmental disorders. *Current Genomics*, *8*(7), 429–444. doi:10.2174/138920207783591717 PMID:19412416

McNamara, R. K., & Strawn, J. R. (2013). Role of long chain omega-3 fatty acids in psychiatric practice. *PharmaNutrition*, *1*(2), 41–49. doi:10.1016/j.phanu.2012.10.004 PMID:23607087

McNeil, S. E. (2017). Editorial: Disorders in children and adolescents: Challenges in diagnosis and treatment with an emphasis on neurodevelopmental disorders. The *American Journal of Psychiatry. Resident's Journal*, *12*(9), 2–2. doi:10.1176/appi.ajp-rj.2017.120901

Meyerson, B. J., Wilkins, S. E., & Sawyer, C. H. (1969). Effects of estrogen on self-stimulation behavior in ovariectomized rats. *Physiology & Behavior*, *4*(3), 291–296. doi:10.1016/0031-9384(69)90177-2

Micheletti, S., Palestra, F., Martelli, P., Accorsi, P., Alli, J., Glordano, L., ... Fazzi, E. (2016). Neurodevelopmental profile in Angelman syndrome: More than low intelligence quotient. *Italian Journal of Pediatrics*, *42*(1), 91. doi:10.118613052-016-0301-4 PMID:27769316

Norbury, C. F., & Sparks, A. (2013). Difference or disorder? Cultural issues in understanding neurodevelopmental disorders. *Developmental Psychology*, *49*(1), 45–58. doi:10.1037/a0027446 PMID:22390668

O' Shea, S., & McInnis, M. G. (2016). Neurodevelopmental origins of bipolar disorder: IPSC models. *Molecular and Cellular Neurosciences*, *73*, 63–73. doi:10.1016/j.mcn.2015.11.006 PMID:26608002

O'Haire, M. E., McKenzie, S. J., Beck, A. M., & Slaughter, V. (2013). Social behaviors increase in children with autism in the presence of animals compared to toys. *PLoS One*, *68*(2), e57010. doi:10.1371/journal.pone.0057010 PMID:23468902

Pearson, N. (1962). Self-stimulation in the goat. *Acta Physiologica (Oxford, England)*, *55*(2-3), 276–285. doi:10.1111/J.1748-1716.1962.tb02441.x PMID:14485613

Peshawaria, R., & Venkatesan, S. (1992a). *Behavioral approaches to teaching mentally handicapped children: A manual for teachers*. National Institute for the Mentally Handicapped.

Peshawaria, R., & Venkatesan, S. (1992b). *Behavioral assessment scales for Indian children with mental retardation (BASIC-MR)*. National Institute for the Mentally Handicapped.

Peshawaria, R., Venkatesan, S., & Menon, D. K. (1988). Consumer demand for services by parents of mentally handicapped individuals. *Indian Journal of Disability & Rehabilitation*, *2*(2), 43–57.

Peshawaria, R., Venkatesan, S., & Menon, D. K. (1990). Behavior problems in mentally handicapped persons: An analysis of parent needs. *Indian Journal of Clinical Psychology*, *17*(2), 63–70.

Peshawaria, R., Venkatesan, S., Mohapatra, B., & Menon, D. K. (1990). Teachers' perception of problem behaviors among mentally handicapped persons in special school settings. *Indian Journal of Disability & Rehabilitation*, *4*(1), 23–30.

Ploeger, A., & Galis, F. (2011). Evolutionary approaches to autism: An overview and integration. *McGill Journal of Medicine*, *13*(2), 38. PMID:22363193

Racine, E., Caron, R., & Stanton-Jean, M. (2018). Justice and neurodevelopmental disorders: Moral-political philosophies, policies, and their outcomes. *Seminars in Pediatric Neurology*, *25*, 1. doi:10.1016/j.spen.2018.03.006 PMID:29735107

Read, J., Fosse, R., Moskowitz, A., & Perry, B. (2014). The traumagenic neurodevelopmental model of psychosis revisited. *Neuropsychiatry*, *4*(1), 65–79. doi:10.2217/npy.13.89

Reiss, S., Levitan, G., & Szyszko, G. W. (1982). Emotional disturbance and mental retardation: Diagnostic overshadowing. *American Journal of Mental Deficiency*, *86*(6), 567–574. PMID:7102729

Reiss, S., & Szyszko, J. (1983). Diagnostic overshadowing and professional experience with mentally retarded persons. *American Journal of Mental Deficiency*, *87*(4), 396–402. PMID:6829617

Riva, D., Bellugi, U., & Denckla, M. B. (2005). *Neurodevelopmental disorders: cognitive/behavioral phenotypes*. Montrouge, France: John Libbey Eurotext.

Romano, E., Cosentino, L., Laviola, G., & De Filippis, B. (2016). Genes and sex hormones interaction in neurodevelopmental disorders. *Neuroscience and Biobehavioral Reviews*, *67*, 9–24. doi:10.1016/j.neubiorev.2016.02.019 PMID:26952805

Rosenberg, D. R., & Keshavan, M. S. (1998). Toward a neurodevelopmental model of obsessive-compulsive disorder. *Biological Psychiatry*, *43*(9), 623–640. doi:10.1016/S0006-3223(97)00443-5 PMID:9582996

Rubenstein, J. L., & Merzenich, M. M. (2003). Model of autism: Increased ratio of excitation/inhibition in key neural systems. *Genes Brain & Behavior*, *2*(5), 255–267. doi:10.1034/j.1601-183X.2003.00037.x PMID:14606691

Russell, V. A. (2007). Neurobiology of animal models of attention-deficit hyperactivity disorder. *Journal of Neuroscience Methods*, *161*(2), 185–198. doi:10.1016/j.jneumeth.2006.12.005 PMID:17275916

Russell, V. A., Sagvolden, T., & Johansen, E. B. (2005). Animal models of attention-deficit hyperactivity disorder. *Behavioral and Brain Functions*, *1*(1), 9. doi:10.1186/1744-9081-1-9 PMID:16022733

Sadowski, B., & Dembiriska, M. (1973). Some characteristics of self-stimulation behavior of dogs. *Acta Neurobiologiae Experimentalis*, *33*(4), 757–769. PMID:4205636

Salvador-Carulla, L., Bertelli, M., & Martinez-Leal, R. (2018). The road to the 11th edition of the International Classification of Diseases: Trajectories of scientific consensus and contested science in the classification of intellectual disability/intellectual developmental disorders. Current Opinions in Psychiatry, 31(2), 79-87. doi: .0000000000000396 doi:10.1097/YCO

Shen, M. D., Nordahi, C. W., Young, G. S., Wotton-Gorges, S. L., Lee, A., Liston, S. E., ... Amarai, D. G. (2013). Early brain enlargement and elevated extra-axial fluid in infants who develop autism spectrum disorder. *Brain*, *136*(Pt9), 2825–2835. doi:10.1093/brain/awt166 PMID:23838695

Solomon, M., Hessl, D., Chiu, S., Olsen, E., & Hendren, R. L. (2009). Towards a neurodevelopmental model of clinical case formulation. *Psychiatria Clinica*, *32*(1), 199–211. PMID:19248925

Srivastava, A. K. (2011). Book Review: Toy kit for kids with developmental disabilities: User manual. *Journal of Disability Management and Special Education*, *1*(1), 87–88.

State, M. W., & Levitt, P. (2011). The conundrums of understanding genetic risks for autism spectrum disorders. *Nature Neuroscience, 14*(12), 1499–1506. doi:10.1038/nn.2924 PMID:22037497

Summers, J. (2012). Neurodevelopmental outcomes in children with Angelman syndrome after 1 year of behavioral intervention. *Developmental Neurorehabilitation, 15*(4), 239–252. doi:10.3109/17518423.2012.676101 PMID:22646082

Temple, G., & Johnson, C. (2005). *Animals in translation. Using the mysteries of autism to decode animal behavior*. New York: Scribner Book Company.

Thapar, A., Cooper, M., Eyre, O., & Langley, K. (2013). Practitioner review: What have we learned about the causes of ADHD? *Journal of Child Psychology and Psychiatry, and Allied Disciplines, 54*(1), 3–16. doi:10.1111/j.1469-7610.2012.02611.x PMID:22963644

Tognini, P. (2017). Gut microbiota: A potential regulator of neurodevelopment. *Frontiers in Cellular Neuroscience, 11*, 25. doi:10.3389/fncel.2017.00025 PMID:28223922

Vallortigara, G., Snyder, A., Kaplan, G., Bateson, P., Clayton, N. S., & Rogers, L. J. (2008). Are animals autistic savants. *PLoS Biology, 6*(2), e42. doi:10.1371/journal.pbio.0060042 PMID:18288892

Varghese, R. T., & Venkatesan, S. (2013). A comparative study of maternal burnout in autism and hearing impairment. *International Journal of Psychology & Psychiatry, 1*(2), 101–108. doi:10.5958/j.2320-6233.1.2.016

Venkatesan, S. (2000). Play activities in children with mental retardation. *Indian Journal of Clinical Psychology, 27*(1), 124–128.

Venkatesan, S. (2004a). Activity log of preschool children with developmental disabilities and autism spectrum disorders. *Disability, CBR and Inclusive Development, 15*(2), 58–66.

Venkatesan, S. (2004b). Efficacy of home training program in skill enhancement of children with developmental disabilities. *Indian Journal of Clinical Psychology, 31*(1), 121–127.

Venkatesan, S. (2004c). *Children with developmental disabilities: A training guide for parents, teachers, and caregivers. New Delhi: Sage* Publications.

Venkatesan, S. (2004d). *Toy Kit for Kids with Developmental Disabilities: User Manual*. Mysore: All India Institute of Speech and Hearing.

Venkatesan, S. (2007). Professional help-seeking behaviors in parents of children with developmental disabilities. *Journal of All India Institute of Speech and Hearing, 26*(1), 72–75.

Venkatesan, S. (2009). Barriers to optimizing home training programs for children with developmental disabilities. *Journal of All India Institute of Speech and Hearing, 28*(1), 128–134.

Venkatesan, S. (2012). Utility analysis of assembled toy kits for kids with developmental disabilities. *Journal of Disability Management and Special Education*, 2(2), 27–37.

Venkatesan, S. (2014). Availability of toys for children with developmental disabilities. *Journal of Disability Management and Special Education*, *4*(1), 58–70.

Venkatesan, S. (2015a). A growing trend in pseudo-diagnosis: A field study on children frequently mistaken for autism in India. *Psychological Studies*, *60*(1), 91–100. doi:10.100712646-015-0302-1

Venkatesan, S. (2015b). *Problem behavior survey schedule*. Bangalore: Psychotronics.

Venkatesan, S. (2015c). Revisiting goal setting for children with developmental disabilities. *Journal of Disability Management and Special Education*, *5*(2), 19–27.

Venkatesan, S. (2015d). Evaluation of teaching objectives earmarked for children with developmental disabilities. *Disabilities & Impairments*, *29*(2), 85–95.

Venkatesan, S. (2016). A concept analysis of learning disability based on research articles published in India. *Indian Journal of Clinical Psychology*, *43*(2), 97–107.

Venkatesan, S. (2017a). Analysis of bibliography on specific learning disability in India. *Disability, CBR and Inclusive Development*, *28*(2), 59–73. doi:10.5463/dcid.v28i2.540

Venkatesan, S. (2017b). Analysis of attributes in the official definitions for learning disability. *The International Journal of Indian Psychology*, *4*(2), 46-57. doi: 18.01.027/20170402

Venkatesan, S. (2017c). Diagnostic decision tree for a specific learning disability. *International Journal of Education and Psychological Research*, *6*(2), 121–127.

Venkatesan, S. (2017d). Consequence mapping of problem behaviors in children with developmental delays. *Disabilities and Impairments*, *31*(1), 47–64.

Venkatesan, S. (2017e). Barriers and facilitators in home-based problem behavior interventions for children. *Indian Journal of Health and Wellbeing*, *8*(5), 345–351.

Venkatesan, S., & Das, A. K. (1994). The reported burden on family members in receiving/implementing home-based training programs for children with mental handicaps. *Journal of Psychological Researches*, *38*(1 & 2), 39–45.

Venkatesan, S., & Purusotham, P. (2008). A profile of etiological and therapeutic searches by netizen parents/caregivers of children on the autism spectrum. *Journal of All India Institute of Speech and Hearing*, *27*(1), 89–94.

Venkatesan, S., & Rao, P. H. (1996). The significance of some birth factors in mental retardation. *Disabilities & Impairments*, *10*(2), 53–64.

Venkatesan, S., & Ravindran, N. (2012). Play behaviors and activities in siblings of children with developmental disabilities. *Journal of the Indian Academy of Applied Psychology*, *38*(1), 69–78.

Venkatesan, S., & Yashodhara Kumar, G. Y. (2016). Leisure and community exposure in persons with disabilities. *Journal of Disability Management and Special Education*, *6*(1), 1–14.

Venkatesan, S., & Yashodhara Kumar, G. Y. (2017a). Toy index of children with or without developmental disabilities. *Indian Journal of Clinical Psychology*, *44*(1), 60–67.

Venkatesan, S., & Yashodhara Kumar, G. Y. (2017b). Parent opinions and attitudes on toys for children with or without developmental disabilities. *The International Journal of Indian Psychology, 4*(4), 6–20. doi:10.25215/0404.061

Venkatesan, S., Yashodharakumar, G. Y., Gupta, S. K., & Vasudha, H. H. (2015). Gap analysis for evaluation of individualized education programs for children with developmental disabilities. *International Journal of Psychology and Psychiatry, 13*(2), 64–76. doi:10.5958/2320-6233.2015.00017.6

Weinberger, D. R. (1987). The implication of normal brain development for the pathogenesis of schizophrenia. *Archives of General Psychiatry, 44*(7), 660–669. doi:10.1001/archpsyc.1987.01800190080012 PMID:3606332

Wilska, M. L., & Kaski, M. K. (2001). Why and how to assess the aetiological diagnosis of children with intellectual disability/mental retardation and other neurodevelopmental disorders: Description of the Finnish approach. *European Journal of Paediatric Neurology, 5*(1), 7–13. doi:10.1053/ejpn.2001.0398 PMID:11277365

World Health Organization. (1993). *The ICD-10 Classification of Mental and Behavioural Disorders: Clinical descriptions and diagnostic guidelines*. Geneva: Author.

World Health Organization. (2007). *International Classification of Functioning, Disability, and Health-Children and Youth Version (ICF-CY)*. Geneva: Author.

Yan-bin, W. (2009). Impact of Lev Vygotsky on special education. *Canadian Social Science, 5*(5), 100–103.

KEY TERMS AND DEFINITIONS

Diagnostic Overshadowing: A predilection in a clinician or caregiver to attribute each and every behavior of the child after a brief observation as a reflection of their primary condition.

Epigenetic: Relating to or arising from non-genetic influence on gene expression. It is the study of heritable changes in gene function that does not involve a change in the DNA sequence.

Helicopter Parenting: Also called cosset-parenting, it explains a parent who pays extremely close attention to a child's or children's experiences and problems.

Hyper-Parenting: A style of child rearing that inadvertently over schedules and overpacks activities for a given day with the sole intention of making them perfect to guarantee a successful adulthood in the contemporary competitive e-world.

Latchkey Child: A child who is at home without any supervision for some part of the day, especially after school until a parent returns from work.

Microbiome: Refers to a community of microorganisms such as bacteria, fungi, and viruses that inhabit a particular environment, especially within the human body.

Molar-Molecular: They are not different theories or levels of analysis. They are different paradigms of viewing human behavior as inherently extended in time and composed of activities that have integrated parts versus the view that behavior is composed of discrete units occurring at moments of time and strung together to make up a complex phenomenon.

Neuroimaging: The process of producing images of the structure or activity of the brain or another part of the nervous system by techniques such as magnetic resonance imaging or computerized tomography.

Neuroscience: Any or all the sciences, such as neurochemistry, experimental psychology and others which deal with the structure or function of the nervous system.

Stimming: Or self-stimulatory behavior, this involves the repetition of physical movements or sounds indulged by persons to calm or stimulate themselves.

Synaptogenesis: Refers to the formation of synapses between neurons in the nervous system. Although a lifelong process, an explosion of synapse formation occurs especially during early brain development.

Zone of Proximal Development: It is the difference between what a learner can do without help and what they cannot do.

Chapter 2
Auditory Profile of Children With Some Rare Neurodevelopmental Disorders

Saransh Jain
JSS Institute of Speech and Hearing, India

Vijaya Kumar Narne
South Denmark University, Denmark

ABSTRACT

Neurodevelopmental disorder is an umbrella term comprising many muscular, skeletal, metabolic, endocrinal, systemic, and immune-related diseases, which are caused due to the improper/inaccurate development of the central nervous system. Most of these disorders are highly prevalent, but some express rarely in human beings. Such disorders with least prevalence rates are known as rare neurodevelopmental disorders. The sensory system is affected in all individuals with these rare neurodevelopmental disorders, although to a varying extent. Sensory processing in terms of hearing loss is reported by many researchers in many rare neurodevelopmental disorders, but the pathophysiology of audiological findings are seldom investigated. In this chapter, the authors highlight the possible relationship between underlying cause and the resultant audiological symptoms in some of the rare neurodevelopmental disorders. Further, the research studies on the audiological profiling in such disorders are discussed.

INTRODUCTION

The present chapter is a review of the hearing loss in children with neurodevelopmental disorders. The chapters focus on the incidence and prevalence of hearing impairment/auditory processing disorders; and pathophysiology of hearing impairment in such disorders. Available research literature explains the relationship between hearing loss and some common neurodevelopmental disorders. However, such researches with reference to some of the rare neurodevelopmental disorders are limited. In the present chapter, the authors attempted to list the nature and pathophysiology of hearing loss in some of the rare neurodevelopmental disorders. Such information is essential for appropriate assessment and timely and adequate rehabilitation of children with some rare neurodevelopmental disorders.

DOI: 10.4018/978-1-5225-7004-2.ch002

Neurodevelopmental disorders (NDD) are a heterogeneous group of diseases which affects the development of the central nervous system (Sontheimer, 2015). According to DSM-5 classification (American Psychiatric Association, 2013), the neurodevelopmental disorders may be classified into intellectual developmental disorders, communication disorders, autism spectrum disorders, attention deficit hyperactive disorder, specific learning disorder, and motor disorder (Grohol, 2013). The cognitive, behavioral and sensory processing may be affected in these disorders (Ataalla, 2015).

Cognitive impairments are central to all NDD (Gathercole & Alloway, 2006). Tranel and Haan (2007) stated that impairments of attention are common in a wide array of these disorders. Inhibition control, orientation and selective attention were reported to be impaired in children with such disorders (Cornish, Scerif, & Karmiloff-Smith, 2007). Memory impairment is also common in children with NDD (Alloway & Gathercole, 2006). Other domains of cognition including thinking, reasoning, meta-cognitive abilities, learning, etc., are also affected in most of the children with NDD, although to a varying degree. Because of the cognitive, motor, sensory and intellectual impairment, socio-behavioral development is also affected in children with NDD. Such children are at greater risk of developing anxiety-emotional problems and have the poor peer relationship, lower social esteem, and interpersonal problems (Arim, Kohen, Garner, Lach, Brehaut, MacKenzie, & Rosenbaum, 2015). Academic underachievement is secondary to socio-behavioral impairments in children with NDD (Bruce, 2011).

Sensory processing in terms of visual, somatosensory, proprioceptive, kinesthetic, and hearing abilities are affected in children suffering from most of these disorders to a varying extent. Hearing function in terms of absolute hearing sensitivity and auditory processing abilities are impaired in children with NDD (Katbamna & Crumpton, 2011). Profuse research literature addressing the presence of hearing impairment in children with different neurodevelopmental disorders like autism (Lachowska, Pastuszka, Łukaszewicz-Moszyńska, Mikołajewska, & Niemczyk, 2016; Rosenhall, Nordin, Sandström, Ahlsén, & Gillberg, 1999; Worley, Matson, & Kozlowski, 2011), Asperger's syndrome (Kancherla, Van Naarden Braun, & Yeargin-Allsopp, 2013), William's syndrome (Marler, Elfenbein, Ryals, Urban, & Netzloff, 2005), Alstrom syndrome (Frölander, Möller, Rudner, Mishra, Marshall, Piacentini, & Lyxell, 2015), Rett syndrome (Pillion, Rawool, Bibat, & Naidu, 2003), other pervasive developmental disorders (Cruz, Vicaria, Wang, Niparko, & Quittner, 2012; Psillas & Daniilidis, 2003; Tanaka, Adachi, Asanuma, & Sakata, 2011), attention deficit hyperactive disorders (Kelly, Kelly, Jones, Moulton, Verhulst, & Bell, 1993; Mueller & Tomblin, 2012; Munir, 2016; Redmond, Ash, & Hogan, 2015; Riccig & Hynd, 1996; Schmithorst, Plante, & Holland, 2014), and specific learning disability (Edwards, 2010; Hersher, 1980; Keller, Tillery, & McFadden, 2006; Miller & Kiani, 2008; Yeates, 1998), is available.

Researchers found that around 10-15% of the children with high-risk neurological factors develop hearing loss (Vashistha, Aseri, Singh, & Verma, 2016). In one of the epidemiological study, it was found that 7.9% of autistic children have unilateral hearing loss, and 3.5% children develop bilateral hearing loss (Rosenhall, Nordin, Sandström, Ahlsén, & Gillberg, 1999). Kancherla et al. (2013) also reported the prevalence of hearing loss in 6.7% of children with autism spectrum disorders. Kelly et al. (1993) found that hearing loss is prevalent in 14.1% of students with attention deficit hyperactive disorders. These epidemiological data indicate that hearing loss is a common problem in all neurodevelopmental disorders. The hearing disorders in children with NDD's may be directly due to neuro-sensory/ neuromuscular disease/ disorder, or it may be secondary to the drugs, surgery or other complications that may arise during the course of the disorder. Since hearing requires neurological processing of the sound signal, many neural organs including auditory nerve, cochlear nucleus, superior olivary complex, lateral lemniscus, inferior colliculus, medial geniculate body, auditory thalamus, auditory cortex, and association areas, corpus callosum, etc., are actively involved. The NDD's affecting any or all of these neural centers, either directly, or indirectly, affects the hearing and the processing of speech in the auditory system..

However, as stated earlier, NDD's are the set of a heterogeneous group of disorders, some of the neurodevelopmental disorders are rare and being given less attention in the past. A neurodevelopmental disorder is considered as rare when it affects a very small percentage of the population. There is no consensus among literates about the cut-off point, for which a disease can be considered as rare. Any disease may be rare in one part of the world, or for one set of the population, but may be common in another. According to World Health Organization, the rare diseases are deliberating and lifelong diseases with the prevalence rate of less than/equal to 1 per 1000 ("WHO | World Health Organization," n.d.). The rare disease act of United States ("Rare Diseases Act of 2002 (2002 - H.R. 4013)," n.d.), proposed that a disease or condition affecting less than 200,000 people in United States, or about 1 in 1500 affected people, should be considered as rare. In Japan, the prevalence rate of less than 1 in 2500 affected people, whereas European Commission suggested that diseases with low prevalence (1 in 2000 affected people) should be considered as rare (Baldovino, Moliner, Taruscio, Daina, & Roccatello, 2016). But such strict definitions about rare diseases have not been defined while considering the Indian perspective. As per the Indian government policy on rare diseases, submitted to Delhi High Court recently (Bhuyan, 2017), there are around 450 rare diseases prevalent in India. In a report published by the foundation for research on rare diseases and disorders ("Rare Diseases India," n.d.), India has more than 7 billion individuals suffering from rare diseases and disorders. With the consideration that many rare diseases are neurodevelopmental in nature, the research review on specific sensory processing in children with rare neurodevelopmental disorders is sparse.

In this chapter, the authors attempted to review the auditory perceptual characteristics of children with some rare neurodevelopmental disorders. The single or small group case-control studies published in the indexed peer-reviewed reputed journals were selected for the review. As a part of the preliminary assemblage of necessary information, a total of 7000 rare diseases have been identified from the database of various healthcare agencies like World Health Organization, National Organization for Rare Disorders (USA), National Institute of Health (UK), Orphanet (Europe), EPA Science Inventory (USA), Institute of Rare Diseases (Bulgaria), Rare Voices (Australia), National Disease Research Interchange (USA), Cleiss (France), Foundation of Research on Rare Disease and Disorders (India), and Organization for Rare Diseases (India). The brief review of available studies showed that 15 rare neurodevelopmental diseases cause significant hearing loss. These diseases have significant research support for hearing loss. It may be noted that individuals with other rare diseases/disorders may also have the sensorineural hearing loss, but for those children, hearing loss is not a characteristic feature or it may be secondary to some other related complication, but not directly to the disease process. Hence, those diseases were not reviewed here. All the selected syndromes are neurodevelopmental, congenital and genetic in nature. These syndromes are divided into two types on the basis of their pathophysiology. Firstly, the disorders directly affecting the inner ear structures and higher centers of auditory processing, as in some of the musculoskeletal disorders and/or congenital malformations; secondly, the disorders of metabolic, endocrine, systemic and/or infectious origin directly/ indirectly affecting the auditory functioning either by depriving the nutritional supply to the auditory structures or because of the viral/ bacterial/ fungal/ parasitic or related infection/ inflammation, are considered. Only those syndromes which have resulted in hearing loss and/or significant auditory processing disorders are included. The detailed description of such syndromes, their pathophysiology for hearing loss and the audiological findings in individuals diagnosed as having those disorders are as follows:

MUSCULOSKELETAL/CONGENITAL MALFORMATIONS

Musculoskeletal disorders are a set of diseases which affects the body's musculoskeletal system, viz., muscles, tendons, ligaments, nerves, discs, blood vessels, etc. Congenital malformation account for around 2.4% of the total children born ("Congenital Anomalies," n.d.). In the Indian context, Bhide, Gund, and Kar (2016) reported that total prevalence of congenital musculoskeletal anomalies was 231/10,000 live births. Other researchers also reported a prevalence of 179/10,000 live births (Taksande, Vilhekar, Chaturvedi, & Jain, 2010) to 286/10,000 live birth (Sarkar, Patra, Dasgupta, Nayek, & Karmakar, 2013). Among these congenital musculoskeletal malformations, 8.53% of these diseases are rare (Coi, Santoro, Pierini, Marrucci, Pieroni, & Bianchi, 2017), but such prevalence estimate with reference to Indian context is not available. As per the data obtained from the world health organization, congenital anomalies are the single largest cause of infant mortality. Around 11.3% of the 2.68 million children worldwide died because of congenital anomalies from the year 2000-2015. The sensory impairment in terms of hearing loss is common in children with most of the congenital musculoskeletal malformations. Below are some such rare congenital musculoskeletal disorders, where hearing loss is commonly reported.

1. **Acrocallosal Syndrome:** It is an autosomal recessive disorder significantly characterized by partial or complete agenesis of corpus callosum, multiple dysmorphic features, and mental retardation (Schinzel, 1979). Other brain abnormalities like the growth of multiple cysts in the brain tissue are also reported (Ramteke, Darole, Shaikh, Padwal, Agrawal, Shrivastava, & Kamath, 2011). Physical symptoms like syndactyly, polydactyly, hypertelorism and macrocephaly have also been seen in these individuals (Singal, Pandit, Saini, Singh, & Dhawan, 2014).

Bilateral sensorineural hearing loss and cortical auditory processing disorders are common in these children (Cataltepe & Tuncbilek, 1992; Gulati, Menon, Kabra, & Kalra, 2003). Cataltepe and Tuncbilek (1992) first reported that apart from the other common features of Acrocallosal syndrome, their patient (2 year old Turkish boy) also showed the features of bilateral sensorineural hearing loss. Later Courtens and his co-researchers (Courtens, Vamos, Christophe, & Schinzel, 1998) also reported the presence of bilateral mixed hearing loss in a 17-month-old boy with Acrocallosal syndrome. Gulati et al. (2003) also reported of congenital bilateral sensorineural hearing loss in a 5-year-old child with Acrocallosal syndrome. Other otologic manifestations include mild conductive hearing loss, narrow external auditory canal, and pre-auricular skin tags (National Organization for Rare Disorders, 2003). The exact patho-physiology of sensorineural hearing loss in such individuals is unknown, but it is thought to be genetic in origin. Poor oral and aural hygiene may contribute to the middle ear infections causing conductive/mixed hearing loss in these children.

Since individuals with Acrocallosal syndrome are significantly characterized by partial or complete agenesis of corpus callosum, higher auditory processing and inter-hemispheric transfer of language information may be highly affected in them. However, no such published case study restricts the authors to comment on the higher auditory processing abilities in their individuals, but auditory processing disorders in terms of auditory closure and hemispheric lateralization of language impairment are seen in other cases with corpus callosum agenesis (Jain & Dinesh, 2016).

2. **Cornelia De-Lange Syndrome:** It is a severe genetic disorder affecting the physical and intellectual development of children (Chatfield, Schrier, Li, Clark, Kaur, Kline, … Krantz, 2012). Marked growth retardation is the characteristic feature of Cornelia De-Lange syndrome. Other limb malformations, dysmorphic facial features like low anterior hairline, arched eyebrow, synophrys and long philtrum are common physical features in these children (Kline, Krantz, Sommer, Kliewer, Jackson, FitzPatrick, … Selicorni, 2007).

Auditory symptoms are seen in many cases of De-Lange syndrome (Egelund, 1987; Janek, Smith, Kline, Benke, Chen, Kimball, & Ishman, 2016). Marchisio et al. (2008) did the auditory profiling of 50 cases with Cornelia De-Lange syndrome and reported that 94% such children had otitis media with effusion. The conductive hearing loss was detected in 60% of the children, whereas 20% children had sensorineural hearing loss. Structural ear abnormality was also reported in on such child (Moretto, Pereira, & Aguiar, 2012). While Marchisio et al. (2008) reported the low prevalence of sensorineural hearing loss in these individuals. Other researchers have reported relatively high prevalence of sensorineural hearing loss in children with Cornelia De-Lange syndrome.

In a clinical review of 310 children with De Lange syndrome, Jackson, Kline, Barr, and Koch (1993) found that hearing loss of mild to severe degree may be present in around 50-60% of all the cases. The hearing loss was due to sensorineural component in 35-40% of the cases whereas remaining 15-20% cases showed conductive symptoms. Kim et al. (2008) also reported the prevalence of sensorineural hearing loss in 50% of the cases with Cornelia De-Lange syndrome. Hypoplastic cochlea and dysplastic vestibule are found in all the cases with hearing loss. These findings point towards the structural malformation attributing to the sensorineural hearing loss in children with Cornelia De-Lange syndrome.

3. **Hurler Syndrome:** Hurler syndrome, also known as mucopolysaccharidosis type I, is a lysosomal storage disease characterized by progressive deterioration in mental and physical body functioning, dwarfism, and sensory impairment. The disease is caused due to the deficiency of enzyme alpha-L iduronidase which is responsible for the degradation of mucopolysaccharides in lysosome. Without this enzyme, Keratan sulphate and Dermatan sulphate start depositing in the body. Excessive deposition of Keratan sulphate in the cochlear duct, stria vascularis and cochlear nerve disrupts the cochlear function and results in mild to profound sensorineural hearing loss (Friedmann, Spellacy, Crow, & Watts, 1985; Ruckenstein, Macdonald, Clarke, & Forte, 1991).

Researchers reported the high prevalence of conductive and sensori-neural hearing loss in children with Hurler's syndrome (Gökdoğan, Altinyay, Gökdoğan, Tutar, Gündüz, Okur, … Kemaloğlu, 2016; Kiely, Kohler, Coletti, Poe, & Escolar, 2017; Oghan, Harputluoglu, Guclu, Guvey, Turan, & Ozturk, 2007). Gökdoğan et al. (2016) reported severe mixed hearing loss in two cases with Hurlers syndrome, whereas one patient showed moderate to moderately severe conductive hearing loss. For all the three patient, the tympanogram showed type 'B' indicative of otitis media with effusion. Poor ear ventilation due to consistent upper respiratory tract infection and poor hygiene may be attributed to middle ear infection in these cases. Oghan et al. (2007) inserted permanent T-tubes in two patients with Hurler's syndrome and found an improvement of around 20 dB in their hearing sensitivity post-operatively.

4. **Morquio Syndrome:** Morquio syndrome (also known as mucopolysaccharidosis type IV) is an autosomal recessive lysosomal storage disorder (James, Berger, Elston, & Odom, 2006) where the body cannot process certain types of mucopolysaccharidosis resulting in the accumulation of keratan sulphate (Prat, Lemaire, Bret, Zabraniecki, & Fournié, 2008). As discussed in the Hurlers syndrome, excessive deposition of the keratan sulphate has devastating effect on cochlea and cochlear nerve. Significant skeletal and sensory deficits may be observed in individuals with this syndrome (Prat, Lemaire, Bret, Zabraniecki, & Fournié, 2008).

Hearing patterns in Morquio syndrome was first described by Riedner and Levin (1977). The researchers reported that 3/18 children with Morquio syndrome in their study had conductive hearing loss, whereas remaining 15/18 children had mixed or sensorineural hearing loss. Bilateral moderate conductive hearing loss was observed in one child with Morquio's syndrome (Santos, López, González, & Domínguez, 2011). But many other researchers reported sensorineural hearing loss in such children (Martell, Lau, Mei, Burnett, Decker, & Foehr, 2011; Taksande & Vilhekar, 2008). Auditory nerve disorder was also reported in a child with MPS IVA (Jain, Dwarakanath, & Suresh, 2014).

5. **Sanfilippo Syndrome:** The diseases was first described by Sylvester Sanfilipo (Sanfilippo, Podosin, Langer, & Good, 1963) as a lysosomal storage disorder, characterized by sensory, motor and behavioral deficits (Heldermon, Hennig, Ohlemiller, Ogilvie, Herzog, Breidenbach, … Sands, 2007). The disorder is caused due to the deficiency of glycosaminoglycan 'heparan sulphate' resulting in storage of sulphates and glycolipids (gangloisides) in the extracellular matrix and on cell surface glycoproteins. Heparan sulphate regulates the hair cell morphogenesis and homeostasis (Coulson-Thomas, Gesteira, Esko, & Kao, 2014) which is very important for normal cochlear hair cell functioning.

Since hair cells are directly affected in heparin sulphate deficiency, sensorineural hearing loss is reported in some cases of Sanfilippo's disease (Simmons, Bruce, Penney, Wraith, & Rothera, 2005). In a retrospective review of 46 children with Sanfillipo's syndrome, severe sensorineural hearing loss and speech delay was present in all the children (Buhrman, Thakkar, Poe, & Escolar, 2014). The conductive hearing loss in these individuals is also reported and thought to be secondary to upper respiratory tract infection (Mesolella, Cimmino, Cantone, Marino, Cozzolino, Casa, … Iengo, 2013).

6. **Keutel Syndrome:** Keutal syndrome is an autosomal recessive disorder caused due to the loss of functioning of matrix Gla protein gene (MGP). MGP inhibits the calcification in the soft tissue cartilages. Loss of MGP causes excessive calcification in the soft tissues of the body. This results in cartilaginous calcification, pulmonary stenosis, psychomotor delay and sensory abnormalities in children with Keutal disease (Ziereisen, De Munter, & Perlmutter, 1993). Calcification in the soft tissues of the cochlea and of the arteries supplying to the inner ear structures results in sensorineural hearing loss in individuals with Keutal syndrome (Keutel, Jörgensen, & Gabriel, 1971). Ossification of the basal and apical turns of cochlea is reported by Parmar and his colleagues (Parmar, Blaser, Unger, Yoo, Papsin, Parmar, … Yoo, 2006).

Sensorineural hearing loss is often seen in children with Keutel syndrome (Khosroshahi, Sahin, Akyuz, & Ede, 2014; Meier, Weng, Alexandrakis, Rüschoff, & Goeckenjan, 2001). Acar, Yilmaz, Sekercioglu, and Yuksel (2010) presented the audiological findings of a 35 year old female diagnosed with Keutel syndrome. Pure tone audiometry thresholds showed moderate sensorineural hearing loss in right ear and severe mixed hearing loss in the left ear. The mixed hearing loss was due to the calcification of the soft tissues in the middle ear. Hur et al. (2005) reviewed the molecular and clinical characteristics of 17 patients with Keutel syndrome and found that 12/17 patients were having the mixed hearing loss.

7. **Lenz-Majewski Syndrome:** Lenz-Majewski syndrome is the only known human disease to be caused by disrupted phosphatidylserine metabolism (Sousa, Jenkins, Chanudet, Tasseva, Ishida, Anderson, … Moore, 2014). Phosphatidylserine synthesis increase in cell fibroblast, which disrupts its regulatory functioning. Phosphatidylserine is present in the apical plasma membrane of the organ of corti (Shi, Gillespie, & Nuttall, 2007). Increased phosphatidylserine causes cell apoptosis and necrosis. This may be etiological factor of sensorineural hearing loss in individuals with Lenz-Majewski syndrome. Other symptoms of the disorder include craniodiaphyseal dysplasia, mental retardation and hypertelorism (James, Berger, Elston, & Odom, 2006; pp 571).

Sensorineural hearing loss is common but poorly documented in this syndrome (Toriello, Reardon, Gorlin, & Gorlin, 2004). Gorlin, Toriello and Cohen (1995) reported the possible sensorineural hearing loss in cases with Lenz-Majewski syndrome. The dysgenesis of the corpus callosum and the involvement of cortical auditory structures in Lenz-Majewski syndrome (Saraiva, 2000) point towards the possible higher-order auditory processing deficit in such children.

8. **Alpha-Mannosidosis Syndrome:** An autosomal recessive lysosomal storage disorder of alpha-manosidosis is caused by the deficit activity of enzyme alpha-mannosidase (Roces, Lüllmann-Rauch, Peng, Balducci, Andersson, Tollersrud, … von Figura, 2004). Alpha and Beta mannosidosis enzyme are richly present in the bone cells of the body. The defective alpha-manosidosis enzyme reduces the breakdown of sugar derived from glycoproteins in the lysosome which results in lysosomal accumulation in the cell. This impairs the cellular functioning and cell apoptosis (Shimmin, Ramirez, Matheson, & Dennis, 1989).

Hearing loss is seen in both alpha and beta mannosidosis (Beck, Olsen, Wraith, Zeman, Michalski, Saftig, … Malm, 2013; Malm & Nilssen, 2008; Michalski & Klein, 1999). Individuals with alpha-manosidosis syndrome typically develop ear infection probably due to bony abnormalities leading to eustachian tube closure (Malm & Nilssen, 2008). In some cases of alpha-manosidosis syndrome, sensorineural hearing loss was also observed which is thought to be due to skull bone abnormalities affecting the bony labyrinth of the inner ear (Autio, Louhimo, & Helenius, 1982).

ENDOCRINAL, METABOLIC, SYSTEMIC, INFECTIOUS AND OTHER DISEASES

The endocrine system consists of hormones secreted by various glands of the body directly into the circulatory system. Hypo secretion or hyper secretion of hormones and benign/malignant tumors of the glands results in endocrinal disorders. Metabolic system or metabolism comprise of catabolism, i.e. breaking down the organic matter (glucose, lipids, carbohydrates, etc.); and building up of organic components (proteins, nucleic acids, etc.) inside the cell body. The basic function of the metabolic system is to provide nutrition to the cells and removal of nitrogenous waste from the cell body. The metabolism occurs through various chemical transformations within the cell. Abnormal chemical reactions inside the cell body cause metabolic disorders (Graef, Wolfsdorf, & Greenes, 2008). The term 'Systemic' means affecting the entire body rather than a single organ. The systemic diseases affect a number of body organs and tissues. All the metabolic, infectious and endocrinal disorders ultimately affect the body circulatory system and are systemic in nature.

There are no published studies to estimate the incidence and prevalence of endocrinal, metabolic, systemic, infectious and other rare diseases probably due to co-morbidity of these disorders with other musculoskeletal, neural, and related diseases. However, the incidence and prevalence of individual syndromes are available to some extent and described below. All the syndromes mentioned below are rare and exhibits the symptoms of hearing loss and auditory processing disorders.

1. **Cockayne Syndrome:** It is a rare autosomal recessive neurodegenerative disorder characterized by impaired development of nervous system, photosensitivity, ear and eye abnormalities and sensorineural hearing loss (Neill & Dingwall, 1950). The incidence of Cockayne syndrome is estimated to be 2.77 per million live births in Japan (Kubota, Ohta, Ando, Koyama, Terashima, Kashii, … Hayashi, 2015). In United States, the incidence is less than 1 per 250,000 live births. As of 1992, only 140 cases of Cockayne syndrome were reported (National Organization for Rare Disorders, 2003). Mutation of CSA and CSB genes causes Cockayne syndrome. The annual incidence is about 1/200,000 live births in European countries ("Orphanet: Cockayne syndrome," 2011). However, such incidence and prevalence rate with reference to Indian context is not available and needs to be investigated.

Cockayne syndrome is caused due to mutation of ERCC8 (CSA) and ERCC6 (CSB) genes. The proteins made up of CSA and CSB genes are responsible for DNA repair. However, the altered expression of these genes causes non-repair of the damaged DNA. Thus the damage accumulates and this leads to malfunctioning of the cells and cell death (Rapin, Weidenheim, Lindenbaum, Rosenbaum, Merchant, Krishna, & Dickson, 2006; Wilson, Stark, Sutton, Danda, Ekbote, Elsayed, … Wilson, 2016). This is systemic and may result in inner ear hair cell necrosis and finally apoptosis. Shemen, Mitchell, and Farkashidy (1984) reported bilateral symmetrical sensorineural hearing loss in three patients with Cockayne syndrome. Laugel (2013) stated that sensorineural deafness should be considered as the characteristic feature of Cockayne syndrome. In a large-scale study on 102 patients, 44% patients were found to have conductive or mixed hearing loss whereas remaining 56% had sensorineural hearing loss (Wilson, Stark, Sutton, Danda, Ekbote, Elsayed… Wilson, 2016). Whatever may be a type of hearing loss, all the patients exhibited bilateral symmetrical hearing loss with severe to profound degree for those having sensorineural hearing loss.

2. **Dyekeratosis Congenita:** Dyskeratosis congenital (also known as Zinsser-Cole-Engman syndrome) is a progressive bone marrow failure syndrome characterized by hyper pigmentation of skin, oral leukoplakia and nail dystrophy (James, Berger, Elston, & Odom, 2006). The prevalence of dyekeratosis congenital is estimated to be 1/1,000,000 in Europe ("Orphanet: Dyskeratosis Congenita," 2011).

Vullimay et al. (2001) found that RNA component of telomerase is mutated in dyskeratosis congenital. This gives rise to ribosomopathy, i.e. an abnormal ribosomal function in the cells. Ultimately, the telomerase RNA component (TERC) is affected. TERC maintains the sequencing of DNA during the developmental period (Greider, 1996). Affected TERC inactivated most cell types soon after the development (Wong & Collins, 2006). This results in sensory degeneration in the early stages of life. Despite sensory degeneration, the reports investigating the hearing sensitivity in children with dyskeratosis congenital reported that hearing loss is rare in these individuals (Kalejaiye, Giri, Brewer, Zalewski, King, Adams, … Alter, 2016). Kalejaiye et al (2016) reviewed the otological manifestation of inherent bone marrow failure syndromes and stated that hearing loss was not present in any of the 37 children with dyskeratosis congenital. However single case studies on dyskeratosis congenital indicated the presence of sensorineural hearing loss in these individuals (García & Teruya-Feldstein, 2014; Hall, Prentice, Smiley, & Werkhaven, 1995; Savage, 2013).

3. **Fabry Disease:** It is a rare X-linked lysosomal storage disease which is associated with the sphingolipidosis, i.e. dysfunctional metabolism of sphingolipids. It is a circulatory disorder caused due to the deposition of globotriaosylceramide (a glycolipid) in the blood vessels (Karen, Hale, & Ma, 2005). This accumulation leads to the improper/insufficient blood supply to the organs of the body which causes impairment of the concerned organs. Localized pain in the body extremities (Hoffmann, Beck, Sunder-Plassmann, Borsini, Ricci, & Mehta, 2007), with nephrological, cardiac and skin diseases(Chew, Ghosh, & McCulloch, 1982) are common symptoms of Fabry disease. The prevalence of Fabry disease range from 1/10,000 to 1/100,000 Caucasian males (Branton, Schiffmann, Sabnis, Murray, Quirk, Altarescu, … Kopp, 2002; Houge & Skarbøvik, 2005; Meikle, Hopwood, Clague, & Carey, 1999). The exact prevalence of Fabry disease in Indian scenario is unknown, however, Verma, Ranganathan, Dalal, and Phadke (2012) estimated that lysosomal storage disorder occurs in 1/7000-8000 individuals.

Tinnitus, vertigo, nausea and hearing loss are often reported in children with Fabry disease (Germain, Avan, Chassaing, & Bonfils, 2002; Keilmann, Hegemann, Conti, & Hajioff, 2006; Suntjens, Dreschler, Hess-Erga, Skrunes, Wijburg, Linthorst, … Biegstraaten, 2017). Germain et al. (2002) investigated the cochlear involvement in 22 patients with Fabry disease. A test battery approach was adapted, including pure tone audiometry, tympanometry, oto-acoustic emissions and auditory brainstem responses, to assess the auditory functioning. It was reported that hearing sensitivity was affected in as many as 86.36% of patients. Among the affected individuals, 32% of the patients experienced sudden deafness and 37% of the individuals had high-frequency sensorineural hearing loss. All the patients had sensorineural hearing loss with no conductive involvement (bilateral 'A' type tympanogram in all patients). Using the neuropathological findings, the authors found the evidence of glycosphingolipid accumulation in the vascular endothelial and ganglion cells of the inner ear. Atrophy of stria vascularis and the spiral ligaments due to glycosphingolipid accumulation is also reported to the causative factor for sensorineural involvement in these individuals. Ototoxicity due to related nephorological disorder may be another causative factor for cochlear hearing loss in these individuals.

4. **Johanson-Blizzard Syndrome:** It is a rare autosomal recessive disorder caused by the mutation of UBR1 gene which encodes the ubiquitin ligase enzyme (Alkhouri, Kaplan, Kay, Shealy, Crowe, Bauhuber, & Zenker, 2008; Zenker, Mayerle, Lerch, Tagariello, Zerres, Durie, … Reis, 2005). Ubiquitin ligase regulated the production of ubiquitin protein, which helps in cell division, cell signaling, cell surface receptor function, DNA maintenance and homeostasis (Ciechanover, 1994; Ciechanover & Iwai, 2004). The disorder involves multiple systems featuring abnormal pancreatic, nasal, and skeletal development associated with cognitive and sensory impairment (Alkhouri, Kaplan, Kay, Shealy, Crowe, Bauhuber, & Zenker, 2008). According to NORD (National Organization for Rare Disorders, 2003), the frequency of Johanson-Blizzard syndrome is estimated to be 1/250,000 live births. In a recent report published by orphaned on rare diseases ("Prevalence and Incidence of Rare Diseases: Bibilographic Data," 2016), it is estimated that the prevalence of Johanson-Blizzard syndrome is estimated to be 0.4/100,000 live births in Europe. But such incidence/prevalence report with reference to Indian context is unavailable.

Congenital aplasia (absence of cochlea) (Johanson & Blizzard, 1971) and bilateral cystic dilation of the cochlea (Braun, Lerner, & Gershoni-Baruch, 1991) is seen in children with Johanson-Blizzard syndrome. Rosanowski, Hoppe, Hies, and Eysholdt (1998) reported dystopic ears in one such female. Recent case reports also reported the presence of sensorineural hearing loss in such individuals (Almashraki, Abdulnabee, Sukalo, Alrajoudi, Sharafadeen, & Zenker, 2011; Ellery & Erdman, 2014; Ramos, Ramos, Ramos, Peixoto, & Ramos, 2010). Johanson and Blizzard related the hearing loss with hypothyroidism, but later researchers found the hearing loss in patients with normal thyroid functioning also (Sismanis, Polisar, Ruffy, & Lambert, 1979). Ectodermal deficits are also attributed to the underlying cause of sensorineural hearing loss. Since the otic capsule of the inner ear develops from the midline ectoderm, ectodermal dysplasia syndrome can cause dysplasia, aplasia and other structural and functional deficits of the inner ear (Shin & Hartnick, 2004).

5. **Kearns-Sayre Syndrome:** Kearns-Sayre syndrome is a mitochondrial myopathy occurs due to the large-scale deletion of mitochondrial DNA. The loss of mitochondrial DNA occurs in the embryonic period, at the germ cell level (López-Gallardo, López-Pérez, Montoya, & Ruiz-Pesini, 2009). According to Ding et al. (2013), mutation in the mitochondrial DNA is an important cause of hearing loss. Mitochondrial DNA is also associated with presbycusis (age-related hearing loss) (Yamasoba, Someya, Yamada, Weindruch, Prolla, & Tanokura, 2007). The prevalence of Kearns-Sayre syndrome is approximately 2/100,000 in Europe ("Prevalence and Incidence of Rare Diseases: Bibilographic Data," 2016).

The major symptom of Kearns-Sayre syndrome is that involving the eye muscles (Harvey & Barnett, 1992). Sensorineural hearing loss in Kearns-Sayre syndrome (Kornblum, Broicher, Walther, Herberhold, Klockgether, Herberhold, & Schröder, 2005) and other mitochondrial myopathies has been reported in the literature (Chinnery, Elliott, Green, Rees, Coulthard, Turnbull, & Griffiths, 2000; Zwirner & Wilichowski, 2001). Kornblum et al. (2005) reported that as many as 10/17 patients with Kearns-Sayre syndrome showed mild to moderate high-frequency sensorineural hearing loss. Profound hearing loss in both ears has been reported by many researchers in individuals with Kearns-Sayre syndrome (Bahmad, Costa, Teixeira, de Barros Filho, Viana, & Marshall, 2014; Chinnery, Elliott, Green, Rees, Coulthard,

Turnbull, & Griffiths, 2000; Oliveira, Brosco, Oliveira, Alvarenga, Oliveira, Brosco, ... Alvarenga, 2017; Pijl & Westerberg, 2008).

6. **Noorie Syndrome:** Noorie disease is an X-linked autosomal recessive disorder caused by the mutation of Noorie disease protein (NDP) gene. The NDP gene regulates the vascular development of retina and some important blood vessels of the inner ear (Ye, Smallwood, & Nathans, 2011). This is the reason that despite it being a congenital ocular disorder, many people with Noorie disease develop progressive hearing loss which starts mostly by the second decade of life (Halpin, Owen, Gutiérrez-Espeleta, Sims, & Rehm, 2005). The incidence and prevalence of Noorie disease in unknown.

While profiling the audiological characteristics of 12 individuals with Noorie disease, Halpin et al. (2005) found severe sensorineural hearing loss in all of them. The authors attributed stria vascularis involvement causing hearing loss in these individuals. The primary reason of stria vascularis involvement in Noorie disease is that it houses the main vasculature of the cochlea. Rehm et al. (2002) analyzed the relationship between vascular deficits and sensorineural hearing loss in a mouse model of Norrie disease. The histological analysis of the cochlea revealed significantly enlarged vessels of the stria vascularis at the apex of the cochlea. As the hearing loss progressed, the hair cells also started degenerating. In the advanced stages, there was a significant loss of inner hair cells as well.

7. **Refsum Disease:** It is an autosomal recessive neurological disease caused due to over-accumulation of phytanic acid in body cells and tissues (Kahlert, Schönfeld, & Reiser, 2005). The role of phytanic acid is unclear in humans, however, it regulates the metabolism of the fatty acids in mice (Nogueira, Meehan, & O'Donoghue, 2014). The effect of increased generation of phytanic acid in the inner ear is unexplored, but it is thought to affect the insulin production causing immune deficiency and hearing loss. The prevalence of Refsum disease is around 0.1/100,000 in the European population ("Prevalence and Incidence of Rare Diseases: Bibilographic Data," 2016).

Audiological examination of many patients with Refsum's disease revealed cochlear involvement in most of them (Bamiou, Spraggs, Gibberd, Sidey, & Luxon, 2003; Bergsmark & Djupesland, 1968; Oysu, Aslan, Basaran, & Baserer, 2001). Bamiu et al. (2003) investigated the site of origin of hearing loss in nine individuals with Refsum's disease. The researchers reported that the hearing loss ranged from mild to moderate degree predominantly in high frequencies. They also found subtle auditory nerve involvement in 8/9 such patients. Auditory neuropathy was reported in one case with Refsum's disease (Oysu, Aslan, Basaran, & Baserer, 2001).

To summarize, a range of rare neurodevelopmental disorders were reviewed derived from the most popular healthcare agencies of the world, and the disorders were categorized into musculoskeletal disorders and/or congenital malformations; and the disorders of metabolic, endocrine, systemic and/or infectious origin, on the basis of their pathophysiology. Among these diseases/disorders, 15 rare NDD's which causes significant hearing impairment are reviewed. Diseases of musculoskeletol/congenital malformations were those which affect the body's musculoskeletol system, viz., muscles, tendons, ligaments, nerves, discs, blood vessels, etc. Acrocallosal syndrome is one such musculoskeletol disorder where sensorineural hearing loss and auditory processing disorders are prevalent and are due to genetic disturbances and agenesis of corpus callosum. Hearing loss in Cornelia De-Lange syndrome is due to the structural deformity of the auditory mechanism. Hurler's, Morquio, Sanfillipo, and Alpha-Mannosidosis syndromes are lysosomal storage disorders and are thought to affect the cellular composition of the inner ear. Keutel and Lenz-Majewski syndrome is protein deficiency disease and results in cellular disruption in the cochlea. The disorders of metabolic, endocrine, systemic and/or infectious origin included Cockayne, Noorie, and Johanson-Blizzard syndrome, which is also a protein deficiency disease. Dyekeratosis congenital is a progressive bone marrow failure syndrome, which can result in ribosomopathy. Farby is also lysosomal storage disorder affecting the vascular supply to the cochlea. Kearns-Sayre is a mitochondrial myopathy causing mitochondrial hearing loss. Lastly, Refsum disease is a phytanic acid storage disorder, which disturbs the metabolism of the inner ear resulting in hearing loss.

The above review indicated that despite different pathophysiologies, hearing loss of sensorineural type and moderate to profound degree is prevalent in many children with rare neurodevelopmental disorders. Thus, detailed assessment of hearing sensitivity in children with rare NDD's is warranted. In the presence of hearing loss in children with rare NDD's, timely management is essential not only for hearing function but also for speech, language, psychological, social, emotional and personality development. The auditory rehabilitation varies from individual to individuals ranging from medical/surgical management for conductive/mixed hearing loss and hearing aids, cochlear implants and other assistive listening devices for sensorineural hearing impairment. The choice of auditory rehabilitation also depends upon the severity of hearing loss and associated problems.

CONCLUSION

The present chapter highlighted the pathophysiological features causing hearing loss in some rare neurodevelopmental disorders. As for most of the disorders, the pathophysiology causing hearing loss was unavailable, the authors tried to correlate the underlying cause/deficit due to the specific pathology and its relationship with auditory structures. Further, the studies reporting hearing loss and other audiological symptoms in individuals with some rare neurological disorders are discussed.

REFERENCES

Acar, G. O., Yilmaz, M., Sekercioğlu, N., & Yüksel, A. (2010). Keutel syndrome in a patient presenting with hearing loss. *B-ENT*, *6*, 201–204. PMID:21090163

Alkhouri, N., Kaplan, B., Kay, M., Shealy, A., Crowe, C., Bauhuber, S., & Zenker, M. (2008). Johanson-Blizzard syndrome with mild phenotypic features confirmed by UBR1 gene testing. *World Journal of Gastroenterology*, *14*(44), 6863–6866. doi:10.3748/wjg.14.6863 PMID:19058315

Alloway, T. P., & Gathercole, S. E. (Eds.). (2006). *Working memory and neurodevelopmental disorders*. Hove, UK: Psychology Press.

Almashraki, N., Abdulnabee, M. Z., Sukalo, M., Alrajoudi, A., Sharafadeen, I., & Zenker, M. (2011). Johanson-Blizzard syndrome. *World Journal of Gastroenterology*, *17*(37), 4247–4250. doi:10.3748/wjg.v17.i37.4247 PMID:22072859

American Psychiatric Association. (2013). *Diagnostic and statistical manual of mental disorders: DSM-5* (5th ed.). Washington, DC: American Psychiatric Association.

Arim, R. G., Kohen, D. E., Garner, R. E., Lach, L. M., Brehaut, J. C., MacKenzie, M. J., & Rosenbaum, P. L. (2015). Psychosocial functioning in children with neurodevelopmental disorders and externalizing behavior problems. *Disability and Rehabilitation*, *37*(4), 345–354. doi:10.3109/09638288.2014.919361 PMID:24840026

Ataalla, M. (2015). Behavioral, mental health issues and neurodevelopmental disorders. In O. Naga (Ed.), *Pediatric Board Study Guide* (pp. 29–43). Cham: Springer; doi:10.1007/978-3-319-10115-6_2

Autio, S., Louhimo, T., & Helenius, M. (1982). The clinical course of mannosidosis. *Annals of Clinical Research*, *14*, 93–97. PMID:7149616

Bahmad, F. Jr, Costa, C. S. A., Teixeira, M. S., de Barros Filho, J., Viana, L. M., & Marshall, J. (2014). Familial Alström syndrome: A rare cause of bilateral progressive hearing loss. *Revista Brasileira de Otorrinolaringologia (English Ed.)*, *80*(2), 99–104. doi:10.5935/1808-8694.20140023 PMID:24830966

Baldovino, S., Moliner, A. M., Taruscio, D., Daina, E., & Roccatello, D. (2016). Rare diseases in Europe: From a wide to a local perspective. *The Israel Medical Association Journal*, *18*, 359–363. PMID:27468531

Bamiou, D. E., Spraggs, P. R. D., Gibberd, F. B., Sidey, M. C., & Luxon, L. M. (2003). Hearing loss in adult Refsum's disease. *Clinical Otolaryngology and Allied Sciences*, *28*(3), 227–230. doi:10.1046/j.1365-2273.2003.00694.x PMID:12755761

Beck, M., Olsen, K. J., Wraith, J. E., Zeman, J., Michalski, J. C., Saftig, P., ... Malm, D. (2013). Natural history of alpha mannosidosis a longitudinal study. *Orphanet Journal of Rare Diseases*, *8*(1), 88. doi:10.1186/1750-1172-8-88 PMID:23786919

Bergsmark, J., & Djupesland, G. (1968). Heredopathia Atactica Polyneuritiformis (Refsum's Disease) An Audiological Examination of two Patients. *European Neurology*, *1*(2), 122–130. doi:10.1159/000113655 PMID:4177049

Bhide, P., Gund, P., & Kar, A. (2016). Prevalence of congenital anomalies in an Indian maternal cohort: Healthcare, prevention, and surveillance implications. *PLoS One*, 11. PMID:27832123

Bhuyan, A. (2017, May 26). *Government submits rare disease policy to Delhi HC, recommends Rs 100 Crore for genetic diseases*. Retrieved from https://thewire.in/140229/rare-disease-policy/

Branton, M. H., Schiffmann, R., Sabnis, S. G., Murray, G. J., Quirk, J. M., Altarescu, G., ... Kopp, J. B. (2002). Natural history of Fabry renal disease: Influence of alpha-galactosidase: A activity and genetic mutations on clinical course. *Medicine*, *81*(2), 122–138. doi:10.1097/00005792-200203000-00003 PMID:11889412

Braun, J., Lerner, A., & Gershoni-Baruch, R. (1991). The temporal bone in the Johanson-Blizzard syndrome. *Pediatric Radiology*, *21*(8), 580–583. doi:10.1007/BF02012603 PMID:1815181

Bruce, S. K. (2011). Academic underachievement: A neurodevelopmental perspective. *Revista Médica Clínica Las Condes*, *22*(2), 211–217. doi:10.1016/S0716-8640(11)70415-1

Buhrman, D., Thakkar, K., Poe, M., & Escolar, M. L. (2014). Natural history of Sanfilippo syndrome type A. *Journal of Inherited Metabolic Disease*, *37*(3), 431–437. doi:10.100710545-013-9661-8 PMID:24271936

Cataltepe, S., & Tuncbilek, E. (1992). A family with one child with acrocallosal syndrome, one child with anencephaly-polydactyly, and parental consanguinity. *European Journal of Pediatrics*, *151*(4), 288–290. doi:10.1007/BF02072231 PMID:1499582

Chatfield, K. C., Schrier, S. A., Li, J., Clark, D., Kaur, M., Kline, A. D., ... Krantz, I. D. (2012). Congenital heart disease in Cornelia de Lange syndrome: Phenotype and genotype analysis. *American Journal of Medical Genetics. Part A*, *158A*(10), 2499–2505. doi:10.1002/ajmg.a.35582 PMID:22965847

Chew, E., Ghosh, M., & McCulloch, C. (1982). Amiodarone-induced cornea verticillata. *Canadian Journal of Ophthalmology. Journal Canadien D'ophtalmologie*, *17*, 96–99. PMID:7116220

Chinnery, P. F., Elliott, C., Green, G. R., Rees, A., Coulthard, A., Turnbull, D. M., & Griffiths, T. D. (2000). The spectrum of hearing loss due to mitochondrial DNA defects. *Brain*, *123*(1), 82–92. doi:10.1093/brain/123.1.82 PMID:10611123

Ciechanover, A. (1994). The ubiquitin-mediated proteolytic pathway: Mechanisms of action and cellular physiology. *Biological Chemistry Hoppe-Seyler*, *375*, 565–581. PMID:7840898

Ciechanover, A., & Iwai, K. (2004). The ubiquitin system: From basic mechanisms to the patient bed. *IUBMB Life*, *56*(4), 193–201. doi:10.1080/1521654042000223616 PMID:15230346

Coi, A., Santoro, M., Pierini, A., Marrucci, S., Pieroni, F., & Bianchi, F. (2017). Prevalence estimates of rare congenital anomalies by integrating two population-based registries in Tuscany, Italy. *Public Health Genomics*, *20*(4), 229–234. doi:10.1159/000481358 PMID:29045944

Congenital Anomalies: Prevalence and Risk Factors. (n.d.). Retrieved March 31, 2018, from https://www.researchgate.net/publication/259526843_Congenital_Anomalies_Prevalence_and_Risk_Factors

Cornish, K., Scerif, G., & Karmiloff-Smith, A. (2007). Tracing syndrome-specific trajectories of attention across the lifespan. *Cortex*, *43*(6), 672–685. doi:10.1016/S0010-9452(08)70497-0 PMID:17710820

Coulson-Thomas, V. J., Gesteira, T. F., Esko, J., & Kao, W. (2014). Heparan sulfate regulates hair follicle and sebaceous gland morphogenesis and homeostasis. *The Journal of Biological Chemistry*, *289*(36), 25211–25226. doi:10.1074/jbc.M114.572511 PMID:25053416

Courtens, W., Vamos, E., Christophe, C., & Schinzel, A. (1998). Acrocallosal syndrome in Algerian boy born to consanguineous parents: Review of the literature and further delineation of the syndrome. *American Journal of Medical Genetics*, *69*(1), 17–22. doi:10.1002/(SICI)1096-8628(19970303)69:1<17::AID-AJMG4>3.0.CO;2-Q PMID:9066878

Cruz, I., Vicaria, I., Wang, N.-Y., Niparko, J., & Quittner, A. L. (2012). Language and behavioral outcomes in children with developmental disabilities using cochlear implants. *Otology & Neurotology*, *33*(5), 751–760. doi:10.1097/MAO.0b013e3182595309 PMID:22699986

Ding, Y., Leng, J., Fan, F., Xia, B., & Xu, P. (2013). The role of mitochondrial DNA mutations in hearing loss. *Biochemical Genetics*, *51*(7-8), 588–602. doi:10.100710528-013-9589-6 PMID:23605717

Edwards, L. (2010). Learning Disabilities in Deaf and Hard-of-Hearing Children. In M. Marschark & P. E. Spencer (Eds.), *The Oxford handbook of deaf studies, language and education* (Vol. 2). Oxford University Press. doi:10.1093/oxfordhb/9780195390032.013.0028

Egelund, E. P. (1987). Congenital hearing loss in patients with Cornelia de Lange syndrome (a report of two cases). *The Journal of Laryngology and Otology*, *101*(12), 1276–1279. doi:10.1017/S0022215100103652 PMID:3323381

Ellery, K. M., & Erdman, S. H. (2014). Johanson-Blizzard Syndrome: Expanding the Phenotype of Exocrine Pancreatic Insufficiency. *Journal of the Pancreas*, *15*(4), 388–390. PMID:25076350

Friedmann, I., Spellacy, E., Crow, J., & Watts, R. W. (1985). Histopathological studies of the temporal bones in Hurler's disease. *The Journal of Laryngology and Otology*, *99*(01), 29–41. doi:10.1017/S0022215100096250 PMID:3918131

Frölander, H. E., Möller, C., Rudner, M., Mishra, S., Marshall, J. D., Piacentini, H., & Lyxell, B. (2015). Theory-of-mind in individuals with Alström syndrome is related to executive functions, and verbal ability. *Frontiers in Psychology*, *6*, 1426. doi:10.3389/fpsyg.2015.01426 PMID:26441796

García, F. M. S., & Teruya-Feldstein, J. (2014). The diagnosis and treatment of dyskeratosis congenita: A review. *Journal of Blood Medicine*, *5*, 157–167. PMID:25170286

Gathercole, S. E., & Alloway, T. P. (2006). Practitioner review: Short-term and working memory impairments in neurodevelopmental disorders: Diagnosis and remedial support. *Journal of Child Psychology and Psychiatry, and Allied Disciplines*, *47*(1), 4–15. doi:10.1111/j.1469-7610.2005.01446.x PMID:16405635

Germain, D. P., Avan, P., Chassaing, A., & Bonfils, P. (2002). Patients affected with Fabry disease have an increased incidence of progressive hearing loss and sudden deafness: An investigation of twenty-two hemizygous male patients. *BMC Medical Genetics*, *3*(1), 10. doi:10.1186/1471-2350-3-10 PMID:12377100

Gökdoğan, Ç., Altinyay, Ş., Gökdoğan, O., Tutar, H., Gündüz, B., Okur, İ., ... Kemaloğlu, Y. K. (2016). Audiologic evaluations of children with mucopolysaccharidosis. *Revista Brasileira de Otorrinolaringologia (English Ed.)*, *82*(3), 281–284. doi:10.1016/j.bjorl.2015.05.007 PMID:26601996

Gorlin, R. J., Toriello, H. V., & Cohen, M. M. (1995). *Hereditary hearing loss and its syndromes*. New York: Oxford University Press.

Graef, J. W., Wolfsdorf, J. I., & Greenes, D. S. (Eds.). (2008). *Manual of pediatric therapeutics* (7th ed.). Philadelphia: Lippincott Williams & Wilkins.

Greider, C. W. (1996). Telomere length regulation. *Annual Review of Biochemistry*, *65*(1), 337–365. doi:10.1146/annurev.bi.65.070196.002005 PMID:8811183

Grohol, J. M. (2013). *DSM-5 Changes: Neurodevelopmental Disorders*. Retrieved November 14, 2017, from pro.psychcentral.com/dsm-5-changes-neurodevelopmental-disorders/004366.html

Gulati, S., Menon, S., Kabra, M., & Kalra, V. (2003). Schinzel Acrocallosal syndrome. *Indian Journal of Pediatrics*, *70*(2), 173–176. doi:10.1007/BF02723749 PMID:12661815

Hall, J. W., Prentice, C. H., Smiley, G., & Werkhaven, J. (1995). Auditory dysfunction in selected syndromes and patterns of malformations : Review and case findings. *Journal of the American Academy of Audiology*, *6*, 80–92. PMID:7696681

Halpin, C., Owen, G., Gutiérrez-Espeleta, G. A., Sims, K., & Rehm, H. L. (2005). Audiologic features of Norrie disease. *The Annals of Otology, Rhinology, and Laryngology*, *114*(7), 533–538. doi:10.1177/000348940511400707 PMID:16134349

Harvey, J. N., & Barnett, D. (1992). Endocrine dysfunction in Kearns-Sayre syndrome. *Horumon To Rinsho*, *37*, 97–103. PMID:1424198

Heldermon, C. D., Hennig, A. K., Ohlemiller, K. K., Ogilvie, J. M., Herzog, E. D., Breidenbach, A., ... Sands, M. S. (2007). Development of sensory, motor and behavioral deficits in the murine model of sanfilippo syndrome type B. *PLoS One*, *2*(8), e772. doi:10.1371/journal.pone.0000772 PMID:17712420

Hersher, L. (1980). Hearing loss and learning disability. *American Journal of Diseases of Children*, *134*, 94. PMID:7350794

Hoffmann, B., Beck, M., Sunder-Plassmann, G., Borsini, W., Ricci, R., & Mehta, A. (2007). Nature and prevalence of pain in Fabry disease and its response to enzyme replacement therapy: A retrospective analysis from the Fabry Outcome Survey. *The Clinical Journal of Pain*, *23*(6), 535–542. doi:10.1097/AJP.0b013e318074c986 PMID:17575495

Houge, G., & Skarbøvik, A. J. (2005). [Fabry disease--a diagnostic and therapeutic challenge]. *Tidsskrift for Den Norske Laegeforening: Tidsskrift for Praktisk Medicin. Ny Raekke*, *125*, 1004–1006.

Hur, D. J., Raymond, G. V., Kahler, S. G., Riegert-Johnson, D. L., Cohen, B. A., & Boyadjiev, S. A. (2005). A novel MGP mutation in a consanguineous family: Review of the clinical and molecular characteristics of Keutel syndrome. *American Journal of Medical Genetics. Part A*, *135A*(1), 36–40. doi:10.1002/ajmg.a.30680 PMID:15810001

Jackson, L., Kline, A. D., Barr, M. A., & Koch, S. (1993). de Lange syndrome: A clinical review of 310 individuals. *American Journal of Medical Genetics*, *47*(7), 940–946. doi:10.1002/ajmg.1320470703 PMID:8291537

Jain, S., & Dinesh, N. (2016). A rare manifestation of specific learning disability in a child with Aicardi syndrome. *Acta Oto-Laryngologica Case Reports*, *1*(1), 17–23. doi:10.1080/23772484.2016.1192949

Jain, S., Dwarakanath, V. M., & Suresh, S. (2014). Audiological profile of a patient with MPS type IVA. *Rare Diseases and Orphan Drugs*, *1*. Retrieved from http://rarejournal.org/rarejournal/article/view/30

James, W. D., Berger, T. G., Elston, D. M., & Odom, R. B. (2006). *Andrews' diseases of the skin: Clinical dermatology* (10th ed.). Philadelphia: Saunders Elsevier.

Janek, K. C., Smith, D. F., Kline, A. D., Benke, J. R., Chen, M. L., Kimball, A., & Ishman, S. L. (2016). Improvement in hearing loss over time in Cornelia de Lange syndrome. *International Journal of Pediatric Otorhinolaryngology*, *87*, 203–207. doi:10.1016/j.ijporl.2016.06.032 PMID:27368472

Johanson, A., & Blizzard, R. (1971). A syndrome of congenital aplasia of the alae nasi, deafness, hypothyroidism, dwarfism, absent permanent teeth, and malabsorption. *The Journal of Pediatrics*, *79*(6), 982–987. doi:10.1016/S0022-3476(71)80194-4 PMID:5171616

Kahlert, S., Schönfeld, P., & Reiser, G. (2005). The Refsum disease marker phytanic acid, a branched chain fatty acid, affects Ca2+ homeostasis and mitochondria, and reduces cell viability in rat hippocampal astrocytes. *Neurobiology of Disease*, *18*(1), 110–118. doi:10.1016/j.nbd.2004.08.010 PMID:15649701

Kalejaiye, A., Giri, N., Brewer, C. C., Zalewski, C. K., King, K. A., Adams, C. D., ... Alter, B. P. (2016). Otologic manifestations of Fanconi anemia and other inherited bone marrow failure syndromes. *Pediatric Blood & Cancer*, *63*(12), 2139–2145. doi:10.1002/pbc.26155 PMID:27428025

Kancherla, V., Van Naarden Braun, K., & Yeargin-Allsopp, M. (2013). Childhood vision impairment, hearing loss and co-occurring autism spectrum disorder. *Disability and Health Journal*, *6*(4), 333–342. doi:10.1016/j.dhjo.2013.05.003 PMID:24060256

Karen, J. K., Hale, E. K., & Ma, L. (2005). Angiokeratoma corporis diffusum (Fabry disease). *Dermatology Online Journal*, *11*, 8. PMID:16403380

Katbamna, B., & Crumpton, T. (2011). Impact of Neurodevelopmental Disorders on Hearing in Children and Adolescents. In D. R. Patel, D. E. Greydanus, H. A. Omar, & J. Merrick (Eds.), *Neurodevelopmental Disabilities* (pp. 297–320). Dordrecht: Springer Netherlands. doi:10.1007/978-94-007-0627-9_19

Keilmann, A., Hegemann, S., Conti, G., & Hajioff, D. (2006). Fabry disease and the ear. In A. Mehta, M. Beck, & G. Sunder-Plassmann (Eds.), *Fabry Disease: Perspectives from 5 Years of FOS*. Oxford, UK: Oxford PharmaGenesis. Retrieved from http://www.ncbi.nlm.nih.gov/books/NBK11606/

Keller, W. D., Tillery, K. L., & McFadden, S. L. (2006). Auditory processing disorder in children diagnosed with nonverbal learning disability. *American Journal of Audiology*, *15*(2), 108–113. doi:10.1044/1059-0889(2006/014) PMID:17182875

Kelly, D. P., Kelly, B. J., Jones, M. L., Moulton, N. J., Verhulst, S. J., & Bell, S. A. (1993). Attention deficits in children and adolescents with hearing loss: A survey. *American Journal of Diseases of Children*, *147*(7), 737–741. doi:10.1001/archpedi.1993.02160310039014 PMID:8322743

Keutel, J., Jörgensen, G., & Gabriel, P. (1971). Ein neues autosomal-rezessiv vererbbares Syndrom. *Deutsche Medizinische Wochenschrift*, *96*(43), 1676–1681, passim. doi:10.1055-0028-1110200 PMID:5099199

Khosroshahi, H. e., Sahin, S., Akyuz, Y., & Ede, H. (2014). Long term follow-up of four patients with Keutel syndrome. *American Journal of Medical Genetics. Part A*, *164*(11), 2849–2856. doi:10.1002/ajmg.a.36699 PMID:25123378

Kiely, B. T., Kohler, J. L., Coletti, H. Y., Poe, M. D., & Escolar, M. L. (2017). Early disease progression of Hurler syndrome. *Orphanet Journal of Rare Diseases*, *12*(1), 32. doi:10.118613023-017-0583-7 PMID:28193245

Kim, J., Kim, E. Y., Lee, J. S., Lee, W. S., & Kim, H. N. (2008). Temporal bone CT findings in Cornelia de Lange syndrome. *AJNR. American Journal of Neuroradiology*, *29*(3), 569–573. doi:10.3174/ajnr.A0888 PMID:18065514

Kline, A. D., Krantz, I. D., Sommer, A., Kliewer, M., Jackson, L. G., FitzPatrick, D. R., ... Selicorni, A. (2007). Cornelia de Lange syndrome: Clinical review, diagnostic and scoring systems, and anticipatory guidance. *American Journal of Medical Genetics. Part A*, *143A*(12), 1287–1296. doi:10.1002/ajmg.a.31757 PMID:17508425

Kornblum, C., Broicher, R., Walther, E., Herberhold, S., Klockgether, T., Herberhold, C., & Schröder, R. (2005). Sensorineural hearing loss in patients with chronic progressive external ophthalmoplegia or Kearns-Sayre syndrome. *Journal of Neurology*, *252*(9), 1101–1107. doi:10.100700415-005-0827-7 PMID:15827867

Kubota, M., Ohta, S., Ando, A., Koyama, A., Terashima, H., Kashii, H., ... Hayashi, M. (2015). Nationwide survey of Cockayne syndrome in Japan: Incidence, clinical course and prognosis. *Pediatrics International*, *57*(3), 339–347. doi:10.1111/ped.12635 PMID:25851792

Lachowska, M., Pastuszka, A., Łukaszewicz-Moszyńska, Z., Mikołajewska, L., & Niemczyk, K. (2016). Cochlear implantation in autistic children with profound sensorineural hearing loss. *Revista Brasileira de Otorrinolaringologia (English Ed.)*, *84*(1), 15–19. doi:10.1016/j.bjorl.2016.10.012 PMID:27939998

Laugel, V. (2013). Cockayne syndrome: The expanding clinical and mutational spectrum. *Mechanisms of Ageing and Development*, *134*(5-6), 161–170. doi:10.1016/j.mad.2013.02.006 PMID:23428416

López-Gallardo, E., López-Pérez, M. J., Montoya, J., & Ruiz-Pesini, E. (2009). CPEO and KSS differ in the percentage and location of the mtDNA deletion. *Mitochondrion*, *9*(5), 314–317. doi:10.1016/j.mito.2009.04.005 PMID:19410662

Malm, D., & Nilssen, Ø. (2008). Alpha-mannosidosis. *Orphanet Journal of Rare Diseases*, *3*(1), 21. doi:10.1186/1750-1172-3-21 PMID:18651971

Marchisio, P., Selicorni, A., Pignataro, L., Milani, D., Baggi, E., Lambertini, L., ... Principi, N. (2008). Otitis media with effusion and hearing loss in children with Cornelia de Lange syndrome. *American Journal of Medical Genetics. Part A*, *146A*(4), 426–432. doi:10.1002/ajmg.a.32183 PMID:18203151

Marler, J. A., Elfenbein, J. L., Ryals, B. M., Urban, Z., & Netzloff, M. L. (2005). Sensorineural hearing loss in children and adults with Williams syndrome. *American Journal of Medical Genetics. Part A*, *138*(4), 318–327. doi:10.1002/ajmg.a.30970 PMID:16222677

Martell, L., Lau, K., Mei, M., Burnett, V., Decker, C., & Foehr, E. D. (2011). Biomarker analysis of Morquio syndrome: Identification of disease state and drug responsive markers. *Orphanet Journal of Rare Diseases*, *6*(1), 84. doi:10.1186/1750-1172-6-84 PMID:22176730

Meier, M., Weng, L. P., Alexandrakis, E., Rüschoff, J., & Goeckenjan, G. (2001). Tracheobronchial stenosis in Keutel syndrome. *The European Respiratory Journal*, *17*(3), 566–569. doi:10.1183/09031936.01.17305660 PMID:11405537

Meikle, P. J., Hopwood, J. J., Clague, A. E., & Carey, W. F. (1999). Prevalence of lysosomal storage disorders. *Journal of the American Medical Association*, *281*(3), 249–254. doi:10.1001/jama.281.3.249 PMID:9918480

Mesolella, M., Cimmino, M., Cantone, E., Marino, A., Cozzolino, M., Casa, R., ... Iengo, M. (2013). Management of otolaryngological manifestations in mucopolysaccharidoses: Our experience. *Acta Otorhinolaryngologica Italica*, *33*, 267–272. PMID:24043915

Michalski, J.-C., & Klein, A. (1999). Glycoprotein lysosomal storage disorders: A- and β-mannosidosis, fucosidosis and α-N-acetylgalactosaminidase deficiency. *Biochimica et Biophysica Acta (BBA) -. Molecular Basis of Disease*, *1455*(2-3), 69–84. doi:10.1016/S0925-4439(99)00077-0 PMID:10571005

Miller, H., & Kiani, R. (2008). Inter-relationships between hearing impairment, learning disability services and mental health: Are learning disability services 'deaf' to hearing impairments? *Advances in Mental Health and Learning Disabilities*, *2*(2), 25–30. doi:10.1108/17530180200800014

Moretto, M. J., Pereira, T. de S., & de Aguiar, S. M. H. C. Á. (2012). Case Report: Cornelia de Lange Syndrome (CDLS). *Archives of Health Investigation*, *1*, 78.

Mueller, K. L., & Tomblin, J. B. (2012). Examining the comorbidity of language disorders and ADHD. *Topics in Language Disorders*, *32*, 228–246. doi:10.1097/TLD.0b013e318262010d PMID:25505812

Munir, K. M. (2016). The co-occurrence of mental disorders in children and adolescents with intellectual disability/intellectual developmental disorder. *Current Opinion in Psychiatry*, *29*(2), 95–102. doi:10.1097/YCO.0000000000000236 PMID:26779862

National Organization for Rare Disorders (Ed.). (2003). *NORD guide to rare disorders*. Philadelphia: Lippincott Williams & Wilkins.

Neill, C. A., & Dingwall, M. M. (1950). A Syndrome Resembling Progeria: A Review of Two Cases. *Archives of Disease in Childhood*, *25*(123), 213–223. doi:10.1136/adc.25.123.213 PMID:14783428

Nogueira, C., Meehan, T., & O'Donoghue, G. (2014). Refsum's Disease and Cochlear Implantation. *The Annals of Otology, Rhinology, and Laryngology*, *123*(6), 425–427. doi:10.1177/0003489414526846 PMID:24690989

Oghan, F., Harputluoglu, U., Guclu, E., Guvey, A., Turan, N., & Ozturk, O. (2007). Permanent t-tube insertion in two patients with Hurler's syndrome. *International Journal of Audiology*, *46*(2), 94–96. doi:10.1080/14992020600975287 PMID:17365060

Oliveira, L. S., de, Brosco, K. C., Oliveira, E. B., Alvarenga, K. de F., Oliveira, L. S., de, & Brosco, K. C., … Alvarenga, K. de F. (2017). Cochlear implant in Kearns-Sayre syndrome: Case study of twin sisters. *Audiology - Communication Research*, 22.

Orphanet: Cockayne syndrome. (2011). Retrieved April 12, 2018, from http://www.orpha.net/consor/cgi-bin

Orphanet: Dyskeratosis congenita. (2011). Retrieved April 12, 2018, from http://www.orpha.net/consor/cgi-bin

Oysu, C., Aslan, I., Basaran, B., & Baserer, N. (2001). The site of the hearing loss in Refsum's disease. *International Journal of Pediatric Otorhinolaryngology*, *61*(2), 129–134. doi:10.1016/S0165-5876(01)00559-6 PMID:11589979

Parmar, H., Blaser, S., Unger, S., Yoo, S.-J., Papsin, B., Parmar, H., ... Yoo, S.-J. (2006). Petrified ears in a patient with Keutel syndrome: Temporal bone CT findings. *Pediatric Radiology*, *36*(3), 241–243. doi:10.100700247-005-0036-7 PMID:16328322

Pijl, S., & Westerberg, B. D. (2008). Cochlear implantation results in patients with Kearns-sayre syndrome. *Ear and Hearing*, *29*(3), 472–475. doi:10.1097/01.aud.0000310791.83193.62 PMID:18382375

Pillion, J. P., Rawool, V. W., Bibat, G., & Naidu, S. (2003). Prevalence of hearing loss in Rett syndrome. *Developmental Medicine and Child Neurology*, *45*(5), 338–343. doi:10.1111/j.1469-8749.2003.tb00405.x PMID:12729148

Prat, C., Lemaire, O., Bret, J., Zabraniecki, L., & Fournié, B. (2008). Morquio syndrome: Diagnosis in an adult. *Joint, Bone, Spine. Revue du Rhumatisme*, *75*, 495–498. PMID:18456538

Prevalence and incidence of rare diseases: Bibilographic data. (2016). Retrieved on April 17, 2018, from http://www.orphadata.org/cgi-bin/index.php/

Psillas, G., & Daniilidis, J. (2003). Low-frequency hearing assessment by middle latency responses in children with pervasive developmental disorder. *International Journal of Pediatric Otorhinolaryngology*, *67*(6), 613–619. doi:10.1016/S0165-5876(03)00071-5 PMID:12745154

Ramos, S., Ramos, H. F., Ramos, R. F., Peixoto, C. A. M., & Ramos, B. F. (2010). Johanson-Blizzard syndrome. *Revista Brasileira de Otorrinolaringologia (English Ed.)*, *76*, 794–794. PMID:21180950

Ramteke, V. V., Darole, P. A., Shaikh, Z. F., Padwal, N. J., Agrawal, B., Shrivastava, M. S., & Kamath, S. (2011). Acrocallosal syndrome in a young hypertensive male. *BMJ Case Reports*, *2011*(apr27 1), bcr1220103648. doi:10.1136/bcr.12.2010.3648 PMID:22696705

Rapin, I., Weidenheim, K., Lindenbaum, Y., Rosenbaum, P., Merchant, S. N., Krishna, S., & Dickson, D. W. (2006). Cockayne syndrome in adults: Review with clinical and pathologic study of a new case. *Journal of Child Neurology*, *21*(11), 991–1006. doi:10.1177/08830738060210110101 PMID:17092472

Rare Diseases Act of 2002 (2002 - H.R. 4013). (n.d.). Retrieved November 14, 2017, from https://www.govtrack.us/congress/bills/107/hr4013

Rare Diseases India. (n.d.). Retrieved November 14, 2017, from http://www.rarediseasesindia.org/

Redmond, S. M., Ash, A. C., & Hogan, T. P. (2015). Consequences of co-occurring attention-deficit/hyperactivity disorder on children's language impairments. *Language, Speech, and Hearing Services in Schools*, *46*(2), 68–80. doi:10.1044/2014_LSHSS-14-0045 PMID:25381450

Rehm, H. L., Zhang, D. S., Brown, M. C., Burgess, B., Halpin, C., Berger, W., ... Chen, Z. Y. (2002). Vascular defects and sensorineural deafness in a mouse model of Norrie disease. *The Journal of Neuroscience*, *22*(11), 4286–4292. doi:10.1523/JNEUROSCI.22-11-04286.2002 PMID:12040033

Riccig, C. A., & Hynd, G. W. (1996). Relationship between ADHD and central auditory processing disorder: A review of the literature. *School Psychology International*, *17*(3), 235–252. doi:10.1177/0143034396173001

Riedner, E. D., & Levin, L. S. (1977). Hearing patterns in Morquio's syndrome (mucopolysaccharidosis IV). *Archives of Otolaryngology*, *103*(9), 518–520. doi:10.1001/archotol.1977.00780260048003 PMID:409383

Roces, D. P., Lüllmann-Rauch, R., Peng, J., Balducci, C., Andersson, C., Tollersrud, O., ... von Figura, K. (2004). Efficacy of enzyme replacement therapy in alpha-mannosidosis mice: A preclinical animal study. *Human Molecular Genetics*, *13*(18), 1979–1988. doi:10.1093/hmg/ddh220 PMID:15269179

Rosanowski, F., Hoppe, U., Hies, T., & Eysholdt, U. (1998). Das Johanson-Blizzard- Syndrom. *HNO*, *46*(10), 876–878. doi:10.1007001060050328 PMID:9846268

Rosenhall, U., Nordin, V., Sandström, M., Ahlsén, G., & Gillberg, C. (1999). Autism and hearing loss. *Journal of Autism and Developmental Disorders*, *29*(5), 349–357. doi:10.1023/A:1023022709710 PMID:10587881

Ruckenstein, M. J., Macdonald, R. E., Clarke, J. T., & Forte, V. (1991). The management of otolaryngological problems in the mucopolysaccharidoses: A retrospective review. *The Journal of Otolaryngology*, *20*, 177–183. PMID:1908026

Sanfilippo, S. J., Podosin, R., Langer, L., & Good, R. A. (1963). Mental retardation associated with acid mucopolysacchariduria (heparitin sulfate type). *The Journal of Pediatrics*, *63*(4), 837–838. doi:10.1016/S0022-3476(63)80279-6

Santos, S., López, L., González, L., & Domínguez, M. J. (2011). Hearing loss and airway problems in children with Mucopolysaccharidoses. *Acta Otorrinolaringologica Espanola*, 411–417. doi:10.1016/j.otorri.2011.05.003 PMID:21757178

Saraiva, J. M. (2000). Dysgenesis of corpus callosum in Lenz-Majewski hyperostotic dwarfism. *American Journal of Medical Genetics*, *91*(3), 198–200. doi:10.1002/(SICI)1096-8628(20000320)91:3<198::AID-AJMG8>3.0.CO;2-4 PMID:10756342

Sarkar, S., Patra, C., Dasgupta, M. K., Nayek, K., & Karmakar, P. R. (2013). Prevalence of congenital anomalies in neonates and associated risk factors in a tertiary care hospital in eastern India. *Journal of Clinical Neonatology*, *2*(3), 131–134. doi:10.4103/2249-4847.119998 PMID:24251257

Savage, S. A. (2013). Dyskeratosis Congenita. In *Gene Review* (1st ed.). Seattle, WA: University of Washington, Seattle.

Schinzel, A. (1979). Postaxial polydactyly, hallux duplication, absence of the corpus callosum, macrencephaly and severe mental retardation: A new syndrome? *Helvetica Paediatrica Acta*, *34*, 141–146. PMID:457430

Schmithorst, V. J., Plante, E., & Holland, S. (2014). Unilateral deafness in children affects development of multi-modal modulation and default mode networks. *Frontiers in Human Neuroscience*, *8*, 164. doi:10.3389/fnhum.2014.00164 PMID:24723873

Shemen, L. J., Mitchell, D. P., & Farkashidy, J. (1984). Cockayne syndrome: An audiologic and temporal bone analysis. *The American Journal of Otology*, *5*, 300–307. PMID:6720882

Shi, X., Gillespie, P. G., & Nuttall, A. L. (2007). Apical phosphatidylserine externalization in auditory hair cells. *Molecular Membrane Biology*, *24*(1), 16–27. doi:10.1080/09687860600926883 PMID:17453410

Shimmin, L. C., Ramirez, C., Matheson, A. T., & Dennis, P. P. (1989). Sequence alignment and evolutionary comparison of the L10 equivalent and L12 equivalent ribosomal proteins from archaebacteria, eubacteria, and eucaryotes. *Journal of Molecular Evolution*, *29*(5), 448–462. doi:10.1007/BF02602915 PMID:2515294

Shin, J. J., & Hartnick, C. J. (2004). Otologic manifestations of ectodermal dysplasia. *Archives of Otolaryngology--Head & Neck Surgery*, *130*(9), 1104–1107. doi:10.1001/archotol.130.9.1104 PMID:15381599

Simmons, M. A., Bruce, I. A., Penney, S., Wraith, E., & Rothera, M. P. (2005). Otorhinolaryngological manifestations of the mucopolysaccharidoses. *International Journal of Pediatric Otorhinolaryngology*, *69*(5), 589–595. doi:10.1016/j.ijporl.2005.01.017 PMID:15850680

Singal, R., Pandit, S., Saini, A., Singh, P., & Dhawan, N. (2014). The Acrocallosal syndrome in a neonate with further widening of phenotypic expression. *Iranian Journal of Child Neurology*, *8*, 60–64. PMID:24949054

Sismanis, A., Polisar, I. A., Ruffy, M. L., & Lambert, J. C. (1979). Rare congenital syndrome associated with profound hearing loss. *Archives of Otolaryngology*, *105*(4), 222–224. doi:10.1001/archotol.1979.00790160056015 PMID:426713

Sontheimer, H. (2015). *Diseases of the nervous system*. Amsterdam: Elsevier Academic Press.

Sousa, S. B., Jenkins, D., Chanudet, E., Tasseva, G., Ishida, M., Anderson, G., ... Moore, G. E. (2014). Gain-of-function mutations in the phosphatidylserine synthase 1 (PTDSS1) gene cause Lenz-Majewski syndrome. *Nature Genetics*, *46*(1), 70–76. doi:10.1038/ng.2829 PMID:24241535

Suntjens, E., Dreschler, W. A., Hess-Erga, J., Skrunes, R., Wijburg, F. A., Linthorst, G. E., ... Biegstraaten, M. (2017). Hearing loss in children with Fabry disease. *Journal of Inherited Metabolic Disease*, *40*(5), 725–731. doi:10.100710545-017-0051-5 PMID:28567540

Taksande, A., & Vilhekar, K. (2008). Hurler syndrome or Morquio syndrome: Intelligence required for diagnosing the case. *The Indian Journal of Radiology & Imaging*, *18*(2), 175. doi:10.4103/0971-3026.40306

Taksande, A., Vilhekar, K., Chaturvedi, P., & Jain, M. (2010). Congenital malformations at birth in Central India: A rural medical college hospital based data. *Indian Journal of Human Genetics*, *16*(3), 159–163. doi:10.4103/0971-6866.73412 PMID:21206705

Tanaka, M., Adachi, N., Asanuma, S., & Sakata, H. (2011). Characteristics of cases with comorbid profound deafness and pervasive developmental disorders. *Pediatric Otorhinolaryngology Japan*, *32*, 91–95.

Toriello, H. V., Reardon, W., Gorlin, R. J., & Gorlin, R. J. (Eds.). (2004). *Hereditary hearing loss and its syndromes* (2nd ed.). Oxford, UK: Oxford University Press.

Tranel, D., & de Haan, E. (2007). Selective developmental neuropsychological disorders. *Cortex*, *43*(6), 667–671. doi:10.1016/S0010-9452(08)70496-9 PMID:17710819

Vashistha, I., Aseri, Y., Singh, B. K., & Verma, P. C. (2016). Prevalence of hearing impairment in high risk infants. *Indian Journal of Otolaryngology and Head and Neck Surgery*, *68*(2), 214–217. doi:10.100712070-015-0869-9 PMID:27340640

Verma, P. K., Ranganath, P., Dalal, A. B., & Phadke, S. R. (2012). Spectrum of Lysosomal storage disorders at a medical genetics center in northern India. *Indian Pediatrics*, *49*(10), 799–804. doi:10.100713312-012-0192-4 PMID:22791670

Vulliamy, T., Marrone, A., Goldman, F., Dearlove, A., Bessler, M., Mason, P. J., & Dokal, I. (2001). The RNA component of telomerase is mutated in autosomal dominant dyskeratosis congenita. *Nature*, *413*(6854), 432–435. doi:10.1038/35096585 PMID:11574891

WHO. (n.d.). Retrieved November 14, 2017, from http://www.who.int/en/

Wilson, B. T., Stark, Z., Sutton, R. E., Danda, S., Ekbote, A. V., Elsayed, S. M., ... Wilson, I. J. (2016). The Cockayne Syndrome Natural History (CoSyNH) study: Clinical findings in 102 individuals and recommendations for care. *Genetics in Medicine*, *18*(5), 483–493. doi:10.1038/gim.2015.110 PMID:26204423

Wong, J. M. Y., & Collins, K. (2006). Telomerase RNA level limits telomere maintenance in X-linked dyskeratosis congenita. *Genes & Development*, *20*(20), 2848–2858. doi:10.1101/gad.1476206 PMID:17015423

Worley, J. A., Matson, J. L., & Kozlowski, A. M. (2011). The effects of hearing impairment on symptoms of autism in toddlers. *Developmental Neurorehabilitation*, *14*(3), 171–176. doi:10.3109/17518423.2011.564600 PMID:21548858

Yamasoba, T., Someya, S., Yamada, C., Weindruch, R., Prolla, T. A., & Tanokura, M. (2007). Role of mitochondrial dysfunction and mitochondrial DNA mutations in age-related hearing loss. *Hearing Research*, *226*(1-2), 185–193. doi:10.1016/j.heares.2006.06.004 PMID:16870370

Ye, X., Smallwood, P., & Nathans, J. (2011). Expression of the Norrie disease gene (Ndp) in developing and adult mouse eye, ear, and brain. *Gene Expression Patterns*, *11*(1-2), 151–155. doi:10.1016/j.gep.2010.10.007 PMID:21055480

Yeates, S. (1998). Hearing Loss in People with Learning Disabilities. *Tizard Learning Disability Review*, *3*(2), 20–28. doi:10.1108/13595474199800014

Zenker, M., Mayerle, J., Lerch, M. M., Tagariello, A., Zerres, K., Durie, P. R., ... Reis, A. (2005). Deficiency of UBR1, a ubiquitin ligase of the N-end rule pathway, causes pancreatic dysfunction, malformations and mental retardation (Johanson-Blizzard syndrome). *Nature Genetics*, *37*(12), 1345–1350. doi:10.1038/ng1681 PMID:16311597

Ziereisen, F., De Munter, C., & Perlmutter, N. (1993). The Keutel syndrome. Report of a case and review of the literature. *Pediatric Radiology*, *23*(4), 314–315. doi:10.1007/BF02010925 PMID:8414764

Zwirner, P., & Wilichowski, E. (2001). Progressive sensorineural hearing loss in children with mitochondrial encephalomyopathies. *The Laryngoscope*, *111*(3), 515–521. doi:10.1097/00005537-200103000-00024 PMID:11224785

KEY TERMS AND DEFINITIONS

Auditory Processing: Auditory processing is set of processes which are essential for the perception of acoustic stimuli through the auditory system.

Hearing: Hearing is a process of receiving, extracting and interpreting the acoustic signal through the auditory mechanism.

Hearing Loss: Any loss in the hearing ability due to any pathology in the peripheral or central auditory system is known as hearing loss.

Neurodevelopmental Disorders: Neurodevelopmental disorders are set of diseases/disorders which affects the nervous system during the developmental period.

Pathophysiology: An illustration of the causative factor of a particular symptom and its relationship with the underlying pathology.

Rare Diseases: A disease is considered to be rare if its incidence and prevalence are very less in comparison to other diseases/disorders of same/similar origin.

Syndrome: A syndrome is a set of symptoms co-occurring in an individual due to some underlying pathology.

Chapter 3
Feeding and Swallowing Issues in Children With Neuro-Developmental Disorders

Srushti Shabnam
All India Institute of Speech and Hearing, India

Sunil Kumar Ravi
Shravana Institute of Speech and Hearing, India

Swapna N.
All India Institute of Speech and Hearing, India

ABSTRACT

The chapter highlights the feeding and swallowing issues seen in children with neuro-developmental disorders, types, and extent of the problem across different disorders; its relation with the neuro-development of the child; effect on the quality of life of the parents/caregivers along with the child, specifically in the Indian context. It also focuses on the importance of assessment, team approach, and review of available tests for the assessment of feeding and swallowing problems in these children. The chapter is also going to give a few insights into the challenges faced by speech-language pathologists during the assessment of the feeding and swallowing issues in these children in the Indian scenario. The chapter will also include a section on applications of ICF model to feeding and swallowing issues in children with neurodevelopmental disorders.

INTRODUCTION

The Diagnostic and Statistical Manual of Mental Disorders, Fifth Edition (DSM-5; American Psychiatric Association, 2013) describes Neuro-developmental disorders (NDDs) as a group of conditions, which have their onset in the developmental period. The diversity and extent of developmental deficits vary from very specific limitations of learning or control of executive functions to global impairments of social skills or intelligence, which can affect speech, language, and cognitive abilities. The conditions such as Intellectual Disability, Autism Spectrum Disorders, Cerebral Palsy, Attention-Deficit/ Hyperactivity Disorders and Global developmental delay are a few of the common NDDs.

DOI: 10.4018/978-1-5225-7004-2.ch003

It is well known that in these developmental disorders, the deficits can be seen in either one or multiple domains such as cognition, motor, speech, and language, or social skills. However, very little is known about the commonly associated feeding and swallowing issues in these children with NDD, which occurs due to various underlying deficits. The objective of the present chapter is to provide an overview of the feeding and swallowing issues reported in children with cerebral palsy, intellectual disability, and autism spectrum disorders. Further, the chapter includes a review of the available assessment tests or tools for feeding and swallowing and the need for developing feeding/swallowing assessment scales based on International Classification of Functioning, Disability, and Health (ICF; WHO, 2001). The chapter also includes a brief note on the importance of early intervention of feeding and swallowing issues in children with NDD, highlighting the role of speech-language pathologists (SLPs), with a few future directions.

INTRODUCTION TO FEEDING AND SWALLOWING

Feeding, in general, is a basic skill which exists from the beginning of infancy. It provides nutrition for normal growth and development; satisfies hunger and maintains the homeostasis, gives opportunities for sensory and motor stimulation, and oro-motor skill development, etc., thus serving to fulfill the biological functions of the body. Feeding also has a deep impact on the psychological aspect of a developing child. The behaviors of both parent/caregiver and child during feeding contribute significantly to the overall success of the feeding interaction as well as feeding performance, which in turn strengthen the mother-child bonding. Mealtimes with the family as well as outside the family play an important role in the social life of the child (Morris & Klein, 1987; Kummer, 2008).

The development of feeding in infancy depends on the maturation of gut, lungs and neural system. The functional and anatomic development of gut includes improvement in esophageal and intestinal motility, the functioning of the lower esophageal sphincter (LES), the process of ejection of stomach contents and development of the absorptive surface area of the gut. The respiration becomes more efficient by 32 to 34 weeks of gestation and continues to develop until two years of age. Our central nervous system matures in a peripheral to central sequence and our brainstem begins to mature by the second trimester. The brainstem controls our vital functions such as heart rate, blood pressure, digestion and sleep; and cerebral cortex regulates our functional life such as voluntary actions, thought process, memory etc. During early infancy, brainstem plays a major role in controlling all our life-sustaining reflexes (including breathing, suckling etc.) (Kliegman & Stanton, 2011; Kenner & McGrath, 2010; Gardner & Merenstein, 2002; Stiles & Jernigan, 2010).

Physiologically, the stages of feeding are divided into four main components: (a) oral phase (inclusive of oral preparatory and oral transport); (b) triggering of the swallow reflex; (c) pharyngeal phase, and; (d) esophageal phase. The process of feeding includes the placement of food in the mouth, the manipulation of food in the oral cavity prior to the initiation of the swallow, including mastication (oral preparatory phase), and the oral transport stage of the swallow when the bolus is propelled backwards by the tongue. When the food substance reaches the anterior faucial arch at the rear of the mouth, the pharyngeal swallow reflex is triggered. Following this, the pharyngeal phase occurs in which the base of the tongue and the pharyngeal wall move toward each another to create the pressure that is needed to project the bolus into the pharynx. The pharynx contracts and squeezes the bolus down. The pharyngeal phase is complete when the cricopharyngeal sphincter opens and the food or liquid moves into the esophagus. The esophageal phase follows, when the muscles of the esophagus move the bolus in peristaltic or rhythmic, wavelike contractions from the top of the esophagus into the stomach. The act of swallowing is, therefore, just one process in the broader context of feeding, which allows the transfer of food and liquid from the back of the mouth to the stomach. It is a complex behavior emerging from interacting cranial nerves of the brainstem and governed by neural regulatory mechanisms in the medulla, as well as in sensorimotor and limbic cortical systems (Logemann, 1998).

At early infancy, all these four components of feeding are involuntary and as a result, they display numerous brainstem-mediated oral reflexes. These oral reflexes are broadly divided into two groups, i.e., adaptive and protective reflexes. The adaptive reflexes consist of rooting and suckling and protective reflexes consist of tongue protrusion, tongue lateralization, phasic bite, gag reflex, and cough. The swallow reflex comes under both adaptive and protective reflex and this reflex begins at the third trimester and continues into adulthood (Morris & Klein, 2000; Stiles & Jernigan, 2010; Wolf & Glass, 1992).

From being completely dependent on the feeder at early infancy through semi-dependency, children learn to be completely independent for feeding. The early neurologic development is one of the major prerequisites which allow the transition from brainstem-mediated suckling reflexes to complex, voluntary oral movement during feeding. The anatomical changes such as enlargement of the oral cavity provide more space for food to be manipulated within the mouth. Another major prerequisite for feeding is postural support, as infants mature, their trunk control, neck control, and jaw control matures in a sequence. This gross motor control is required to support the fine motor control which includes chewing and biting. The gradual development in oral motor skills helps the child to move from breastfeeding to bottle feeding, intake of solid items using spoon, then on to mashed and soft pieces that can be broken with the tongue, and later soft- and hard food textures that require biting and chewing; drinking using bottle, straw and open cup (Morris & Klein, 2000; Dodrill, 2014).

Followed by learning to eat solid food, the next stage is mature mealtime behavior, which is subsequent to improvements in their cognitive development. According to Piaget's theory of cognitive development, from birth to 2 years of age (sensorimotor stage), infants understand the world through movements and sensation, meanwhile, during feeding they may be predisposed to refuse the food items which they cannot manage from a sensory or motor prospective; at 2-7 years of age (preoperational stage), children likely to be egocentric, and see things from their point of view; in the mealtime, they have a tendency to like food prepared in a particular manner and usually dislike if there is any change is made. In concrete operation stage (7-11 years), children begin to think logically and they also understand that they can alter foods to suit their preferences; in formal operational stage (above 12 years), children's thinking becomes more rational and they understand that the consumption of few food items is necessary to maintain good health irrespective of their likes or dislikes.

DEVELOPMENT OF FEEDING AND SWALLOWING

During infancy, swallowing is more associated with primitive reflexes which are controlled by specific cranial nerves; phasic bite reflex, rooting response, gag reflex, rooting response transverse tongue response, and tongue protrusion etc. As these reflexes diminish gradually over a period of time; it leads to the onset of chewing, swallowing of solids and handling of the spoon for feeding. Furthermore, the development of feeding is associated with the maturity of oral structures, upper limbs, and other skills which determines the pattern of feeding. In their earlier days of life, infants can only suck and swallow liquids, but as they grow, the sucking and swallowing actions are followed by more mature feeding skills i.e., biting, chewing, eating from a spoon, drinking from a cup and a straw (Arvedson & Brodsky, 1993). The summary of the development of feeding and swallowing skills from birth to two years of age is listed in Table 1.

The development of feeding and swallowing is associated with anatomical changes and neural maturation. In infants, feeding is more reflexive in nature and is under brainstem control; with maturation, these reflexive functions gradually become voluntary in nature. Similarly, during infancy swallow does not engage voluntary oral-preparatory phase and oral phase, while with maturation, swallow consists of voluntary oral-preparatory phase, voluntary oral phase, and involuntary pharyngeal and esophageal phases which is supported by the sensory afferent nerve fibers, motor efferent fibers, paired brainstem swallowing centers and supra-bulbar neural inputs (Stevenson & Allaire,1991).

FEEDING AND SWALLOWING PROBLEMS

Feeding and swallowing problems are common in neonates, toddlers, and preschoolers; both in typically developing and in those with developmental disorders. Reau, Senruria, Lebailly, and Christoffel (1996) reported that 25 to 40% of the typical infants and toddlers were found to have feeding issues such as colic, vomiting, slow feeding and refusal to eat. Other problems include agitation and distress while feeding, poor social reciprocity between child and caregiver while feeding, refusal to eat food, preference of certain food textures etc. There can be wide variation in the type of feeding problems seen in infants and young children. Feeding and swallowing problems can also be seen in 80% of the children with developmental delay (Lindberg, Bohlin, & Hagekull, 1991; Reilly, Skuse, Wolke, & Stevenson, 1999).

According to DSM-IV-TR (American Psychiatric Association, 2000), feeding problems grossly can be due to neurological impairments, structural abnormalities and behavioral problems. The maturation of central and peripheral nervous systems and proper coordination among muscles of oral cavity, pharynx, and esophagus have a crucial role in the acquisition of normal swallowing and feeding skills (Miller, 1982). Therefore, any kind of anomaly in the developing brain and/or structural or functional deficits in the oral, pharyngeal or esophageal region can lead to a spectrum of cognitive, communicative, behavioral, and motor abnormalities which in turn can result in feeding and swallowing problems. There are several conditions which can lead to feeding and swallowing issues, such as cleft lip and/or palate, congenital malformations, cardiorespiratory problems, motor disabilities, neurologic dysfunction,

Table 1. Summary of feeding and swallowing development from birth to two years.

Age (Months)	Skill Level
0-4	Hand to mouth feeding, hand on the bottle during feeding
4-7	Spoon feeding and cup drinking begins, munching, chewing, semi-solids from a spoon
6-8	Sucking of liquid from the cup, assisting with a spoon
9-10	Drinks from the cup held by the caregiver, Pincer grasp for finger feeding
11-12	Self-feeding by grasping spoon with whole hands holds a cup with 2 hands; 4-5 consecutive swallows holds and tips bottle by self
15-24	Skills refined for independent self-feeding

brain injury, prematurity, liver function problems, gastrointestinal disorders, metabolic disorders, autism and a variety of developmental syndromes. In the subsequent sections, an attempt has been made to describe the feeding and swallowing problems in the children with cerebral palsy, intellectual disability and autism spectrum disorders.

1. Cerebral Palsy

Cerebral Palsy (CP) has been defined as a group of permanent disorders of the development of movement and posture, balance and coordination causing activity limitation, that is attributed to non-progressive deficits, that occur in the developing fetal or infant brain (Rosenbaum, Paneth, Leviton, Goldstein, Bax, Damiano, … Jacobsson, 2007). Cerebral palsy is a motor disorder which is often associated with disturbances of sensation, perception, cognition, communication, and behavior; epilepsy, secondary musculoskeletal problems and feeding and swallowing problems. CP can result from maldevelopment of the brain; nervous system anomalies such as anencephaly, hydrocephaly etc. and injuries to the brain at various stages from several weeks after conception (prenatal period), through birth (perinatal period), to early childhood (postnatal period). Hence, depending on the site of lesion in the brain, the symptoms will vary, i.e. abnormal muscle tone, disturbance of balance mechanisms, muscle weakness and loss of selective motor control lead to an inability to stretch the muscles, involuntary movements etc.

Respiratory problems such as recurrent aspiration, poor cough and airway clearance, respiratory muscle weakness, and sleep apnea, are often seen in the children with neurological impairment. Recurrent aspiration results due to weakness and poor coordination between the muscles of mouth, pharynx, larynx, esophagus and diaphragm; likewise, weakness and poor coordination in expiratory abdominal, intercostal muscles and glottic muscles lead to a poor cough and airway clearance (Seddon & Khan, 2003). Similarly, the abnormalities in oral muscle tone and strength and general body posture lead to feeding and swallowing problems in children with CP. Chewing and swallowing are relatively complex motor behaviors in the repertoire of infant motor activity, and hence are extremely sensitive to neurologic dysfunction. Lack of tongue lateralization, instability of the lower jaw, restricted temporo-mandibular joint and phasic biting can severely limit the individual's ability to chew, position, and swallow a food bolus safely. Also, the prolonged retention of the reflexes could be another cause of feeding problems; the persistence of the primitive reflexes such as suckle-swallowing, rooting, gagging, biting, asymmetrical tonic neck reflex etc. can interfere with a child's eating skills. Further, the swallowing reflex may be completely absent or more often delayed. This could lead to aspiration due to poor coordination of swallowing. When the neuromotor coordination of swallowing is deficient, there may be gagging in some cases with associated vomiting or aspiration, choking, and pneumonia (Rogers, Arvedson, Buck, Smart, & Msall, 1994; Ottenbacher, Bundy, & Short, 1983; Morris, 1989).

The most commonly seen feeding and swallowing problems in these children are difficulty in sucking and swallowing, difficulty in chewing and biting, difficulty in getting food off spoon with lips, failure to self-feed, spillage of food from corners of the mouth, drooling, prolong feeding time, improper feeding positions, coughing and choking during feeding, vomiting and/or nasal regurgitation, constipation and recurrent chest infections (Gangil, Patwari, Aneja, Ahuja, & Anand, 2001; Ghayas, Naz, Fazil, & Sulman, 2014; Diwan & Diwan, 2013). All these issues can lead to longer mealtime duration of more than 30 minutes. If this occurs on a regular basis, it suggests the presence of feeding and/or swallowing problems (Arvedson, 2013).

Case Vignette #1

BH was brought to the clinic with a complaint of limited speech and language output. Consequent to the speech and language evaluation, he was diagnosed with Global developmental delay and was enrolled in regular speech therapy. On one fortunate day, the speech therapist happened to see the mealtime behavior of the child. The child had severe coughing and nasal regurgitation, he was only on liquid diet and feeding was done in the supine position. The child was fed using a spoon. Though the mother poured the milk or juice to the back of the mouth, the child was able to swallow the only 1/3rd of the liquid; the rest of it was ejected out. The mealtime time extended up to 45 minutes, as there was a cough, liquid loss, nasal regurgitation, cleaning up the mess and feeding the child again. The mealtime was equally uncomfortable for the child as well as for the mother.

2. Intellectual Disabilities

Intellectual disabilities (ID) are described as limitations in intellectual functioning, deficient social behaviors or skills, and inadequate daily living skills (American Association on Intellectual and Developmental Disabilities, 2008). Intellectual disability is diagnosed when Intelligence quotient (IQ) is less than 70. ID can be caused by environmental, genetic, behavioral, social and/or other multiple factors such as poverty; malnutrition, maternal drugs and alcoholism; severe stimulation deficit; congenital malformation of the brain and/or any injury to the brain during pre-, peri-, and post-natal period (McLaren & Bryson, 1987; Campbell, Morgan, & Jackson, 2004). The common genetic conditions such as Down (trisomy 21) syndrome, Klinefelter's (47, XXY) syndrome, Digeorge syndrome, Prader-Willi syndrome, Angelman syndrome, Williams syndrome, Phelan-McDermid (22q13del) syndrome, Mowat-Wilson syndrome, genetic ciliopathy are associated with ID (Badano, Mitsuma, Beales, & Katsanis, 2006).

Feeding and swallowing problems seen in these children are tantrums while feeding, bizarre food habits, multiple food dislikes, food selectivity based on texture, delay or difficulty in chewing, difficulty in sucking or swallowing, delay and/or lack of self-feeding, disruptive behavior, inappropriate amount of food intake; pica, malnutrition, rumination, vomiting, regurgitation, eating too fast, food stealing and poor appetite (Linscheid, 1983; O'Brien, Repp, Williams, & Christophersen, 1991; Matson, Gardner, Coe, & Sovner, 1991). Studies also have reported that 50-80% of the individuals with Down syndrome have associated feeding and swallowing problems (Van Dyke, Peterson, & Hoffman, 1990).

The feeding problems in children with ID could have resulted from various organic and environmental factors such as physical obstructions and deficits (deformities in oral musculature, food allergies, cleft palate, muscular dystrophy, and paralysis); and lack of opportunities for skill development and aversive feeding experiences respectively (Riordan, Iwata, Finney, Wohl, & Stanley, 1984; Siegel, 1982). The feeding problem in children with Down syndrome could result from immature chewing pattern, poor bolus control and manipulation, primitive backward and forward movement of tongue against the palate, tongue thrust, poor lateralization of tongue, pooling of food in lateral and anterior sulcus, swallowing of large, poorly chewed morsels, esophageal obstruction and gastroesophageal reflux (Malavika, 2015).

Case Vignette#2

AJ, a 4-year-old boy was brought to our clinic with the complaint of limited speech and language output, poor mental abilities, inadequate biting and chewing; difficulty in blowing and sucking; open mouth posture and drooling. Results of examination of his oral peripheral mechanism suggested poor lip closure, poor tongue and jaw movements; and inadequate intra-oral breath pressure. Parents reported that he took the longer time to chew and swallow the food. A mealtime observation revealed frequent food pocketing and he had difficulty in clearing the food using the tongue. The self-feeding skills were poor and he needed assistance to hold a spoon, cup, glass etc.

3. Autism Spectrum Disorder

Autism spectrum disorder (ASD) has been described as NDD that is characterized by deficits in social communication and social interaction, as well as the presence of restricted repetitive and stereotyped patterns of behavior, interests, and activities (American Psychiatric Association, 2013). Although etiology behind ASD has not been firmly established, speculations have been made by different researchers; for instance, Trottier, Srivastava, and Walker (1999) proposed that etiology of ASD is complex in nature and can be because of both genetic and environmental factors. Frequently observed genetic causes are multifactorial inheritance, fragile X syndrome and tuberous sclerosis (Freitag, 2007); and the commonly reported environmental causes are categorized into three categories i.e., *pre-natal* (congenital rubella syndrome, teratogen exposure, etc.) *factors, peri-natal factors* (low birth weight, premature delivery, etc.) and *post-natal factors* (autoimmune diseases, viral infection, vitamin D deficiency, controversial MMR Vaccine etc. (Wakefield, Murch, Anthony, Linnell, Casson, Malik, … Harvey, 1998; Ashwood & van de Water, 2004; Davidson, Myers, & Weiss 2004; Schultz, 2005; Kern & Jones, 2006; Kolevzon, Gross, & Reichenberg, 2007; Cannel, 2008).

The feeding issues discovered in children with ASD are usually categorized into three types: (1) food selectivity; (2) food refusal, and; (3) disruptive mealtime behaviors (Cermak, Curtin, & Bandini, 2010; Schreck, Smith, & Williams 2004; Rogers, Magill-Evans, & Rempel, 2012). There is a tendency to have confined dietary variety, food neophobia, food denial, restricted diet based on texture, unusual food preferences (e.g., specific food colors, shapes, textures, presentation, or specific arrangement of food on the plate), insistence on eating food with specific utensils/dishes, poor mealtime social behavior, unusual posturing during meals, and oral motor problems, and a tendency towards being overweight were the most often found feeding issues in these children (Badalyan & Schwartz, 2011; Marshall, Hill, Ziviani, & Dodrill, 2014).

The feeding issues in these children can be because of the presence of perseveration, impulsivity, neophobia, sensory impairments, social noncompliance, and biological food intolerance in these children. Also, parental anxiety, reinforcement of negative feeding patterns, and communication deficits can be considered as additional factors which hamper the feeding skills in these children (Cumine, Leach, & Stevenson, 2000; Shaw, Garcia, Thorn, Farley, & Flanagan, 2003). The behavioral, social, communicative and cognitive deficits in these children can disrupt the feeding and learning of mealtime behaviors. The ritualistic and repetitive behaviors and behavioral inflexibility in them can lead to rigid mealtime routine. Tactile and oral defensiveness and presence of sensory oversensitivity in the oral region are commonly seen in these children, which lead to food selectivity in them (Baranek, Boyd, Poe, David, & Watson, 2007; Tomchek & Dunn 2007; Williams, Dalrymple, & Neal, 2000; Lane, Young, Baker, & Angley, 2010).

Case Vignette #3

PS was brought to us with a complaint limited speech and language output, poor social communication and few behavior issues. He was diagnosed with Autism spectrum disorder. The parents were asked about his mealtime behavior and eating patterns. It was found that although he was 3 years 5 months old, he was still on liquid and semi-solid diet, had poor biting and chewing skills and he preferred eating only soft and sweet food items such as idli with sugar, rice porridge, milk etc. He generally refused to eat any kind of fresh fruits or vegetables and milk was the only thing which he would take without creating any fuss. For feeding other food items, the mother had to seat the child near a water tap and every time she fed him, the tap had to be opened. The mealtime would usually extend from 25-35 minutes.

ASSESSMENT OF FEEDING AND SWALLOWING SKILLS

Feeding and swallowing assessment in children should include a detailed case history specific to feeding, observation of eating and drinking with different consistencies along with the assessment of neuromotor development and oral sensory motor skills. The case history information should include details of medical history; reports from other health professionals, and information provided by parents/ caregivers specific to the feeding skills of the child. Additionally, the observation of eating and drinking with different consistencies should be done along with child's mealtime behavior assessment, parent-child interaction and usage of any compensatory feeding strategies. Objective evaluation can be done using videofluoroscopic swallow study (VFSS) or a flexible endoscopic evaluation of swallowing (FEES), in case there is any concern about safe swallowing (Logemann, 1995). Various subjective assessment tools have been developed to evaluate the feeding and swallowing skills in children with NDD, with a few tools being disease/disorder-specific, while others being common for all disorders.

Multidisciplinary Feeding Profile (Kenny, Koheil, Greenberg, Reid, Milner, Moran, & Judd, 1989) is one of the scales developed specifically for assessing feeding issues in children with neurological deficits. The profile includes a numerical rating scale to assess physical/neurologic factors, oral-facial structure, oral-facial sensory inputs, oral-facial motor function, ventilation/phonation, and a functional feeding assessment for children with neurologic deficits. Few questionnaires have been developed specifically to assess feeding behaviors and patterns, specifically in children with ASD and one such commonly used tool is the *Brief Autism Mealtime Behavior Inventory* (BAMBI; Lukens & Linscheid, 2008) which consists of 18 items. The objective of this inventory is to assess mealtime behavior problems in children with autism under three domains: limited variety (8 items), food refusal (5 items) and features of autism (5 items).

Few subjective feeding assessment scales have been developed for children in various age ranges and these are categorized into scales that can be used for children from birth to two years of age and for children above two years of age. *Neonatal Oral Motor Assessment Scale* (NOMAS; Palmer, Crawley, & Blanco, 1993) is a checklist to evaluate the behaviors in categories of normal, disorganized and dysfunction of tongue and jaw movement in the age range of birth to 8 weeks; *Schedule for Oral motor Assessment* (SOMA; Skuse, Stevenson, Reilly, & Mathisen, 1995) is an objective scale used widely to rate oral-motor skills and recognize the areas of the dysfunction which might lead to feeding difficulties for the children in the age range of 8-24 months.

The *Child Eating Behavior Inventory* (CEBI; Archer, Rosenbaum, & Streiner, 1991) is a parent perception rating scale used to assess feeding problems and how the parent-child relationship is influenced and is developed for children in 2-12 years of age range; *Behavioral Pediatrics Feeding Assessment Scale-Child behaviors subscale* (Crist, McDonnell, Beck, Gillespie, Barrett, & Mathews, 1994), developed to find out the child behavior associated with poor nutritional intake. *Mealtime Behavior Questionnaire* (Berlin, Davies, Silverman, Woods, Fischer, & Rudolph, 2010) is yet another tool primarily used to evaluate mealtime behavior problems under the following domains: food refusal/ avoidance (12 items), food manipulation (7 items), mealtime aggression/ distress (9 items), and choking/ gagging/vomiting (3 items). Some of the other tools for feeding and swallowing assessment used across the countries for children include *About Your Child's Eating- Revised* (Davies, Ackerman, Davies, Vannatta, & Noll, 2007), *Montreal Children's Hospital Feeding Scale* (Ramsay, Martel, Porporino, & Zygmuntowicz, 2011), *Screening Tool of Feeding Problems Applied to Children* (STEP-CHILD; Seiverling, Hendy, & Williams, 2011), *Pediatric Eating Assessment tool* (Pedi-EAT; Thoyre, Pados, Park, Estrem, Hodges, McComish, … Murdoch, 2014), etc.

Table 2 provides a comprehensive review of the available tests/tools used for assessment of feeding and swallowing skills in children which were developed in Western countries. Few of the subjective tests are specific to the assessment of structures involved in feeding and swallowing, while others assist in examining the behavioral, functional, social and emotional aspects of the children. It can also be noted that few of the tests include the assessment by professionals only, while others depend on parental perceptions about feeding problems in their children. However, there is limited number of assessment tools which considers the assessment by both the professionals as well as parental perspectives. As the majority of these tests are specific to certain aspects of feeding and swallowing, professionals depend upon multiple numbers of tests to understand the exact nature and extent of the feeding and swallowing problems in children. Further, many of these available tests or scales do not provide information regarding feeding and swallowing problems in children as per ICF classification which emphasizes on understanding the disorder in terms of body structures and functions; activities, and participation.

According to International Classification of Functioning, Disability, and Health (ICF; WHO, 2001), the feeding and swallowing assessment should include information about mealtime environment (participation), child's behavior and activities during mealtime (activities) and motor skills, neuromotor development and neuromuscular condition (body function and structures). The various factors related to impairment, disability and handicap dimensions for feeding and swallowing assessment according to ICF has been mentioned in Table 3.

Feeding Handicap Index for children (FHI-C; Swapna & Srushti, 2017) was developed on the basis of ICF classification and standardized and validated in Indian context that measures the handicapping effect of feeding problems in children in the age range of 2-10 years. The FHI was prepared by collecting information from the literature and from the complaints concerning feeding received from the parents of children with communication disorders. FHI-C has a total of 38 items with 21 in the physical domain, 12 in the functional domain and 5 in the emotional domain. The items in the FHI-C focused on the physical problems encountered by the children during feeding and swallowing, i.e. problems related to the oral, pharyngeal and esophageal phase of feeding and swallowing and its impact on the day to day functioning and emotional aspects of the child. In this tool, a three-point rating scale is used to rate the responses obtained from the parents so as to obtain a quantitative score. Each statement is accompanied with response choice of "never" (a score of zero), "sometimes" (a score of 1) or "always" (a score of 2) resulting in a maximum score of 76. At the end of the administration of FHI, the parents/caregivers

Table 2. Summary of tools available for feeding and swallowing assessment in children.

Test	Authors	Age Range	Description
Developmental Pre-feeding checklist	Morris and Klein (1987)	Birth to 24 months	The developmental pre-feeding checklist was developed to assess feeding skill. It provides a description of the skill observed in accordance with the age equivalencies provided.
Multidisciplinary Feeding Profile	Kenny et al. (1989)	Age not specified	Multidisciplinary Feeding Profile is a protocol for the quantitative assessment of feeding disorders developed for the children with neurologic deficits.
Oral-motor Feeding Rating Scale	Jelm (1990)	1 year to adulthood	Oral-motor Feeding Rating Scale is record keeping form that helps you screen and categorize the many varieties of oral-motor movements and note specific patterns. As the client eats a typical meal, the clinician can analyze lip/cheek movement, tongue movement, and jaw movement.
Child Eating Behavior Inventory (CEBI)	Archer, Rosenbaum, and Streiner (1991)	2-12 years	CEBI was developed to understand the parent-child relationships during mealtime.
Neonatal Oral Motor Assessment Scale (NOMAS)	Palmer, Crawley, and Blanco (1993)	Birth to 8 weeks	NOMAS has a 28-item checklist that divides a neonate's oral motor feeding patterns into normal, disorganized, or dysfunctional.
Schedule for Oral motor Assessment (SOMA)	Skuse, Stevenson, Reilly, and Mathisen (1995)	8-24 months	SOMA is used to assess oral-motor function is assessed across a range of food textures and fluids.
Behavioral pediatric feeding Assessment Scale (BPFAS)	Crist & Napier-Phillips (2001)	Age not specified	BPFAS is a parent survey tool with 35 items, which assesses feeding and mealtime behavior.
Children's eating behavior Questionnaire (CEBQ)	Wardle, Guthrie, Sanderson, and Rapoport (2001)	Age not specified	CEBQ was developed for young children are a parent-report measure comprised of 35 items. It is made up of eight scales: food responsiveness, emotional over-eating, and enjoyment of food, the desire to drink, satiety responsiveness, Slowness in eating, emotional under-eating, and food fussiness.
Early feeding skills (EFS) Assessment for Preterm Infants	Thoyre, Shaker, and Pridham, (2005)	Age not specified	EFS is a checklist developed for assessing infant readiness for and tolerance of feeding and for profiling the infant's developmental stage regarding specific feeding skills, i.e., the abilities to remain engaged in feeding, organize oral-motor functioning, coordinate swallowing with breathing, and maintain physiologic stability.
Brief Autism Mealtime Behavior Inventory (BAMBI)	Lukens and Linscheid (2008)	3-11 years	BAMBI was developed as a standardized informant report measure to assess the mealtime and feeding behaviors in children with ASD
The Screening tools of feeding Problems applied to children (STEP-CHILD)	Seiverling, Hendy, and Williams (2011)	24 months to 18 years	STEP-CHILD was developed to identify feeding problems in children. It has 15 items divided under 6 subscales i.e., chewing problems, rapid eating, food refusal, food selectivity, vomiting, and stealing food.
Montreal Children's Hospital Feeding Scale	Ramsay, Martel, Porporino, and Zygmuntowicz (2011)	6 months to 6 years	The MCH-Feeding Scale is a bilingual 14-item parent report tool can be used by pediatricians and other health care professionals for quick identification of feeding problems.
Dysphagia Disorder Survey (DDS)	Sheppard, Hochman, and Baer (2014)	8-82 years	DDS was developed for identifying and describing swallowing and feeding function for eating and drinking in children and adults with developmental disability.
Pediatric Eating Assessment tool (Pedi-EAT)	Thoyre et al. (2014)	6 months to 7 years	Pedi-EAT is a parent-report instrument developed to assess symptoms of feeding problems in children.

Table 3. Body structure and function, Activities and Participation and Environmental and personal factors related to feeding and swallowing

Body Structure and Function	Activities and Participation	Environmental and Personal Factors
Structure: Structures involved in oral, oral preparatory, pharyngeal and esophageal stages; neural structures. *Functions:* Vegetative skills, swallowing process, digestive functions, neuromotor functions.	*Eating:* Expressing the need, execution of the coordinated tasks (both fine and gross motor) required for eating, hand to mouth coordination. *Drinking:* Expressing the need, execution of the coordinated tasks (both fine and gross motor) required for drinking such as holding the cup or bottle, drinking through a straw, and/or breastfeeding.	Products or substances for personal consumption; Support from immediate family, personal care providers, and health professionals; Individual attitudes of immediate family members, personal care providers, health professionals, societal attitudes; availability of health services.

of the children have to be instructed to self-rate the overall severity of the feeding problem on a 7 point rating scale where '1' suggests normal feeding skills and '7' suggests severely affected feeding skills.

As a part of clinical validation, the tool was administered to three different groups of children with cerebral palsy, autism spectrum disorders and intellectual disability. The results revealed a significant difference between these three groups and the typically developing children. It was found that 75-95% the children with CP had difficulty in using spoon for eating, drinking using straw, using tongue to clear the food particles in the mouth and ability to rinse and spit; and around 25-60% children with CP had difficulty in sucking, chewing, eating with fingers, drinking using glass/cup, inadequate weight gain, inadequate amount of eating, avoidance of solid food and longer feeding time.

Among the group with ASD, 70-80% of the children had difficulty in using finger and spoon for eating, drinking using straw, usage of tongue to clear the food particles in the mouth and ability to rinse and spit; neophobia and avoidance of specific food items, longer mealtime, and avoidance of feeding in social situation. Around 20-30% of the children with ASD had the presence of gag while eating and refusal to eat and temper tantrums while feeding.

It was also found that 50-60% of the children with ID had difficulty in using spoon scooping the food as well as eating independently, drinking using straw, using of the tongue to clear the food particles in the mouth and ability to rinse and spit; inappropriate weight gain and avoidance of specific food items. Around 30-40% of children with ID had difficulty in chewing, using fingers to eat, drink independently; retention of food in the mouth, spillage of food from the mouth, dislike to be dependent on others for feeding, refusal to eat and temper tantrums while feeding.

ETHICAL ISSUES IN FEEDING AND SWALLOWING

With the feeding and swallowing problem, there comes the responsibility of decision making about the food and feeding by the professionals as well as by the caregiver(s). The decisions such as choosing the type of food, the consequences of intake of specific food (allergy to certain food item), route of intake (feeding tubes), and/or consistency of food (Leslie & Crawford, 2017) needs to be made. Also, we know that humans are very emotional toward food and food habits as it connects us with our culture and society, hence due importance also needs to be provided for choosing culture-specific food.

Children with feeding and swallowing problems are a critical population which makes the ethical decision making a complicated time-consuming procedure. This decision making may call for inputs from multiple team members. For SLPs, who deal with the assessment and management of feeding and swallowing problems, it is challenging to balance between the ethical decision making and health care policies.

CHALLENGES IN EARLY INTERVENTION OF FEEDING AND/OR SWALLOWING PROBLEMS

In the Indian scenario, one of the challenges in dealing with feeding issues is the lack of awareness among the parents about the feeding problems faced by their children, due to which it is underreported to the speech-language pathologist. As revealed through the study by Srushti and Swapna (2014), there was a significant difference between the scores obtained from FHI-C and parent/caregiver severity rating scale in children with cerebral palsy. In another study by Swapna and Srushti (2015) too, it was found that parents with ASD and ID underreported the feeding problems. In the group with ASD, 68.8% of the children had feeding issues while parental responses suggested that 79.9% had no feeding issues; only 20% of parents felt that their children have feeding issues. Similarly, in children with ID, FHI-C score indicated that 83% of children had feeding issues, while parental responses suggested that 63.9% had no feeding issues; only 37.2% of parents felt that their children have feeding issues. The results of the above-mentioned studies indicated that parents of these children with communication disorders are not much sensitive towards the feeding issues faced by these children.

Personal interaction with these parents suggested that parents were more concerned about the speech and language deficits and look for speech and language intervention, while some parents although they are concerned about the feeding issues in their children, they are not aware of professionals who are involved in treating these issues. Many parents, due to lack of knowledge of intervention strategies that can be used for their children, have a tendency to use strategies like pinching the nose or shaking the child to swallow; or feeding in the supine position, which can be life-threatening.

NEED FOR EARLY INTERVENTION

As feeding plays an important role in the overall development of physical, functional and psychosocial aspects of life, it is important to intervene the feeding and swallowing difficulties as early as possible. The persistence of feeding and swallowing issues will hamper the normal growth and development of the child. The delay in the introduction of developmentally appropriate food at sensitive period can lead to inadequate oral motor and oral sensory development (Illingworth & Lister, 1964). The long-standing feeding problems in young children increase the frustration and anxiety in child along with the feeder and the entire family and gradually they become more resistant to any kind of change (Archer & Szatmari, 1990; Babbitt, Hoch, Coe, Cataldo, Kelly, Stackhouse, & Perman, 1994; Benoit, 1993). The persistence of feeding and swallowing problems in these children can result in malnutrition in them. Also, unidentified swallowing problem may result in chronic lung disease or aspiration pneumonia (Cloud, Ekvall, & Hicks 2005; Pavan, 1996).

TEAM APPROACH AND THE ROLE OF SPEECH-LANGUAGE PATHOLOGISTS IN INTERVENTION

The complex nature of feeding and swallowing problems in children makes it difficult to remediate through single disciplinary approach; hence there is a need for the multidisciplinary approach for the intervention of children with feeding and swallowing issues. Depending on the nature and etiology of feeding and swallowing problem, the team may vary from client to client, for example, children with CP would require Neurologist, Pediatrician, Gastroenterologist, Speech-Language pathologist, Physiotherapist, Nutritionist, Clinical Psychologist, etc., while team for children with ASD and/or ID might not require Neurologists and Gastroenterologists, instead an Occupational therapist can play an important role in them. Hence, based on the nature and etiology of the problem the team can consist of Neurologist, Pediatrician, Otolaryngologist, Gastroenterologist, Pediatric Dentist, Radiologist, Speech-Language Pathologist, Physiotherapist, Occupational therapist, Nutritionist, Clinical Psychologist, Clinical Nutritionist, Nurse, Social worker, family and other health professionals.

Speech-language pathologists play a major in the evaluation, diagnosis, and intervention of infants and children with swallowing and feeding difficulties. They provide information about feeding and swallowing difficulties to parents/caregivers of children who have feeding problems or who are at risk for developing feeding problems. They also educate other medical and non-medical professionals about the needs of children with feeding and swallowing issues and their role in the diagnosis and intervention of these issues. Speech-language pathologists conduct comprehensive assessment using both subjective and objective tests to recognize normality and abnormality in the anatomy and physiology of feeding; they take decisions regarding the instrument to be used for evaluation procedures, identify the severity and nature of feeding and swallowing problem, interpret the data obtained from the instrumental evaluation, form treatment plans of individual clients and determine the capability of the child for safe and appropriate food intake. They are also responsible for documenting improvement and determining correct discharge criteria; providing individualized treatment program; counseling parents/caregivers and educating them to prevent further complications related to feeding and swallowing.

CONCLUSION

Even though significant advancements have been made in the assessment and treatment of children with the NDDs, it continues to be challenging for the clients, parents/ caregivers and all health professionals involved in this process. The assessment and intervention of these children require a multidisciplinary approach which can address the physical, functional, emotional and psychosocial needs of the client. Also, there is a need to improve the awareness among the common people as well as among the health professionals regarding the feeding and swallowing problems associated with NDDs; as feeding and swallowing problems can negatively affect the dietary intake and growth and development of the child. It is important that the speech-language pathologists have adequate knowledge about feeding and swallowing problems associated with different NDDs prevailing in the society and are well trained and well equipped to handle these clients.

REFERENCES

American Association on Intellectual and Developmental Disabilities. (2008). *Mental Retardation: Definition, Classification, and Systems of Supports* (10th ed.). Washington, DC: American Association on Intellectual and Developmental Disabilities.

American Psychiatric Association. (2000). *DSM-IV-TR: Diagnostic and statistical manual of mental disorders, text revision*. Washington, DC: American Psychiatric Association.

American Psychiatric Association. (2013). *Diagnostic and statistical manual of mental disorders: DSM-5* (5th ed.). Washington, DC: American Psychiatric Association.

Archer, L. A., Rosenbaum, P. L., & Streiner, D. L. (1991). The children's eating behavior inventory: Reliability and validity results. *Journal of Pediatric Psychology*, *16*(5), 629–642. doi:10.1093/jpepsy/16.5.629 PMID:1744810

Archer, L. A., & Szatmari, P. (1990). Assessment and treatment of food aversion in a four year old boy: A multidimensional approach. *Canadian Journal of Psychiatry*, *35*(6), 501–505. doi:10.1177/070674379003500606 PMID:1698524

Arvedson, J., & Brodsky, L. (1993). Management of swallowing problems. *Pediatric Swallowing and Feeding: Assessment and Management*, 327–387.

Arvedson, J. C. (2013). Feeding children with cerebral palsy and swallowing difficulties. *European Journal of Clinical Nutrition*, *67*(S2), S9–S12. doi:10.1038/ejcn.2013.224 PMID:24301008

Ashwood, P., & Van de Water, J. (2004). Is autism an autoimmune disease? *Autoimmunity Reviews*, *3*(7–8), 557–562. doi:10.1016/j.autrev.2004.07.036 PMID:15546805

Babbitt, R. L., Hoch, T. A., Coe, D. A., Cataldo, M. F., Kelly, K. J., Stackhouse, C., & Perman, J. A. (1994). Behavioral assessment and treatment of pediatric feeding disorders. *Journal of Developmental and Behavioral Pediatrics*, *15*(4), 278–291. doi:10.1097/00004703-199408000-00011 PMID:7798374

Badalyan, V., & Schwartz, R. H. (2011). Feeding problems and GI dysfunction in children with Asperger syndrome or pervasive developmental disorder not otherwise specified; comparison with their siblings. *Open Journal of Pediatrics*, *1*(04), 51–63. doi:10.4236/ojped.2011.14014

Badano, J. L., Mitsuma, N., Beales, P. L., & Katsanis, N. (2006). The ciliopathies: An emerging class of human genetic disorders. *Annual Review of Genomics and Human Genetics*, *7*(1), 125–148. doi:10.1146/annurev.genom.7.080505.115610 PMID:16722803

Baranek, G. T., Boyd, B. A., Poe, M. D., David, F. J., & Watson, L. R. (2007). Hyper-responsive sensory patterns in young children with autism, developmental delay, and typical development. *American Journal of Mental Retardation*, *112*(4), 233–245. doi:10.1352/0895-8017(2007)112[233:HSPIYC]2.0.CO;2 PMID:17559291

Benoit, D. (1993). Failure to thrive and feeding disorders. In C. H. Zeanah (Ed.), *Handbook of Infant Mental Health* (pp. 317–331). New York: Guilford Press.

Berlin, K. S., Davies, W. H., Silverman, A. H., Woods, D. W., Fischer, E. A., & Rudolph, C. D. (2010). Assessing children's mealtime problems with the Mealtime Behavior Questionnaire. *Children's Health Care*, *39*(2), 142–156. doi:10.1080/02739611003679956

Campbell, J. M., Morgan, S. B., & Jackson, J. N. (2004). Autism spectrum disorders and mental retardation. In R. T. Brown (Ed.), *Handbook of pediatric psychology in school settings*. Lawrence Erlbaum Associates.

Cannell, J. J. (2008). Autism and vitamin D. *Medical Hypotheses*, *70*(4), 750–759. doi:10.1016/j.mehy.2007.08.016 PMID:17920208

Cermak, S. A., Curtin, C., & Bandini, L. G. (2010). Food selectivity and sensory sensitivity in children with autism spectrum disorders. *Journal of the Academy of Nutrition and Dietetics*, *110*(2), 238–246. PMID:20102851

Cloud, H., Ekvall, S. W., & Hicks, L. (2005). Feeding problems of the child with special health-care needs. In S. W. Ekvall & V. K. Ekvall (Eds.), *Pediatric Nutrition in Chronic Diseases and Developmental Disorders: Prevention, assessment and treatment* (2nd ed., pp. 172–182). New York: Oxford University Press.

Crist, W., McDonnell, P., Beck, M., Gillespie, C. T., Barrett, P., & Mathews, J. (1994). Behavior at mealtimes and the young child with cystic fibrosis. *Journal of Developmental and Behavioral Pediatrics*, *15*(3), 157–161. doi:10.1097/00004703-199406000-00001

Crist, W., & Napier-Phillips, A. (2001). Mealtime behaviors of young children: A comparison of normative and clinical data. *Journal of Developmental and Behavioral Pediatrics*, *22*(5), 279–286. doi:10.1097/00004703-200110000-00001 PMID:11718230

Cumine, V., Leach, J., & Stevenson, G. (2000). *The pre-school child with autism*. London: David Fulton.

Davidson, P. W., Myers, G. J., & Weiss, B. (2004). Mercury exposure and child development outcomes. *Pediatrics*, *113*(Supplement 3), 1023–1029. PMID:15060195

Davies, W. H., Ackerman, L. K., Davies, C. M., Vannatta, K., & Noll, R. B. (2007). About your child's eating: Factor structure and psychometric properties of a feeding relationship measure. *Eating Behaviors*, *8*(4), 457–463. doi:10.1016/j.eatbeh.2007.01.001 PMID:17950934

Diwan, S., & Diwan, J. (2013). A study of feeding problems in children with cerebral palsy. *National Journal of Integrated Research in Medicine*, *4*, 78–86.

Dodrill, P. (2014). Feeding problems and oropharyngeal dysphagia in children. *Journal of Gastroenterology and Hepatology Research*, *3*(5).

Freitag, C. M. (2007). The genetics of autistic disorders and its clinical relevance: A review of the literature. *Molecular Psychiatry*, *12*(1), 2–22. doi:10.1038j.mp.4001896 PMID:17033636

Gangil, A., Patwari, A. K., Aneja, S., Ahuja, B., & Anand, V. K. (2001). Feeding problems in children with cerebral palsy. *Indian Pediatrics*, *38*(8), 839–846. PMID:11520994

Ghayas, N., Naz, S., Fazil, H., & Sulman, N. (2014). Identification of oromotor impairments perceived by parents related to feeding difficulties in children with cerebral palsy. *International Journal of Physical and Social Sciences*, *4*(7), 229.

Glass, R. P., & Wolf, L. S. (1992). *Feeding and swallowing disorders in infancy: Assessment and management*. San Antonio, TX: Therapy Skill Builders.

Illingworth, R. S., & Lister, J. (1964). The critical or sensitive period, with special reference to certain feeding problems in infants and children. *The Journal of Pediatrics*, *65*(6), 839–848. doi:10.1016/S0022-3476(64)80006-8 PMID:14244090

Jelm, J. M. (1990). Oral-motor/feeding rating scale. Tucson, AZ: Therapy skill builders.

Kenner, C., & McGrath, J. M. (Eds.). (2010). *Developmental care of newborns and infants: A guide for health professionals* (2nd ed.). St. Louis, MO: Mosby.

Kenny, D. J., Koheil, R. M., Greenberg, J., Reid, D., Milner, M., Moran, R., & Judd, P. L. (1989). Development of a multidisciplinary feeding profile for children who are dependent feeders. *Dysphagia*, *4*(1), 16–28. doi:10.1007/BF02407398 PMID:2534818

Kern, J. K., & Jones, A. M. (2006). Evidence of toxicity, oxidative stress, and neuronal insult in autism. *Journal of Toxicology and Environmental Health. Part B*, *9*(6), 485–499.

Kliegman, R., & Stanton, R. (2011). *Nelson textbook of pediatrics*. Philadelphia, PA: Elsevier Saunders.

Kolevzon, A., Gross, R., & Reichenberg, A. (2007). Prenatal and perinatal risk factors for autism: A review and integration of findings. *Archives of Pediatrics & Adolescent Medicine*, *161*(4), 326–333. doi:10.1001/archpedi.161.4.326 PMID:17404128

Kummer, A. (2008). *Cleft palate & craniofacial anomalies: Effects on speech and resonance* (2nd ed.). New York, NY: Cengage Learning.

Lane, A. E., Young, R. L., Baker, A. E., & Angley, M. T. (2010). Sensory processing subtypes in autism: Association with adaptive behavior. *Journal of Autism and Developmental Disorders*, *40*(1), 112–122. doi:10.100710803-009-0840-2 PMID:19644746

Leslie, P., & Crawford, H. (2017). *The Concise Guide to Decision Making and Ethics in Dysphagia*. Guildford, UK: J&R Press Ltd.

Lindberg, L., Bohlin, G., & Hagekull, B. (1991). Early feeding problems in a normal population. *International Journal of Eating Disorders*, *10*(4), 395–405. doi:10.1002/1098-108X(199107)10:4<395::AID-EAT2260100404>3.0.CO;2-A

Linscheid, T. R. (1983). Eating problems in children. In C. E. Walker & M. C. Roberts (Eds.), *Handbook of clinical child psychology*. New York: Wiley.

Logemann, J. (1998). Mechanisms of normal and abnormal swallowing. In *Otolaryngology Head and Neck Surgery* (pp. 1844–1849). St. Louis, MO: Mosby.

Logemann, J. A. (1995). Dysphagia: Evaluation and treatment. *Folia Phoniatrica et Logopaedica*, *47*(3), 140–164. doi:10.1159/000266348 PMID:7640720

Lukens, C. T., & Linscheid, T. R. (2008). Development and validation of an inventory to assess mealtime behavior problems in children with autism. *Journal of Autism and Developmental Disorders, 38*(2), 342–352. doi:10.100710803-007-0401-5 PMID:17578658

Malavika, A. (2015). *An Investigation of the Feeding Problems in Children with Down Syndrome* (Unpublished Master's dissertation). University of Mysore, Mysore.

Marshall, J., Hill, R. J., Ziviani, J., & Dodrill, P. (2014). Features of feeding difficulty in children with Autism Spectrum Disorder. *International Journal of Speech-Language Pathology, 16*(2), 151–158. doi:10.3109/17549507.2013.808700 PMID:24001171

Matson, J. L., Gardner, W. I., Coe, D. A., & Sovner, R. (1991). A scale for evaluating emotional disorders in severely and profoundly mentally retarded persons development of the diagnostic assessment for the severely handicapped (DASH) scale. *The British Journal of Psychiatry, 159*(3), 404–409. doi:10.1192/bjp.159.3.404 PMID:1958951

McLaren, J., & Bryson, S. E. (1987). Review of recent epidemiological studies of mental retardation: Prevalence, associated disorders, and etiology. *American Journal of Mental Retardation, 92*(3), 243–254. PMID:3322329

Merenstein, G. B., & Gardner, S. L. (2002). *Handbook of Neonatal Intensive Care*. St. Louis, MO: Mosby.

Miller, A. J. (1982). Deglutition. *Physiological Reviews, 62*(1), 129–184. doi:10.1152/physrev.1982.62.1.129 PMID:7034008

Morris, S. E. (1989). Development of oral-motor skills in the neurologically impaired child receiving non-oral feedings. *Dysphagia, 3*(3), 135–154. doi:10.1007/BF02407132 PMID:2517923

Morris, S. E., & Klein, M. D. (1987). Pre-feeding skills: A comprehensive resource for feeding development. Tucson, AZ: Therapy Skill Builders.

Morris, S. E., & Klein, M. D. (2000). *Pre-feeding skills: A comprehensive resource for mealtime development*. San Antonio, TX: Therapy Skill Builders.

O'Brien, S., Repp, A. C., Williams, G. E., & Christophersen, E. R. (1991). Pediatric feeding disorders. *Behavior Modification, 15*(3), 394–418. doi:10.1177/01454455910153007 PMID:1953626

Ottenbacher, K., Bundy, A., & Short, M. A. (1983). The development and treatment of oral-motor dysfunction: A review of clinical research. *Physical & Occupational Therapy in Pediatrics, 3*(2), 1–13. PMID:27541087

Palmer, M. M., Crawley, K., & Blanco, I. A. (1993). Neonatal Oral-Motor Assessment scale: A reliability study. *Journal of Perinatology, 13*(1), 28–35. PMID:8445444

Pavan, M. H. (1996). Disorders of feeding and swallowing in infants and children: Pathophysiology, diagnosis, and treatment. *Archives of Pediatrics & Adolescent Medicine, 150*(8), 886–886. doi:10.1001/archpedi.1996.02170330112028

Ramsay, M., Martel, C., Porporino, M., & Zygmuntowicz, C. (2011). The Montreal Children's Hospital Feeding Scale: A brief bilingual screening tool for identifying feeding problems. *Paediatrics & Child Health*, *16*(3), 147–e17. doi:10.1093/pch/16.3.147 PMID:22379377

Reau, N. R., Senturia, Y. D., Lebailly, S. A., & Christoffel, K. K. (1996). Infant and toddler feeding patterns and problems: Normative data and a new direction. *Journal of Developmental and Behavioral Pediatrics*, *17*(3), 149–153. doi:10.1097/00004703-199606000-00002 PMID:8783060

Reilly, S. M., Skuse, D. H., Wolke, D., & Stevenson, J. (1999). Oral-motor dysfunction in children who fail to thrive: Organic or non-organic? *Developmental Medicine and Child Neurology*, *41*(2), 115–122. doi:10.1017/S0012162299000225 PMID:10075097

Riordan, M. M., Iwata, B. A., Finney, J. W., Wohl, M. K., & Stanley, A. E. (1984). Behavioral assessment and treatment of chronic food refusal in handicapped children. *Journal of Applied Behavior Analysis*, *17*(3), 327–341. doi:10.1901/jaba.1984.17-327 PMID:6239853

Rogers, B., Arvedson, J., Buck, G., Smart, P., & Msall, M. (1994). Characteristics of dysphagia in children with cerebral palsy. *Dysphagia*, *9*(1), 69–73. doi:10.1007/BF00262762 PMID:8131428

Rogers, L. G., Magill-Evans, J., & Rempel, G. R. (2012). Mothers' challenges in feeding their children with autism spectrum disorder-Managing more than just picky eating. *Journal of Developmental and Physical Disabilities*, *24*(1), 19–33. doi:10.100710882-011-9252-2

Rosenbaum, P., Paneth, N., Leviton, A., Goldstein, M., Bax, M., Damiano, D., ... Jacobsson, B. (2007). A report: The definition and classification of cerebral palsy April 2006. *Developmental Medicine and Child Neurology*, *109*(suppl 109), 8–14. PMID:17370477

Schreck, K. A., Williams, K., & Smith, A. F. (2004). A comparison of eating behaviors between children with and without autism. *Journal of Autism and Developmental Disorders*, *34*(4), 433–438. doi:10.1023/B:JADD.0000037419.78531.86 PMID:15449518

Schultz, R. T. (2005). Developmental deficits in social perception in autism: The role of the amygdala and fusiform face area. *International Journal of Developmental Neuroscience*, *23*(2–3), 125–141. doi:10.1016/j.ijdevneu.2004.12.012 PMID:15749240

Seddon, P. C., & Khan, Y. (2003). Respiratory problems in children with neurological impairment. *Archives of Disease in Childhood*, *88*(1), 75–78. doi:10.1136/adc.88.1.75 PMID:12495971

Seiverling, L., Hendy, H. M., & Williams, K. (2011). The screening tool of feeding problems applied to children (STEP-CHILD): Psychometric characteristics and associations with child and parent variables. *Research in Developmental Disabilities*, *32*(3), 1122–1129. doi:10.1016/j.ridd.2011.01.012 PMID:21316919

Shaw, R. J., Garcia, M., Thorn, M., Farley, C. A., & Flanagan, G. (2003). Treatment of feeding disorders in children with Down syndrome. *Clinical Child Psychology and Psychiatry*, *8*(1), 105–117. doi:10.1177/1359104503008001010

Sheppard, J. J., Hochman, R., & Baer, C. (2014). The dysphagia disorder survey: Validation of an assessment for swallowing and feeding function in developmental disability. *Research in Developmental Disabilities, 35*(5), 929–942. doi:10.1016/j.ridd.2014.02.017 PMID:24637033

Siegel, L. J. (1982). Classical and operant procedures in the treatment of a case of food aversion in a young child. *Journal of Clinical Child and Adolescent Psychology, 11*(2), 167–172. doi:10.120715374424jccp1102_12

Skuse, D., Stevenson, J., Reilly, S., & Mathisen, B. (1995). Schedule for oral-motor assessment (SOMA): Methods of validation. *Dysphagia, 10*(3), 192–202. doi:10.1007/BF00260976 PMID:7614861

Srushti, S., & Swapna, N. (2014). *Development and validation of feeding handicap index in children* (Unpublished Master's dissertation). University of Mysore, Mysore.

Stevenson, R. D., & Allaire, J. H. (1991). The development of normal feeding and swallowing. *Pediatric Clinics of North America, 38*(6), 1439–1453. doi:10.1016/S0031-3955(16)38229-3 PMID:1945550

Stiles, J., & Jernigan, T. L. (2010). The basics of brain development. *Neuropsychology Review, 20*(4), 327–348. doi:10.100711065-010-9148-4 PMID:21042938

Swapna, N., & Srushti, S. (2015). Validation of Feeding handicap index in children with Intellectual Disability and Autism Spectrum Disorder. Unpublished ARF Project funded by the All India Institute of Speech and Hearing, Mysore.

Swapna, N., & Srushti, S. (2017). *Manual of Feeding Handicap Index for Children (FHI-C)*. Mysore: All India Institute of Speech and Hearing.

Thoyre, S. M., Pados, B. F., Park, J., Estrem, H., Hodges, E. A., McComish, C., ... Murdoch, K. (2014). Development and content validation of the pediatric eating assessment tool (Pedi-EAT). *American Journal of Speech-Language Pathology, 23*(1), 46–59. doi:10.1044/1058-0360(2013/12-0069) PMID:24097795

Thoyre, S. M., Shaker, C. S., & Pridham, K. F. (2005). The early feeding skills assessment for preterm infants. *Neonatal Network: The Journal of Neonatal Nursing, 24*(3), 7–16. doi:10.1891/0730-0832.24.3.7 PMID:15960007

Tomchek, S. D., & Dunn, W. (2007). Sensory processing in children with and without autism: A comparative study using the short sensory profile. *The American Journal of Occupational Therapy, 61*(2), 190–200. doi:10.5014/ajot.61.2.190 PMID:17436841

Trottier, G., Srivastava, L., & Walker, C.-D. (1999). Etiology of infantile autism: A review of recent advances in genetic and neurobiological research. *Journal of Psychiatry & Neuroscience, 24*(2), 103–115. PMID:10212552

Van Dyke, D. C., Peterson, L. L., & Hoffman, M. N. (1990). Problems in feeding. In *Clinical Perspectives in the Management of Down Syndrome* (pp. 102–106). New York, NY: Springer. doi:10.1007/978-1-4613-9644-4_8

Wakefield, A. J., Murch, S. H., Anthony, A., Linnell, J., Casson, D. M., Malik, M., ... Harvey, P. (1998). RETRACTED: Ileal-lymphoid-nodular hyperplasia, non-specific colitis, and pervasive developmental disorder in children. *Lancet, 351*(9103), 637–641. doi:10.1016/S0140-6736(97)11096-0 PMID:9500320

Wardle, J., Guthrie, C. A., Sanderson, S., & Rapoport, L. (2001). Development of the children's eating behaviour questionnaire. *Journal of Child Psychology and Psychiatry, and Allied Disciplines*, *42*(7), 963–970. doi:10.1111/1469-7610.00792 PMID:11693591

Williams, P. G., Dalrymple, N., & Neal, J. (2000). Eating habits of children with autism. *Pediatric Nursing*, *26*(3), 259–264. PMID:12026389

World Health Organization. (2001). *International Classification of Functioning, Disability and Health: ICF*. World Health Organization.

KEY TERMS AND DEFINITIONS

Autism Spectrum Disorder: Autism spectrum disorder is a group of disorders characterized by deficits in social and communication functioning along with behavioral and sensory issues.

Cerebral Palsy: Cerebral palsy is a motor disorder that occurs due to damage in the developing brain resulting in issues with the development of movement, posture, balance and coordination that in turn affects the execution of activities of daily living.

Feeding: This refers to the process of placing food in the mouth, manipulation of food, and the propulsion of food backward by the tongue.

Feeding Handicap Index for Children: This is a 38-item parent/caregiver reported tool designed to assess the nature of feeding problems and their impact on different domains of life (physical, functional, and emotional) in children with developmental disabilities in the age group of 2-10 years.

Intellectual Deficit: Intellectual deficit refers to the limitations in intellectual functioning leading to inadequate social and daily living skills.

Oral Reflexes: These are reflex actions originating in the central nervous system that are exhibited by normal infants at birth, in response to particular stimuli. These reflexes are later suppressed due to the development of higher centers in the brain during the first three to twelve months of postnatal life. The oral reflexes include rooting, sucking/suckling, swallowing, tongue protrusion, tongue lateralization, phasic bite, gag, and cough.

Swallowing: It is one process in the broader context of feeding, which allows the safe transfer of food and liquid from the mouth to the stomach.

Chapter 4
Application of Advanced Hearing Aid Technology in Pediatric Hearing Aid Fitting

Prashanth Prabhu
All India Institute of Speech and Hearing, India

ABSTRACT

Pediatric hearing aid fitting has always been a challenge for an audiologist. There are lots of technological advances in the field of hearing aids which are yet to be verified and used in the pediatric population. The chapter focuses on reviewing the recent advancements in hearing aid technology which can benefit children with hearing impairment. It is attempted to determine the application of these technology in pediatric hearing aid fitting. The lack of translational research to provide empirical evidence in this area is highlighted. It is stressed in the chapter that audiologists should use their clinical knowledge and use appropriate verification methods to make appropriate recommendations in pediatric hearing aid fitting.

INTRODUCTION

As there are advancements in hearing aid technology, audiologists should be aware of the efficacy of these technologies especially in children with hearing impairment. Literature is limited especially in pediatric population regarding the usefulness of advanced hearing aid features such as directional microphones, noise reduction algorithms, open fit hearing aids and Receiver in the ear (RITE) hearing aids, frequency transposition and ChannelFree™ hearing aids. The listening needs of children are different from that of adults, and assessment of their needs plays an important role in the selection of appropriate advanced hearing aid technology. Studies are essential which accurately examines the benefit with these advanced technologies, especially in children.

In this chapter, it has been attempted to review some of the hearing aid technological advancements and its benefit in the pediatric population:

DOI: 10.4018/978-1-5225-7004-2.ch004

DIRECTIONAL MICROPHONES

Directional microphone technology was developed to improve speech perception in noise. The directional microphones amplify only the sounds which arrive from the front and reduce the noise from the surroundings. This technology is especially useful in one to one conversations and improves speech perception in noise. Previous studies on adults have reported that directional microphones improve speech perception in noise (Bentler, 2005). Gravel, Fausel, Liskow, and Chobot (1999) have reported that speech perception in noise was better among children between 4 to 11 years of age. The speech was presented directly in front (0 degrees) and noise was presented directly behind (180 degrees). Signal to noise ratio (SNR) – 50 was determined using multi-talker babble in an adaptive manner. The results of their study clearly showed improved aided performance with directional microphones compared to the omnidirectional condition.

Ricketts, Galster, and Tharpe (2007) simulated different classroom environments and determined speech perception in 26 children in the age range of 10-17. Omnidirectional and directional microphones were used to determine speech understanding abilities in presence of noise. Speech perception was better only when the speaker was in front of the child. Directional microphones do no improve speech perception when the speaker was behind or towards the side of the child. The review of the studies on the efficacy of directional hearing aids in children suggests that they help in improving speech when presented from the front and suppresses the surrounding environmental noise. However, for younger children and infants, incidental learning happens a lot and their attention moves from one speaker to another very fast. Studies have shown that children who are less than 2 years old learn to communicate by overhearing the surrounding speech in addition to direct communication (Akhtar, 2005). There are limited studies which have attempted to assess the effects of directional microphones on incidental learning in children with hearing impairment. In addition, there is a dearth of literature on the effect of directional microphones on localization abilities, which has direct implication for safety, especially in children.

Based on the literature, it is well reported that directional microphones can be recommended for older children in specific situations where the speaker is in the front and noise are from the surroundings. Frequency modulated (FM) systems provide better SNRs compared to directional microphones. However, it is not always practical when the child listens to speech babble (multiple speakers). Parents should have the option of switching between omnidirectional and directional mode depending on the listening situation. Adaptive directionality is reported to be better compared to fixed directionality. However, there are limited studies on the efficacy of adaptive directionality in children (Auriemmo, Kuk, Lau, Dornan, Sweeton, Marshall,... Stenger, 2009). The option of activating or deactivating directional microphones should be thoroughly discussed with the parents. They should also be oriented regarding the application of these hearing aids and its benefits in real life situations.

DIGITAL NOISE REDUCTION ALGORITHMS

One of the main aims of advancement in hearing aid technology was to reduce the negative impact of speech perception in noise in individuals with hearing loss using noise reduction algorithms (Bentler & Chiou, 2006). Noise reduction algorithms work on automatically identifying speech and noise. The hearing aid would reduce noise and amplify only speech. The algorithms work on identifying if the signal is continuous or fluctuating by calculating the amount of modulations. The gain would be reduced for steady noise and fluctuating speech signal would be amplified. Bentler (2005) conducted an in-depth review and reported that digital noise reduction algorithms do not improve or degrade speech perception in presence of noise. Mueller and Bentler (2005) reported that there was an improvement in acceptable noise level (ANL) for adult hearing aid users with the use of noise reduction algorithms. However, they reported that there was no improvement in speech understanding with this technology. But the enhancement in comfort in presence of noise even without improvement in speech understanding may result in increased acceptance of hearing aids.

Studies on assessment of the efficacy of noise reduction algorithms in children are limited. Furthermore, these strategies are company specific and hence it is difficult to generalize the results (Bentler & Chiou, 2006). There are differences across companies in terms of gain reduction algorithms and onset/offset times of activation. It is well reported that audibility and bandwidth requirement is greater for in children (Stelmachowicz, Hoover, Lewis, Kortekaas, & Pittman, 2000; Stelmachowicz, Pittman, Hoover, Lewis, & Moeller, 2004) compared to adult listeners. There is a requirement of appropriate hearing aid verification method to evaluate the gain and bandwidth of the hearing aid when the noise reduction feature is activated. Hence, digital noise reduction algorithms can be used only in older school going children who might have difficulty listening in presence of noise.

OPEN FIT AND RECEIVER IN THE EAR (RITE) DEVICES FOR CHILDREN

Most of the adults with hearing impairment would prefer small or invisible hearing aids considering the cosmetic appearance. The same hold good even in children and for parents of children with hearing impairment. With the advanced feedback cancellation algorithms, open fit hearing aids are reported to be beneficial (Byrne, Sinclair, & Noble, 1998; Kuk, Keenan, & Ludvigsen, 2005; Magnusson, Claesson, Persson, & Tengstrand, 2013). In addition, open fit hearing aids also lead to increased comfort and fewer rejections of hearing aids (Gnewikow & Moss, 2006; Johnson, 2006; Taylor, 2006). The reduced occlusion effect is reported to provide better comfort in individuals using open fit hearing aids (Johnson, 2006; Taylor, 2006).

Similarly, attempts are also done to combine in the ear (ITE) coupled to receiver in the ear canal (RIC) hearing aids to provide additional gain with RIC hearing aids. The separation of receiver and microphone also reduces the size of the hearing aid which improves the cosmetic appeal and better fitting of the hearing aid. The benefit with RIC over a behind the ear (BTE) is demonstrated by few studies reported in the literature (Alworth, Plyler, Reber, & Johnstone, 2010; Conrad & Rout, 2013). Audiologists, who have succeeded with adults using open fit and RITE have logically considered using them even for children. However, there are no studies which have actually attempted to verify the benefit of these hearing aids in children. Open fit hearing aids are of smaller size and can be fitted without custom ear molds. These are the major advantages of such hearing aids over traditional hearing aids. However, additional factors with respect to the individual child should be carefully verified before prescribing such hearing aids to children.

Considering the small size of these hearing aids, it is difficult to use telecoil or direct audio input or FM technology in low-end hearing aids. In addition, domes for children are not available in different sizes to fit all the children appropriately. In addition, the thin wiring usually gets broken because of rough use of hearing aids by children. In RITE, replacement of ITE shell of RITE as the child grows can be costly. Considering the miniature nature of the hearing aids, the durability of such hearing aids can be a concern. In addition, because of the smaller battery size, the life of the battery is less which requires frequent replacement of the batteries. These are some of the limitations of such hearing aids which should be kept in mind before prescribing these hearing aids. Thus, open fit hearing aids and RITE can be recommended for children only after careful verification and validation of the efficacy of these hearing aids.

FREQUENCY LOWERING TECHNOLOGY

Individuals with severe to profound hearing loss or individuals with steeply sloping hearing loss encounter several communication challenges since they cannot use high-frequency information. Most of the speech sounds are at high frequencies and affects the normal speech and language development in children (Boothroyd, 1984; Elfenbein, Hardin-Jones, & Davis, 1994; Stelmachowicz, Pittman, Hoover, Lewis, & Moeller, 2004). This can further impair their academic performance in future (Sterne & Goswami, 2000). This lead to exploration of the new technology called frequency lowering techniques where low frequencies were transposed or compressed within the audibility range of an individual.

Previous studies have reported that linear frequency transposition technology can be successfully used in children with steeply sloping sensorineural hearing loss (Auriemmo, Kuk, & Stenger, 2008; Smith, Dann, & Brown, 2009). Auriemmo, Kuk, and Stenger (2008) reported improvement in perception of vowels and consonants in 10 school going children with steeply sloping hearing loss after 6 weeks of usage of frequency lowering technology. Smith et al. (2009) reported improved speech perception and also production in six children after using frequency lowering technology for 24 weeks. Thus, studies do report improvement in speech perception with this technology. However, the technology varies across companies and generalization is difficult. Also, it requires training with this technology for improvement in speech perception. With the advancement in cochlear implants and hybrid implants, this technology is rarely recommended for children since more benefit is obtained from cochlear implants.

ChannelFree™ HEARING AIDS

The digital filtering that is done across channels in a multi-channel hearing aid can lead to unnecessary distortions which can further impair the speech perception. There is a loss of differences in levels across speech sounds when the number of compression channels increases. These cues are very important for both individuals with normal hearing and individuals with hearing impairment (Moore & Glasberg, 1986). The studies on multi-channel hearing aids show that vowel recognition is poorer because of the loss of level difference cues that occur with increase in the number of channels (Franck, van Kreveld-Bos, Dreschler, & Verschuure, 1999). The probable solution for this could be with the use of ChannelFree™ hearing aids which tries to overcome the negative effects of a multi-channel hearing aid.

ChannelFree™ hearing aids were introduced to overcome the adverse effect of multichannel compression on the perception of spectral contrasts in speech. The perception of phonemes especially vowels is identified based on spectral contrast. The signal that comes to the hearing aid is applied a frequency gain curve based on the overall level amplitude of the signal and does not split the signal into different channels. For each client, based on the audiogram a family of frequency curves is determined. Based on the input signal, appropriate frequency gain curve is selected by the synchronizer in the circuit. Since the signal is not divided into different compression channels, the spectral contrasts of the input speech signal are retained (Schaub, 2009). ChannelFree™ hearing aids also reduce distortion compared to a multi-channel hearing aid (Schaub, 2009).

Dillon, Keidser, O'Brien, and Silberstein (2003) studied the differences in perception of quality of speech using ChannelFree™ hearing aids and other multi-channel hearing aids. They reported that ChannelFree™ hearing aids were preferred by the majority of the participants for perception of speech and music. Kodiyath, Mohan, and Bellur (2017) compared aided performance and hearing aid preference between multi-channel and ChannelFree™ hearing aids. They reported that the performance was better with ChannelFree™ hearing aids compared to multi-channel hearing aids. They suggested that ChannelFree™ hearing aids retain the spectral contrasts and enhance the temporal cues. Most of the participants of the study preferred ChannelFree™ hearing aids rather than multi-channel hearing aids. DeSilva, Kooknoor, Shetty, and Thontadarya (2016) also reported that consonant identification scores in presence of noise was better with ChannelFree™ hearing aids compared to multichannel hearing aids in individuals with cochlear hearing loss. Considering all these advantages, it can be assumed that it can benefit even children with hearing impairment. However, there are no studies which have attempted to determine the efficacy of ChannelFreeTM hearing aids in pediatric population.

Apart from the above mentioned technologies, there are other advancements too which may be beneficial in pediatric hearing aid fitting. For an audiologist to recommend the technology to the child there has to be sufficient concrete evidence. Most of the studies are company funded and the studies lag behind in the level of evidences. Thus, it is high time that evidence-based practice is incorporated in pediatric hearing aid fitting.

EVIDENCE-BASED PRACTICE

The need of the hour is the use of evidence-based approaches in proper assessment and intervention of children with hearing impairment. However, the practical scenario is different where there is a clear dearth of good quality studies on the efficacy of hearing aid technologies especially in children. The speed of technological innovation is more than actual time for translation research on the technology. By the time studies regarding efficacy are published, devices may have undergone significant modification or may no longer be available in the market. Studies of the effects of advanced hearing aid technologies, such as noise reduction and directional microphones, in children are not widespread in the literature.

Traditionally, evidence-based practice only referred to evaluation of peer-reviewed research published in scholarly journals and relied mainly on external evidences. However, as Dollaghan (2007) suggests, evidence-based practice should also encompass clinician's experience and expertise regarding the hearing aid technology and it should also consider the preferences of technology by the patient or the family members. Thus, it is essential to have a broader perspective of evidence-based practice for evaluating technological advancements for paediatric hearing aid users. Audiologists should be careful in not blindly believing the false claims (sometimes) by the hearing aid manufacturers. The research evidence published by the companies alone may not be valid sources of external evidence.

Palmer and Grimes (2005) did an in-depth review of the efficacy of signal processing technology in hearing aids for pediatric patients. They considered 226 studies which were relevant to the study. Out of these, only 8 studies had sufficient levels of evidence which could be included for in-depth review. They concluded that wide dynamic range compression (WDRC) strategy results in better speech understanding in quiet and in the noise surrounding for pediatric hearing aid users (Marriage & Moore, 2003;

Jenstad, Seewald, Cornelisse, & Shantz, 1999). Although studies like these are important for audiologists, the studies are very limited regarding advanced hearing aid fitting technologies in children. Many audiologists have questioned if these technological advances are appropriate to use with children, and, if so, what methods should be used to verify their function. Unfortunately, guidelines or other forms of external validation are not readily available for clinicians making these important clinical decisions. Thus, considering the limited evidence-based research in children, audiologists should attempt to verify pediatric hearing aid fitting and make an attempt to collect evidence for the efficacy of the technology.

The present book chapter highlights the need for adopting an evidence-based approach to verify these advanced hearing aid technologies for pediatric hearing aid fitting.

FUTURE DIRECTIONS

Despite multiple advances in research related to pediatric amplification, a lot of research is yet to be done to determine the effectiveness of advanced hearing aid technology. There is a need for translational studies evaluating the benefit of children with these technologies. This would definitely help an audiologist to choose appropriate technology for pediatric hearing aid fitting. In addition to hearing aid technology, there is also a boom in the technological advancement of assistive listening devices (ALDs) and there is a need to carry out empirical studies to assess the efficacy of the same. Independent studies should validate these advanced features should be promoted to ensure appropriate benefit to hearing aid users of all ages.

CONCLUSION

Pediatric hearing aid fitting has always been a challenge for an audiologist. Appropriate verification of hearing aid for young children is very important for understanding the effectiveness of hearing aid fitting. Selection of an appropriate hearing aid technology is vital in the development of communication skills. Considering the rapid technological advancement and lack of evidence-based research, audiologists should use their clinical knowledge and use appropriate verification methods to make appropriate recommendations in pediatric hearing aid fitting.

ACKNOWLEDGMENT

The author acknowledges Dr. Savithri, Director, All India Institute of Speech and Hearing, Mysuru for providing the support.

REFERENCES

Akhtar, N. (2005). The robustness of learning through overhearing. *Developmental Science*, *8*(2), 199–209. doi:10.1111/j.1467-7687.2005.00406.x PMID:15720377

Alworth, L. N., Plyler, P. N., Reber, M. B., & Johnstone, P. M. (2010). The effects of receiver placement on probe microphone, performance, and subjective measures with open canal hearing instruments. *Journal of the American Academy of Audiology, 21*(4), 249–266. doi:10.3766/jaaa.21.4.4 PMID:20388451

Auriemmo, J., Kuk, F., Lau, C., Dornan, B. K., Sweeton, S., Marshall, S., & Stenger, P. (2009). Efficacy of an adaptive directional microphone and a noise reduction system for school-aged children. *Journal of Educational Audiology, 15*, 15–27.

Auriemmo, J., Kuk, F., & Stenger, P. (2008). Criteria for evaluating the performance of linear frequency transposition in children. *The Hearing Journal, 61*(4), 50–52. doi:10.1097/01.HJ.0000315831.15143.9f

Bentler, R., & Chiou, L. K. (2006). Digital noise reduction: An overview. *Trends in Amplification, 10*(2), 67–82. doi:10.1177/1084713806289514 PMID:16959731

Bentler, R. A. (2005). Effectiveness of directional microphones and noise reduction schemes in hearing aids: A systematic review of the evidence. *Journal of the American Academy of Audiology, 16*(7), 473–484. doi:10.3766/jaaa.16.7.7 PMID:16295234

Bentler, R. A. (2005). Effectiveness of directional microphones and noise reduction schemes in hearing aids: A systematic review of the evidence. *Journal of the American Academy of Audiology, 16*(7), 473–484. doi:10.3766/jaaa.16.7.7 PMID:16295234

Boothroyd, A. (1984). Auditory perception of speech contrasts by subjects with sensorineural hearing loss. *Journal of Speech, Language, and Hearing Research: JSLHR, 27*(1), 134–144. doi:10.1044/jshr.2701.134 PMID:6716999

Byrne, D., Sinclair, S., & Noble, W. (1998). Open earmold fittings for improving aided auditory localization for sensorineural hearing losses with good high-frequency hearing. *Ear and Hearing, 19*(1), 62–71. doi:10.1097/00003446-199802000-00004 PMID:9504273

Conrad, S., & Rout, A. (2013). Perceived Occlusion and Comfort in Receiver-in-the-Ear Hearing Aids. *American Journal of Audiology, 22*(2), 283–290. doi:10.1044/1059-0889(2013/11-0025) PMID:23824427

DeSilva, M. D. K., Kooknoor, V., Shetty, H. N., & Thontadarya, S. (2016). Effect of multichannel and channels free hearing aid signal processing on phoneme recognition in quiet and noise. *International Journal of Health Sciences and Research, 6*(3), 248–257.

Dillon, H., Keidser, G., O'Brien, A., & Silberstein, H. (2003). Sound quality comparisons of advanced hearing aids. *The Hearing Journal, 56*(4), 30–40. doi:10.1097/01.HJ.0000293908.50552.34

Dollaghan, C. A. (2007). *The handbook for evidence-based practice in communication disorders*. Paul H. Brookes Pub.

Elfenbein, J. L., Hardin-Jones, M. A., & Davis, J. M. (1994). Oral communication skills of children who are hard of hearing. *Journal of Speech, Language, and Hearing Research: JSLHR, 37*(1), 216–226. doi:10.1044/jshr.3701.216 PMID:8170125

Franck, B. A., van Kreveld-Bos, C. S., Dreschler, W. A., & Verschuure, H. (1999). Evaluation of spectral enhancement in hearing aids, combined with phonemic compression. *The Journal of the Acoustical Society of America, 106*(3 Pt 1), 1452–1464. doi:10.1121/1.428055 PMID:10489703

Gnewikow, D., & Moss, M. (2006). Hearing aid outcomes with open and closed canal fittings. *The Hearing Journal*, *59*(11), 66–72. doi:10.1097/01.HJ.0000286220.14835.13

Gravel, J. S., Fausel, N., Liskow, C., & Chobot, J. (1999). Children's speech recognition in noise using omni-directional and dual-microphone hearing aid technology. *Ear and Hearing*, *20*(1), 1–11. doi:10.1097/00003446-199902000-00001 PMID:10037061

Jenstad, L. M., Seewald, R. C., Cornelisse, L. E., & Shantz, J. (1999). Comparison of linear gain and wide dynamic range compression hearing aid circuits: Aided speech perception measures. *Ear and Hearing*, *20*(2), 117–126. doi:10.1097/00003446-199904000-00003 PMID:10229513

Johnson, E. E. (2006). Segmenting dispensers: Factors in selecting open-canal fittings. *The Hearing Journal*, *59*(11), 58–64. doi:10.1097/01.HJ.0000286219.07211.99

Kodiyath, G. K., Mohan, K. M., & Bellur, R. (2017). Influence of channel and ChannelFree™ processing technology on the vocal parameters in hearing-impaired individuals. *Indian Journal of Otology*, *23*(1), 21–26. doi:10.4103/0971-7749.199506

Kuk, F., Keenan, D., & Ludvigsen, C. (2005). Efficacy of an open fitting hearing aid. *Hearing Review*, *12*(4), 26–32.

Magnusson, L., Claesson, A., Persson, M., & Tengstrand, T. (2013). Speech recognition in noise using bilateral open fit hearing aids: The limited benefit of directional microphones and noise reduction. *International Journal of Audiology*, *52*(1), 29–36. doi:10.3109/14992027.2012.707335 PMID:22928919

Marriage, J. E., & Moore, B. C. (2003). New speech tests reveal benefit of widedynamic-range, fast-acting compression for consonant discrimination in children with moderate-to-profound hearing loss. *International Journal of Audiology*, *42*(7), 418–425. doi:10.3109/14992020309080051 PMID:14582638

Moore, B. C., & Glasberg, B. R. (1986). A comparison of two-channel and single-channel compression hearing aids. *Audiology*, *25*(5), 210–226. doi:10.3109/00206098609078387 PMID:3566630

Mueller, G. H., & Bentler, R. A. (2005). Fitting hearing aids using clinical measures of loudness discomfort levels: An evidence-based review of effectiveness. *Journal of the American Academy of Audiology*, *16*(7), 461–472. doi:10.3766/jaaa.16.7.6 PMID:16295233

Palmer, C. V., & Grimes, A. M. (2005). Effectiveness of signal processing strategies for the pediatric population: A systematic review of the evidence. *Journal of the American Academy of Audiology*, *16*(7), 505–514. doi:10.3766/jaaa.16.7.10 PMID:16295237

Ricketts, T., Galster, J., & Tharpe, A. M. (2007). Directional benefit in simulated classroom environments. *American Journal of Audiology, 16*(2), 130-144. doi:(2007/017 doi:10.1044/1059-0889

Smith, J., Dann, M., & Brown, P. M. (2009). An evaluation of frequency transposition for hearing-impaired school-age children. *Deafness & Education International*, *11*(2), 62–82. doi:10.1179/146431509790559633

Stelmachowicz, P. G., Hoover, B. M., Lewis, D. E., Kortekaas, R. W., & Pittman, A. L. (2000). The relation between stimulus context, speech audibility, and perception for normal-hearing and hearing-impaired children. *Journal of Speech, Language, and Hearing Research: JSLHR*, *43*(4), 902–914. doi:10.1044/jslhr.4304.902 PMID:11386477

Stelmachowicz, P. G., Pittman, A. L., Hoover, B. M., Lewis, D. E., & Moeller, M. P. (2004). The importance of high-frequency audibility in the speech and language development of children with hearing loss. *Archives of Otolaryngology--Head & Neck Surgery*, *130*(5), 556–562. doi:10.1001/archotol.130.5.556 PMID:15148176

Sterne, A., & Goswami, U. (2000). Phonological awareness of syllables, rhymes, and phonemes in deaf children. *Journal of Child Psychology and Psychiatry, and Allied Disciplines*, *41*(5), 609–625. doi:10.1111/1469-7610.00648 PMID:10946753

Taylor, B. (2006). Real-world satisfaction and benefit with opencanal fittings. *The Hearing Journal*, *59*(11), 74–82. doi:10.1097/01.HJ.0000286222.91963.39

KEY TERMS AND DEFINITIONS

Assistive Listening Device: They are special amplification devices which would be beneficial in adverse listening conditions.

Digital Noise Reduction: Automatic reduction of noise in a noisy environment. Hearing aid algorithm separates speech and noise and it suppresses noise and enhances the speech.

Directional Hearing Aids: Hearing aids which amplify the sounds originating only from the front and reduce gain for surrounding sounds.

Evidence-Based Practice: Use of any form of assessment/rehabilitation approach/tool on patients which is verified through empirical studies.

Hearing Aids: Amplification device to amplify the soft sounds. It is used as a management strategy for individuals with the sensorineural hearing loss.

Chapter 5
Neurodevelopmental Disorders From a Clinical Linguistics Perspective

Brajesh Priyadarshi
All India Institute of Speech and Hearing, India

B. V. M. Mahesh
All India Institute of Speech and Hearing, India

ABSTRACT

The chapter attempts at bringing out an overview of linguistic-based deficits in neurodevelopmental disordered (NDD) population. Clinical linguistics as a discipline has provided a different dimension to view each patient as a distinctive case and has brought out the utilization of comprehensive depiction of individual skill patterns and deficits. As the NDDs are heterogeneous in nature, understanding their language deficits using achievement tests might not provide a clear description of these disorders. Hence, controlled experimental investigations using varied methodological designs could help in tapping their common linguistic variations which may augment key professionals to better identify, assess, and rehabilitate these individuals. While appreciating all these factors, the chapter provides first-hand information on some of the neuro-developmental disorders and also the language-based diagnostic markers to identify them.

INTRODUCTION

Neurodevelopmental disorders (NDD) is an umbrella term used for a group of disorders that includes impairments of cognition, communication, motor skills and general behavior. According to World Health Organization (2002), 1.4% of the world's population has developmental disabilities and among these 80% of them lives in the developing countries (Morrison & Cosden, 1997). As there are no proven pharmacological treatments for these set of disorders, a variety of early rehabilitation strategies are advocated. These are classified under the disorders of intellectual functioning, communication disorders (Language and speech) and motoric disorders. These may also be able to coexist along with a syndrome

DOI: 10.4018/978-1-5225-7004-2.ch005

where developmental disorders form a part of the symptom cluster, for instance, Down's syndrome. According to Diagnostic and Statistical Manual of Mental Disorders, 5th edition (American Psychiatric Association, 2013), NDD is broadly classified into intellectual disability (ID)/(Intellectual Developmental Disorders), Specific Learning Disorder, Communication Disorders, Autism Spectrum Disorders (ASD), Motor Disorders and Attention Deficit Hyperactivity Disorder (ADHD).

According to Crystal (1986), Clinical Linguistics is the application of the theories, methods, and findings of linguistics (including Phonetics) to the study of those situations where all language handicaps are diagnosed and treated. It is a sub-discipline of Linguistics which involves the application of linguistic theory to the field of Speech-Language Pathology. In other words, it is a branch of Applied Linguistics, used to describe, analyze, and treat language disabilities. Clinical Linguistics has provided a new dimension to view each NDD patient as a unique case and it has brought out the necessity of making full and detailed descriptions of individual patterns of skills and deficits. It has been applied for certain clinical purposes such as helping in revealing the communicative status of the patient's linguistic patterns. According to the different identifiable types of the linguistic deficit/disorder, it aids in differential diagnosis and categorization of the NDD patient's behaviors. According to Jakobson (1971) the pathology of language, far from being a random disturbance, obeys a set of rules; the rules underlying the regression of language cannot be elicited without the consistent use of linguistic techniques and methodology. An explicit knowledge of the nature of language, its grammar, and its functioning would be helpful in providing adequate therapies to individuals who are suffering from NDD.

Crystal (1984) and Grunwell (1985, 1993) argues that the careful and systematic description of the patient's communication behavior provides a means of assessing that behavior in relation to linguistic and developmental areas. They suggest that linguistic analysis can reveal the systematic and communicative status of the patient's linguistic patterns on their own, regardless of considerations of target norms. The insights of linguistic theory and methods also facilitate the formulation of specific treatment aim and strategies for NDD patients. Linguistic analysis at different points during assessment and management process allows the identification and evaluation of changes in the patient's communicative behavior and it helps to find out which component of language is affected in this kind of population. In a nutshell, Clinical Linguistics can help a professional in effective assessment, description, and management of a wide range of multifaceted disorders such as NDD. The following are some of the disorders which come under the preview of NDD.

1. Intellectual Disability (ID)

Intellectual disability (ID) is known to be an impairment of general mental abilities that influence adaptive functioning, conceptual understanding, and social domains. If these deficits are observed to be found in the younger age group, with less than 5 years of age, they are generally termed as Developmentally Delayed (DD). The term ID more suits for the other group who are older than 5 years and who can reliably undergo a test of intelligence quotient (IQ). The severity of the intellectual disability is based on a combination of the level of intellectual functioning, adaptive functioning, and intensity of supports needed. When individuals with ID show difficulty to undergo IQ test then a diagnosis is made without labeling the level of functioning. Whether an individual is termed as ID/DD, they show up significant deficits in the developmental milestones across speech/language, motoric, social, emotional and adaptive behaviors. Intellectual Disability is more common in males compared to females and the majority of the prevalence data on this population agree that 85% of this population has mild Intellectual Disability and percentage of ID in the severe category is static and have been less than 0.5% from several decades.

The connotation of DD needs to be carefully applied as the diagnosis of DD pertains to the fact that these individuals would generally overcome their impediments with reasonable assistance of rehabilitation specialists. A team approach with a focus on rehabilitating the major developmental milestones would help these individuals to join the mainstream population. The earlier term referring to these disorders - 'Mental Retardation' is obsolete which is replaced by the terminology of Intellectual Disability (ID) according to Rosa's law that is elucidated in the 11th version of the InternationalClassification of Diseases. DD/ID can be seen as an isolated condition or can coexist as a part of syndrome clusters such as Autism, Down's syndrome or any type of X-linked syndromes. Regarding etiological factors, environmental risk factors along with a specified etiology can be identified in the majority of the individual's Mild intellectual disability. In individuals with a severe disability, it is possible to identify the etiology in at least two-thirds of the affected individuals. Some of the commonly identified etiological factors linked to ID include chromosomal disorders, genetic syndromes, congenital brain malformations, neurodegenerative diseases, congenital infections, inborn errors of metabolism, and birth injury.

From the clinical linguistics perspective, the prominent phonological characteristics of NDD population with Intellectual disabilities can be observed as deletion of consonants and typically inconsistent occurrences of errors. The frequent processes seen in this population are cluster reduction and final consonant deletion. The severity of phonological problems increases with the degree of cognitive deficits. Fricatives are most frequently affected followed by laterals and aspirated stops (Shriberg & Widder, 1990). The syntax of children with Intellectual disabilities is reduced both expressively and receptively. They master syntactic constructions as typically developing children do, but at a slower pace. They use short and simple structures and have difficulty understanding long and complex utterances. In young ID children, the production of grammatical words is reduced i.e. use of articles (is, are), prepositions (on, in, at), pronouns (he, she), modal verbs (can, must, may, might, will, would, should), auxiliaries (will, shall, may, might, can, could, must, ought to, should, would, used to, need) and conjunctions. This gives their utterances a telegraphic character (Brown, 1973). ID children reach MLU2 around 4-5 years CA, MLU 3 around 7-8 years and MLU 6 around 14 or 15 years. According to Rondal (2013), themorphosyntactical limitations in the language development and functioning of ID stem from a lesser ability in implicit learning, which is very much important in the grammatical development. Significant delays and specific impairments in the expressive language of children with ID have been noted. These deficits have been directly linked to specific deficits in acquiring grammatical aspects of language. Studies of young children with ID have found widely varying rates of changes in the mean length of utterance (MLU) within the population. Their rate of development is very slow and these children may never develop beyond the early stages of grammatical development. However, in general, the complexity of their sentences is in proportion to their MLU. Although they use the same range of two-word phrases as all children, they have difficulty in mastering the many rules for talking in grammatically correct sentences (Rondal, 2009). It was also observed that older ID children and adolescents more frequently omit free and bound grammatical morphemes than MLU matched typically developing controls in the narrative speech sample (Chapman, Schwartz, & Bird, 1991; Chapman, Seung, Schwartz, & Bird, 1998).

Among the several subgroups of Intellectual Disability (ID), Down Syndrome (DS) is a common focused group wherein several investigations on phonetic and phonological behaviors have been studied. However, several inconsistencies in the findings have led investigators confused on whether the errors observed in this population are phonetic or phonologic. As reported by few studies, the early phonetic behaviors of individuals with DS may overlap with that of typically developing children (TD) in terms of vowel and consonants approximations of babbling (Smith & Stoel-Gammon, 1996). However, those children with DS who did not receive intervention at early years is known to produce late onset babbling who continue to show a delay in their productions even till the end of the first year which was attributed to their generalized hypotonicity of muscles (Lynch, Oller, Steffens, & Levine, 1995; Stoel-Gammon, 2001). Phonological development after the first year of life shows comparable development in the order of acquisition of speech sounds to that of TD children which is consistent with the notion of phonological delay (Stoel-Gammon, 1980). Some studies refute these claims on the basis that DS children have difficulty in producing the nonsense words despite they can differentiate these from real words in a perceptual judgment task which supports for a motoric deficit and not a phonological acquisition delay (Dodd, 1975). Hence, it is yet to be known whether the speech sound errors in children with Down syndrome occur due to phonetic or phonological delay. Some of the common phonological processes operating in children with DS include, but not limited to, Cluster Reduction, Fronting, Final consonant deletion and Deaffrication.

Regarding the acquisition of syntax, children with DS always fall below in their expressive syntax in comparison to their comprehension and cognitive abilities. This has been hypothesized to be a deficit in coordinating various syntactic structures such as word order, pronouns, and adverbs (Miles & Chapman, 2002). In non-DS groups, studies have shown that individuals with intellectual disability might follow the same developmental pattern of syntax but with a slower rate of acquisition. The statement is true on a range of parameters such as utterance length and syntactic complexity (Graham & Graham, 1971); mastery of bound morphemes (Newfield & Schlanger, 1968) and phrase structure acquisition (McLeavey, Toomey, & Dempsey, 1982).

Cognitive assessment of individuals with ID includes those tests that measure an individual's Attention (divided and shared), Memory, Speed of processing the verbal and nonverbal stimuli and Executive functions (Organization, flexibility, problem-solving, planning, sequencing, judgement etc). Several standardized tools are available to check cognition and selection of the tool is dictated by needs of testing environment (children versus adults) and type of testing required (Norm references versus criterion based). An exemplary table of the most commonly used cognitive tests is provided in Table 1.

2. Specific Learning Disorder

According to DSM-5 (American Psychiatric Association, 2013), specific learning disorder refers to an umbrella term of reading, writing and mathematical difficulties. The term specific learning disorder assumes that reading, writing and other academic difficulties commonly co-occur together and hence justifies the usage of a single entity rather than identifying these disorders separately. Specific learning disorders were identified based on the area of learning deficit such as reading disability (dyslexia), mathematics disability (dyscalculia/acalculia), a disorder of written expression (dysgraphia), and Non-Verbal Learning Disability (NVLD). The specific learning disorder is generally diagnosed when an individual has significant difficulties in their academic performances despite having age-appropriate teaching and learning experiences with normal cognition and sociocultural factors. Early identification is the key as it prevents academic failure, psychosocial disturbances and lifelong implications for academic success, occupation, socioeconomic well–being, and consequently health. Reading disability is one of the most commonly diagnosed categories of specific learning disorder that occurs with several co-morbid disorders such as Language impairments, motor, and behavioral deficits. Mathematical learning difficulties

Table 1. Commonly used assessment tools for children with ID

Test Name	Age of Testing	Tested Items
Wechsler Intelligence Scale for Children – 4th edition (WISC-IV)	6 years–16 years,	15 subtests; yields IQ, verbal comprehension, reasoning, working memory, and processing speed.
Wechsler Adult Intelligence Scale – 3rd edition (WAIS-III)	16 years–adulthood	14 subtests; yields IQ, comprehension, organization, working memory, and processing speed
Kaufman Brief Intelligence Test –2nd edition	4–90 years	Verbal and non-verbal domain scores based on Verbal knowledge, riddles and matrices
Non-Verbal Performance Tests		
Ravens Standard Progressive Matrices	Child-adult norms	Measures abstract reasoning
Comprehensive Test of Nonverbal Intelligence (CTONI)	6–89 years	Six subtests; yields non-verbal IQ, picture non-verbal IQ, and geometric non-verbal IQ indices
Memory Scales		
Children's Memory Scale (CMS)	5–16 years	Yields immediate and delayed scores for both verbal memory and visual memory, general memory, delayed recognition, learning, and attention/concentration
Wechsler Memory Scale – 3rd edition (WMS-III)	16 years–adulthood	Six core and five optional subtests; yields three domain scores: Immediate memory, general memory (delayed), and working memory

are fairly common and the prevalence of which is higher in girls than in boys due to environmental and biological, factors. Dyscalculia is commonly associated with medical and psychiatric syndromes such as epilepsy and fragile X syndrome hence these conditions need to be assessed before arriving at a final diagnosis. Among the specific learning disorders, understanding dysgraphia which is the difficulty in associating the phonemes of a language to its corresponding written form is least researched.

Linguistically, it can be characterized that their major problem is in deducing the language rules, resulting in delays in morphological rule acquisition and in the development of syntactic complexity. These children have problems in the area of inflectional morphology, specifically, they omit functional words, bound morphemes encoding case, gender, number, person etc. or, they use them incorrectly. It also seems that in these children, the development of inflectional morphology comes to a standstill at an early stage and beyond that point, the acquisition process cannot advance without difficulties. These children, with the given deficits in syntax and semantics, produce shorter, less cohesive stories that are syntactically simple and contain frequent errors of syntax, semantics, and morphology.

Morphological difficulties are known to impact the literacy as these acts as pre-requisites to successfully encode classroom-based instructions. Morphologically complex forms, for instance, a combination of free morpheme with a prefix/suffix could make the decoding process in a child with learning disability difficult (Green, 2009; Jarmulowicz & Hay, 2009). Utterance length and complexity acquisition are observed to increase in a linear yet slowed fashion in children with a learning disability compared to typically developing peers who show a rapid increase in utterance length and complexity. Some studies have shown no known grammatical deficit in children with learning disability, however, a careful analysis of the subjection selection of these studies indicate that the investigators had chosen the population with higher IQ ranges compared to the routine studies of children with learning difficulties (Scott & Windsor, 2000).

3. Communication Disorders

According to DSM-5 (American Psychiatric Association, 2013), classification of NDDs, communication disorder includes language disorder, speech sound disorders, social pragmatic disorder and childhood-onset fluency disorders. If carefully observed, the classification system of DSM-5 includes several of the communication disorders into one, for instance, expressive and mixed receptive language disorders is represented by a single entity called language disorders. Additionally, the diagnostic label of stuttering has been replaced as childhood-onset fluency disorder and those individuals who were earlier classified as Pervasive-Developmental Disorders- not otherwise specified are categorized into social pragmatic disorder without accompanying the stereotypic behaviors. The previously used term of phonological disorder is replaced with speech sound disorders.

Individuals with language disorders are known to have marked difficulties in morphosyntax compared to other domains of language. Within the domain of morphosyntax, aspects such as verb ending (e.g.,-ed forms), plurals (e.g.–s), articles (e.g., the, a) and verb denoting the tenses (e.g., is/was sleeping) are known to be the problem areas (Bortolini, Caselli, Deevy, & Leonard, 2002; Leonard, 2014). Some investigators explain the aberrations at the level of morphosyntax using syntax and pragmatic competency deficits (Rice, Wexler, & Cleave, 1995; van der Lely, 2003; Wexler, 1994). On contrary, these deficits are explained as to the core cognitive issues operating in these populations which are further boosted by studies which have shown the influence of time pressure on storage and processing capabilities in children with language disorders (Montgomery, 2003; Weismer, 2000). Furthermore, other studies have shown slower reaction time in children with language disorders which are attributed to their speed of cognitive processing (Kail, 1994).

The term 'speech sound disorder' is certainly new to the profession of Speech-Language Pathology as in terms of its usage, however, it is a cover term classically referred for phonological or articulation disorders. Speech sound disorder is a neutral term which does not presuppose the causative factors for the behavioural outcomes that was otherwise assumed while using the diagnostic labels of phonological/articulation disorder. It is characterized by Substitutions, Omissions, Deletions and Additions of speech sounds which could be generally tested using an imitation based norm/criterion referenced standardized articulation tests generally at the word and/or connected speech level. Some of the commonly used tests to analyze speech sound disorders in English are provided in Table 2.

Childhood-onset fluency disorder has replaced the terms of stuttering and Cluttering in DSM-5. There is only a change in the diagnostic label but the characteristic features remain the same. Childhood-onset fluency disorder is characterized by the core features of sound/syllable repetition, prolongations and blocks. Additionally few individuals with the above disorder may also show revisions, hesitations/pauses and interjections which affects the smooth and continuous flow of speech but these are classified as typical disfluencies and the sole presence of these symptoms does not qualify for a diagnosis of childhood-onset fluency disorder. Many individuals also show physical tension, negative reactions and avoidance of sounds, and situations. Although childhood-onset fluency disorder is known to begin

Table 2. Commonly used assessment tools for speech sound disorders in English

Test Name	Age of Testing	Tested Items
Diagnostic Evaluation of Articulation and Phonology (DEAP)	3.0 to 8.11 years	Screening, articulation, phonological assessment, and oral motor screening.
Arizona Articulation Proficiency Scale (AAPS – 3rd edition)	1.5 to 18 years	Tests sound in words and connected speech. Outcome measures include percentile and standard scores.
Goldman-Fristoe Test of Articulation (GFTA-2)	2 -21 years	Checks sound in single words, connected speech, stimulability in syllables, words and sentences. Outcome measure includes percentiles and standard scores.
Bankson-Bernthal Test of Phonology	3-9 years	Uses picture stimuli to assess the accuracy of consonants, clusters and phonological processes.

around 21/2 years of age, 95% of the children show the disfluencies within the age of 5 years (Yairi & Ambrose, 2005). Another category included under the childhood-onset fluency disorder is Cluttering. Cluttering is characterized by rapid/irregular speech rate accompanied by typical disfluencies (revisions, interjections). Individuals with cluttering may have cognitive and linguistic deficits which include poor attention and concentration, lack of awareness towards their problem, word finding difficulties and prosodic difficulties. Childhood-onset fluency disorders can coexist with other related disorders such as intellectual disabilities, speech sound disorders and languages disorders (Healey, Reid, & Donaher, 2005; Ntourou, Conture, & Lipsey, 2011; Wolk, Edwards, & Conture, 1993). A history regarding the child's problem, medical history and the presence/absence of a positive family history, negative reactions and analysis of speech fluency (frequency of disfluencies, duration, secondary behaviours) is generally undertaken. Additionally, if warranted, help from other professionals such as a psychologist would be sought to address the avoidance and negative reaction associated with the speaking behaviours in children with fluency disorders. Several norm-referenced tests are available to check the dysfluent speech symptoms of children. Stuttering Severity Instrument (SSI-3; Riley, 1994) evaluates the child's disfluencies using reading and conversations tasks in terms of frequency of stuttering, duration of the stuttered moments and Physical concomitants. For non-readers, picture description tasks are generally used and scores of all these domains are added up to arrive at a final score which would be used to categorize an individual into various categories of stuttering severity. Other tests such as Stuttering Prediction Instrument (Riley, 1981), Test of Childhood Stuttering (Gilliam, Logan & Pearson, 2009) are also in use to quantify the dysfluent behaviors. For the disorder of cluttering, a checklist by Daly and Cantrell (2006) called 'Predictive Cluttering Inventory' (PCI) is used which is a 7-point rating scale that assess the behaviors in the domains of pragmatics, speech-motor, language-cognition and Motor Coordination-Writing Problems. Although subjective tests are a quick way of measuring the fluency disorders, objective analysis of disfluent symptoms are analysed using acoustic measures. A valuable addition to the current acoustic measure is kinematic analysis, which provides quantifiable data with fluent speech samples of children with stuttering. Incorporating kinematic analysis as a short duration measures would also provide further insights into the slightest changes provided by the behavioural treatments in the enhancement of speech fluency behaviours.

4. Autism Spectrum Disorders (ASD)

Autism spectrum disorders (ASD) is a group of disorders which share deficits across social, communication, and behavioral domains. According to DSM-5 (American Psychiatric Association, 2013), this category includes four specific disorders viz., autistic disorder (autism), childhood disintegrative disorder, Asperger's syndrome and pervasive developmental disorder not otherwise specified. These disorders include deficits in: a) social communication and interaction, and; b) Restrictive and repetitive behaviors. The degree of communication impairment depends on which category a given individual would fall into the groups of ASDs. Males are 4 times more common to be diagnosed to have autism than females and it has been noted that the prevalence rate has neither increased nor decreased from the past few decades. While focussing on the Asperger's syndrome, one needs to assess behavioral and social domains as these are deficit areas which need attention. They are not reported to have obvious deficits in spoken language comprehension or production. PDD-NOS shares the characteristic features of both autistic disorder and Asperger's syndrome, nevertheless, it does not meet the criteria for both. There is a high overlap of ASDs with ID and when it co-occurs it poses a significant challenge to the rehabilitation specialists as affected individuals become less functional overall across various domains of development. Although causes for ASD are yet to be known, there are some known syndromes that are most likely to cause ASDs (including Down syndrome and Fragile-X syndrome). The lack of social justice and acceptable social skills most often prevents persons with autism to independently participate in the community. They may have intense emotions but may fail to understand how to express the same in social situations. Brook and Bowler (1992) listed some of the pragmatic deficits presented by children with autism: a) Problems in encoding meaning relevant to conversation; b) Difficulty in understanding verbal /nonverbal cues of partner; c) Problem in initiating and responding to questions; d) Literal interpretations of verbal messages, and; e) Poor turn-taking and topic maintenance. From the clinical linguistics perspective, the prominent disability pointers related to speech and language of children with autism are as follows:

1. Faster learning of concrete than abstract words, including more ready learning of words that refer to objects as opposed to emotions.
2. Lack of understanding of relationships between words.
3. Pronoun reversal (use of *you* for *I* and *I* for *you*; referring to self as he, she etc).
4. Use of short and less complex sentences than age-matched typically developing peers; occasional use of incorrect word order.
5. The omission of grammatical features such as plural inflections and conjunctions.
6. These children involve more deficits in surface morphology and phonology rather than deep syntax (Eigsti & Bennetto, 2009).

Other pragmatic related deficits include:

1. Public behavior tends to be the same as private behavior.
2. Conventional behavior will seem startling. Those with autism may see conventional behavior as inappropriate and unconventional behavior as normal or reasonable because they do not share a common perspective.

3. They are unable to organize and manage themselves appropriately at parties, during free time, breaks and vacations.
4. They cannot read the subtle body language or cues indicating that others are bored, embarrassed and have the desire to change the subject.
5. Friendly overtures, humor and jokes are misunderstood and difficulty in understanding sarcasm.
6. Very little or no eye contact.
7. Tends to get too close when speaking to someone (lack of personal space).
8. Talks excessively about one or two topics (cricket, movies, etc.).
9. Difficulty understanding group interactions.

Among the ASDs, Asperger's disorder has relatively received focused attention due to its unique deficit in social use of language. Koning and Magill-Evans (2001) have reported social skills difficulties in adolescents with Asperger's syndrome using social skill rating system. The study reported significant differences between individuals with Asperger's syndrome and typical adolescents across social perception, social skills, number of friends, the frequency of contact and social competence. Another study analyzed individuals with Aspergers' and individuals with high functioning autism for their narration abilities while answering the questions related to a short video clip played back to the groups. Interestingly, both the groups performed similarly across a range of language functions whereas differed only in terms of the usage of verb markers (Sueng, 2007). Other studies have also echoed pragmatic difficulties in individuals with Asperger syndrome (Bartlett, Armstrong, & Roberts, 2005; Landa, 2000). Although several other syndromes do share the characteristics feature of ASDs (e.g. Fragile-X syndrome, Williams Syndrome), providing a detailed account of cognitive-linguistic characteristics of these syndromes is beyond the aim and scope of the current chapter.

5. Motor Disorders

According to DSM-5 classification (American Psychiatric Association, 2013), motor disorders are referred to a group of disorders which includes developmental coordination disorders, specified/ unspecified tic disorders, stereotypic movement disorders and cerebral palsy. As the role of movement based rehabilitation specialists (Physiotherapists/Occupation therapists/Orthopaedic specialists) is of prime importance in the majority of the above-listed disorders, the focus is more on Cerebral Palsy as clinical linguists have an important role in understanding and characterizing the speech deficits in this population.

According to American Academy of Cerebral Palsy and Developmental Medicine, cerebral palsy (CP) described a group of permanent disorders of the development of movement and posture, causing activity limitation that is attributed to progressive disturbances that occurred in the developing fetal or infant brain. Cerebral Palsy is classified as spastic (hemiplegia, diplegia, quadriplegia), dyskinetic (choreathetoid, dystonia), hypotonic, or mixed. The estimated worldwide prevalence rate of CP is to be 2–3 per 1,000 live births. Prevalence of CP is higher during infancy and later it reduces the signs and symptoms may resolve in due course of time. Several risk factors are identified to cause CP but the issues of prematurity and low birth weight are significant risk factors to develop CP and multiple disabilities. While analyzing the communication deficits one needs to focus on all the subsystems of speech that includes respiration, phonation, resonation, and articulation. Articulatory deficits are the most common and easily identified pattern of individuals with CP. Therefore, a sound knowledge of linguistics especially, phonetics and phonology are required while doing assessment and treatment with these patients. Additionally, the usage of perceptual measures in transcribing the speech samples forms a significant step while analyzing the speech intelligibility patterns post the treatment in these individuals also falls under the purview of clinical linguistics. The phonological characteristics of this population include the errors in the production of fricatives and affricates, distortion of consonants as well as vowel productions and/or inconsistent sound substitutions and omissions. Certain phonological processes as depicted below are also evident:

1. **Related to Temporal Coordination:** Voicing difficulties including devoicing of initial consonants, or voicing of unvoiced sounds, the variable realization of voiced-voiceless cognates, prevocalic voicing, consonant cluster reductions, and final consonant deletions, stopping of fricatives or friction of stops, weak syllable deletions.
2. **Related to Motor Control:** Fronting, backing, stopping, gliding, the lateral realization of apical and coronal fricatives, vowelization of /l/ and /r/, nasalization.
3. Phonological awareness in CP population has been a focus of an investigation by many studies. Card and Dodd (2006) compared the phonological awareness abilities in children with CP who could and could not speak. It was observed that children with CP who could speak outnumbered those who could not speak on tasks such as segmenting syllables and phoneme manipulation tasks. Additionally CP children who could speak also performed relatively better when judging written words for rhyme. It was concluded that an ability to speak would facilitate phonological awareness in children with CP compared to their non-speaking counterparts. Recent studies have confirmed the earlier findings that individuals with CP with limited speech output are also at a significant risk for limited literacy development (Peeters, Verhoeven, de Moor, & van Balkom, 2009).
4. Platt, Andrews, and Howie (1980) showed that adults with congenital cerebral palsy had frequent errors in fricatives wherein the word-initial and final positions were substituted and devoicing of affricates in the word final position was also observed. The omission of consonants was observed to be three times more common in word-final than in initial positions.
5. Some of the recent articulatory kinematic studies have reported spatial and temporal variability patterns as indexed using STI (Spatiotemporal Index) in individuals with mild Spastic cerebral palsy indicated poor movement control across these domains leading to perceptual based articulatory errors (Chen, Chen, Hong, Yang, Yang, & Wu, 2010; Hong, Chen, Yang, & Chen, 2007).

6. Attention Deficit Hyperactivity Disorder (ADHD)

Developmentally inappropriate levels of attention, hyperactivity and impulsivity are the hallmarks of individuals with ADHD. Behavioural issues occur in the absence of delay/deviance in cognitive or psychiatric conditions. Individuals with ADHD have significant communication difficulties, particularly the expression of communication via the verbal modality. Majority of individuals with ADHD have the delay in language development and they may also show residual language expression difficulties. In some individuals with ADHD despite showing commendable levels at other aspects of language, pragmatic usage of the same could be a significant difficulty. For instance, they may show communication breakdown while narrating an incident that requires the coherent production of related ideas in a context. Pragmatic difficulties are far more common in this population wherein they may fail to answer simple questions or requests and at times they fail to acknowledge feedbacks to their listeners. Difficulty in varying their language structure depending on the change in communication context or the speaker is also a marked difficulty witnessed in individuals with ADHD (Tannock, Purvis, & Schachar, 1993). Working memory and Executive function deficits have long been hypothesized for the communication difficulties evidenced in ADHD population. A clinical linguist could help a child with ADHD in profiling their language behaviours with the help of a Speech Language Pathologists (SLPs). Although less standardized tools are available to understand their language deficits, norm referenced or criterion referenced tests developed on typical children may help in analysing these behaviors. While examining the child's language abilities, pragmatic behaviours need greater attention and this could be a primary focus of intervention for children with ADHD by SLPs.

7. Sensory Impairment

To acquire spoken language, normal functioning of the auditory and visual modality is a pre-requisite. Normal hearing individuals can hear a wide range of audible frequencies beginning from 20 to 20,000 Hz. Although the perceptual dynamic range is higher, not all the frequencies in this range are used to hear human speech. The majority of the sound pattern of the spoken language would lie anywhere between 250–6,000 Hz range. These include the energy carriers of speech – vowels lying in the low-frequency region whereas consonants – meaning carriers of speech have a mixture of low and high-frequency sounds; occupy a wide spoken frequency range. The hearing could be classified into mild, severe and profound hearing losses which could be either conductive, sensory-neural and mixed hearing loss. Developmental disabilities are more common in individuals with hearing loss and approximately 30% of children have intellectual disabilities, cerebral palsy, vision impairment, or epilepsy. Individuals with hearing loss are at increased risk for spoken language delay which promotes early identification and rehabilitation of the same which reduces the academic, social and economic burden of the society. Hearing loss can affect a child's ability to learn both to speak and to understand spoken language. Auditory Verbal Therapy (AVT) along with spoken language therapy is the key to overcome the deficits in language learning of these individuals. Although the oral mode of communication is the preferred choice, sometimes when there is a limited benefit, other forms of communication is also promoted. These include a manual form of communication such as finger spelling or sign language forms. Visual impairment may also affect certain domains of cognitive linguistic behaviors, for instance, these individuals may have a peculiar difficulty in expressing abstract semantic terminologies (for instance colors). With the notion that these individuals may have normal hearing acuity, their language development may not be significantly different from their typically developing peers.

The prominent disability pointers related to speech and language of children with hearing impairment who are orally educated, syntactic development is delayed, and the end point of syntactic development falls far short of normal language competence (Mogford, 1993). Various syntactic errors are characteristic of the language produced by orally educated children with HI, even after the age of 10 years (Quiegley & King, 1980). The type of syntactic errors made by these adolescents suggests that most individuals with HI do not fully acquire the grammar of the spoken language. Bamford and Saunders (1992), in their study on children with hearing loss, showed that these children were more likely to use content words such as nouns and verbs in their speech, while grammatical words such as prepositions, conjunctions, and pronouns were less likely to be observed in their speech. Children with hearing loss face problems in learning and usage of lexical and functional morphemes such as adverbs, prepositions, pronouns, along with using relative clauses, complex sentences, and verb inflections. The sentences formed by people with hearing loss are simple, with frequent use of nouns and a shorter mean length utterance compared with that of people with normal hearing. They often have verbal errors in their speech, and their sentences are characterized by disagreement between subject and verb (Kricoss & Seyfried, 1996).

Some of the grammatical deficits observed in children with Hearing Impairment are - the omission of function words such as 'a', 'an' 'the' and conjunctions; difficulty in plural markers; regularizing the irregular plurals; and omission of auxiliary verbs. If not all, the majority of children with HI show Telegraphic speech wherein one omits the functional words leading to the production of only the content words. The above mentioned syntactic and morphological difficulties of children with HI has been studied in older age groups which also correlated well with their degree of hearing loss and hence wide variations could be expected in the symptom cluster depending on the severity of hearing loss (Levitt, 1987; Russell, Power, & Quigley, 1976). The above-described deficits in syntax and morphology may continue to be present in children with HI due to slow intervention process which ultimately also have a bearing on child's academic success. Poor academic performance in children with HI occurs due to inadequate auditory-oral language skills which impact reading and writing the language and it is reported that their reading level hardly ever crosses the fourth grade.

CONCLUSION AND FUTURE DIRECTIONS

Neurodevelopmental disorders are a group of disorders wherein most of the population shows a wide range of deficits across the domains of speech and language. The current chapter brings out an overview of linguistic-based deficits in populations such as Intellectual Disability, Autism Spectrum Disorders, Hearing Impairment, Learning Disability and other significant entities. In these disorders, components of language such as phonetics, phonology, syntax, morphology, semantics, and pragmatics may be differentially affected. Although most of these domains are affected in these NDDs, there are increased possibilities that anyone or few of the above-mentioned domains could be prominently exhibited. These sensitive domains need to be assessed in greater details to get a better understanding of the disorder itself. In the review, speech/language deficits were provided separately for each NDDs for the sake of clarity but increasing number of studies have identified the co-existence of NDDs, for instance, individuals with Down syndrome may also have hearing loss which can aggravate their language-based deficits. This kind of pattern can itself be explored on a large group of samples which might help in future to understand their common behavioral patterns. As the NDDs are a heterogeneous group of disorders, understanding this population with limited exploration of methodologies on various domains of speech and language might not provide a clear depiction of the disorders. Therefore, with carefully controlled methodology one can always tap the common patterns of linguistic variations which could further augment some of the professionals such as Speech-Language Pathologists (SLP) to better assess and rehabilitate these disorders.

Majority of the studies which has been reviewed have assessed the language achievement across different disorders but language achievement tests do not evaluate the dynamic processing of language in real time. As there is a possibility to carry out such procedures using Reaction Time (RT) paradigms and Event-Related Potential (ERP) studies, one can always correlate the language achievement scores with these tasks which can help to identify common behavioral patterns of language among these disorders which have hardly been ever explored in recent times.

REFERENCES

American Psychiatric Association. (2013). Diagnostic and statistical manual of mental disorders (5th ed.). Arlington, VA: American Psychiatric Publishing.

Bamford, J., & Saunders, E. (1992). Hearing impairment, auditory perception and language disability. *Child Language Teaching and Therapy*, *8*(2), 227–228. doi:10.1177/026565909200800218

Bartlett, S. C., Armstrong, E., & Roberts, J. (2005). Linguistic resources of individuals with Asperger syndrome. *Clinical Linguistics & Phonetics*, *19*(3), 203–213. doi:10.1080/02699200410001698634 PMID:15823956

Bortolini, U., Caselli, M. C., Deevy, P., & Leonard, L. B. (2002). Specific language impairment in Italian: The first steps in the search for a clinical marker. *International Journal of Language & Communication Disorders*, *37*(2), 77–93. doi:10.1080/13682820110116758 PMID:12012618

Brook, S. L., & Bowler, D. M. (1992). Autism by another name? Semantic and pragmatic impairments in children. *Journal of Autism and Developmental Disorders*, *22*(1), 61–81. doi:10.1007/BF01046403 PMID:1592765

Brown, R. (1973). *A first language: The early stages*. Oxford, UK: Harvard University Press. doi:10.4159/harvard.9780674732469

Card, R., & Dodd, B. (2006). The phonological awareness abilities of children with cerebral palsy who do not speak. *Augmentative and Alternative Communication*, *22*(3), 149–159. doi:10.1080/07434610500431694 PMID:17114160

Chapman, R. S., Schwartz, S. E., & Bird, E. K. R. (1991). Language skills of children and adolescents with Down syndrome: I. Comprehension. *Journal of Speech and Hearing Research*, *34*(5), 1106–1120. doi:10.1044/jshr.3405.1106 PMID:1836243

Chapman, R. S., Seung, H. K., Schwartz, S. E., & Bird, E. K. R. (1998). Language skills of children and adolescents with Down syndrome: II. Production deficits. *Journal of Speech, Language, and Hearing Research: JSLHR*, *41*(4), 861–873. doi:10.1044/jslhr.4104.861 PMID:9712133

Chen, C., Chen, H., Hong, W., Yang, F. G., Yang, L., & Wu, C. (2010). Oromotor variability in children with mild spastic cerebral palsy: A kinematic study of speech motor control. *Journal of Neuroengineering and Rehabilitation*, *7*(1), 54. doi:10.1186/1743-0003-7-54 PMID:20979638

Crystal, D. (1984). *Linguistic Encounters with language handicapped*. Oxford, UK: Blackwell.

Crystal, D. (1986). Pasado, presente y futuro de la linguïsticaclinica [The past, present and future of clinical linguistics]. In M. Montfort (Ed), Investigaccion y logopedia (pp. 34-42). Madrid: Ciencias de la EducacionPreescolar y Especial, III LogopedicsCongess, Madrid.

Daly, D. A., & Cantrell, R. P. (2006). *Cluttering: Characteristics labelled as diagnostically significant by 60 fluency experts*. Paper presented at the 6th IFA world congress on disorders of fluency, Dublin, Ireland.

Dodd, B. (1975). Recognition and reproduction of words by Down's syndrome and non-Down's syndrome retarded children. *American Journal of Mental Deficiency*, *80*(3), 306–311. PMID:127529

Eigsti, I. M., & Bennetto, L. (2009). Grammaticality judgments in autism: Deviance or delay. *Journal of Child Language, 36*(5), 999–1021. doi:10.1017/S0305000909009362 PMID:19224652

Gillam, R. B., Logan, K. J., & Pearson, N. A. (2009). *Test of Childhood Stuttering (TOCS).* Pearson Inc.

Graham, J. T., & Graham, L. W. (1971). Language behaviour of the mentally retarded: Syntactic characteristics. *American Journal of Mental Deficiency, 75*(5), 623–629. PMID:5551507

Green, L. (2009). Morphology and literacy: Getting our heads in the game. *Language, Speech, and Hearing Services in Schools, 40*(3), 283–285. doi:10.1044/0161-1461(2009/08-0091)

Grunwell, P. (1985). *Phonological Assessment of Child Speech (PACS).* Windsor: NFER-Nelson.

Grunwell, P. (1993). *Analysing cleft palate speech.* London: Whurr Publishers Ltd.

Healey, E. C., Reid, R., & Donaher, J. (2005). Treatment of the child who stutters with co-existing learning, behavioral, and cognitive challenges. In R. Lees & C. Stark (Eds.), *The treatment of stuttering in the young school-aged child* (pp. 178–196). London: Whurr Publishers.

Hong, W. H., Chen, C. L., Yang, L. Y., & Chen, H. C. (2007). Kinematic analysis of speech motor control in children with cerebral palsy. In F. Ibrahim, N. A. A. Osman, J. Usman, & N. A. Kadri (Eds.), *Third Kuala Lumpur International Conference on Biomedical Engineering 2006. IFMBE Proceedings,* Vol 15. Berlin: Springer. 10.1007/978-3-540-68017-8_52

Jakobson, R. (1971). Linguistics in relation to other sciences. In *Selected writings, Word and language* (pp. 655–696). Mouton.

Jarmulowicz, L., & Hay, S. E. (2009). Derivational morphophonology: Exploring errors in third graders' productions. *Language, Speech, and Hearing Services in Schools, 40*(3), 299–311. doi:10.1044/0161-1461(2008/08-0006)

Kail, R. A. (1994). A method for studying the generalized slowing hypothesis in children with specific language impairment. *Journal of Speech Language and Hearing Research, 37*(2), 418–421. doi:10.1044/jshr.3702.418 PMID:8028323

Koning, C., & Magill-Evans, J. (2001). Social and Language Skills in Adolescent Boys with Asperger Syndrome. *Autism, 5*(1), 23–36. doi:10.1177/1362361301005001003 PMID:11708387

Kricoss, B. P., & Seyfried, D. N. (1996). Speech and language characteristics, assessment and management issues. In R. L. Schow & M. A. Nerbonne (Eds.), *Introduction to aural rehabilitation* (pp. 168–229). Boston: Allyn & Bacon.

Landa, R. (2000). Social language use in Asperger syndrome and high-functioning autism. In A. Klin, F. R. Volkmar, & S. S. Sparrow (Eds.), *Asperger syndrome* (pp. 125–155). New York: Guilford Press.

Leonard, L. B. (2014). *Children with specific language impairment.* Cambridge, MA: MIT Press.

Levitt, H. (1987). Interrelationships among the speech and language measures. *ASHA Monographs, 26*, 123–139. PMID:3509665

Lynch, M. P., Oller, D. K., Steffens, M. L., & Levine, S. L. (1995). Onset of speech-like vocalizations in infants with Down syndrome. *American Journal of Mental Retardation*, *100*(1), 68–86. PMID:7546639

McLeavey, B. C., Toomey, J. F., & Dempsey, P. J. (1982). Nonretarded and mentally retarded children's control over syntactic structures. *American Journal of Mental Deficiency*, *86*(5), 485–494. PMID:7124802

Miles, S., & Chapman, R. S. (2002). Narrative content as described by individuals with Down syndrome and typically developing children. *Journal of Speech, Language, and Hearing Research*, *45*(1), 175–189. doi:10.1044/1092-4388(2002/013)

Mogford, K. (1993). Oral Language acquisition in the prelinguistically deaf. In D. Bishop & K. Mogford (Eds.), *Language Development in Exceptional Circumstances* (pp. 110–131). Hove, UK: Erlbaum.

Montgomery, J. (2003). Working memory and comprehension in children with SLI: What do we know so far? *Journal of Communication Disorders*, *36*, 221–231. doi:10.1016/S0021-9924(03)00021-2 PMID:12742669

Morrison, G. M., & Cosden, M. A. (1997). Risk, resilience, and adjustment of individuals with learning disabilities. *Learning Disability Quarterly*, *20*(1), 43–60. doi:10.2307/1511092

Newfield, M. U., & Schlanger, B. B. (1968). The acquisition of English morphology by normal and educable mentally retarded children. *Journal of Speech, Language, and Hearing Research: JSLHR*, *11*(4), 693 706. doi:10.1044/jshr.1104.693 PMID:5719224

Ntourou, K., Conture, E. G., & Lipsey, M. W. (2011). Language abilities of children who stutter: A meta-analytical review. *American Journal of Speech-Language Pathology*, *20*(3), 163–179. doi:10.1044/1058-0360(2011/09-0102) PMID:21478281

Peeters, M., Verhoeven, L., de Moor, J., & van Balkom, H. (2009). Importance of speech production for phonological awareness and word decoding: The case of children with cerebral palsy. *Research in Developmental Disabilities*, *30*(4), 712–726. doi:10.1016/j.ridd.2008.10.002 PMID:19026521

Platt, L. J., Andrews, G., & Howie, P. M. (1980). Dysarthria of adult cerebral palsy: II. Phonemic analysis of articulation errors. *Journal of Speech and Hearing Research*, *23*(1), 41–55. doi:10.1044/jshr.2301.41 PMID:7442183

Quiegley, S. P., & King, C. M. (1980). Syntactic performance of Hearing Impaired and normal hearing individuals. *Applied Psycholinguistics*, *1*(4), 329–356. doi:10.1017/S0142716400000990

Rice, M. L., Wexler, K., & Cleave, P. L. (1995). Specific language impairment as a period of extended optional infinitive. *Journal of Speech and Hearing Research*, *38*(4), 850–863. doi:10.1044/jshr.3804.850 PMID:7474978

Riley, G. (1981). *SPI: Stuttering Prediction Instrument*. Austin, TX: Pro-Ed.

Riley, G. (1994). *SSI-3: Stuttering Severity Instrument* (3rd ed.). Austin, TX: Pro-Ed.

Rondal, J. A. (2009). Spoken language in persons with Down syndrome: A life span perspective. *International Journal of Early Childhood Special Education*, *1*(2), 138–155.

Rondal, J. A. (2013). Explaining grammatical difficulties in intellectual disabilities. *Revista de Logopedia, Foniatría y Audiología, 33*(2), 64–68. doi:10.1016/j.rlfa.2013.04.002

Russell, W., Power, D., & Quigley, S. P. (1976). Linguistics and deaf children. Washington, DC: A. G. Bell Association for the deaf.

Scott, C. M., & Windsor, J. (2000). General language performance measures in spoken and written narrative and expository discourse of school-age children with language learning disabilities. *Journal of Speech, Language, and Hearing Research: JSLHR, 43*(2), 324–339. doi:10.1044/jslhr.4302.324 PMID:10757687

Seung, H. K. (2007). Linguistic characteristics of individuals with high functioning autism and Asperger syndrome. *Clinical Linguistics & Phonetics, 21*(4), 247–259. doi:10.1080/02699200701195081 PMID:17453867

Shriberg, L. D., & Widder, C. J. (1990). Speech and prosody characteristics of adults with mental retardation. *Journal of Speech and Hearing Research, 33*(4), 627–653. doi:10.1044/jshr.3304.627 PMID:2273880

Smith, B. L., & Stoel-gammon, C. (1996). A quantitative analysis of reduplicated and variegated babbling in vocalizations by Down syndrome infants. *Clinical Linguistics & Phonetics, 10*(2), 119–129. doi:10.3109/02699209608985166

Stoel-Gammon, C. (1980). Phonological analysis of four Down's syndrome children. *Applied Psycholinguistics, 1*(01), 31–48. doi:10.1017/S0142716400000710

Stoel-Gammon, C. (2001). Down syndrome phonology: Developmental patterns and intervention strategies. *Down's syndrome, Research, and Practice. The Journal of the Sarah Duffen Centre, 7*(3), 93–100. PMID:11721538

Tannock, R., Purvis, K. L., & Schachar, R. J. (1993). Narrative abilities in children with attention deficit hyperactivity disorder and normal peers. *Journal of Abnormal Child Psychology, 21*(1), 103–117. doi:10.1007/BF00910492 PMID:8463500

van der Lely, H. K. J. (2003). Do heterogeneous deficits require hetero-geneous theories? SLI subgroups and the RDDR hypothesis. In Y. Levy & J. Schaeffer (Eds.), *Language competence across populations: Toward a definition of specific language impairment* (pp. 97–133). Mahwah, NJ: Lawrence Erlbaum Associate.

Weismer, E. S. (2000). Intervention for children with developmental language delay. In D. V. M. Bishop & L. B. Leonard (Eds.), *Specific language impairments in children: Causes, characteristics, intervention and outcome* (pp. 157–176). Hove, UK: Psychology Press.

Wexler, K. (1994). Optional infinitives, head movement and the economy of derivations. In N. Hornstein & D. Lightfoot (Eds.), *Verb movement* (pp. 305–350). New York: Cambridge University Press. doi:10.1017/CBO9780511627705.016

Wolk, L., Edwards, M. L., & Conture, E. G. (1993). Coexistence of stuttering and disordered phonology in young children. *Journal of Speech, Language, and Hearing Research: JSLHR, 36*(5), 906–917. doi:10.1044/jshr.3605.906 PMID:8246479

World Health Organization. (2002). *ICF: The international classification of functioning, disability, and health. Towards a common language for functioning, disability, and health.* Retrieved May 9, 2018. from: http://www.who.int/classifications/icf/training/icfbeginnersguide.pdf

Yairi, E., & Ambrose, N. (2005). *Early childhood stuttering for clinicians by clinicians.* Austin, TX: PRO-ED.

KEY TERMS AND DEFINITIONS

Clinical Linguistics: This is a branch of applied linguistics which deals with identifying, describing, and treating individuals with language-based disabilities. This applies linguistic theories to provide solutions for communication disorders.

Grammatical Morphology: A component of language that studies the formation of words, the relationship of each word with other and grammatical rules of word order.

Hearing Impairment: It is defined as the partial or total inability to hear in one or both the ears due to congenital and acquired causes.

Intellectual Disability: This is one of the major neurodevelopmental disorders which are characterized by significantly impaired mental functioning. They show significant deficits in mental abilities, social skills, and adaptive functioning. These individuals may score less than 70 across a range of IQ tests.

Language Impairment: An impairment of conceptual formulation and expression of language-based components of morphophonology, syntax, semantics, and pragmatics.

Mean Length of Utterance: An indicator of grammatical complexity which is derived by counting the total number of morphemes by a total number of utterances.

Neuro-Developmental Disorders: These are a group of developmental disorders that occur due to high-risk factors during pre, peri, and postnatal time periods. They are known to cause significant disability across language, motor, cognitive, social, and adaptive domains.

Chapter 6
Recent Advances and Neural Connectivity in Autism

Kiran Srivastava
Amity University, India

Lalit Kumar Singh
Lucknow University, India

ABSTRACT

The current chapter has reviewed the functional and structural brain connectivity in children with autism spectrum disorders (ASD). Neuropathological studies of the cerebral cortex in autism indicate abnormalities of synaptic and columnar structure and of neuronal migration. The MRI morphometry in young children with autism reveals excessive volume of cerebrum or cerebral white matter or increased total brain volume. The absence of such a volume difference in adults suggests that early hyperplasia in autism is followed by a plateau during which brain growth in normal subjects catches up. The developmental course of brain connectivity and the categorization potential of different connectivity process are important topics that are investigated by different studies. Finally, several studies contribute to a better understanding of the links between cellular abnormalities in the autistic cortex (both cerebral and cerebellar) and disturbances in network connectivity.

INTRODUCTION

Autism spectrum disorders (ASDs) are a family of neurodevelopmental syndromes with the prevalence of roughly 0.5–1.5% (Brugha, McManus, Bankart, Scott, Purdon, Smith, & Meltzer, 2011). ASDs are very common in males than in females, with a gender ratio of around 4:1 (Maenner & Durkin, 2010). ASD is a contemporary term which takes into account older concept of 'autism' or 'childhood autism', but in addition covers cases which, while sharing many of the symptoms of autism, do not cover the strict criteria for this disorder (Geschwind, 2009). ASDs are diagnosed on the basis of impairments in mainly three domains of behavior: social contact and relationships, verbal communication and repetitive, limited interests and behaviors (Robinson, Koenen, McCormick, Munir, Hallett, Happé, & Ronald, 2012). These symptoms are in attendance from early life (before 36 months of age). ASDs are clinically

DOI: 10.4018/978-1-5225-7004-2.ch006

diverse, with the severity of the variety of symptoms, and the impairment they cause, varying extensively (Geschwind, 2009). Some community with an ASD also have an intellectual disability (low intelligence quotient; IQ), but at least 25% of those with 'classic' autism, and advanced proportion of those with milder ASDs, show normal or superior intellectual function (Rutter, 1983).

Autism Spectrum Disorder featuring both average range IQ and a history of ordinary language acquisition is called Asperger's syndrome (Sharma, Woolfson, & Hunter, 2010). Nonetheless, it is debated whether Asperger's is strictly a syndrome separate from autism (Wing, Gould, & Gillberg, 2011) and future DSM-5 diagnostic criteria would eliminate it as a separate diagnosis as well as be introducing additional changes to ASD diagnosis. ASDs are acknowledged to be highly genetic, with estimates of heritability ranging from roughly 0.5 to 0.9 (Ronald & Hoekstra, 2011). However, environmental factors, including perinatal and obstetric problems, also play a role (Gardener, Spiegelman, & Buka, 2011). First-degree relatives of affected persons are at augmented risk of an ASD, and also of milder social and communication impairments dubbed the 'broader autism phenotype' (Whitehouse, Coon, Miller, Salisbury, & Bishop, 2010). These studies provided a diverse picture. Clear cut abnormalities were identified in some individual cases of ASD, however, there was immense inconsistency in these researches outcome, with a range of diverse focal and generalized pathologies being reported in a wide range of studies.

The majority of persons with an ASD showed no qualitative abnormalities noticeable with such methods, although some quantitative differences were found, for example, reduced size of the corpus callosum and cerebellum, and amplified volume of the caudate nucleus in ASD, on standard, compared with controls, although with small or average effect sizes for a review and meta-analysis (Stanfield, McIntosh, Spencer, Philip, Gaur, & Lawrie, 2008). For example, near the beginning case reports recognized cerebellar hypoplasia and ventricular bulge in ASD cases (Courchesne, Hesselink, Jernigan, & Yeung-Courchesne, 1987) but other investigators reported no magnetic resonance imaging (MRI) malformation in nearly all cases, and normal cerebellar development (Garber, Ritvo, Chiu, Griswold, & Kashanian, 1989). In Asperger's syndrome, many case reports of left temporal (Jones & Kerwin, 1990) left frontal and bilateral opercular cortical abnormalities (Berthier, Starkstein, & Leiguarda, 1990) were reported, with little consistency. MRI findings did not present a single pattern. Autism is a mixed disease entity containing various clinical subgroups, which do not demonstrate similar radiologic pictures (Nowell, Hackney, Muraki, & Coleman 1990).

Early positron emission tomography (PET) review likewise produced contradictory findings. Early findings reported widespread increases in glucose metabolism crossways in the brain of some autistic adults (Rumsey, Duara, Grady, Rapoport, Margolin, Rapoport, & Cutler, 1985) but another study found no dissimilarity (Herold, Frackowiak, Le Couteur, Rutter, & Howlin, 1988). These studies inferred that, while some cases of ASD are connected with qualitative neurological abnormalities, there is no clear localization of exact areas of the brain, with a variety of cortical, subcortical and cerebellar regions all having been involved in different cases. In addition, abnormalities in the mean volume of diverse areas have been found, these are of modest magnitude, with considerable overlap between ASD and control groups. Hence, in order to understand the neurobiology of autism, an understanding of the whole brain, rather than individual areas of interest, is required.

NEURODEVELOPMENTAL PROCESS

The previous analysis of data typically divided gestation somewhat at random into trimesters, with little consideration of brain development. (Otake, Schull, & Yoshimaru, 1991). The studies have revealed that, based on what happens from a neurodevelopmental viewpoint, it makes far greater sense to divide the gestational period into four "vital" periods. During the first few weeks of gestation, neural cells embark on to thrive at an exponential rate, peaking at a rate of roughly two hundred and fifty thousand per minute. At approximately the eighth week, neurons begin to relocate from the deepest layer of the brain out towards the periphery or cortex. Each neuron has a definite address and it has to reach that final target if it is to perform the functions for which it was intended and to execute their functions correctly. They cannot perform appropriate functions if they are not in the right place at the right time. In this regard, brain operations (and consequently early behavior) are critically dependent on the arrangement of neurons in the brain or the structural symphony of neuronal networks (brain matter). Therefore, if the normal progression of development is disrupted in any way, the aftermath can be far-reaching. This is especially the case when neural movement is disrupted.

After about the fifteenth week of gestation, when nearly all of the neural brain matter is already laid down, the neural cells commence to set apart or branch out. At around thirty weeks the neurons in the cerebellum start to connect with other areas. The cerebellum is decisively important for coordinating many aspects of brain processing. It is the absolute relay station, linking with all other important brain areas. Thirty weeks is a vital period for the all important Purkinje cells to complete their complicated connections with other neural fibers. Purkinje cells in the cerebellum are very outsized neurons that form widespread parallel networks with other neurons from numerous regions of the brain, thus allowing coordination of functions essential and important for the survival of the newborn. Although developing later in the gestational phase, the cerebellum is usually fully shaped at birth, even though not yet completely mature. Basically, the neurons begin to bond with others through additional development and maturation. This period of divergence continues as the process of myelination (insulation of nerve fibers) starts and continues until birth and well after, into the early childhood phase of development.

From the point of genesis until birth, neural brain cells migrate and develop at different times, progress to different sites, and do so at diversified but quite rapid rates. It is important to keep in mind that many functions are underway during gestation-neural cells proliferate and migrate, then set apart, dendrites (the end branches of neural cells) and axons (the stem of neural cells) grow at different rates, synapses (the gaps between the neural cells which contain transmitter substances) shape and some are lost, and myelin (a white fatty tissue) insulates axons and process transmission of signals.

NEURODEVELOPMENTAL COURSE OF AUTISM

It has been reported that autism is caused by disturbance of the Central Nervous System (CNS) just former to birth, i.e at the perinatal or in the postnatal stage. (Bachevalier, 1994; Kemper & Baumann, 1993). When viewed from a neurodevelopmental standpoint, this is very heartening because it means that nearly all of the neurons have already been recognized and therefore very little neural tissue would be damaged or affected. It follows from what was said earlier about the timing of a disruptive event that later disruption will produce poor neural tissue contribution if any at all. This absolutely authenticates the findings by Tsai (1989) and Kemper and Bauman (1993) that there is no obvious neuroanatomical contribution in autism. It may also offer much greater hope for altering the behavioral disturbances that occur with the different set of symptoms of autism.

Most fascinatingly, statistics from some of the most carefully documented studies (Kemper & Baumann, 1993; Coleman, Romano, Lapham, & Simon, 1985) suggests that the cortex or outer layer of the brain in autism is unblemished and has no structural abnormalities. Their conclusion also suggested that any disturbance in the developing brain of someone with autism occurs before the thirty-week period of gestation and exclusively disrupts associations in the midbrain and brainstem areas. This is a period when neurons are primarily setting apart and making associations with each other from one region of the brain to another. Such interconnections are important for the successful assimilation of information that accompanies distinctive brain information processing and adaptive behavior. Kemper and Bauman's (1993) did a study which states that the crucial areas of malformation in autism occur in two areas, the limbic system and the cerebellum and its circuits. The limbic system plays an important role in various facets of emotion, memory and learning, and motivation. It includes multiple areas of the brain-the hippocampus, amygdala, mammillary bodies, anterior cingulate gyrus and nuclei of the septum.

Kemper and Bauman's (1993) in their study designated that the neural cells of the limbic system in autism are small in size and compactly packed per unit volume as equated with age and sex-matched controls. Such a picture is reliable with a chronologically younger brain where the limbic system is truncated in its development. The fact that the brain cells are so tightly packed that the normal formation of some of the cells was disrupted. As a result, the consequence of such a condition results in poor information processing as well as in executive functioning by brain.

The second foremost area of abnormality found by Kemper and Bauman (1993) was in the cerebellum and its many circuits and interconnections. Moreover, they came up with a significant loss of Purkinje cells all through the cerebellum, in particular in the posterior regions. The degeneration of Purkinje cells helps determine the timing of the abnormalities. During gestation, climbing fibers begin from the olivary nucleus, located in the brainstem, and migrate to connect posteriorly with Purkinje cells. Research studies in humans advise that these connections occur at thirty weeks of gestation. Also, once the associations are made, the system becomes one single unit (olivary nucleus, climbing fibers and Purkinje cells).

If anything happen to the Purkinje cells after the connections have been made, the entire system degenerates and decay. However, in the brains of people with autism Kemper and Bauman (1993) found that, even though there was a chief loss of Purkinje cells, the olivary nuclei were preserved. This reflects that whatever happened to the Purkinje cells had to have happened just preceding to thirty weeks of gestation. Furthermore, they also found that many of the neurons penetrated deep in the nuclei of the cerebellum, those accountable for input and output of information and communication with other portions of the brain were atypical. In the younger cases, the neurons were abnormally large ("hypertrophied") whereas in their older cases the same neurons were minimized in size in every case and there was substantial cell loss.

Hudspeth and Pribram (1992) hypothesized that, because of the degeneration of Purkinje cells, the normal circuit (i.e. olivary nucleus, connecting fibers and Purkinje cells) was not organised and the autistic person had to depend on to the more primal circuit as the central means of neuronal communication. Furthermore, they hypothesize that because the more primitive fetal circuit was not considered for adult life, they become bigger (hypertrophied) in response to extended demand and may ultimately "burn out" and die. This would especially be the case if there was no effort to alter the stimuli reaching the young autistic brain and cause it to become overtaxed and difficult to handle peripheral demands. On the other hand, a program intended to deliver stimuli or information in a carefully modulated manner would give the autistic brain a greater opportunity to process the information more adaptively without the overload.

It would give the developing brain an opportunity to establish additional normal circuitry through the brain anatomy like brain function with its inter-relationship. It is well known that brain structure initiates the function, but then such structures develop appropriately only if they are in turn triggered by external environmental events (Hudspeth & Pribram, 1992). The structure and function cycle is pivotal for the growth and maturation of the brain and, consequently, adaptive behavior.

However, any program planned to improve the more normal growth and development of the brain increases the possibility for more normative brain-behavior functioning. How much can be done to establish normal brain development and functioning in someone with autism, from an entirely neuroscientific viewpoint, still remains to be seen. More investigations are needed in this area to categorically answer this question. Nevertheless, the findings reviewed in this paper advocates that much can be gained if the suitable program is used with autistic children, starting at a very tender age and applying the appropriate technique intensively for the duration of many years.

PROFILING OF NEURAL CONNECTIVITY IN AUTISM

Damasio and Maurer (1978) stated in their study that autism results due to anatomical and functional changes at mesolimbic (dopaminergic) brain areas (ventromedial prefrontal cortex, medial temporal lobes, limbic striatum and thalamus), as detrimental effect to these brain regions can cause features of autism (impaired social and emotional functioning, stereotyped behaviours, mannerisms and obsessionality). This assumption is supported by studies in animals and human (Critchley, Daly, Bullmore, Williams, Van Amelsvoort, Robertson, & Murphy, 2000). Areas outside the limbic system, such as the parietal lobes, are related to autism. The poor attention about indulgent significant social cues in autism is similar to negligence and attention deficiency in the parietal lobe damage (Bryson, Wainwright-Sharp, & Smith, 1990). In addition to structural abnormalities in the cerebellum, another aetiological factor related with autism is the functional decline in cerebellar-cortical serotonergic pathways due to acquired cerebellar lesions, which can lead to poor performance in social and emotional behaviour and dysfunctioning in executive functions and obsessions (Chugani, Muzik, Rothermel, Behen, Chakraborty, Mangner, & Chugani, 1997). Brain imaging methods are used in the investigation of these proposed structural and functional changes in autistic spectrum disorders itself.

Magnetic Resonance Imaging (MRI) Studies

1. Head Circumference and Total Brain Volume

Atypical head circumference growth curve in the first two years of life is a phenotypical risk factor for autism (Courchesne & Pierce, 2005; Redcay & Courchesne, 2005). In the case of autism, head circumference that is normal or near normal size at birth follows a rapid growth pattern at about four months (Dawson, Munson, Webb, Nalty, Abbott, & Toth, 2007; Hazlett, Poe, Gerig, Smith, Provenzale, Ross, & Piven, 2005). It has been shown that 37% of autistic children between the ages of two and four meet the criteria for developmental macrocephaly (Lainhart, Piven, Wzorek, Landa, Santangelo, Coon, & Folstein, 1997). In one of the studies reported by (Webb, Nalty, Munson, Brock, Abbott, & Dawson, 2007) where 28 children with autism from birth up to 36 months were involved, has shown accelerated growth of the head circumference and previous studies have indicated that repeatedly. This head circumference growth pattern occurs independently from autistic regression. In autism, head circumference growth rate has been compared to the period from birth to 12 months; after the 12th month, these findings show that unusually rapid head growth is limited to the 1st year of life (Dawson, 2008). Many research findings have shown that symptoms of autism become easily understandable during the first 8 to 12 months. (Dawson, Osterling, Meltzoff, & Kuhl, 2000; Klin, Chawarska, Paul, Rubin, Morgan, Wiesner, & Volkmar, 2004). Consequently, the onset of acceleration in head circumference growth between 4 and 12 months leads to significant behavioral symptoms and an overlap between these symptoms. Interestingly, Dawson et al. (2007) reported a decline in the rate of head circumference growth in the subsequent 12 months to be associated with a loss of or deceleration in the acquisition of new skills. Another study by Dawson et al. (2007) reported that rapid growth in head circumference from birth to 12-months, followed by a deceleration in growth after 12 months to be a threat marker for the development of autistic features by 24 months (Elder, Dawson, Toth, Fein, & Munson, 2008).

The MRI is used in order to determine the size and outline of brain structures. The outcomes of research conducted using the MRI technique has been reliable with results obtained by head circumference studies in terms of autism. It has been reported that children aged 3-4 years with autism had a considerably larger total brain volume compared to normally developing peers or those with developmental delayed (Sparks, Friedman, Shaw, Aylward, Echelard, Artru, & Dager, 2002). Another study by Courchesne et al. (1994) showed that 90% of autistic children aged between two and four years had bigger brain volumes than usual. Using the MRI investigation, the size of the brain among autistic children aged between one-and-a-half and four years old revealed to be abnormally increased (about 5-10%). However, it has not been clearly determined whether the growth pattern of young children (four years old) is everlasting among older children and adolescents (Aylward, Minshew, Field, Sparks, & Singh, 2002). It has been found that the size of the brain in autistic children at birth was 13% smaller than the control group, reached a 10% bigger size at the age of one and was at the onset of puberty only 2% larger than the control group; these results were obtained by the estimation of head circumference and brain weight using MRI brain volume and autopsy studies (Redcay & Courchesne, 2005). It has been mentioned earlier that in a large proportion of persons with autism in adulthood, the volume of the brain did not differ much from healthy controls. Moreover, if the size of the brain is larger than normal in developmental disorders such as autism, it leads to a reduction in long-distance structural and functional connections (Lewis & Elman, 2008).

2. White and Grey Matter Changes

Unusual brain growth in autistic children mostly stems from cerebral white and grey matter. However, studies reported that this growth originates from the disproportionate increase of white matter, not grey matter (Herbert, Ziegler, Deutsch, O'brien, Lange, Bakardjiev, & Kennedy, 2003). Differences in white matter volume can be associated with abnormalities in axonal density and organization, myelination abnormalities or the abnormal multiplication of glial cells (O'hearn, Asato, Ordaz, & Luna, 2008). In two different studies with autistic children (between one-and-a-half and four years old) has been shown to significantly increase white matter rather than grey matter (Hazlett, Poe, Gerig, Smith, Provenzale, Ross, & Piven, 2005; Courchesne, Karns, Davis, Ziccardi, Carper, Tigue, & Lincoln, 2001). However, it is not obvious whether this increase in older children and adolescents is for life long or not (Palmen, Pol, Kemner, Schnack, Durston, Lahuis, & Van Engeland, 2005; Lotspeich, Kwon, Schumann, Fryer, Goodlin-Jones, Buonocore, ... & Reiss, 2004). Even though the growth rate of grey matter has been shown to be smaller than that of white matter in early life, it is reported to remain persistent in the adulthood phase also (Courchesne, Karns, Davis, Ziccardi, Carper, Tigue, & Lincoln, 2001; Palmen, Pol, Kemner, Schnack, Durston, Lahuis, & Van Engeland, 2005).

Diffusion tensor imaging (DTI), also known as diffusion tensor magnetic resonance imaging (DTMRI) is a technique used to determine the integrity of white brain matter. One of the important parameters determined by this method, which actually helps to identify the movement of water molecules in the brain, is fractional anisotropy, which reflects the asymmetry in fluid movement (Taylor, Hsu, Krishnan, & MacFall., 2004). High fractional anisotropy values project a more intense or more appropriate structure of the brain. Two different studies in children and adults with autism have shown a decrease in the cerebral white matter using fractional anisotropy. A reduction in the temporal cortex among adults with autism has also been indicated using fractional anisotropy (Lee, Bigler, Alexander, Lazar, DuBray, Chung, & Lu, 2007), as well as on the ventromedial prefrontal cortex, anterior cingulate, temporal lobe, amygdala and cortical and along subcortical regions containing the corpus callosum in autistic children and adolescents (Barnea-Goraly, Kwon, Menon, Eliez, Lotspeich, & Reiss, 2004). The most consistent findings reflecting the reduction in brain size using anisotropy has been reported for the corpus callosum (Barnea-Goraly, Kwon, Menon, Eliez, Lotspeich, & Reiss, 2004; Keller, Kana, & Just, 2007). In one of the study, a 14% reduction in the volume of the corpus callosum was shown, which is associated with decreased in fractional anisotropy on genu and splenium (Alexander, Lee, Lazar, Boudos, DuBray, Oakes,... & Bigler, 2007).

In contrast to these findings, Ben-Bashat et al. (2007) observed a connection or association between amplified fractional anisotropy values and white matter maturity in autistic children at younger ages. These findings have been allied with abnormal increases in brain volume during the early ages of children with autism In recent times, impairment in corpus callosum are found to be associated with the theory of inadequate universal functional connectivity in adults with autism (Just, Cherkassky, Keller, Kana, & Minshew, 2006). Functional brain imaging findings have shown a decline in the activation of the synchronization of many brain areas concerning different functions like social content interpretation (Castelli, Frith, Happe, & Frith, 2002) working memory (Koshino, Carpenter, Minshew, Cherkassky, Keller, & Just, 2005), executive functions (Just, Cherkassky, Keller, Kana, & Minshew, 2006) and visual imagery (Kana, Keller, Cherkassky, Minshew, & Just, 2006). These findings have led to the proposition that inadequate cortical connections may be associated with autistic disorders (Belmonte, Allen, Beckel-Mitchener, Boulanger, Carper, & Webb, 2004). The decrease in white matter along with structural coalition in the context of autism may cause differences in functional connectivity, while the theory of mind deficits (Baron-Cohenet, Leslie, & Frith, 1985) within the autism context can potentially be accountable for weak central coherence as well as social and cognitive symptoms

3. Cerebral Cortex

The largest and most constant increase has been reported for the frontal lobe, in spite of a grey and white matter increase having been in the frontal, temporal and parietal lobes in many other studies (Hazlett, Poe, Gerig, Smith, & Piven, 2006; Carper & Courchesne, 2002). In autism, there exists an opposite growth rate from the norm subsequent to the period of accelerated growth in cerebral and cerebellar regions. For example, it has been found that frontal lobe, grey and white matter volume shows increase by 19% at two- and four years of age and 46% between the ages of nine and 12 in normal children, while in autistic children, these rates are 1% and 14%, respectively (Carper & Courchesne, 2002; Carper & Courchesne, 2000).

In autism, abnormal asymmetry patterns in the frontal and temporal areas related to language have been reported. Herbert et al. (2002) have shown that lateral inferior frontal cortex language (Broca's area is associated with pars opercularis) has invalidated asymmetry in children with autism. It has also been found an increase in the right side of the frontal language area by 27% when compared to controls' with 17% larger volume on the left side of the frontal language region. In relation to these findings, planum temporal asymmetry has been reported to be fairly dissimilar between the two groups; autistic males reported a 25% left dominance, while this rate was only 5% for the control group. Differences in terms of right-sided symmetry at the supramarginal posterior gyrus have been acknowledged between autistic (39% greater) and control groups (greater than 2%). Another asymmetry area is the posterior superior temporal cortex in the Wernicke's area, although this is not statistically significant. Structural abnormalities like abnormal asymmetry found in autistic males in language regions may be in relation to abnormalities in language skills (Kim, Lee, Shin, Cho, & Lee, 2002).

4. Cerebellum

The cerebellum plays a pivotal role in coordinating between voluntary movements and complex movements. Findings obtained from animal and human studies have shown that the cerebellum may be important in cognitive processes, in language use and emotion (Kim, Lee, Shin, Cho, & Lee, 2002; Acosta & Pearl, 2004). Several MRI studies have determined that when patients suffering from autism in different age groups are compared with a control group, there is a noteworthy increase in cerebellar volume. This increase in cerebellar volume function is typically proportional to the total brain volume (Minshew, Sweeney, Bauman, & Webb, 2005). Rarest findings reported by Hazlett et al. (2005) states that there was no disparity in terms of cerebellum size in autistic children below the age of three (18-35 months). In contrast to the increase in the total volume of the cerebellum, some autistic children reflected a relatively small volume vermis (Kaufmann, Cooper, Mostofsky, Capone, Kates, Newschaffer, & Lanham, 2003; Courchesne, Saitoh, Yeung-Courchesne, Press, Lincoln, Haas, & Schreibman,1994). Vermis hypoplasia in autism is in connection with deficits in automatically attention directing and research behavior.

Courchesne et al. (1994) proposed that autistic disorders have two subtypes related to cerebellum pathology: a. vermis hypoplasia and b. vermis hyperplasia. However, no differences have been suggested concerning IQ levels of the subjects being affected by cerebellar volume in different study groups matched for IQ (Garber & Ritvo, 1992). It has been reported that increases in the volume of the frontal lobe is associated with a reduction in cerebellar vermis volume. It has been shown that patients with normal vermis volume have functional frontal cortex volume, while patients with vermis hypoplasia have greater frontal cortex volume and are dysfunctional.

Abnormal neuronal signals from subcortical structures can affect the overall development of the cerebral cortex and increased in the neuronal activity can in this way lead to growth among neuronal elements. Therefore, it has been claimed that abnormal neuronal activity in the cerebelloretinal-thalamocortical projections (probably associated with the decrease in inhibitor signals as a consequence of the premature reduction in the number of cerebellar Purkinje cells) can lead to developmental failure in the frontal lobe and in the other input regions (Carper & Courchesne, 2000). These changes in the volume are not specific to autism and are also commonly found in various developmental and psychiatric disorders (Courchesne, Saitoh, Yeung-Courchesne, Press, Lincoln, Haas, & Schreibman, 1994; Okugawa, Sedvall, & Agartz, 2003). Mostly in autism, hypoplasia at the composition of the brain stem has been identified by Hashimoto et al. (1995) in a study that evaluated cerebellum and brain stem structures.

5. Amygdala

Amygdala volume shows an increase in the proportion to the total cerebral volume in children with autism. Sparks et al. (2002) found that autistic children (aged between 36-56 months) had an atypical amygdala growth rate (13-16%). It has been reported that an increased amygdala volume (without increasing total cerebral volume) at three years of age is seen in children aged between three and six years old (Munson, Dawson, Abbott, Faja, Webb, Friedman, & Dager, 2006). An increase in amygdala volume has been found to be in association with more severe anxiety (Juranek, Filipek, Berenji, Modahl, Osann, & Spence, 2006) and with poor communication skills and social skills. In a study with autistic males aged between the 8 and 18 years compared with a healthy control group, it was reported that there have been changes in the volume of amygdala, which had grown up to 15% between 8-12 age period, but in the period between the ages of 13-18 there were found to be no much difference at the amygdala volume.

Changes in volume in amygdala among men with healthy development increased by about 40% between the ages of 8 and 18; but, this was not the case for males with autism. These findings are significant for the understanding of amygdala volume initially being larger than normal in autistic children, and also important to indicate that children diagnosed with autitm have no age-related changes in the overall volume of the amygdala in the healthy controls (Schumann, Hamstra, Goodlin-Jones, Lotspeich, Kwon, Buonocore, & Amaral, 2004). These findings are authenticated by some MRI studies, including those belonging to autistic adolescents and adults where results showed an amygdala volume not significantly different or smaller as compared to those in control groups (Aylward, Minshew, Goldstein, Honeycutt, Augustine, Yates, ... & Pearlson, 1999). It has been reported that amygdala abnormalities in autism spectrum disorders play a very important role in social symptoms (Nacewicz, Dalton, Johnstone, Long, McAuliff, Oakes, & Davidson, 2006).

6. Hippocampus

In autism, research findings are ambiguous regarding the volume of the hippocampus. MRI study by Schumann et al. (2004) showed an increase in the volume of the hippocampus and this increase is constant during adolescence of autistic children. A study that incorporated autistic adolescents and young adults reported a decrease in hippocampal volume (Aylward, Minshew, Goldstein, Honeycutt, Augustine, Yates, ... & Pearlson, 1999). Where autism is concerned, many research findings have shown no significant differences in hippocampal volume (Piven, Bailey, Ranson, & Arndt,1998; Saitoh, Courchesne, Egaas, Lincoln, & Schreibman, 1995).

7. Corpus Callosum

The corpus callosum is highly responsible for transferring cortical and subcortical information between homologous regions of the cerebral hemisphere. It is in association with bilateral sensory and motor combination such as bimanual motor coordination, visual attention scrolling and procedural memory processes. In autism, especially in the subsequent region of the corpus callosum, a decline in volume was noted (Egaas, Courchesne, & Saitoh, 1995). These findings are in relation to interhemispheric weakness in autism (O'hearn, Asato, Ordaz, & Luna, 2008).

8. Caudate Nucleus

It has been revealed that there has been an increase in the volume of the caudate nucleus in autism. This increase in volume may be interconnected with observed repetitive and ritualistic behavior in adolescents and adults with autism (Hollander, Anagnostou, Chaplin, Esposito, Haznedar, Licalzi, & Buchsbaum, 2005; Sears, Vest, Mohamed, Bailey, Ranson, & Piven, 1999).

PET and SPECT Studies

In the context of autism, functional neuroimaging studies were conducted at rest or during various activities. Injected or inhaled radiopharmaceuticals were applied in positron emission tomography (PET) methods of investigation. Dissolved radioactive isotopes emit positrons that are identified by the PET camera. Some PET techniques determine blood flow, while others compute cerebral metabolic rate (Bush, Valera, & Seidman, 2005). In PET studies performed with autistic children at rest, it has been found that a decline in blood flow occurred in the temporal lobes. Poor Functionality in the temporal lobe was determined within the auditory associative cortex and superior temporal sulcus. Functional damage in the auditory cortex of autistic children may clarify initial diagnoses of going deaf and experiencing the serious worsening in communication. It has been recommended that functional deterioration in the superior temporal sulcus might take into account an emotional and cognitive components of autistic symptoms indirectly, due to these being closely associated with the fronto-parietal and limbic areas of the multimodal organization (Zilbovicius, Boddaert, Belin, Poline, Remy, Mangin, & Samson, 2000).

A study using PET scan conducted with autistic adults found an increase in glucose utilization in the brain at rest (Rumsey, Duara, Grady, Rapoport, Margolin, Rapoport, & Cutler, 1985). Despite these conclusions, unconventional results during the interpretations of different tasks have also been reported. Haznedar et al. (2000) documented a poor glucose metabolism in the anterior and posterior cingulate gyrus right through a verbal learning test for autism and Asperger's syndrome. Similarly, in a diverse PET study, a decline in relative glucose metabolism was determined for frontal lobe medial/cingulate regions during verbal memory operations. The same study exhibited an increase in relative glucose metabolism in the occipital and parietal regions (Hazlett, Buchsbaum, Hsieh, Haznedar, Platholi, & LiCalzi, 2004).

Neuronal activation regions in auditory cortical processing were also analysed using the PET technique. Activation in the superior temporal gyrus was scrutinized while listening to the complex speech-like sounds of adults with autism, which was parallel to the control group (Boddaert, Chabane, Belin, Bourgeois, Royer, Barthelemy, & Zilbovicius, 2004). However, while this activation was discerned for the right superior temporal gyrus in the autistic group, the opposite pattern was the monitor in the control group. It has been shown that even though there is less activation in the left temporal areas, where there is noticeable activation pattern at the right middle frontal gyrus among autistic individuals (Boddaert, Belin, Chabane, Poline, Barthélémy, Mouren-Simeoni, & Zilbovicius, 2003). In one of the studies involving children with autism, lower activation patterns in the left superior temporal gyrus (in the auditory-related field) has been acknowledged when listening to speech-like sounds, similar to what was found in adults. According to these conclusions, it is recommended that abnormalities in auditory cortical processing are in sync with defects in language skills and that they result in a poor response to the voice among those suffering from autism (Boddaert, Belin, Chabane, Poline, Barthélémy, Mouren-Simeoni, & Zilbovicius, 2003). Study using a PET scan with high functioning autistic adults who practiced during instruction the tasks of theory of mind also identified decrease in the activity of medial prefrontal cortex, bilateral superior temporal sulcus and basal temporal area, which are the apparatus of the mentalization network (Castelli, Frith, Happe, & Frith, 2002).

In several PET studies, the connection between neurotransmitter systems and autism has been probed. In a PET study with autistic children showed a decrease in the binding capacity of serotonin transporter protein in the entire brain (Nakamura, Sekine, Ouchi, Tsujii, Yoshikawa, Futatsubashi, & Matsuzaki, 2010). In autistic individuals, decreased serotonin transporter protein binding capacity in the anterior and posterior cingulate cortex has been related with deterioration in social cognition, parallel to decreased serotonin transporter protein binding capacity in the thalamus is associated with persistent and obsessive behaviours. It has also been reported that dopamine transporter protein (the dopamine transporter = DAT) binding correlates in the opposite way with serotonin transporter binding protein in the orbitofrontal cortex. These findings sustain the relationship between autism and serotonergic/dopaminergic systems.

In accord with several PET studies, reduced regional blood flow in the temporal cortex (George, Costa, Kouris, Ring, & Ell,1992; Mountz, Tolbert, Lill, Katholi, & Liu, 1995; Gillberg, Bjure, Uvebrant, Vestergren, & Gillberg, 1993), frontal cortex parietal cortex, occipital cortex, thalamus, basal ganglia and cerebellar hemisphere (Ryu, Lee, Yoon, Kim, Lee, & Shin, 1999) has been detected in Single-photon emission computed tomography (SPECT) studies with autistic children and adults. In a study of children and adolescents with high-functioning autism, confirmation has been provided in the presence of abnormal neuronal network lateralization. In this study, it has been found lower blood flow at the right angular region than the left angular region and also lower blood flow at left pericallosal, thalamic and hippocampal areas than right pericallosal, thalamic and hippocampal regions (Ito, Mori, Hashimoto, Miyazaki, Hori, Kagami, & Kuroda, 2005).

A decrease in regional cerebral blood flow in the bilateral insula, superior temporal gyrus and left prefrontal cortex have been documented by Ohnishi et al. (2000) in a SPECT study with autistic children. Autistic symptoms are in association with perfusion patterns in the limbic system and the medial prefrontal cortex. In one of the SPECT study done by Ohnishi et al. (2000) assistance is provided for impairments in communication and social skills that is thought to be related to the theory of mind deficits in association with perfusion changes in the medial prefrontal cortex and anterior cingulate gyrus, as well as the obsessive desire for similarity, which is associated with the right medial temporal lobe. Regional blood flow patterns are vital in terms of representing the possible location of abnormalities in brain function that determine abnormal behavior within the context of autism (Ohnishi, Matsuda, Hashimoto, Kunihiro, Nishikawa, Uema, & Sasaki, 2000). Makkonen et al. (2008) investigated the association between neurotransmitter systems and autism using SPECT. SPECT displayed a reduction of serotonin transporter protein binding capacity in the medial frontal cortex in accordance with PET studies in this area; however, DAT binding capacity did not differ in autistic individuals.

Functional MRI (fMRI) Studies

According to the SPECT and PET techniques, the fMRI method has better spatial and temporal resolution, is not an intrusive procedure and does not involve ionizing radiation (Bush, Valera, & Seidman, 2005). Autistic individuals have degraded cognitive processing, both in a self-referential and other referential context. In another recent study, healthy individuals were compared to autistic patients for self-other reference tasking. The results stated that autistic patients responded more to other metallization as opposed to self-referential mentalization at the middle cingulate cortex, while these two apparatus respond equally at the ventromedial prefrontal cortex (Lombardo, Chakrabarti, Bullmore, Sadek, Pasco,

Wheelwright, & Baron-Cohen, 2009). This finding is consistent with earlier studies which reported that decreased activity in the middle cingulate cortex while high-functioning autism making their decisions the social condition (Chiu, Kayali, Kishida, Tomlin, Klinger, Klinger, & Montague, 2008). These atypical responses only occur in areas that chiefly process self-knowledge and do not influence the area that primarily responds to other-referential information. The other difference at the ventromedial prefrontal cortex is closely related with the degree of social impairment in autism in early childhood. It has been found that individuals whose ventromedial prefrontal cortex reflect dissimilarity between self- and others have had the least social disruption during early childhood, while persons whose ventromedial prefrontal cortex makes little or any differences between self- and other mentalizing are more likely to have qualified maximum social disruption during early childhood. These findings are important in terms of showing the atypical organization of neural circuits, basically in self-information encoding, in the context of autism (Lombardo, Chakrabarti, Bullmore, Sadek, Pasco, Wheelwright, & Baron-Cohen, 2009).

Brain regions such as the medial prefrontal cortex, rostral anterior cingulate, posterior cingulate and the precuneus have pretty high metabolic movement during resting states. Within managed processes like self-trial thought as well as higher-level social and emotional processes. Persistently activate the medial cortical network, which includes the medial prefrontal cortex, rostral anterior cingulate, posterior cingulate and precuneus. This metabolic activity is censored during tasks that require cognitive effort. The suppression during the process, which is observed as "deactivations" using the fMRI method, is due to interrupted mental activity during rest. Kennedy et al. (2006) proposed that this deactivation does not appear in autistic individuals. These findings have been reported due to the absence or abnormal mental processes in autism. The absence of this deactivation in autism has shown abnormalities in an internally managed process and these findings have been suggested to be associated with social and emotional deficits in terms of autism.

Individuals suffering from autistic disorders and Asperger's syndrome also experience difficulties in the perception of faces. It has been shown that healthy individuals have increased activation in the fusiform gyrus during face processing and increased activation in the inferior temporal gyrus during processing object activation, while individuals with autistic disorders or Asperger's syndrome have less activation in the right fusiform gyrus and more activation during face discrimination (this is not the case for objects). The autism group is likely to use more of the inferior temporal gyrus during face processing when compared to the control group. This finding shows that they process faces like objects (Schultz, Gauthier, Klin, Fulbright, Anderson, Volkmar, & Gore, 2000). The basic zone associated with face processing in healthy individuals is the lateral fusiform gyrus (called as "fusiform face area"). It has been reported to decrease activation in the fusiform gyrus and other areas associated with processing face detection such as the inferior occipital gyrus, superior temporal gyrus and amygdala in individuals with autism during face detection tasks. It has also been documented that autistic individuals use distinct neuronal systems for seeing faces and have individual-specific, scattered activation patterns when compared to normal individuals.

Findings on fMRI when administered on high-functioning autistic adults, reported decreased activation in the fusiform gyrus during the identification of the person who has been seen before, in contrast to the earlier studies. Social dysfunction in autism has been in relation to most general abnormalities depicted in the social brain network (Pierce, Müller, Ambrose, Allen, & Courchesne, 2001). The severity of impairment in social functioning is related to a reduction in the connections between fusiform face area and amygdala and also increment in the connections between fusiform face area and right inferior frontal cortex. This result reflects neuronal abnormalities in the limbic system to be related to a prevalence of poor social impairment in autism (Kleinhans, Johnson, Richards, Mahurin, Greenson, Dawson, & Aylward, 2009).

Neuronal activation fields associated with working memory have been studied using the fMRI technique. Luna et al. (2002) documented lower activation in the dorsolateral prefrontal cortex and posterior cingulate regions during spatial working memory. Koshino et al. (2007) showed that individuals with autism, had lower activation in the inferior left prefrontal area (verbal processing and working memory-related) and right posterior temporal are (related to the theory of mind) when involved in working memory task that used photographic facial stimuli. The same study reflected findings like activation in the different division of the fusiform area in autistic individuals. It has also been identified that fusiform activation is in the lower and lateral division and also displaced from the typical region activated during face detection when compared to the region activated during object detection in an autistic group. These findings assist the notion that face processing in autism analyzes features of the face as an object in terms of humanitarian significance. Abnormal fusiform activation depicted a lower-level link with the frontal area associated with the presence of the neuronal communication network, which has reduced synchronization (Koshino, Kana, Keller, Cherkassky, Minshew, & Just, 2007).

The mirror neuron system (the pars opercularis in the inferior frontal gyrus) is dynamic during observation, imitation and understanding the actions of others. Therefore, it is supposed to provide a neuronal mechanism for a complete understanding of the purpose and actions of others. Along with the limbic system, it is thought to reconcile a better understanding of emotions or facilitating sympathy with someone else's feelings. Thus, the feelings of others are supposed to be real and not simply at a cognitive level but understood at an emotional level (empathy). It has been shown that there is no activation of mirror neurons on the pars opercularis during the imitation of emotional expression in children with autism. Activation in this region is inversely proportional to the severity of the symptoms shown. Early functional defects that emerge in the mirror neuron system have been considered as the primary cause of poor social and emotional functioning in autistic disorders (Minshew & Williams, 2007).

In fMRI studies when done on autistic individuals, a significant reduction has been seen in the timing of the activation or synchronization between cortical areas in association with memory functioning, language, problem-solving and social cognition. These findings supported the theory of "insufficient functional connectivity" (underconnectivity) within and between neocortical systems (Minshew & Williams, 2007).

CONCLUSION

In autism, neuroanatomical defects during the early stages of brain development such as hypoplasia at specific areas as well as excessive cerebral growth lead to abnormalities in the development of functional systems. If in the process of developing the brain, is traumatized by genetic or environmental factors, the functional structures and hence, functional activities, are disrupted. Abnormal functional activity and organization disturb different structures in different ways because autism is associated with neural defects in many types and locations. Functional imaging studies state various limitations, where patients diagnosed with autism and Asperger's syndrome are studied together, thus study groups have the heterogeneous diagnostic measurement. It is proposed that in future studies, working groups can be formed to be a homogeneous diagnostic measurement consisting of different age groups and different levels of mental development when testing different tasks.

REFERENCES

Acosta, M. T., & Pearl, P. L. (2004, September). Imaging data in autism: From structure to malfunction. *Seminars in Pediatric Neurology*, *11*(3), 205–213. doi:10.1016/j.spen.2004.07.004 PMID:15575415

Alexander, A. L., Lee, J. E., Lazar, M., Boudos, R., DuBray, M. B., Oakes, T. R., ... Bigler, E. D. (2007). Diffusion tensor imaging of the corpus callosum in Autism. *NeuroImage*, *34*(1), 61–73. doi:10.1016/j.neuroimage.2006.08.032 PMID:17023185

Amaral, D. G., Schumann, C. M., & Nordahl, C. W. (2008). Neuroanatomy of autism. *Trends in Neurosciences*, *31*(3), 137–145. doi:10.1016/j.tins.2007.12.005 PMID:18258309

Aylward, E. H., Minshew, N. J., Field, K., Sparks, B. F., & Singh, N. (2002). Effects of age on brain volume and head circumference in autism. *Neurology*, *59*(2), 175–183. doi:10.1212/WNL.59.2.175 PMID:12136053

Aylward, E. H., Minshew, N. J., Goldstein, G., Honeycutt, N. A., Augustine, A. M., Yates, K. O., ... Pearlson, G. D. (1999). MRI volumes of amygdala and hippocampus in non–mentally retarded autistic adolescents and adults. *Neurology*, *53*(9), 2145–2145. doi:10.1212/WNL.53.9.2145 PMID:10599796

Bachevalier, J. (1994). Medial temporal lobe structures and autism: A review of clinical and experimental findings. *Neuropsychologia*, *32*(6), 627–648. doi:10.1016/0028-3932(94)90025-6 PMID:8084420

Barnea-Goraly, N., Kwon, H., Menon, V., Eliez, S., Lotspeich, L., & Reiss, A. L. (2004). White matter structure in autism: Preliminary evidence from diffusion tensor imaging. *Biological Psychiatry*, *55*(3), 323–326. doi:10.1016/j.biopsych.2003.10.022 PMID:14744477

Baron-Cohen, S., Leslie, A. M., & Frith, U. (1985). Does the autistic child have a "theory of mind"? *Cognition*, *21*(1), 37–46. doi:10.1016/0010-0277(85)90022-8 PMID:2934210

Bashat, D. B., Kronfeld-Duenias, V., Zachor, D. A., Ekstein, P. M., Hendler, T., Tarrasch, R., & Sira, L. B. (2007). Accelerated maturation of white matter in young children with autism: A high b value DWI study. *NeuroImage*, *37*(1), 40–47. doi:10.1016/j.neuroimage.2007.04.060 PMID:17566764

Belmonte, M. K., Allen, G., Beckel-Mitchener, A., Boulanger, L. M., Carper, R. A., & Webb, S. J. (2004). Autism and abnormal development of brain connectivity. *The Journal of Neuroscience*, *24*(42), 9228–9231. doi:10.1523/JNEUROSCI.3340-04.2004 PMID:15496656

Berthier, M. L., Starkstein, S. E., & Leiguarda, R. (1990). Developmental cortical anomalies in Asperger's syndrome: Neuroradiological findings in two patients. *The Journal of Neuropsychiatry and Clinical Neurosciences*, *2*(2), 197–201. doi:10.1176/jnp.2.2.197 PMID:2136076

Boddaert, N., Belin, P., Chabane, N., Poline, J. B., Barthélémy, C., Mouren-Simeoni, M. C., & Zilbovicius, M. (2003). Perception of complex sounds: Abnormal pattern of cortical activation in autism. *The American Journal of Psychiatry*, *160*(11), 2057–2060. doi:10.1176/appi.ajp.160.11.2057 PMID:14594758

Boddaert, N., Chabane, N., Belin, P., Bourgeois, M., Royer, V., Barthelemy, C., & Zilbovicius, M. (2004). Perception of complex sounds in autism: Abnormal auditory cortical processing in children. *The American Journal of Psychiatry*, *161*(11), 2117–2120. doi:10.1176/appi.ajp.161.11.2117 PMID:15514415

Brugha, T. S., McManus, S., Bankart, J., Scott, F., Purdon, S., Smith, J., & Meltzer, H. (2011). Epidemiology of autism spectrum disorders in adults in the community in England. *Archives of General Psychiatry*, *68*(5), 459–465. doi:10.1001/archgenpsychiatry.2011.38 PMID:21536975

Bryson, S. E., Wainwright-Sharp, J. A., & Smith, I. M. (1990). Autism: A developmental spatial neglect syndrome? *Advances in Psychology*, *69*, 405–427. doi:10.1016/S0166-4115(08)60468-9

Bush, G., Valera, E. M., & Seidman, L. J. (2005). Functional neuroimaging of attention-deficit/hyperactivity disorder: A review and suggested future directions. *Biological Psychiatry*, *57*(11), 1273–1284. doi:10.1016/j.biopsych.2005.01.034 PMID:15949999

Carper, R. A., & Courchesne, E. (2000). Inverse correlation between frontal lobe and cerebellum sizes in children with autism. *Brain*, *123*(4), 836–844. doi:10.1093/brain/123.4.836 PMID:10734014

Carper, R. A., Moses, P., Tigue, Z. D., & Courchesne, E. (2002). Cerebral lobes in autism: Early hyperplasia and abnormal age effects. *NeuroImage*, *16*(4), 1038–1051. doi:10.1006/nimg.2002.1099 PMID:12202091

Castelli, F., Frith, C., Happé, F., & Frith, U. (2002). Autism, Asperger syndrome and brain mechanisms for the attribution of mental states to animated shapes. *Brain*, *125*(8), 1839–1849. doi:10.1093/brain/awf189 PMID:12135974

Chiu, P. H., Kayali, M. A., Kishida, K. T., Tomlin, D., Klinger, L. G., Klinger, M. R., & Montague, P. R. (2008). Self responses along cingulate cortex reveal quantitative neural phenotype for high-functioning autism. *Neuron*, *57*(3), 463–473. doi:10.1016/j.neuron.2007.12.020 PMID:18255038

Chugani, D. C., Muzik, O., Rothermel, R., Behen, M., Chakraborty, P., Mangner, T., & Chugani, H. T. (1997). Altered serotonin synthesis in the dentatothalamocortical pathway in autistic boys. *Annals of Neurology*, *42*(4), 666–669. doi:10.1002/ana.410420420 PMID:9382481

Coleman, P. D., Romano, J., Lapham, L., & Simon, W. (1985). Cell counts in cerebral cortex of an autistic patient. *Journal of Autism and Developmental Disorders*, *15*(3), 245–255. doi:10.1007/BF01531496 PMID:4030660

Courchesne, E., Hesselink, J. R., Jernigan, T. L., & Yeung-Courchesne, R. (1987). Abnormal neuroanatomy in a nonretarded person with autism: Unusual findings with magnetic resonance imaging. *Archives of Neurology*, *44*(3), 335–341. doi:10.1001/archneur.1987.00520150073028 PMID:3827686

Courchesne, E., Karns, C. M., Davis, H. R., Ziccardi, R., Carper, R. A., Tigue, Z. D., & Lincoln, A. J. (2001). Unusual brain growth patterns in early life in patients with autistic disorder an MRI study. *Neurology*, *57*(2), 245–254. doi:10.1212/WNL.57.2.245 PMID:11468308

Courchesne, E., & Pierce, K. (2005). Brain overgrowth in autism during a critical time in development: Implications for frontal pyramidal neuron and interneuron development and connectivity. *International Journal of Developmental Neuroscience*, *23*(2-3), 153–170. doi:10.1016/j.ijdevneu.2005.01.003 PMID:15749242

Courchesne, E., Saitoh, O., Yeung-Courchesne, R., Press, G. A., Lincoln, A. J., Haas, R. H., & Schreibman, L. (1994). Abnormality of cerebellar vermian lobules VI and VII in patients with infantile autism: Identification of hypoplastic and hyperplastic subgroups with MR imaging. *AJR. American Journal of Roentgenology*, *162*(1), 123–130. doi:10.2214/ajr.162.1.8273650 PMID:8273650

Critchley, H. D., Daly, E. M., Bullmore, E. T., Williams, S. C., Van Amelsvoort, T., Robertson, D. M., & Murphy, D. G. (2000). The functional neuroanatomy of social behaviour: Changes in cerebral blood flow when people with autistic disorder process facial expressions. *Brain*, *123*(11), 2203–2212. doi:10.1093/brain/123.11.2203 PMID:11050021

Damasio, A. R., & Maurer, R. G. (1978). A neurological model for childhood autism. *Archives of Neurology*, *35*(12), 777–786. doi:10.1001/archneur.1978.00500360001001 PMID:718482

Dawson, G. (2008). Early behavioral intervention, brain plasticity, and the prevention of autism spectrum disorder. *Development and Psychopathology*, *20*(3), 775–803. doi:10.1017/S0954579408000370 PMID:18606031

Dawson, G., Munson, J., Webb, S. J., Nalty, T., Abbott, R., & Toth, K. (2007). Rate of head growth decelerates and symptoms worsen in the second year of life in autism. *Biological Psychiatry*, *61*(4), 458–464. doi:10.1016/j.biopsych.2006.07.016 PMID:17137564

Dawson, G., Osterling, J., Meltzoff, A. N., & Kuhl, P. (2000). Case study of the development of an in fant with autism from birth to two years of age. *Journal of Applied Developmental Psychology*, *21*(3), 299–313. doi:10.1016/S0193-3973(99)00042-8 PMID:23667283

Egaas, B., Courchesne, E., & Saitoh, O. (1995). Reduced size of corpus callosum in autism. *Archives of Neurology*, *52*(8), 794–801. doi:10.1001/archneur.1995.00540320070014 PMID:7639631

Elder, L. M., Dawson, G., Toth, K., Fein, D., & Munson, J. (2008). Head circumference as an early predictor of autism symptoms in younger siblings of children with autism spectrum disorder. *Journal of Autism and Developmental Disorders*, *38*(6), 1104–1111. doi:10.100710803-007-0495-9 PMID:18058011

Garber, H. J., & Ritvo, E. R. (1992). Magnetic resonance imaging of the posterior fossa in autistic adults. *The American Journal of Psychiatry*, *149*(2), 245–247. doi:10.1176/ajp.149.2.245 PMID:1734747

Garber, H. J., Ritvo, E. R., Chiu, L. C., Griswold, V. J., & Kashanian, A. (1989). A magnetic resonance imaging study of autism: Normal fourth ventricle size and absence of pathology. *The American Journal of Psychiatry*, *146*(4), 532–534. doi:10.1176/ajp.146.4.532 PMID:2929757

Gardener, H., Spiegelman, D., & Buka, S. L. (2011). Perinatal and neonatal risk factors for autism: A comprehensive meta-analysis. *Pediatrics*, *128*(2), 344–355. doi:10.1542/peds.2010-1036 PMID:21746727

George, M. S., Costa, D. C., Kouris, K., Ring, H. A., & Ell, P. J. (1992). Cerebral blood flow abnormalities in adults with infantile autism. *The Journal of Nervous and Mental Disease*, *180*(7), 413–417. doi:10.1097/00005053-199207000-00002 PMID:1624921

Geschwind, D. H. (2009). Advances in autism. *Annual Review of Medicine*, *60*(1), 367–380. doi:10.1146/annurev.med.60.053107.121225 PMID:19630577

Gillberg, I. C., Bjure, J., Uvebrant, P., Vestergren, E., & Gillberg, C. (1993). SPECT (single photon emission computed tomography) in 31 children and adolescents with autism and autistic-like conditions. *European Child & Adolescent Psychiatry*, *2*(1), 50–59. doi:10.1007/BF02098830 PMID:21590529

Hashimoto, T., Tayama, M., Murakawa, K., Yoshimoto, T., Miyazaki, M., Harada, M., & Kuroda, Y. (1995). Development of the brainstem and cerebellum in autistic patients. *Journal of Autism and Developmental Disorders*, *25*(1), 1–18. doi:10.1007/BF02178163 PMID:7608030

Hazlett, E. A., Buchsbaum, M. S., Hsieh, P., Haznedar, M. M., Platholi, J., LiCalzi, E. M., ... Hollander, E. (2004). Regional glucose metabolism within cortical Brodmann areas in healthy individuals and autistic patients. *Neuropsychobiology*, *49*(3), 115–125. doi:10.1159/000076719 PMID:15034226

Hazlett, H. C., Poe, M., Gerig, G., Smith, R. G., Provenzale, J., Ross, A., & Piven, J. (2005). Magnetic resonance imaging and head circumference study of brain size in autism: Birth through age 2 years. *Archives of General Psychiatry*, *62*(12), 1366–1376. doi:10.1001/archpsyc.62.12.1366 PMID:16330725

Hazlett, H. C., Poe, M. D., Gerig, G., Smith, R. G., & Piven, J. (2006). Cortical gray and white brain tissue volume in adolescents and adults with autism. *Biological Psychiatry*, *59*(1), 1–6. doi:10.1016/j.biopsych.2005.06.015 PMID:16139816

Haznedar, M. M., Buchsbaum, M. S., Wei, T. C., Hof, P. R., Cartwright, C., Bienstock, C. A., & Hollander, E. (2000). Limbic circuitry in patients with autism spectrum disorders studied with positron emission tomography and magnetic resonance imaging. *The American Journal of Psychiatry*, *157*(12), 1994–2001. doi:10.1176/appi.ajp.157.12.1994 PMID:11097966

Herbert, M. R., Harris, G. J., Adrien, K. T., Ziegler, D. A., Makris, N., Kennedy, D. N., & Takeoka, M. (2002). Abnormal asymmetry in language association cortex in autism. *Annals of Neurology*, *52*(5), 588–596. doi:10.1002/ana.10349 PMID:12402256

Herbert, M. R., Ziegler, D. A., Deutsch, C. K., O'brien, L. M., Lange, N., Bakardjiev, A., & Kennedy, D. (2003). Dissociations of cerebral cortex, subcortical and cerebral white matter volumes in autistic boys. *Brain*, *126*(5), 1182–1192. doi:10.1093/brain/awg110 PMID:12690057

Herold, S., Frackowiak, R. S. J., Le Couteur, A., Rutter, M., & Howlin, P. (1988). Cerebral blood flow and metabolism of oxygen and glucose in young autistic adults. *Psychological Medicine*, *18*(4), 823–831. doi:10.1017/S0033291700009752 PMID:3270827

Hollander, E., Anagnostou, E., Chaplin, W., Esposito, K., Haznedar, M. M., Licalzi, E., & Buchsbaum, M. (2005). Striatal volume on magnetic resonance imaging and repetitive behaviors in autism. *Biological Psychiatry*, *58*(3), 226–232. doi:10.1016/j.biopsych.2005.03.040 PMID:15939406

Hudspeth, W. J., & Pribram, K. H. (1992). Psychophysiological indices of cerebral maturation. *International Journal of Psychophysiology, 12*(1), 19–29. doi:10.1016/0167-8760(92)90039-E PMID:1740399

Ito, H., Mori, K., Hashimoto, T., Miyazaki, M., Hori, A., Kagami, S., & Kuroda, Y. (2005). Findings of brain 99mTc-ECD SPECT in high-functioning autism-3-dimensional stereotactic ROI template analysis of brain SPECT. *The Journal of Medical Investigation, 52*(1-2), 49-56.

Jones, P. B., & Kerwin, R. W. (1990). Left temporal lobe damage in Asperger's syndrome. *The British Journal of Psychiatry, 156*(4), 570–572. doi:10.1192/bjp.156.4.570 PMID:2386870

Juranek, J., Filipek, P. A., Berenji, G. R., Modahl, C., Osann, K., & Spence, M. A. (2006). Association between amygdala volume and anxiety level: Magnetic resonance imaging (MRI) study in autistic children. *Journal of Child Neurology, 21*(12), 1051–1058. doi:10.1177/7010.2006.00237 PMID:17156697

Just, M. A., Cherkassky, V. L., Keller, T. A., Kana, R. K., & Minshew, N. J. (2006). Functional and anatomical cortical underconnectivity in autism: Evidence from an fMRI study of an executive function task and corpus callosum morphometry. *Cerebral Cortex, 17*(4), 951–961. doi:10.1093/cercor/bhl006 PMID:16772313

Kana, R. K., Keller, T. A., Cherkassky, V. L., Minshew, N. J., & Just, M. A. (2006). Sentence comprehension in autism: Thinking in pictures with decreased functional connectivity. *Brain, 129*(9), 2484–2493. doi:10.1093/brain/awl164 PMID:16835247

Kaufmann, W. E., Cooper, K. L., Mostofsky, S. H., Capone, G. T., Kates, W. R., Newschaffer, C. J., & Lanham, D. C. (2003). Specificity of cerebellar vermian abnormalities in autism: A quantitative magnetic resonance imaging study. *Journal of Child Neurology, 18*(7), 463–470. doi:10.1177/0883073803 0180070501 PMID:12940651

Keller, T. A., Kana, R. K., & Just, M. A. (2007). A developmental study of the structural integrity of white matter in autism. *Neuroreport, 18*(1), 23–27. doi:10.1097/01.wnr.0000239965.21685.99 PMID:17259855

Kemper, T. L., & Bauman, M. L. (1993). The contribution of neuropathologic studies to the understanding of autism. *Neurologic Clinics, 11*(1), 175–187. doi:10.1016/S0733-8619(18)30176-2 PMID:8441369

Kennedy, D. P., Redcay, E., & Courchesne, E. (2006). Failing to deactivate: Resting functional abnormalities in autism. *Proceedings of the National Academy of Sciences of the United States of America, 103*(21), 8275–8280. doi:10.1073/pnas.0600674103 PMID:16702548

Kim, B. N., Lee, J. S., Shin, M. S., Cho, S. C., & Lee, D. S. (2002). Regional cerebral perfusion abnormalities in attention deficit/hyperactivity disorder. *European Archives of Psychiatry and Clinical Neuroscience, 252*(5), 219–225. doi:10.100700406-002-0384-3 PMID:12451463

Kleinhans, N. M., Johnson, L. C., Richards, T., Mahurin, R., Greenson, J., Dawson, G., & Aylward, E. (2009). Reduced neural habituation in the amygdala and social impairments in autism spectrum disorders. *The American Journal of Psychiatry, 166*(4), 467–475. doi:10.1176/appi.ajp.2008.07101681 PMID:19223437

Klin, A., Chawarska, K., Paul, R., Rubin, E., Morgan, T., Wiesner, L., & Volkmar, F. (2004). Autism in a 15-month-old child. *The American Journal of Psychiatry, 161*(11), 1981–1988. doi:10.1176/appi.ajp.161.11.1981 PMID:15514396

Koshino, H., Carpenter, P. A., Minshew, N. J., Cherkassky, V. L., Keller, T. A., & Just, M. A. (2005). Functional connectivity in an fMRI working memory task in high-functioning autism. *NeuroImage, 24*(3), 810–821. doi:10.1016/j.neuroimage.2004.09.028 PMID:15652316

Koshino, H., Kana, R. K., Keller, T. A., Cherkassky, V. L., Minshew, N. J., & Just, M. A. (2007). fMRI investigation of working memory for faces in autism: Visual coding and underconnectivity with frontal areas. *Cerebral Cortex, 18*(2), 289–300. doi:10.1093/cercor/bhm054 PMID:17517680

Lainhart, J. E., Piven, J., Wzorek, M., Landa, R., Santangelo, S. L., Coon, H., & Folstein, S. E. (1997). Macrocephaly in children and adults with autism. *Journal of the American Academy of Child and Adolescent Psychiatry, 36*(2), 282–290. doi:10.1097/00004583-199702000-00019 PMID:9031582

Lask, B., Gordon, I., Christie, D., Frampton, I., Chowdhury, U., & Watkins, B. (2005). Functional neuroimaging in early-onset anorexia nervosa. *International Journal of Eating Disorders, 37*(1), 49–51. doi:10.1002/eat.20117 PMID:15852320

Lee, J. E., Bigler, E. D., Alexander, A. L., Lazar, M., DuBray, M. B., Chung, M. K., & Lu, J. (2007). Diffusion tensor imaging of white matter in the superior temporal gyrus and temporal stem in autism. *Neuroscience Letters, 424*(2), 127–132. doi:10.1016/j.neulet.2007.07.042 PMID:17714869

Lewis, J. D., & Elman, J. L. (2008). Growth-related neural reorganization and the autism phenotype: A test of the hypothesis that altered brain growth leads to altered connectivity. *Developmental Science, 11*(1), 135–155. doi:10.1111/j.1467-7687.2007.00634.x PMID:18171375

Lombardo, M. V., Chakrabarti, B., Bullmore, E. T., Sadek, S. A., Pasco, G., Wheelwright, S. J., & Baron-Cohen, S. (2009). Atypical neural self-representation in autism. *Brain, 133*(2), 611–624. doi:10.1093/brain/awp306 PMID:20008375

Lotspeich, L. J., Kwon, H., Schumann, C. M., Fryer, S. L., Goodlin-Jones, B. L., Buonocore, M. H., ... Reiss, A. L. (2004). Investigation of neuroanatomical differences between autism and Asperger syndrome. *Archives of General Psychiatry, 61*(3), 291–298. doi:10.1001/archpsyc.61.3.291 PMID:14993117

Luna, B., Minshew, N. J., Garver, K. E., Lazar, N. A., Thulborn, K. R., Eddy, W. F., & Sweeney, J. A. (2002). Neocortical system abnormalities in autism An fMRI study of spatial working memory. *Neurology, 59*(6), 834–840. doi:10.1212/WNL.59.6.834 PMID:12297562

Maenner, M. J., & Durkin, M. S. (2010). Trends in the prevalence of autism on the basis of special education data. *Pediatrics, 126*(5), 1018–1025. doi:10.1542/peds.2010-1023 PMID:20974790

Makkonen, I., Riikonen, R., Kokki, H., Airaksinen, M. M., & Kuikka, J. T. (2008). Serotonin and dopamine transporter binding in children with autism determined by SPECT. *Developmental Medicine and Child Neurology, 50*(8), 593–597. doi:10.1111/j.1469-8749.2008.03027.x PMID:18754896

Minshew, N. J., Sweeney, J. A., Bauman, M. L., & Webb, S. J. (2005). Neurologic aspects of autism. In F. R., Volkmar, R. Paul, A. Klin, & D. J. Cohen (Eds.), Handbook of autism and pervasive developmental disorders, diagnosis, development, neurobiology, and behavior (3rd ed.; vol. 1, pp. 473-514). John Wiley & Sons, Inc. doi:10.1002/9780470939345.ch18

Minshew, N. J., & Williams, D. L. (2007). The new neurobiology of autism: Cortex, connectivity, and neuronal organization. *Archives of Neurology*, *64*(7), 945–950. doi:10.1001/archneur.64.7.945 PMID:17620483

Mountz, J. M., Tolbert, L. C., Lill, D. W., Katholi, C. R., & Liu, H. G. (1995). Functional deficits in autistic disorder: Characterization by technetium-99m-HMPAO and SPECT. *Journal of Nuclear Medicine*, *36*(7), 1156–1162. PMID:7790938

Munson, J., Dawson, G., Abbott, R., Faja, S., Webb, S. J., Friedman, S. D., & Dager, S. R. (2006). Amygdalar volume and behavioral development in autism. *Archives of General Psychiatry*, *63*(6), 686–693. doi:10.1001/archpsyc.63.6.686 PMID:16754842

Nacewicz, B. M., Dalton, K. M., Johnstone, T., Long, M. T., McAuliff, E. M., Oakes, T. R., & Davidson, R. J. (2006). Amygdala volume and nonverbal social impairment in adolescent and adult males with autism. *Archives of General Psychiatry*, *63*(12), 1417–1428. doi:10.1001/archpsyc.63.12.1417 PMID:17146016

Nakamura, K., Sekine, Y., Ouchi, Y., Tsujii, M., Yoshikawa, E., Futatsubashi, M., & Matsuzaki, H. (2010). Brain serotonin and dopamine transporter bindings in adults with high-functioning autism. *Archives of General Psychiatry*, *67*(1), 59–68. doi:10.1001/archgenpsychiatry.2009.137 PMID:20048223

Nowell, M. A., Hackney, D. B., Muraki, A. S., & Coleman, M. (1990). Varied MR appearance of autism: Fifty-three pediatric patients having the full autistic syndrome. *Magnetic Resonance Imaging*, *8*(6), 811–816. doi:10.1016/0730-725X(90)90018-W PMID:2266809

O'Hearn, K., Asato, M., Ordaz, S., & Luna, B. (2008). Neurodevelopment and executive function in autism. *Development and Psychopathology*, *20*(4), 1103–1132. doi:10.1017/S0954579408000527 PMID:18838033

Ohnishi, T., Matsuda, H., Hashimoto, T., Kunihiro, T., Nishikawa, M., Uema, T., & Sasaki, M. (2000). Abnormal regional cerebral blood flow in childhood autism. *Brain*, *123*(9), 1838–1844. doi:10.1093/brain/123.9.1838 PMID:10960047

Okugawa, G., Sedvall, G. C., & Agartz, I. (2003). Smaller cerebellar vermis but not hemisphere volumes in patients with chronic schizophrenia. *The American Journal of Psychiatry*, *160*(9), 1614–1617. doi:10.1176/appi.ajp.160.9.1614 PMID:12944335

Otake, M., Schull, W. J., & Yoshimaru, H. (1991). Brain damage among the prenatally exposed. *Journal of Radiation Research*, *32*(1SUPPLEMENT), 249–264. doi:10.1269/jrr.32.SUPPLEMENT_249 PMID:1762113

Palmen, S. J., Pol, H. E. H., Kemner, C., Schnack, H. G., Durston, S., Lahuis, B. E., & Van Engeland, H. (2005). Increased gray-matter volume in medication-naive high-functioning children with autism spectrum disorder. *Psychological Medicine*, *35*(4), 561–570. doi:10.1017/S0033291704003496 PMID:15856726

Pierce, K., Müller, R. A., Ambrose, J., Allen, G., & Courchesne, E. (2001). Face processing occurs outside the fusiformface area in autism: Evidence from functional MRI. *Brain*, *124*(10), 2059–2073. doi:10.1093/brain/124.10.2059 PMID:11571222

Piven, J., Bailey, J., Ranson, B. J., & Arndt, S. (1998). No difference in hippocampus volume detected on magnetic resonance imaging in autistic individuals. *Journal of Autism and Developmental Disorders*, *28*(2), 105–110. doi:10.1023/A:1026084430649 PMID:9586772

Redcay, E., & Courchesne, E. (2005). When is the brain enlarged in autism? A meta-analysis of all brain size reports. *Biological Psychiatry*, *58*(1), 1–9. doi:10.1016/j.biopsych.2005.03.026 PMID:15935993

Robinson, E. B., Koenen, K. C., McCormick, M. C., Munir, K., Hallett, V., Happé, F., & Ronald, A. (2012). A multivariate twin study of autistic traits in 12-year-olds: Testing the fractionable autism triad hypothesis. *Behavior Genetics*, *42*(2), 245–255. doi:10.100710519-011-9500-3 PMID:21927971

Ronald, A., & Hoekstra, R. A. (2011). Autism spectrum disorders and autistic traits: A decade of new twin studies. *American Journal of Medical Genetics. Part B, Neuropsychiatric Genetics*, *156*(3), 255–274. doi:10.1002/ajmg.b.31159 PMID:21438136

Rumsey, J. M., Duara, R., Grady, C., Rapoport, J. L., Margolin, R. A., Rapoport, S. I., & Cutler, N. R. (1985). Brain metabolism in autism: Resting cerebral glucose utilization rates as measured with positron emission tomography. *Archives of General Psychiatry*, *42*(5), 448–455. doi:10.1001/archpsyc.1985.01790280026003 PMID:3872650

Rutter, M. (1983). Cognitive deficits in the pathogenesis of autism. *Journal of Child Psychology and Psychiatry, and Allied Disciplines*, *24*(4), 513–531. doi:10.1111/j.1469-7610.1983.tb00129.x PMID:6630326

Ryu, Y. H., Lee, J. D., Yoon, P. H., Kim, D. I., Lee, H. B., & Shin, Y. J. (1999). Perfusion impairments in infantile autism on technetium-99m ethyl cysteinate dimer brain single-photon emission tomography: Comparison with findings on magnetic resonance imaging. *European Journal of Nuclear Medicine*, *26*(3), 253–259. doi:10.1007002590050385 PMID:10079316

Saitoh, O., Courchesne, E., Egaas, B., Lincoln, A. J., & Schreibman, L. (1995). Cross-sectional area of the posterior hippocampus in autistic patients with cerebellar and corpus callosum abnormalities. *Neurology*, *45*(2), 317–324. doi:10.1212/WNL.45.2.317 PMID:7854533

Schultz, R. T., Gauthier, I., Klin, A., Fulbright, R. K., Anderson, A. W., Volkmar, F., & Gore, J. C. (2000). Abnormal ventral temporal cortical activity during face discrimination among individuals with autism and Asperger syndrome. *Archives of General Psychiatry*, *57*(4), 331–340. doi:10.1001/archpsyc.57.4.331 PMID:10768694

Schumann, C. M., Hamstra, J., Goodlin-Jones, B. L., Lotspeich, L. J., Kwon, H., Buonocore, M. H., & Amaral, D. G. (2004). The amygdala is enlarged in children but not adolescents with autism; the hippocampus is enlarged at all ages. *The Journal of Neuroscience*, *24*(28), 6392–6401. doi:10.1523/JNEUROSCI.1297-04.2004 PMID:15254095

Sears, L. L., Vest, C., Mohamed, S., Bailey, J., Ranson, B. J., & Piven, J. (1999). An MRI study of the basal ganglia in autism. *Progress in Neuro-Psychopharmacology & Biological Psychiatry*, *23*(4), 613–624. doi:10.1016/S0278-5846(99)00020-2 PMID:10390720

Sharma, S., Woolfson, L. M., & Hunter, S. C. (2012). Confusion and inconsistency in diagnosis of Asperger syndrome: A review of studies from 1981 to 2010. *Autism*, *16*(5), 465–486. doi:10.1177/1362361311411935 PMID:21810909

Sparks, B. F., Friedman, S. D., Shaw, D. W., Aylward, E. H., Echelard, D., Artru, A. A., & Dager, S. R. (2002). Brain structural abnormalities in young children with autism spectrum disorder. *Neurology*, *59*(2), 184–192. doi:10.1212/WNL.59.2.184 PMID:12136055

Stanfield, A. C., McIntosh, A. M., Spencer, M. D., Philip, R., Gaur, S., & Lawrie, S. M. (2008). Towards a neuroanatomy of autism: A systematic review and meta-analysis of structural magnetic resonance imaging studies. *European Psychiatry*, *23*(4), 289–299. doi:10.1016/j.eurpsy.2007.05.006 PMID:17765485

Taylor, W. D., Hsu, E., Krishnan, K. R. R., & MacFall, J. R. (2004). Diffusion tensor imaging: Background, potential, and utility in psychiatric research. *Biological Psychiatry*, *55*(3), 201–207. doi:10.1016/j.biopsych.2003.07.001 PMID:14744459

Tsai, L. Y. (1989). Recent neurobiological findings in autism. In *Diagnosis and treatment of autism* (pp. 83–104). Boston, MA: Springer. doi:10.1007/978-1-4899-0882-7_7

Webb, S. J., Nalty, T., Munson, J., Brock, C., Abbott, R., & Dawson, G. (2007). Rate of head circumference growth as a function of autism diagnosis and history of autistic regression. *Journal of Child Neurology*, *22*(10), 1182–1190. doi:10.1177/0883073807306263 PMID:17940244

Whitehouse, A. J., Coon, H., Miller, J., Salisbury, B., & Bishop, D. V. (2010). Narrowing the broader autism phenotype: A study using the Communication Checklist-Adult Version (CC-A). *Autism*, *14*(6), 559–574. doi:10.1177/1362361310382107 PMID:20923891

Wing, L., Gould, J., & Gillberg, C. (2011). Autism spectrum disorders in the DSM-V: Better or worse than the DSM-IV? *Research in Developmental Disabilities*, *32*(2), 768–773. doi:10.1016/j.ridd.2010.11.003 PMID:21208775

Zilbovicius, M., Boddaert, N., Belin, P., Poline, J. B., Remy, P., Mangin, J. F., & Samson, Y. (2000). Temporal lobe dysfunction in childhood autism: A PET study. *The American Journal of Psychiatry*, *157*(12), 1988–1993. doi:10.1176/appi.ajp.157.12.1988 PMID:11097965

KEY TERMS AND DEFINITIONS

Autism: Autism is a severe developmental disability which involves impairments in the social interaction like being unaware of other people's feelings as well as verbal and nonverbal communication. It is first seen within the first three years of life.

Autism Spectrum Disorder: A group with developmental disorders (such as autism and Asperger's syndrome) which is characterized by impairments in the capacity to communicate and interact socially by the occurrence of repetitive behaviors or restricted interests is called autism spectrum disorder. It is also known as pervasive developmental disorder.

Diffusion Tensor Imaging (DTI): It is an MRI-based neuroimaging technique which makes it possible to estimate the location, orientation, and anisotropy of the brain's white matter tracts.

Dorsolateral Prefrontal Cortex (DLPFC or DL-PFC): It is an area in the prefrontal cortex of the brain of humans as well as non-human primates. It is one of the most highly evolved part of the human brain. It undergoes a continuous period of maturation till adulthood. It is expressed like DLPFC or DL-PFC.

Executive Function: The term executive function is used by psychologists and neuroscientists to describe a loosely defined set of brain processes that are liable for planning, cognitive flexibility, abstract thinking, rule acquisition, initiating proper actions and inhibiting inappropriate actions, and selecting appropriate sensory information.

Intelligence: Intelligence is the aggregate or global capacity of the individual to act purposely, to think rationally and to deal effectively with his environment.

Morphometry: Morphometrics is derived from a Greek word *morphe*, "shape, form," *metria*, "measurement." Morphometry refers to the quantitative analysis of form, a concept that includes size and shape.

Neural Connectivity: Connections between neurons where neuron sends information via neurotransmitter.

Occipital: The occipital lobe is one of the lobes of the cerebral cortex in the brain of mammals. It is the visual processing center of the mammalian brain containing most of the anatomical region of the visual cortex. The crucial visual cortex is Brodmann area 17, also known as called V1 (visual one).

Phylogeny: It is the expression of an evolutionary history of a species (and related species) through genes. These studies focuss on the progression and change of species throughout time and how similar species are connected through genetics and evolutionary time.

Precentral Gyrus: The precentral gyrus is a most important structure on the surface of the posterior frontal lobe. It is also the situated in the primary motor cortex known as Brodmann area 4.

Synapse: A synapse is a small gap at the end of a neuron that permits a signal to pass from one neuron to the other neuron.

Chapter 7
Eye Tracker:
An Assistive Tool in Diagnosis of Autism Spectrum Disorder

Tanu Wadhera
Dr. B. R. Ambedkar National Institute of Technology, India

Deepti Kakkar
Dr. B. R. Ambedkar National Institute of Technology, India

ABSTRACT

The high prevalence of autism spectrum disorder (ASD) has provided a spectrum of diagnostic methodologies ranging from screening scales to technological techniques. The technology-based techniques, especially eye trackers, are shifting the traditional subjective approaches to objective, leading to early ASD screening and intervention. The eye gaze deficits marked by eye trackers are the valid biomarkers of ASD, but the trackers are not clinically available. Another reason for non-availability is the limited number of methodologies which can meaningfully analyze gaze data. The assistance of new technologies into eye tracker system explored here can (1) detect gaze patterns and cognitive abilities of individuals at the single platform and (2) analyze eye movements and events automatically using deep learning system rather than manual interpretation of raw data. These types of systems, if implemented, have the potential to assist clinicians for better ASD diagnosis and intervention approaches.

INTRODUCTION

Recently, International Clinical Epidemiology Network Trust (INCLEN) statistics reported that the number of Autism Spectrum Disorder (ASD) affected children has crossed 10 million in India or roughly it is 23 after 10,000 (Rudra, Belmonte, Soni, Banerjee, Mukerji, & Chakrabarti, 2017). ASD is a neuro-developmental disorder principally classified by impairments in the three core domains viz. social interaction, communication, and restricted-repeated behaviors (Bölte & Hallmayer, 2011). It occurs in the early developmental phase of an individual with the appearance of the spectrum of deficits which differentiates them from typically developed individuals. The failure in maintaining proper eye

DOI: 10.4018/978-1-5225-7004-2.ch007

contacts, recognizing vocal effects (Bekele, Wade, Bian, Fan, Swanson, Warren, & Sarkar, 2016), judging and reading other's facial expressions and intentions are the factors leading to poor interaction and communication in ASD (American Psychiatric Association, 2013). The reason for the same is that the neural networks of ASD individuals use different methodologies in monitoring the social information as compared to controls (Wang, Dapretto, Hariri, Sigman, & Bookheimer, 2004). In addition, the attention deficits, imitation and perception deficits co-occur with the disorder. These deficits are generally common in all individuals but their appearance varies from individual to individual (Bekele, Wade, Bian, Fan, Swanson, Warren, & Sarkar, 2016). The heterogeneity in ASD is not only because it has a wide range of symptoms but also due to variations in disorder onset (Ozonoff, Iosif, Young, Hepburn, Thompson, Colombi, & Rogers, 2011). The fact complicating the situation further is that no universally effective ASD diagnostic approach has been found yet. Therefore, ASD detection is based on the identification of visually appealing atypical behavioral traits and the cognitive mechanisms underlying these behaviors. The process of behavior tracing cannot be a robust diagnostic methodology since some individuals may show symptoms in infancy period or some may show in late childhood. The delay in diagnosis period can lead to delay in treatment process resulting in poor growth of ASD individual as compared to normal with the same age-group. The early diagnosis is not only mandatory for the early treatment but also to enhance their IQ so that they can also get involved in regular activities viz. education and social activities similar to normal individuals.

In literature, dozens of techniques have been proposed not only to diagnose ASD but also to help in identifying more cases. It is found that in ASD the behavioral impairments become very much complex with growth so follow-up screenings of the individual are required. The screening of individual from time to time can keep a track of the impairments. The clinicians and experts have invented different screening tools involving screening scales, interview methods, clinical observations, behavioral measures for evaluation and differential diagnosis of disorder (Matson, Nebel-Schwalm, & Matson, 2007). These primary screening techniques play their role after the onset of disorder making them inappropriate in early diagnosis or prognosis of the disorder. Along with this, there are some other limitations reducing the suitability of these techniques:

1. Age-specific as the scales are designed using different age groups and periods involving infants, childhood, and adult.
2. Rater biasing while measuring and diagnosing disorder sometimes shows symptoms of some other problem from the spectrum of disorder which reduces the effectiveness of this approach (Frazier, Klingemier, Beukemann, Speer, Markowitz, Parikh, & Ahuja, 2016).
3. Time-consuming as the expert need to design many questionnaires and to take responses from children as well as parents is a long-lasting process.
4. Subjective in nature as the disorder description is highly dependent on parent's interview and clinician/expert observations (Frazier, Klingemier, Beukemann, Speer, Markowitz, Parikh, & Ahuja, 2016).
5. The administrator whether parents or clinician needs a proper training of tools or scales before applying the same to the children (Frazier, Klingemier, Beukemann, Speer, Markowitz, Parikh, & Ahuja, 2016). Sometimes, only trained administrators or experts/professionals are hired that further poses a restriction.

Basically, these scales firstly, differentiate the disordered children from normal ones and then classify them into different disorder groups by relating their symptoms with a particular disorder such as differentiating individuals with autism from those with Asperger syndrome, attention deficit and other childhood disorders (Coonrod & Stone, 2005). In order to understand the disorder's underlying factors, the diagnosis is taken to next level where one can study the neurological condition in depth.

The neurological techniques such as Electroencephalogram (EEG), Magnetic Resonance Imaging (MRI), Magnetoencephalography (MEG), functional Magnetic Resonance Imaging (fMRI) and Diffusion Tensor Imaging (DTI) have revealed the abnormalities associated with the brain functioning in ASD (Ekinci, Arman, Işık, Bez, & Berkem, 2010; Pardini, Elia, Garaci, Guida, Coniglione, Krueger, & Gialloreti, 2012; Port, Anwar, Ku, Carlson, Siegel, & Roberts, 2015; Sperdin & Schaer, 2016). These abnormalities were considered to provide potential biomarkers for ASD diagnosis. The growth and potential of techniques in diagnosing disorder have led to the integration of these imaging approaches such as EEG and fMRI (Hames, Murphy, Rajmohan, Anderson, Baker, Zupancic... & Richman, 2016) to address ASD brain abnormalities in the more detailed way. The multimodal approaches were used to discover the multiple modalities of individuals which are responsible for ASD. Also, these approaches provided an opportunity to monitor the impact of the intervention on ASD without undergoing the diagnosis process again. Despite this, these techniques have limitations and are not frequently used for diagnosis process. The limitations are:

1. **Physical Restrictions:** The fixation of electrodes or placing individuals in MRI machine has so many pre-requisite conditions such as movement of the head or other body part is not allowed.
2. **Involves a Lot of Circuitry:** Lot of wiring and the systems for capturing the signal is quite a cumbersome process.
3. Sedation is required otherwise handling hyper-active children would be difficult.
4. The signal of the brain is very complex, difficult to understand and contaminates with a lot of noise (Tanu & Kakkar, 2018).
5. Significant preparations are required to be done prior performing the diagnosis process (Frazier, Klingemier, Beukemann, Speer, Markowitz, Parikh, & Ahuja, 2016).
6. Quite expensive due to which diagnosing disorder frequently is very difficult.

These techniques are considered when the initial screening of disorder has been done or when the deficits become much more appealing. These techniques alone cannot act as the standardized diagnostic methods which can target the disorder entirely. Hence, these scales and techniques available are not valid enough to diagnose disorder accurately and independently. In order to find the valid biomarkers, the diagnostic methodologies are shifting towards the technological techniques. The different technology-based approaches involve diagnosis through video-taping, robots, eye tracking and, tablet-based games (Aresti-Bartolome & Garcia-Zapirain, 2014). Among these, the eye tracking has become an additional and important diagnostic tool for ASD, and hence the eye trackers are gaining much more attention (Pierce, Marinero, Hazin, McKenna, Barnes, & Malige, 2016).

Eye tracking process involves the measurement, record, and scanning of eye position and movement in given frame of time (Poole & Ball, 2006). It traces attention of person and depends upon his interest & nature of the assigned task. These trackers have the potential to quantitatively and objectively measure the eye movement and position in real-time, provide insights into mental imagery, cognitive mechanism and to represent functioning of the cerebellum (Vidal, Turner, Bulling, & Gellersen, 2012).

In 1879, Emile Java observed the eye movements with the mirror during text reading and was the first to describe rapid eye movements called 'saccades' and stationary positions called 'fixations'. The eye movements are also related to cognitive processes such as memory recalling, fatigue, personality traits and visual information processing (Hoppe & Bulling, 2016). These can diagnose various other developmental disorders and conditions. The eye data abnormalities are providing better insight into the entire brain of ASD individuals and can become potential biomarker of ASD. The disorders affecting cerebella such as dementia, progressive neurological disorders requiring real-time analysis such as Alzheimer, Parkinson or stroke can be easily diagnosed using eye trackers (Kumar, Dutta, Das, & Lahiri, 2016). The eye movements recorded while watching television diagnosed individuals with attention deficit, fetal alcohol spectrum and Parkinson's neurological disorders (Tseng, Cameron, Pari, Reynolds, Munoz, & Itti, 2013). The trackers provide a non-invasive platform, regular monitoring, and easy diagnosis facility. Consequently, eye trackers not only measure the behavioral traits but also provide a window to the brain. The technological advantages and advancements play a major role in their wide use. Some of the advantages of eye trackers are:

1. Highly objective, portable, faster and accurate in nature.
2. Captures gaze data and gaze span of infants and young children with the same ease and precision as in case of adults without any need of Intelligence Quotient-matching (verbal, non-verbal and performance) (Guillon, Hadjikhani, Baduel, & Rogé, 2014). Hence, this tool is not age-specific and patient-specific.
3. Identify and describe the gaze patterns involving minute variations and spontaneous view with much more precision (Guillon, Hadjikhani, Baduel, & Rogé, 2014) without restricting the natural actions of a subject.
4. Needs less time for capturing signals and can be implemented easily at any functional level.
5. Identify behavioral traits, visual preference patterns, and physiology of the fundamental deficits in ASD.
6. Provide valid biomarkers (objective indicators) that diagnose ASD in infants and children and accelerates the treatment planning (Pierce, Marinero, Hazin, McKenna, Barnes, & Malige, 2016).
7. Adds some more measuring factors such as gaze fixation accuracy and gaze path (Holmqvist, Nyström, Andersson, Dewhurst, Jarodzka, & Van de Weijer, 2011), directly measures visual social attention (Frank, Vul, & Saxe, 2012).
8. Less set-up time requirement and light weight of trackers made it feasible to carry out the experiments for real-world environment and objects.

The eye tracker has a wide range of applications in human-computer interaction (HCI), in understanding the behavior and problem-solving nature of the individuals, in e-learning and mental-health monitoring. The systems are assisted with many other techniques such as computers, virtual and augmented reality environments, and brain-computer interface to give a better and easy life to neuro-disabled people (Balan, Moldoveanu, Moldoveanu, Morar, & Asavei, 2013). The systems allow the abnormal and disabled children to interact directly with interfaces using their gaze as input instead of using external sources viz. mouse and keyboard (Poole & Ball, 2006). It is also used in the research field related to cognitive mechanisms involved in perception, reading and learning mechanism (Lai, Tsai, Yang, Hsu, Liu, Lee, & Tsai, 2013). In India, it is implemented in human-computer interaction design bed for shopping, banking and traveling purposes (Biswas & Langdon, 2014), and in checking alertness of drivers (George & Routray, 2015).

The purpose of this chapter is threefold. Firstly, the surveys of growth in eye tracking systems for ASD diagnosis, eye tracking parameters, and analysis methods have been discussed. Secondly, practical issues due to which these systems are not clinically available to have been elaborated. Thirdly, the assistance of new methodologies in eye tracker systems has been discussed to provide a solution to the validation and availability of eye trackers clinically.

EYE TRACKING SYSTEMS

It has been found that gaze data and visual attention covers a major portion of the cognitive mechanism which is nearly 83 percent (Wästlund, Shams, Löfgren, Witell, & Gustafsson, 2010). It is only the eye gaze that helps in building the comfort level of any conversation or discussion. The neural mechanisms, associated with producing eye movements can be found in (Freedman & Foxe, 2017), failure can cause changes in the eye movement patterns. These patterns highlight the damaged brain region or any neurodevelopmental disorder due to which neural system breakdown occurs (Freedman & Foxe 2017).

The first eye tracker was lens based constructed by *Edmund Huey* to track the pupil and gaze movements (Lupu & Ungureanu, 2013). The idea of recording of eye movements on the film using light beams was first proposed by *Guy Thomas Buswell*. The author also provided the variation in reading styles of an individual. In order to make precise and non-invasive eye tracker, *Dodge and Cline* constructed cornea reflection based tracker that described eye movement velocity in the horizontal direction only. In this manner, the enhancements were made into trackers and the first head-mounted eye tracking system was invented by *Hartridge and Thompson* to remove the constraint in eye data due to head movement (Lupu & Ungureanu, 2013).

The method of measurement of the eye position and movement is called oculography. The invasive techniques used in measurement are: 1.) Electrooculogram (EOG) potential based eye-tracker: The potential can be thought to be generated by a dipole with cornea as positive charge and retina as negative. A pair of skin electrodes is placed near the eye region to measure the eye movements based on the electrical signal potential (Vidal, Turner, Bulling, & Gellersen, 2012). This electrical potential is called as Electrooculogram and the variations in EOG are due to variations in dipole orientation due to movement of the eyes. The EOG signal is steady when the eyes are in origin position and varies with the movement of the eyes. The EOG variations help in tracking the eye movements. 2.) Scleral tracking: The coil-contact lens embedded with magnetic-field sensors is used to measure the eye movements (Duchowski, Driver, Jolaoso, Tan, Ramey, & Robbins, 2010). These special contact lenses are tightly fitted with eyes helping in tracking the eye movements not only in the horizontal and vertical but also in the torsion direction. It is a highly sensitive method as compared to others in detecting eye movements (Chennamma & Yuan, 2013; Poole & Ball, 2006). These methods need a lot of calibration time, head-positioning, involves a lot of circuitry and set-up procedure.

These techniques then shifted to non-invasive techniques such as desktop-based eye-imaging video techniques. It is basically optical tracking methodology and is a non-contact method of measuring eye movements. The eye region is illuminated by infrared light and the amount of light reflected from the eye sensed by video-camera/sensor is used for calculating eye movements. This video-based method measures the person's point of regard by tracing the cornea-reflection or the pupil-center (Hua, Krishnaswamy, & Rolland, 2006). It is less noisy as compared to other techniques and poses fewer restrictions on the individuals.

The tracker's calibration, head movements, interference during testing, sampling rate, accuracy, and testing environment are the major concerns that can affect the tracked data. They need to account for head movements for better accuracy of data rather than stabilizing the head position and removing the head motion related data (Sasson & Elison, 2012) and trackers such as infrared video-based and remote-eye trackers allow head-movements. The temporal and spatial resolution of the tracker depends upon the tracker's type and model (Boraston & Blakemore, 2007). The pupil-corneal reflection has a sampling rate in the range 50 Hz-2 KHz and for direct measurement, it is 200 Hz. The spatial resolution operates in 0.005 degree-0.5 degree range and 0.1 degrees for direct measurement. The accuracy of the tracker depends upon the artifacts free data. The higher sampling rate brings high accuracy but poses restrictions on the head motion. Hence, while selecting the tracker the sampling rate and head motion trade-off should be accounted. The test needs to be conducted in properly illuminated room, with proper sound-effects as some individuals might have audio hypersensitivity and without the intrusion of the experimenter. The task should not be very complex, time-consuming and should have sound effects and gaps to keep the interest of individuals. During the testing session, the individual with ASD need special care and should be accompanied by parents/caretakers, allow vertical adjustments and the individual with ASD should have more patience while tracking their eyes. The experimenter needs to take care of sitting arrangement, height, positioning of the eye at center of screen and distance between screen & individual. These factors should also follow standard rules and needs to be uniform throughout the experiment to avoid any discrepancy in the result. The tracker's calibration points vary with respect to age of the individual such as 2-point for infants, 5-point calibration for children and 9-point calibration for adults (Sasson & Elison, 2012).

1. Tracking Systems for ASD Diagnosis

In ASD individuals, previously the investigation of visual attention and social orientation has been done using home videotapes and computerized-laboratory experiments. The poor accuracy, lot of prior experimental settings, lack of tracing individuals gaze data and gaze span (Zwaigenbaum, Thurm, Stone, Baranek, Bryson, Iverson... & Rogers, 2007) and poor real-world approximations were some of the limitations of these methodologies which lead to designing of eye trackers. The eye trackers widened ASD marker spectrum by measuring their gaze distribution and detecting sensorimotor eye movement abnormalities (Takarae, Minshew, Luna, & Sweeney, 2004). The eye tracking studies differentiated the ASD individuals from normal individuals as they do not pay much attention to the faces, exhibit abnormal gaze behavior and fail in showing involvement in the joint-attention task (Sasson, Turner-Brown, Holtzclaw Lam, & Bodfish, 2008). The sudden increase in ASD diagnosis studies employing eye trackers is due to the accessibility of the eye-tracking technology and the ease offered by these devices in the diagnosis process. The refinements over past fifteen years have improved accuracy, stability of trackers and provided the possibility of tracking eyes during free viewing and in the natural environment without any prior calibration and head fixation requirement. In one such study, a tablet-based eye tracking algorithm for screening ASD in individuals has been proposed (Vargas-Cuentas, Roman-Gonzalez, Gilman, Barrientos, Ting, Hidalgo, ... & Zimic, 2017). The algorithm tracks eye movements without any restriction of head-motion or calibration and is portable as well as cost-effective.

Eye Tracker

Since its first ASD study (Pelphrey, Sasson, Reznick, Paul, Goldman, & Piven, 2002), some of the findings in which eye tracker has explored ASD behavioral traits, in task-dependent situations, have been provided in tabular form in Table 1. The tabular literature provides a list of eye trackers, different eye parameters to differentiate ASD from normal, sub-types and core deficits targeted in ASD.

Table 1. Eye Tracking Systems for ASD Diagnosis

Eye Tracking System	ASD Number	Age	Nature of Stimuli	Parameter Measured	Findings in Asd	Associated Deficit
ISCAN RK-464 remote-eye-tracker *Pelphrey et al., (2002)*	5	25.2 years(mean)	Photographs of facial expressions.	Eye Movements	Scan paths were erratic, unorganized, undirected, unstrategic and less focused on eyes, ears & mouth.	Social information processing deficit
Spectacles mounted with infrared reflection sensors *Takarae et al., (2004)*	46	14-20 years (mean)	Stationary visual targets	Saccades	Saccadic abnormalities, more variations in saccade accuracy.	Cerebellar vermis abnormalities
Head-mounted tracker-501 model *(Speer, Cook, McMahon, & Clark, 2007)*	12	13.6 years(mean age)	Twenty digitized images	Fixation Duration	(i)ASD individuals focused less on eye portion & more on body portion as compared to controls. (ii)Eye fixation time represents processing & understanding social information ability.	Social Responsiveness Deficit.
Eye-tracking equipment *(Klin & Jones, 2008)*	1	15-month-old.	Video & Point-light animations of person's movement.	Eye Velocity, Eyelid Closure, Visual Fixation	More focus on the mouth as compared to eyes of a woman and impaired biological motion recognition.	Social engagement deficit
Tobii-1750 *Sasson et al., (2008)*	29	114.83-months(mean)	12 picture arrays (6 social & object and 6 object-arrays)	Visual Attention	Explored fewer images but their fixation was detail oriented.	Develops repetitive-repeated behavior
Tobii-X50 (Nakano, Kato, & Kitazawa, 2011)	18	29 years (mean)	Three videos (full face, only eyes, only mouth area) of speech giving an actor.	Eye-blink Synchronization	No eye blink synchronization found while viewing at the speaker.	Social communication deficit
SMI iView X™ RED eye tracker (Shic Bradshaw, Klin, Scassellati, & Chawarska, 2011)	28	20.7 months (mean)	30-second video involving an adult female and male child playing with a puzzle.	Gaze Pattern, Blink Rate	ASD individuals were less focused on adult-child playing activities but paid more attention to toys in the background as compared to typically developed.	Observational Learning Deficit, Social Monitoring Deficit, Cognitive Deficit and Higher Autism Severity
IView X RED eye-tracker (Chawarska, Macari, & Shic, 2012)	54	13-25 monthold	A 3-minute video with social (child-directed audio & eye contact) & nonsocial (toys) domain.	Blink detection and region of interest analysis	(i)Reduced attention in case of explicit interaction cues as compared to controls. (ii)Managed to look at the speaker's face and her lip movements for less time as compared to controls.	Social monitoring and attention deficits

continued on following page

Table 1. Continued

Eye Tracking System	ASD Number	Age	Nature of Stimuli	Parameter Measured	Findings in Asd	Associated Deficit
WearCam, Wearable tracker *Magrelli et al., (2013)*	14	2-11 years	Blowing soap bubbles and Play-Doh sessions.	Gaze Behavior	Fails in detecting complex social sounds and facial-speech correlations.	Multi-sensory integration deficit.
Tobii-1750 (Vivanti, Trembath, & Dissanayake, 2014)	24	46.54-months	6 videos	Gaze Monitoring	Abnormalities in monitoring and responding to the goal-directedness behavior of others.	Attention deficit
Electrooculography Electrodes *(Schmitt, Cook, Sweeney, & Mosconi, 2014)*	65	6-44 years(mean age)	Visual targets subtended at 0.5-degree angle	Saccade Latency, Accuracy, and Dynamics	Reduced saccade accuracy with higher variations and prolonged duration.	Sensorimotor control deficit
iView X RED desktop mounted eye-tracker *(Shic, Macari, & Chawarska, 2014)*	High risk=99 and low risk=42	6-month	Facial images: still & moving while expressing and speaking	Gaze Patterns	Less time devoted to the images presented.	Attention deficit in complex social situations.
Tobii X300 *Wang et al., (2015)*	20	30.8 years (mean)	Natural scene images with the pixel, object and semantic features.	Fixations, Saccade Velocity	More preference for image pixel levels, background and center features as compared to object and semantic features in ASD. Slow fixation on face area but fast fixations on objects were found in ASD.	Social Communication
Tobii-T120 *Pierce et al., (2016)*	135	10-49 months.	Movie with social images & geometric patterns.	Eye Fixation, Saccades.	Geometric image preference can be one of the ASD biomarkers.	Social cognition and language deficit
Tobii 1750 non-invasive eye-tracker *(Rigby, Stoesz, & Jakobson, 2016)*	16	27.8 years (mean age)	12 movie clips and still-frame images	Gaze behavior over three areas of interests.	ASD individuals possess more difficulty in processing dynamic social cues as compared to typically developed individuals.	Social attention deficit.
EyeLink-1000 Remote Eye-Tracker *Caruana et al., (2017)*	17	26.47years(mean)	Co-operative Game	Saccade reaction time	Difficulties in responding to joint attention tasks.	Joint attention deficit.
Video-based eye tracker *(Madipakkam, Rothkirch, Dziobek, & Sterzer, 2017)*	17	35.4 years	Three gray scale, female face images with direct and an averted gaze version of each.	Saccades	(i)In ASD adults, atypical responses to eye contact do not depend on other's gaze direction and face perception. (ii) Gaze avoidance in ASD can lead to new diagnostic and intervention strategies.	Social cues sensitivity impairment
Eye Tracker TX300 *(Tsang, 2018)*	8	9.63 years	Human Pictures with different Emotions	Fixation duration and Scan-path	Individuals show atypicalities in judging the complex emotions especially fear emotion.	

This tabular review depicts that the different eye tracking systems such as TX300 or T120 have the advantage of not any interference with the testing sessions (Sasson & Elison, 2012). These systems used different eye parameters for finding the response of the individuals. The selection of the parameter depends upon the nature of the task and experiment such as attention strategies are depicted by fixations and cognitive using scan-paths. These systems have investigated poor orientation to faces, less attention on the eyes, fewer explorations of social images, and abnormal gaze pattern in joint- attention as some of the markers of ASD. The lack of number, as well as real-time based experimental eye tracking studies in ASD, leads to various contradictory results. One such meta-analysis study has favored the conclusion of studies that gaze direction towards the eye region of person is abnormal in ASD, but contradict another one that no atypicalities were found in gaze direction of ASD oriented towards the mouth (Papagiannopoulou, Chitty, Hermens, Hickie, & Lagopoulos, 2014).

The growth in eye tracking studies provided a new dimension to ASD diagnosis and intervention by presenting evidence in favor of unconscious and involuntary gaze avoidance as one of the markers of ASD. The reduced eye gaze fixation on the eye region can be a robust biomarker for ASD as compared to the fixation on mouth area (Boraston & Blakemore, 2007; Papagiannopoulou, Chitty, Hermens, Hickie, & Lagopoulos, 2014). This suggests that although till date eye trackers are not able to directly target the affected brain area for detecting the disorder, but the biomarkers or signatures can differentiate and screen the individuals not only group-wise but also individually.

2. EYE-TRACKING DATA

The eye tracking data involves the eye movement parameters and the different techniques for analyzing the extracted parameters. The following section provides the detailed discussion of eye movement parameters and analysis techniques.

2.1 Eye Movement Parameters

The eye tracking parameters are used to measure the person's attention level, learning rate, behavioral traits, and emotions. As shown in Figure 1, the following are the parameters measured by the eye tracking systems.

1. **Physiological Indices:** These indices provide the value of person's cognitive workload through blink rate and pupil diameter.
    - **Blink Rate:** When the cognitive workload is high the person blinks at the very low rate. The workload tiredness leads to higher blink rate (Bruneau, Sasse, & McCarthy, 2002). The range for blink rate is 100-200 ms (Schiffman, 2001). The blink rate is associated with individual's psychoticism.
    - **Pupil Diameter:** Large pupil diameter may also indicate more cognitive effort (Marshall, 2000; Pomplun & Sunkara, 2003)
2. **Behavioral Indices:** The parameters providing the behavioral index values from the individual's eye movement data. The different indices are:
    a. **Gaze Pattern:** The pattern obtained by summing all the fixation durations over a particular defined area is called gaze pattern. It provides the information about the user's attention

Figure 1. Eye tracking Parameters

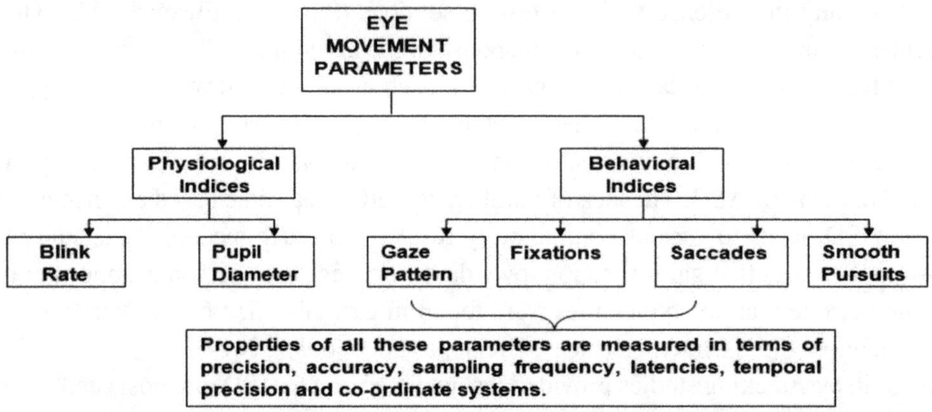

distribution and awareness about their Area of Interest (AOI) (Poole & Ball, 2006). The AOI should be selected in such a way that the AOI's must not overlap with each other else the gaze points would be calculated twice or more number of times. The size of AOI depends upon the accuracy of eye tracker that lies in the range 0.5-1 degree and on human's fovea size which is in 1-2 degree range (Matos, 2010).

b. **Fixations:** The moments where the gaze is stable while visually scanning some static target is known as fixation (Falck-Ytter, Bölte, & Gredebäck, 2013) and is shown in Figure 2. The eyes remain stationary in the process of fixating which indicates that the user is processing the information with greater interest (Poole & Ball, 2006). The information of the visual scene is acquired during fixation. The range of the fixation is from 100ms to 500 ms (Lai, Tsai, Yang, Hsu, Liu, Lee, & Tsai, 2013) and fixation frequency is less than 3Hz. It has been interpreted that longer are the fixations on one area more is the stimulus processing (Falck-Ytter, Bölte, & Gredebäck, 2013) whereas more the overall fixations without any particular AOI lesser is the efficiency. The different fixation parameters required in the analysis of gaze data are (Khachatryan & Rihn, 2014):
   i. **Fixation Count:** It represents the number of fixations.
   ii. **Fixation Duration:** It refers to the processing time implied by the user while fixating on a particular target. The duration is in milliseconds. Longer the fixation duration the more is the difficulty to the user in decoding the fixated object.
   iii. **Total Fixation Duration:** The total fixation duration is the fixation count x fixation duration.
   iv. **Percent Fixated:** It denotes the percentage of subjects fixating on particular AOI.
   v. **Time to First Fixation:** The attention-seeking and interesting properties of the object to be fixated can be measured by calculating the first-fixation time. The faster response in first-fixation indicates that object is much more interesting (Byrne, Anderson, Douglas, & Matessa, 1999).

c. **Saccades:** The fast eye movements which occur rapidly between the fixations are called saccades (Falck-Ytter, Bölte, & Gredebäck, 2013; Poole & Ball, 2006) and are shown in Figure 3. The search frequency depends upon the number of the saccades (Poole & Ball, 2006). The typical value of saccades lies in the range 30-120 ms (Bekele, Wade, Bian, Fan, Swanson, Warren, & Sarkar, 2016). The regressive saccades reveal the confusion and problem a person faces in understanding the visual objects. The saccades are associated with the individual's comprehension difficulties during the reading process. The different saccade parameters are:

i. **Saccade Amplitude:** The attention of the user on particular area/object is measured in terms of the distance/amplitude covered by the eyes (Goldberg & Wichansky, 2003). The saccade amplitude in a range less than 15 or 20 degrees is considered practically (Duchowski, 2007). The succeeding saccade made at higher angles say greater than 90 degrees indicates that the user has changed his direction of looking and may lose his interest.

ii. **Saccade Velocity:** The duration where the neurons acceleration and deceleration leads to the asymmetric waveform is called saccadic velocity. If saccades are small in amplitude then mean velocity is computed, otherwise peak velocity is computed (Di Stasi, Catena, Canas, Macknik, & Martinez-Conde, 2013).

iii. **Saccade Latency:** The time between the target appearance and saccade beginning is called as latency. The latency range is from 100-350 ms but for medium saccade amplitudes, say 5°-10°, it is approximately 200ms.

d. **Smooth Pursuits:** These are the slow eye movements that follow the slowly moving target and stabilize its image on the eye. The spatial attention can be computed from these parameters as the target area is processed properly as compared to other areas besides target. The typical value of the smooth pursuit lies in the range 90-150ms with speed value < 30degree/second. The pattern obtained is asymmetrical in nature when comparing the horizontal and vertical smooth pursuits.

Another parameter like scan-path is also used for measuring the eye movement data and refers to ordered sequential saccades and fixates for particular AOI. In scan-paths fixations are represented in the form of circles and the saccades represent the lines joining the circles (Drusch, Bastien, & Paris, 2014). The desired scan-path needs to be directly aimed at the target with shorter fixation duration (Goldberg & Wichansky, 2003). An efficient scanning is the one in which scan-paths are of more duration and long-lasting (Goldberg & Kotval, 1999). The properties and characteristics which are used to define these parameters are sampling frequency, precision, accuracy, latency, rapidity, temporal precision and co-ordinate system (Freedman & Foxe, 2017).

These parameters are divided into three scales of measurement:

Figure 2. Fixations (Matos, 2010)

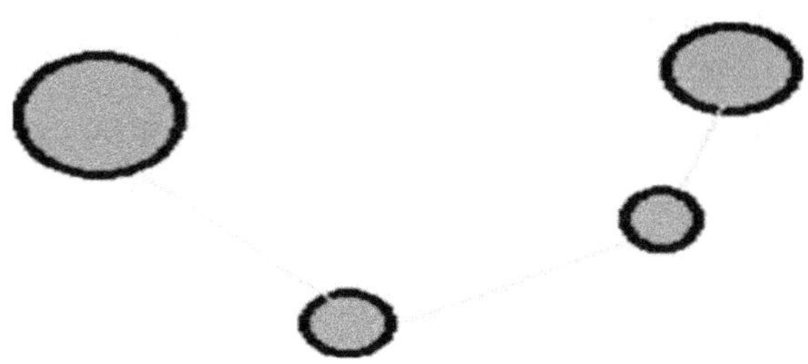

Figure 3. Saccades (Matos, 2010)

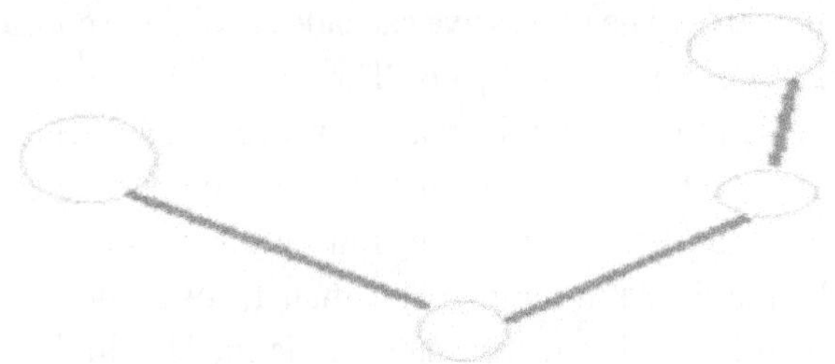

1. **Temporal Scale Measurement:** The measurement of eye movements in time-domain and computing the time duration while performing the reading task. This scale is widely used in the eye tracking studies. The quantitative parameters such as fixation duration, time to the first fixation belong to this measurement scale.
2. **Spatial Scale Measurement:** The measurement of eye movements in space-domain and computing the eyes location, direction, and arrangement in space in visual-perception task. The qualitative parameters belonging to this scale are fixation duration, saccade length. The computation of these parameters is very time consuming and tedious process.
3. **Count Scale Measurement:** The measurement of eye movements on the basis of the frequency of occurrence such as fixation count.

2.2 Eye Movement Data Analysis Techniques

The eye movement parameters described in Figure 1 gives only the numerical values that give only the two-dimensional co-ordinates and distance information failing to extract the complete information about the user. There are algorithms for characterizing fixation density into temporal and spatial information within an area of interest. During analysis, the missing data should be handled properly as it is quite possible to have more amount of missing data in case of disordered individuals. The blinking, head motion and paying less visual attention to stimuli are the possible reasons leading to missing data.

The proper analysis of the described parameters can provide new insights into individual's eye movement physiology. The parameter values need to be filtered prior their analysis with a range of the filter corresponding to their threshold limits. As shown in Figure 4, the eye movement data are analyzed using following methodologies:

1. **Qualitative:** In the qualitative analysis, the eye movement data is analyzed by using the different visualization techniques. The techniques inspect the data visually to distinguish the subjects on the basis of 'where' and for 'how long' they looked.
   a. **Visual Analysis Techniques:** This technique extracts the person's attention distribution from the numerical values and provides the visual representation of the distribution. These techniques are simple, provide a direct view of the eye movement data and are present in all the eye analysis and tracking systems. The different methodologies used for visual analysis are:
      i. **Heat Maps:** These maps can visualize the eye data spatially and visualize fixation counts, absolute and relative gaze duration, and relative gaze duration (Andrienko, Andrienko,

Figure 4. Eye Analysis and Event Detection Methods

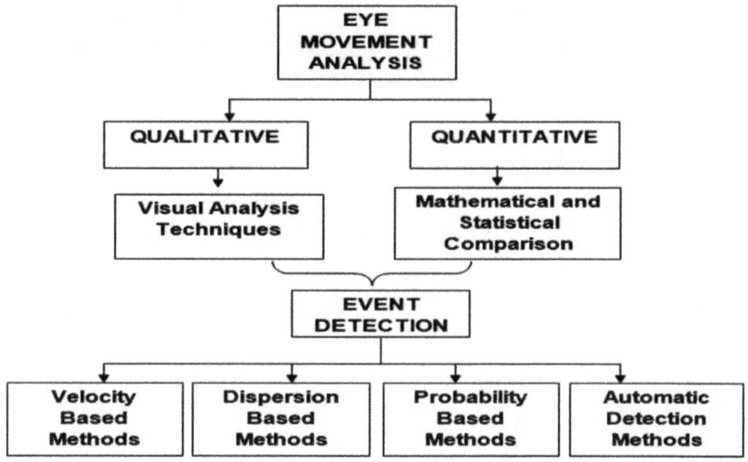

Burch & Weiskopf, 2012). These represent the summation of fixations colors in the heatmap varies with the fixation duration (Drusch, Bastien, & Paris, 2014).

ii. **Gaze-Self Symmetry Plots:** In these plots, the circles are used to represent the fixations and their sizes depend upon the duration of fixation (Andrienko, Andrienko, Burch, & Weiskopf, 2012). The plotting becomes cumbersome when a large amount of eye data appears and hence, is not found very much suitable. The fixations and fixation durations as scan paths can also be represented on these plots. The main problem with this technique is massive overplotting of data.

iii. **Scan Graph:** Two scan paths are compared to calculate their degree of variance (Duchowski, Driver, Jolaoso, Tan, Ramey, & Robbins, 2010). It is chosen in case the tasks are eye movement-focusing tasks.

iv. **Juxtaposed Attention Maps:** It uses different-different display methods to show and compare the attention distribution of a person (Andrienko, Andrienko, Burch, & Weiskopf, 2012).

v. **Density Maps:** The average fixation duration and fixations counts are seen using the density maps. It is helpful in case there are multiple users and provides only aggregate visualizations.

2. **Quantitative:** The mathematical and statistical methodologies are used to analyze the data quantitatively. The raw data is compared statistically for detecting the differences between different groups. For example, comparing number or duration of fixations etc. These methodologies are used for extracting the events from the eye movement data. The simple calculation and comparison of these raw values mathematically and visually do not provide significant results. In order to obtain the suitable and appropriate results, these detected events are then examined properly by using analyzing techniques. The different analysis approaches are:

a. **Velocity Based Methods:** It is one of the simplest methods in which a fixed threshold velocity is chosen for classification of the eye movement data into saccades (fast eye movements) and fixations (slow eye movements). This method is valid if it is limited to two class problem, but introducing any other parameter makes it impossible as one has to handle different threshold levels and real-time task variables (Hoppe & Bulling, 2016). For example, a smooth pursuit, whose velocity varies between fixations and saccades, not only requires a new threshold level setting but also handling other variables like human fatigue and human to human eye velocity variation. The speed and ease with which it can be implemented are the advantages of this method.

b. **Dispersion Based Methods:** In this method, the eye movement data are identified by forming a cluster of the consecutive data around one position in particular dispersion or separation (Hoppe & Bulling, 2016). A moving window spans the data points to check their potential of being clustered together using pre-defined threshold duration/sampling frequency and dispersion threshold parameters. The dispersion of the data points within the window is then investigated using equation given as:

$$D = \{\max(x) - \min(x)\} + \{\max(y) - \min(y)\} \tag{1}$$

where D is a dispersion, x and y represent the coordinates of eye movement data. The window does not group the point say into fixation cluster if D > threshold, and moves to the next point. If D < threshold, the window groups that point to a fixation and this windowing process continues until the end of the protocol. This method is highly robust and provides results with much more accuracy.

c. **Area Based Methods:** In this method, a particular rectangular region is used to identify the eye movement data points say fixations which occur within the specified rectangular target area (Salvucci & Goldberg, 2000). The classification of the data, such as fixations from saccades within the target area is done with the help of duration threshold. The data points lying inside the target area are labeled as fixations and the discarded points are labeled as saccades. Then again, with the help of duration threshold the consecutive fixation points are clustered into groups and groups into fixation tuple.

d. **Probabilistic Methods:** Hidden Markov Model (HMM) uses a probabilistic approach to distinguish between the fixation and saccades (Salvucci & Goldberg, 2000). This model works as two state finite machines and classifies the saccades and fixations on the basis of their probabilistic velocity distributions. The identification of these two parameters is done with the help of the decoding procedure which assigns the fixation and saccade value to the data point. The consecutive points either of saccades or fixations are then transformed into groups. Kalman filters also make use of probabilistic methods to classify the saccades and fixation (Hoppe & Bulling, 2016). It models eye data using velocity and position parameters and estimates the eye state using noisy input data. It also minimizes the error between the estimated and actual state of eye data.

e. **Automatic Detection Methods:** The automatic detection methods are better than traditional methods such as velocity, dispersion and probabilistic methods due to limitations of traditional methods viz. manual thresholding and data pre-segmentation (Hoppe & Bulling, 2016). The rapid increase in data size for more efficient results have made it impossible for the traditional methods to analyze the data efficiently. Machine Learning Techniques: The classifier learns some features during training time and performs automatic event detection on unseen data and categorizes data into fixations, saccades and smooth pursuits. The data is divided into two sets: training and test set. The parameters are first evaluated on the training set and on achieving the optimum performance the evaluation is done on the test set. The advantages are that no need of manual thresholding, stable output free from any noise variation, and can classify the eye parameters using the more information carrying features (Zemblys, Niehorster, Komogortsev, & Holmqvist, 2018). The random tree classifier has been found as the best classifier after comparisons with another classifier (Zemblys, 2016). Recently, Zemblys et al., 2018 used random tree classifier based on 14 feature set to detect the eye parameters and the performance of machine learning algorithm was at the level of an expert.

PRACTICAL ISSUES IN CLINICAL IMPLEMENTATION

The survey of different eye tracking systems has shown that in ASD diagnosis these systems are playing a crucial role. The diagnosis has become very easy with the involvement of trackers, but there are some of the practical issues due to which it is taking time for making them clinically available. The issues are:

- **Parameter Selection:** It has been found that the reliability of the diagnosis depends upon the proper selection of parameters. The parameters might have some limitations and deducing the whole result by relying on single parameter can lead to improper results. The studies surveyed in tabular form have not considered the nature of experiment, parameters compatibility and approach of measuring cognitive load while selecting the eye parameters. For example, pupil diameter has two limitations: sensitivity to luminance and off-axis distortion. In order to obtain better results combination of the different parameters need to be selected and the empirical analysis needs to be based on the integrated parameters to overcome the pitfalls of individual/single parameters and to compute the accuracy values.
- **Analysis Issues:** The event detection algorithms discussed above have some common limitations making them less preferable. The manual thresholding of the eye data points makes it difficult to differentiate between fixations, saccades and smooth pursuits. For example, in case of the area of interest based methods the longer saccades in the target areas are sometimes be considered as fixations (Salvucci & Goldberg, 2000). Hence, the usage of invalid thresholds can bias the result of eye data points (Shic, Scassellati, & Chawarska, 2008). These algorithms are suitable for binary classification of eye data points for example velocity based method find the saccades and rest points are treated as fixations and fail when a third variable needs to be classified in a single step. The data classification turns out to be incorrect if these methods are used with not proposed sampling frequencies (Zemblys, Niehorster, Komogortsev, & Holmqvist, 2018). Various other novel algorithms have been proposed with adaptive thresholding (Mould, Foster, Amano, & Oakley, 2012) but are designed for a specific problem viz. smooth pursuit detection (Larsson, Nystrom, Andersson, & Stridh, 2015), limited noise level ranges (Hessels, Niehorster, Kemner, & Hooge, 2016) and specific purpose viz. detection of microsaccades, separating saccades from smooth pursuit. Due to the disadvantages of these algorithms the eye movement detection systems have shifted to automatic detection methods. The machine learning algorithms make use of handcrafted algorithms which further poses a problem in using them clinically.
- **Validation Challenges:** The validity issue arises due to performing the experiment under controlled situations and without any follow-up studies that can provide the sensitivity and specificity values of the experiment. The studies are limited to the laboratories without considering any real-

world targets for assessing the data of persons. The restriction put on the experiments viz. timing constraints on attention span and the visual pattern is something which is making the study very unreal. Due to this requirement, the studies are limited only to workstations and never reach to real-world clinics.

- **Lack of Collaboration:** Due to lack of assistance of doctors and neurologists the results might be misinterpreted. There is a need for doctors and clinicians collaboration to validate the study and to avoid mistakes.
- **Lack of Correlation:** The eye tracking studies directly indicate the gaze patterns and classify them into normal or abnormal view patterns. The scanning pattern does not correlate with the actual information processing pattern in individuals.
- **Practical Restrictions:** The experts conduct experiments under controlled conditions but for the non-experts, a proper shape and non-manual platform are required to achieve the comparable accuracy. The studies conducted out in the field are very rare, thereby restricting the natural behavioral traits of subjects.
- **Tracker Features:** The infants do have shorter attention and visual spans so the studies conducted on infants will have short designed experiments. The tracker needs to be so fast and accurate so that it can acquire eye movement data in such short duration experiments.
- **Cost:** The cost of the eye trackers is one of the major factors creating hindrance in their clinical availability. Also, in real-time interaction based studies there is a requirement of two or more trackers to understand the social cognitive deficits of individuals. But due to their high cost, these kinds of interaction studies are not feasible.
- **Limitations:** The eye tracking requires intensive calibration, training and holding of the head to reduce artifacts due to head movement. These requirements put few restrictions on natural actions of individuals. This becomes a difficulty in case of disordered individuals such as in case of ASD individuals.
- **Other Issues:** The requirement of an expert, tracing the real-time scope of tools and a large number of samples for generalizing the tool's performance further poses a problem in their clinical availability.

The above-discussed points mainly pose the hindrances in the practical implementation of the eye tracking systems. In addition, the different attributes of the people such as wearing lenses/glasses, pupil color, and long eyelashes can create the problem in recording eye movements accurately. The equipment calibration requires a lot of money, trained users and calibration time are some of the drawbacks of eye tracking systems. The unstructured experimental paradigms such as using animated stimuli or poor presentation of images are the reasons that have led to various contradictory studies. Moreover, the tracker's can involve a single individual in a single slot and do not give the underlying mechanisms related to atypicalities shown by the eye movements.

BRIDGING THE GAPS

The gaps discussed above needs to be filled by providing proper and feasible solutions. The proper analysis of data and customizing eye trackers are the major steps which can solve the clinical issues if done properly. Therefore, some of the solutions are discussed in this section to make the clinical availability of trackers.

1. **Learning-Based Analysis and Proper Feature Set Selection:** Deep Convolutional Neural Networks (CNN) are better because considering sample points, developing features, finding weights and threshold values for classification purpose are all done by themselves in comparison to machine learning theorems where hand-coded algorithms are required to perform all these functions. For CNN implementation accelerators such as Graphics Processing Units (GPUs) are currently deployed to perform parallel computation using a large number of computational cores, provide large data and power to train these models (Lacey, Taylor, & Areibi, 2016). Also, the reproducibility issue of machine learning techniques is resolved by deep learning algorithms.

CNN method provides a signal shape for each eye data point to classify them into fixations, saccades and smooth pursuit within a single learning step. The saccades are recognized from the amplitude variations, fixations have static characteristics with time and smooth pursuits have continuous characteristics along with a smooth change in signal. This approach involves direct learning not only from the continuous eye data values, but also from the eyes of different-different persons (Hoppe & Bulling, 2016; Wang, Wang, & Ji, 2016). The first study to detect saccades, fixations, and smooth pursuits using deep learning is Hoppe (2016) but it does not exploit end-to-end learning approach fully due to use of some handcrafted features. One of the other studies deployed CNN model to find the gaze fixation co-ordinates but did not provide any knowledge about saccades and smooth pursuits. CNN has three layers that select the maximum information carrying features and then reduce the size of features for better classification of the data. All this is done by the network itself without the involvement of frequent human-coded algorithms.

2. **Customize Architecture:** The eye trackers can be customized by integrating them with mobile embedded systems (Motamedi, Gysel, Akella, & Ghiasi, 2016), electronic gadgets and devices with fewer resources (Hailesellasie & Hasan, 2017). In real-world tasks a better hardware which is portable, can process large data and algorithms speedily is mandatory. For customizing these processors with an eye tracker, Field Programmable Gate Array (FPGA) can be a good choice as they are more advantageous than Application Specific Integrated Circuits (ASICs) and can even replace the GPUs in CNN (Motamedi, Gysel, Akella, & Ghiasi, 2016). Some of the advantages are listed below:
    a. Processing of algorithms can be done at much higher speed due to enormous parallelism.
    b. Hardware configuration is flexible and upgradable during model designing.
    c. Fast computation speed leading to better performance.
    d. Easily programmable and reconfigurable.
    e. Can be customized for any special purpose and application (Lacey, Taylor, & Areibi, 2016).
    f. Efficient power consumption.
    g. Performing large-scale operations at a reduced cost.

The motivation behind using FPGA in place of GPU is the emergence of FPGAs in CNN based projects (Ovtcharov, Ruwase, Kim, Fowers, Strauss, & Chung, 2015). Prior studies have utilized FPGA in convolutional layer designing to speed up the performance, less utilization of resources and computation process (Motamedi, Gysel, Akella, & Ghiasi, 2016; Hailesellasie & Hasan, 2017). The block diagram of FPGA based deep learning system for eye tracking has been provided in Figure 5 with FPGA as an alternative to GPUs. The system works as:

A. The subjects are involved in any real-time task viz. interaction or in a classroom environment. During this interaction, the eye tracker is utilized to acquire their eye movement data. The physiological and behavioral eye indices are extracted from the tracked data. In such kind of interactions using more than one eye tracker can provide more accurate data. Feed the eye indices to the CPU where the data is pre-processed before carrying out the data analysis. The filters will remove the noise by removing the invalid points or by reducing the over captured data and interpolating the missing data for better analysis as shown in Figure 6. The fixation filters help in identifying the fixation and saccade at initial stages.
B. Pre-processed data are forwarded to CNN where the features are selected and combined, corresponding to suitable thresholds by the different layers. The feature map is then fed to the classifier. The classifier performance depends upon the importance of the features selected for detection.
C. The sorted feature set which is required for the eye data classification purpose in host processor is sent to the FPGA memory.
D. The processing units in FPGA are designed with the learned parameters to accelerate the operation of CNN will read the data from the memory. The bit-file is compiled offline to define the operations of CNN, which needs to be accelerated. During the runtime, the programming of the FPGA is done in accordance to the bit-file. The offline compiling can be time-consuming but the peculiar nature of CNN to reuse the compile time features in design-phase makes the offline compiling process faster. The data is then processed speedily and the results are placed back on the memory.
E. The results are read from the FPGA memory to CNN on the host processor. The CNN classifiers based on the results fetched from memory will differentiate the ASD subjects from normal with respect to the input eye data features.

Figure 5. Proposed eye tracking system using FPGA for accelerating the data classification

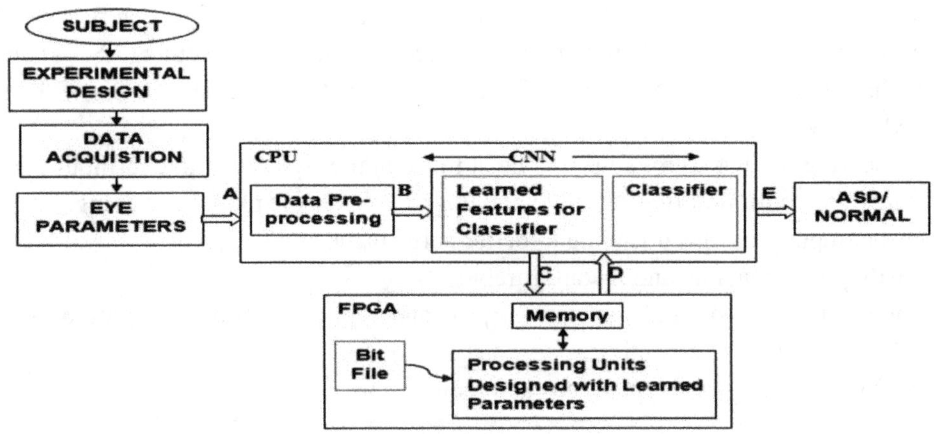

3. **Designing Eye Tracker:** The designing of the new eye trackers can be done with the aim of enhancing the accuracy of the tracking system, without any requirement of intensive calibration, and any restriction on head movement. The trackers can be designed using low processing power platforms viz. mobiles, tablets instead of using computers. These captured signals can be sent through cloud computing to the processors which can analyze the remote data. This kind of thing can even make the eye trackers reach to the less aware places and rural areas. The cost issue and portability of the trackers can be resolved with these kinds of initiatives.
4. **Graphical User Interfaces (GUI):** A GUI can be created to provide a platform to the clinicians that can perform the simple execution of the eye movement data. The GUI can be an integral part of tracking tool by providing separate buttons for displaying stimuli, selecting particular feature set, analyzing data, providing results against selected parameters and plotting gaze curves for much clearer interpretation. One can also keep a record of the individuals by feeding their personal information against their eye diagnostic data.
5. **Open Source Systems:** There should be more and more open source platforms for training the models to provide the results. These systems will allow for reaching the possibility of developing less expensive and processing power hardware. The analysis of the data will be easier with the availability of such systems.
6. **Interdisciplinary Collaboration:** The collaboration among the researchers, clinicians and parents/caretakers of the disordered individuals can provide more user-friendly and an efficient tracker for ASD diagnosis.
7. **Integration with Other Techniques:** The detection accuracy of the trackers can be further enhanced by integrating them with other external electrophysiological signals viz. EEG, Galvanic Skin Response (GSR), Event-Related Potential (ERP) and neuroimaging techniques. This multimodal approach will be reflecting the combined effect of eye-movements with the emotions, perception, attention and cognitive processes that can avoid the overlapping of the disorders diagnosed on the basis of scanning patterns only. This synchronization can provide a holistic view of behavioral traits, individualize the detection and intervention of ASD in real time and can help in correlating person's viewing pattern with his information processing pattern. The problems such as looking at nothing or scanning without meaning can be resolved by this combination. Some integrated systems are available (Bekele, Wade, Bian, Fan, Swanson, Warren, & Sarkar, 2016) but there is a need for more such systems with standardized protocols.

Figure 6. Raw Eye Fixation Data after Filtering

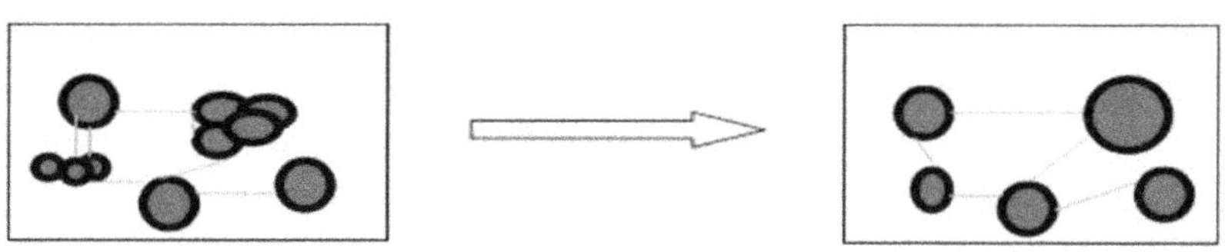

DISCUSSION AND FUTURE SCOPE

The motive of the chapter is to discuss the role of eye trackers in advancing the ASD diagnosis criteria. The advantages of eye trackers make them the perfect substitute for screening scales and neuroimaging techniques. The tracker has dual approach one to diagnose the disorder and another to treat the disorder by being a part of intervention strategies.

Over the years, a lot of changes and advancements have been made in the diagnostic procedure to detect ASD at an early age. Despite these efforts, the age for diagnosis still remains near about 2-2.5 years, which indicates the low availability of gold standard diagnostic tools. The symptoms start appearing right after the birth of a child and demand an initial diagnosis by 12-18 months. The clinical confirmation relies on the lengthy screening scales and expensive medical diagnostic approaches. The screening scales are the preliminary detection techniques that differentiate the atypical individuals from the typically developed. On the basis of scale output, the affected are referred for further medical diagnosis and do not provide any symptom deficit list or their severity levels. The neurological medical techniques study the brain by capturing signals and images using a number of electrodes and seduction methods which in itself is a lengthy and cumbersome process. This is the reason that one cannot follow-up the symptom trajectories and cannot retrace the same. Hence, all these diagnostic methodologies have differences in their opinion making it hard to categorize and detect disorder on even footing. On the other hand, the eye trackers with their objective and quantitative nature of measuring symptoms facilitated us with accurate characterization of disorder and intervention response.

The factors considered while performing eye tracking studies are hypothesis formulation, choosing proper parameters for measuring behavior and associated cognitive mechanism, selecting appropriate tracker and defining the measured data properly for better analysis. Many of the eye tracking studies found using the desktop and electrode based trackers demanding intensive calibration and physical restriction on head and body movement (Shic, Macari, & Chawarska, 2014; Schmitt, Cook, Sweeney, & Mosconi, 2014). These kinds of restrictions can work with adults but in case of children and infants, the tracker should be designed accordingly. The parameters were few and randomly selected by studies, thus failing to validly comment on autism symptoms. The studies have not employed proper fixation filters for data enhancement before carrying out other operations. The fixation filters reduce the data amount by removing invalid and missing data points for efficient analysis. The tracker's high cost and inaccuracies in real-time tasks are some of the factors preventing the universal availability of these systems. Also, various other issues have been discussed that delayed clinical adoption of eye trackers.

The eye movement data provide parameters to consider the different traits of the individuals while tracking eyes. These parameters can provide the entire information about individuals looking criterion, search strategies, and focused area. The parameters should be associated with cognitive processes for a better understanding e.g. fixations are correlated with an individual's attention. The proper familiarization with the eye tracker specifications and the parameter selection is needful before starting the experiment. The parameter analysis is one of the mandatory steps to gain full knowledge about the gaze patterns. Many of the analysis techniques have been discussed and compared on their performance basis. The comparison shows that the detection method should be learning based rather than thresholding for better analysis of the data. Hence, the strength of eye tracking not only lies in its proper calibration but also on the wise selection of integrated parameters and the analysis methodology.

There are plenty of reasons that hinder the eye trackers from being a pervasive technology. When considering these constraints, one needs to remember that the enhancements in trackers can overcome these issues too. Hence, eye trackers have the potential to understand the underlying deficits in ASD and, in turn, help in inventing intervention paradigms for improvement. Also, once the solutions provided in this chapter are implemented, then within no time eye tracker can be the gold-standard diagnostic tool replacing the lengthy and extensive training based techniques. In future, game-based experiments assisted with eye trackers can provide better insights into ASD diagnosis at an early period of individual's life. Such platforms will not only recognized their deficits but will also improve their communicative abilities. The assistance of eye trackers in mobiles and tablets can spread the eye tracking power to everyone's hands.

CONCLUSION

The ideas presented in this chapter have provided a new dimension in the analysis of eye gaze data and in the clinical implementation of the eye tracker. The assistance of eye tracker technology can individualize the ASD diagnosis and intervention in real-time, provide early ASD biomarkers with the possibility of reversing the disorder and can monitor changing symptoms with age. The clinical implementation of eye tracking systems needs full collaboration with the doctors/neurologists for time to time improvement. Learning from looking and generating skills for real-world interaction in ASD is possible with eye tracker as a vital part of different therapies and task evaluation systems, daily activities, robotic diagnosis systems, and virtual reality-based games.

REFERENCES

American Psychiatric Association. (2013). *Diagnostic and statistical manual of mental disorders (DSM-5®)*. American Psychiatric Pub.

Andrienko, G., Andrienko, N., Burch, M., & Weiskopf, D. (2012). Visual analytics methodology for eye movement studies. *IEEE Transactions on Visualization and Computer Graphics*, *18*(12), 2889–2898. doi:10.1109/TVCG.2012.276 PMID:26357198

Aresti-Bartolome, N., & Garcia-Zapirain, B. (2014). Technologies as support tools for persons with autistic spectrum disorder: A systematic review. *International Journal of Environmental Research and Public Health*, *11*(8), 7767–7802. doi:10.3390/ijerph110807767 PMID:25093654

Balan, O., Moldoveanu, A., Moldoveanu, F., Morar, A., & Asavei, V. (2013). Assistive IT for Visually Impaired People. *Journal of Information Systems & Operations Management*, *7*(2), 391–403.

Bekele, E., Wade, J., Bian, D., Fan, J., Swanson, A., Warren, Z., & Sarkar, N. (2016, March). Multimodal adaptive social interaction in a virtual environment (MASI-VR) for children with Autism spectrum disorders (ASD). In Virtual Reality (VR), 2016 IEEE (pp. 121-130). IEEE.

Biswas, P., & Langdon, P. (2014). Eye-gaze Tracking Based Interaction in India. *Procedia Computer Science*, *39*, 59–66. doi:10.1016/j.procs.2014.11.010

Bölte, S., & Hallmayer, J. (Eds.). (2011). *Autism spectrum conditions: FAQs on autism, Asperger syndrome, and atypical autism answered by international experts.* Hogrefe Publishing.

Boraston, Z., & Blakemore, S. J. (2007). The application of eye-tracking technology in the study of autism. *The Journal of Physiology*, *581*(3), 893–898. doi:10.1113/jphysiol.2007.133587 PMID:17430985

Bruneau, D., Sasse, M. A., & McCarthy, J. D. (2002, April).The eyes never lie: The use of eye tracking data in HCI research. *Proceedings of the CHI*, 2, 25.

Byrne, M. D., Anderson, J. R., Douglass, S., & Matessa, M. (1999). Eye tracking the visual search of click-down menus. In *Proceedings of the SIGCHI conference on Human Factors in Computing Systems* (pp. 402-409). ACM. 10.1145/302979.303118

Caruana, N., Stieglitz Ham, H., Brock, J., Woolgar, A., Kloth, N., Palermo, R., & McArthur, G. (2017). Joint attention difficulties in autistic adults: An interactive eye-tracking study. *Autism*, 1362361316676204. PMID:28423919

Chawarska, K., Macari, S., & Shic, F. (2012). Context modulates attention to social scenes in toddlers with autism. *Journal of Child Psychology and Psychiatry, and Allied Disciplines*, *53*(8), 903–913. doi:10.1111/j.1469-7610.2012.02538.x PMID:22428993

Chennamma, H. R., & Yuan, X. (2013). *A survey on eye-gaze tracking techniques.* arXiv preprint arXiv:1312.6410

Coonrod, E. E., & Stone, W. L. (2005). Screening for autism in young children. In F. R. Volkmar, R. Paul, A. Klin, & D. Cohen (Eds.), Handbook of Autism and Pervasive Developmental Disorders (pp. 707–729). New York: Wiley; doi:10.1002/9780470939352.ch1

Di Stasi, L. L., Catena, A., Canas, J. J., Macknik, S. L., & Martinez-Conde, S. (2013). Saccadic velocity as an arousal index in naturalistic tasks. *Neuroscience and Biobehavioral Reviews*, *37*(5), 968–975. doi:10.1016/j.neubiorev.2013.03.011 PMID:23541685

Drusch, G., Bastien, J. C., & Paris, S. (2014). Analysing eye-tracking data: From scanpaths and heatmaps to the dynamic visualization of areas of interest. *Advances in Science, Technology. Higher Education and Society in the Conceptual Age: STHESCA*, *20*, 205.

Duchowski, A. T. (2007). Eye tracking methodology. *Theory into Practice*, 328.

Duchowski, A. T., Driver, J., Jolaoso, S., Tan, W., Ramey, B. N., & Robbins, A. (2010). Scanpath comparison revisited. In *Proceedings of the 2010 symposium on eye-tracking research & applications* (pp. 219-226). ACM. 10.1145/1743666.1743719

Ekinci, O., Arman, A. R., Işık, U., Bez, Y., & Berkem, M. (2010). EEG abnormalities and epilepsy in autistic spectrum disorders: Clinical and familial correlates. *Epilepsy & Behavior*, *17*(2), 178–182. doi:10.1016/j.yebeh.2009.11.014 PMID:20042370

Falck-Ytter, T., Bölte, S., & Gredebäck, G. (2013). Eye tracking in early autism research. *Journal of Neurodevelopmental Disorders*, *5*(1), 28. doi:10.1186/1866-1955-5-28 PMID:24069955

Frank, M. C., Vul, E., & Saxe, R. (2012). Measuring the Development of Social Attention Using Free-Viewing. *Infancy*, *17*(4), 355–375. doi:10.1111/j.1532-7078.2011.00086.x

Frazier, T. W., Klingemier, E. W., Beukemann, M., Speer, L., Markowitz, L., Parikh, S., & Ahuja, V. (2016). Development of an objective autism risk index using remote eye tracking. *Journal of the American Academy of Child and Adolescent Psychiatry*, *55*(4), 301–309. doi:10.1016/j.jaac.2016.01.011 PMID:27015721

Freedman, E. G., & Foxe, J. J. (2017). Eye movements, sensorimotor adaptation and cerebellar-dependent learning in autism: Toward potential biomarkers and subphenotypes. *The European Journal of Neuroscience*, *47*(6), 549–555. doi:10.1111/ejn.13625 PMID:28612953

George, A., & Routray, A. (2015). *Design and Implementation of Real-time Algorithms for Eye Tracking and PERCLOS Measurement for on board Estimation of Alertness of Drivers.* arXiv preprint arXiv:1505.06162

Goldberg, H. J., & Kotval, X. P. (1999). Computer interface evaluation using eye movements: Methods and constructs. *International Journal of Industrial Ergonomics*, *24*(6), 631–645. doi:10.1016/S0169-8141(98)00068-7

Goldberg, H. J., & Wichansky, A. M. (2003). Eye tracking in usability evaluation: A practitioner's guide. In J. Hyönä, R. Radach, & H. Deubel (Eds.), *The mind's eye: Cognitive and applied aspects of eye movement research* (pp. 493–516). Amsterdam: Elsevier. doi:10.1016/B978-044451020-4/50027-X

Guillon, Q., Hadjikhani, N., Baduel, S., & Rogé, B. (2014). Visual social attention in autism spectrum disorder: Insights from eye tracking studies. *Neuroscience and Biobehavioral Reviews*, *42*, 279–297. doi:10.1016/j.neubiorev.2014.03.013 PMID:24694721

Hailesellasie, M., & Hasan, S. R. (2017, May). A fast FPGA-based deep convolutional neural network using pseudo-parallel memories. In *Circuits and Systems (ISCAS), 2017 IEEE International Symposium on* (pp. 1-4). IEEE. 10.1109/ISCAS.2017.8050317

Hames, E. C., Murphy, B., Rajmohan, R., Anderson, R. C., Baker, M., Zupancic, S., ... Richman, D. (2016). Visual, Auditory, and Cross Modal Sensory Processing in Adults with Autism: An EEG Power and BOLD fMRI Investigation. *Frontiers in Human Neuroscience*, *10*, 167. doi:10.3389/fnhum.2016.00167 PMID:27148020

Hessels, R. S., Niehorster, D. C., Kemner, C., & Hooge, I. T. (2017). Noise-robust fixation detection in eye movement data: Identification by two-means clustering (I2MC). *Behavior Research Methods*, *49*(5), 1802–1823. doi:10.375813428-016-0822-1 PMID:27800582

Holmqvist, K., Nyström, M., Andersson, R., Dewhurst, R., Jarodzka, H., & Van de Weijer, J. (2011). *Eye tracking: A comprehensive guide to methods and measures.* Oxford, UK: Oxford University.

Hoppe, S., & Bulling, A. (2016). *End-to-end eye movement detection using convolutional neural networks.* arXiv preprint arXiv:1609.02452

Hua, H., Krishnaswamy, P., & Rolland, J. P. (2006). Video-based eyetracking methods and algorithms in head-mounted displays. *Optics Express*, *14*(10), 4328–4350. doi:10.1364/OE.14.004328 PMID:19516585

Khachatryan, H., & Rihn, A. L. (2014). *Eye-tracking methodology and applications in consumer research.* Retrived from https://edis.ifas.ufl.edu/pdffiles/FE/FE94700.pdf

Klin, A., & Jones, W. (2008). Altered face scanning and impaired recognition of biological motion in a 15-month-old infant with autism. *Developmental Science, 11*(1), 40–46. doi:10.1111/j.1467-7687.2007.00608.x PMID:18171365

Kumar, D., Dutta, A., Das, A., & Lahiri, U. (2016). SmartEye: Developing a novel eye tracking system for quantitative assessment of oculomotor abnormalities. *IEEE Transactions on Neural Systems and Rehabilitation Engineering, 24*(10), 1051–1059. doi:10.1109/TNSRE.2016.2518222 PMID:26780816

Lacey, G., Taylor, G. W., & Areibi, S. (2016). *Deep learning on FPGAS: Past, present, and future.* arXiv preprint arXiv:1602.04283

Lai, M. L., Tsai, M. J., Yang, F. Y., Hsu, C. Y., Liu, T. C., Lee, S. W. Y., & Tsai, C. C. (2013). A review of using eye-tracking technology in exploring learning from 2000 to 2012. *Educational Research Review, 10*, 90–115. doi:10.1016/j.edurev.2013.10.001

Larsson, L., Nyström, M., Andersson, R., & Stridh, M. (2015). Detection of fixations and smooth pursuit movements in high-speed eye-tracking data. *Biomedical Signal Processing and Control, 18*, 145–152. doi:10.1016/j.bspc.2014.12.008

Lupu, R. G., & Ungureanu, F. (2013). A survey of eye tracking methods and applications. *Buletinul Institutului Politehnic din Iaşi,* 71-86.

Madipakkam, A. R., Rothkirch, M., Dziobek, I., & Sterzer, P. (2017). Unconscious avoidance of eye contact with autism spectrum disorder. *Scientific Reports, 7*(1), 13378. doi:10.103841598-017-13945-5 PMID:29042641

Magrelli, S., Jermann, P., Basilio, N., Ansermet, F., Hentsch, F., Nadel, J., & Billard, A. (2013). Social orienting of children with autism to facial expressions and speech: A study with a wearable eye-tracker in naturalistic settings. *Frontiers in Psychology, 4*, 840. doi:10.3389/fpsyg.2013.00840 PMID:24312064

Marshall, S. P. (2000, July). *Method and apparatus for eye tracking and monitoring pupil dilation to evaluate cognitive activity.* U.S. Patent 6,090,051.

Matos, R. (2010). *Designing eye-tracking experiments to measure human behavior.* Retrived from http://www.measuringbehavior.org/files/tutorials/Tobii_MB2010_tutorial_handouts.pdf

Matson, J. L., Nebel-Schwalm, M., & Matson, M. L. (2007). A review of methodological issues in the differential diagnosis of autism spectrum disorders in children. *Research in Autism Spectrum Disorders, 1*(1), 38–54. doi:10.1016/j.rasd.2006.07.004

Motamedi, M., Gysel, P., Akella, V., & Ghiasi, S. (2016). Design space exploration of -based deep convolutional neural networks. In *Design Automation Conference (ASP-DAC), 2016 21st Asia and South Pacific*(pp. 575-580). IEEE. 10.1109/ASPDAC.2016.7428073

Mould, M. S., Foster, D. H., Amano, K., & Oakley, J. P. (2012). A simple nonparametric method for classifying eye fixations. *Vision Research, 57*, 18–25. doi:10.1016/j.visres.2011.12.006 PMID:22227608

Nakano, T., Kato, N., & Kitazawa, S. (2011). Lack of eyeblink entrainments in autism spectrum -disorders. *Neuropsychologia, 49*(9), 2784–2790. doi:10.1016/j.neuropsychologia.2011.06.007 PMID:21699907

Ovtcharov, K., Ruwase, O., Kim, J. Y., Fowers, J., Strauss, K., & Chung, E. S. (2015). Accelerating deep convolutional neural networks using specialized hardware. *Microsoft Research Whitepaper, 2*(11).

Ozonoff, S., Iosif, A. M., Young, G. S., Hepburn, S., Thompson, M., Colombi, C., & Rogers, S. J. (2011). Onset patterns in autism: Correspondence between home video and parent report. *Journal of the American Academy of Child and Adolescent Psychiatry, 50*(8), 796–806. doi:10.1016/j.jaac.2011.03.012 PMID:21784299

Papagiannopoulou, E. A., Chitty, K. M., Hermens, D. F., Hickie, I. B., & Lagopoulos, J. (2014). A systematic review and meta-analysis of eye-tracking studies in children with autism spectrum disorders. *Social Neuroscience, 9*(6), 610–632. PMID:24988218

Pardini, M., Elia, M., Garaci, F. G., Guida, S., Coniglione, F., Krueger, F., & Gialloreti, L. E. (2012). Long-term cognitive and behavioral therapies, combined with augmentative communication, are related to uncinate fasciculus integrity in autism. *Journal of Autism and Developmental Disorders, 42*(4), 585–592. doi:10.100710803-011-1281-2 PMID:21573693

Pelphrey, K. A., Sasson, N. J., Reznick, J. S., Paul, G., Goldman, B. D., & Piven, J. (2002). Visual scanning of faces in autism. *Journal of Autism and Developmental Disorders, 32*(4), 249–261. doi:10.1023/A:1016374617369 PMID:12199131

Pierce, K., Marinero, S., Hazin, R., McKenna, B., Barnes, C. C., & Malige, A. (2016). Eye tracking reveals an abnormal visual preference for geometric images as an early biomarker of an autism spectrum disorder subtype associated with increased symptom severity. *Biological Psychiatry, 79*(8), 657–666. doi:10.1016/j.biopsych.2015.03.032 PMID:25981170

Pomplun, M., & Sunkara, S. (2003, June). Pupil dilation as an indicator of cognitive workload in human-computer interaction. *Proceedings of the International Conference on HCI.*

Poole, A., & Ball, L. J. (2006). Eye tracking in HCI and usability research. Encyclopedia of Human-Computer Interaction, 1, 211-219.

Port, R. G., Anwar, A. R., Ku, M., Carlson, G. C., Siegel, S. J., & Roberts, T. P. (2015). Prospective MEG biomarkers in ASD: Pre-clinical evidence and clinical promise of electrophysiological signatures. *The Yale Journal of Biology and Medicine, 88*(1), 25. PMID:25745372

Rigby, S. N., Stoesz, B. M., & Jakobson, L. S. (2016). Gaze patterns during scene processing in typical adults and adults with autism spectrum disorders. *Research in Autism Spectrum Disorders, 25*, 24–36. doi:10.1016/j.rasd.2016.01.012

Rudra, A., Belmonte, M. K., Soni, P. K., Banerjee, S., Mukerji, S., & Chakrabarti, B. (2017). Prevalence of autism spectrum disorder and autistic symptoms in a school-based cohort of children in Kolkata, India. *Autism Research, 10*(10), 1597–1605. doi:10.1002/aur.1812 PMID:28544637

Salvucci, D. D., & Goldberg, J. H. (2000). Identifying fixations and saccades in eye-tracking protocols. In *Proceedings of the 2000 Symposium on Eye Tracking Research & Applications* (pp. 71-78). ACM. 10.1145/355017.355028

Sasson, N. J., & Elison, J. T. (2012). Eye tracking young children with autism. *Journal of Visualized Experiments*, *61*, 3675. PMID:22491039

Sasson, N. J., Turner-Brown, L. M., Holtzclaw, T. N., Lam, K. S., & Bodfish, J. W. (2008). Children with autism demonstrate circumscribed attention during passive viewing of complex social and nonsocial picture arrays. *Autism Research*, *1*(1), 31–42. doi:10.1002/aur.4 PMID:19360648

Schiffman, H. R. (2001). Fundamental visual functions and phenomena. *Sensation and Perception*, 89-115.

Schmitt, L. M., Cook, E. H., Sweeney, J. A., & Mosconi, M. W. (2014). Saccadic eye movement abnormalities in autism spectrum disorder indicate dysfunctions in cerebellum and brainstem. *Molecular Autism*, *5*(1), 47. doi:10.1186/2040-2392-5-47 PMID:25400899

Shic, F., Bradshaw, J., Klin, A., Scassellati, B., & Chawarska, K. (2011). Limited activity monitoring in toddlers with autism spectrum disorder. *Brain Research*, *1380*, 246–254. doi:10.1016/j.brainres.2010.11.074 PMID:21129365

Shic, F., Macari, S., & Chawarska, K. (2014). Speech disturbs face scanning in 6-month-old infants who develop autism spectrum disorder. *Biological Psychiatry*, *75*(3), 231–237. doi:10.1016/j.biopsych.2013.07.009 PMID:23954107

Shic, F., Scassellati, B., & Chawarska, K. (2008, March). The incomplete fixation measure. In *Proceedings of the 2008 Symposium on Eye Tracking Research & Applications* (pp. 111-114). ACM. 10.1145/1344471.1344500

Speer, L. L., Cook, A. E., McMahon, W. M., & Clark, E. (2007). Face processing in children with autism: Effects of stimulus contents and type. *Autism*, *11*(3), 265–277. doi:10.1177/1362361307076925 PMID:17478579

Sperdin, H. F., & Schaer, M. (2016). Aberrant development of speech processing in young children with autism: New insights from neuroimaging biomarkers. *Frontiers in Neuroscience*, *10*, 393. doi:10.3389/fnins.2016.00393 PMID:27610073

Takarae, Y., Minshew, N. J., Luna, B., & Sweeney, J. A. (2004). Oculomotor abnormalities parallel cerebellar histopathology in autism. *Journal of Neurology, Neurosurgery, and Psychiatry*, *75*(9), 1359–1361. doi:10.1136/jnnp.2003.022491 PMID:15314136

Tanu, W., & Kakkar, D. (2018). A Study on Machine Learning Based Generalized Automated Seizure Detection System. In *Proceedings of 8th International Conference on Cloud Computing, Data Science and Engineering. CONFLUENCE 2018*. (pp. 20), IEEE.

Tsang, V. (2018). Eye-tracking study on facial emotion recognition tasks in individuals with high-functioning autism spectrum disorders. *Autism*, *22*(2), 161–170. doi:10.1177/1362361316667830 PMID:29490486

Tseng, P. H., Cameron, I. G., Pari, G., Reynolds, J. N., Munoz, D. P., & Itti, L. (2013). High-throughput classification of clinical populations from natural viewing eye movements. *Journal of Neurology*, *260*(1), 275–284. doi:10.100700415-012-6631-2 PMID:22926163

Vargas-Cuentas, N. I., Roman-Gonzalez, A., Gilman, R. H., Barrientos, F., Ting, J., Hidalgo, D., ... Zimic, M. (2017). Developing an eye-tracking algorithm as a potential tool for early diagnosis of autism spectrum disorder in children. *PLoS One*, *12*(11), e0188826. doi:10.1371/journal.pone.0188826 PMID:29190703

Vidal, M., Turner, J., Bulling, A., & Gellersen, H. (2012). Wearable Eye Tracking for Mental Health Monitoring. *Computer Communications*, *35*(11), 1306–1311. doi:10.1016/j.comcom.2011.11.002

Vivanti, G., Trembath, D., & Dissanayake, C. (2014). Atypical monitoring and responsiveness to goal-directed gaze in autism spectrum disorder. *Experimental Brain Research*, *232*(2), 695–701. doi:10.100700221-013-3777-9 PMID:24292493

Wang, A. T., Dapretto, M., Hariri, A. R., Sigman, M., & Bookheimer, S. Y. (2004). Neural correlates of facial affect processing in children and adolescents with autism spectrum disorder. *Journal of the American Academy of Child and Adolescent Psychiatry*, *43*(4), 481–490. doi:10.1097/00004583-200404000-00015 PMID:15187809

Wang, K., Wang, S., & Ji, Q. (2016, March). Deep eye fixation map learning for calibration-free eye gaze tracking. In *Proceedings of the Ninth Biennial ACM Symposium on Eye Tracking Research & Applications* (pp. 47-55). ACM. 10.1145/2857491.2857515

Wang, S., Jiang, M., Duchesne, X. M., Laugeson, E. A., Kennedy, D. P., Adolphs, R., & Zhao, Q. (2015). Atypical visual saliency in autism spectrum disorder quantified through model-based eye tracking. *Neuron*, *88*(3), 604–616. doi:10.1016/j.neuron.2015.09.042 PMID:26593094

Wästlund, E., Shams, P., Löfgren, M., Witell, L., & Gustafsson, A. (2010). Consumer perception at point of purchase: Evaluating proposed package designs in an eye-tracking lab. *Journal of Business and Retail Management Research*, *5*(1), 41–50.

Zemblys, R. (2016). Eye-movement event detection meets machine learning. *Biomedical Engineering*, *20*(1).

Zemblys, R., Niehorster, D. C., Komogortsev, O., & Holmqvist, K. (2018). Using machine learning to detect events in eye-tracking data. *Behavior Research Methods*, *50*(1), 160–181. doi:10.375813428-017-0860-3 PMID:28233250

Zwaigenbaum, L., Thurm, A., Stone, W., Baranek, G., Bryson, S., Iverson, J., ... Rogers, S. (2007). Studying the emergence of autism spectrum disorders in high-risk infants: Methodological and practical issues. *Journal of Autism and Developmental Disorders*, *37*(3), 466–480. doi:10.100710803-006-0179-x PMID:16897376

KEY TERMS AND DEFINITIONS

Assistance: The support provided by any system to help another system.

Autism: An early childhood atypical condition characterized by impairment in social interaction and communication.

Autism Spectrum Disorder: Wide range of symptoms leading to individual's brain disability.

Deep Learning: A learning algorithm using a number of layers for extracting and learning feature hierarchies before providing an output for any input.

Diagnosis: Process of studying the symptoms for identifying any disorder or atypical condition.

Eye Tracker: A device that can measure eye movement data viz. fixations and saccades.

Field Programmable Gate Array (FPGA): A programmable semiconductor device allowing designers to configure any design using its logic blocks.

Technology: A tool for investigating and discovering the solution for a problem.

Chapter 8
Eye Tracking as a Tool for Diagnosing Specific Learning Disabilities

Azeez Rizwana
St. Paul's School, India

ABSTRACT

The chapter intends to highlight the use of eye tracker, a tool that tracks eye movements, as a potential tool to aid diagnosis of specific learning disabilities along with psychometric tests. The issue of identifying and assessing children for specific learning disabilities is very difficult and crucial for the psychological, social, and personal wellbeing of the child growing into an adult. A common technique for diagnosing specific learning disabilities is the need of the hour. The eye is considered to be the window to the brain. Any differences in the eye movement can reflect disorders or diseases in the functional areas of cerebral cortex, brain stem, cerebellum, and other areas of the brain. The most important contribution of eye tracking research is it allows examination of different aspects of cognitive performance in moment-to-moment details on very simple tasks and infer the neurobiological basis of cognitive processes. Therefore, the chapter focuses on studies related to use of eye trackers as a futuristic technique in the diagnosis of specific learning disabilities.

INTRODUCTION

The school failure and school dropouts have most of the time been the reason for children not being diagnosed with specific learning disabilities. Therefore, accurate diagnosis during early years of growth, though not an easy task, becomes the need of the hour. The traditional paper-based diagnostic tests for dyslexia are used in different parts of the world such as Diagnostescher Rechtschrieb test (Grund, Naumann, & Haug, 2004) for German, Wide-Range Achievement Test (Wilkinson, 1993) for English, and NIMHANS index of specific learning disabilities (Kapur, John, Rozario, & Oommen, 2002), analyze mostly reading and writing skills and confirm the diagnosis for dyslexia. These tests seem to have limitations because:

DOI: 10.4018/978-1-5225-7004-2.ch008

- They test the behavioral component, that is, the performance to predict the cognitive potential of the child.
- Need unbiased expert knowledge in interpreting results.
- Testing environment may affect the child's level of functioning that may result in discrepancies in findings.
- They are language specific.
- Focus more on reading and the mathematical ability for diagnosis questioning the severity of cognitive dysfunction.

Eye tracking can be an important tool to aid diagnosis of learning disability for a diverse population. Eye trackers record eye movements to predict the cognitive skill/ability of the individual. One can observe and understand the pattern of eye movement through scan path and maps, the duration of time with fixations and saccades while moving the eye along the stimuli. It provides detailed data on the ease and difficulty of reading a text even the subtle difference of whether the text is given was difficult or the individual is finding it difficult and the level or extent of difficulty to read is very clear. It also gives detailed data as to the difference between reading a linguistic or non-linguistic task. Eye trackers are user-friendly and come in various forms from head-mounted to mobile eye trackers making it tailor-made for the specific use. One has to be trained for using and handling data collection for a couple of months to be able to use eye trackers as an aid for diagnosis. The data thus collected may be analyzed by expert psychologists thereby saving a lot of time for experts and providing time-locked online measurements for analysis of the specific level of cognitive functioning.

Research in the field of eye tracking as a tool for diagnosis has been picking up in western countries and has proven to be useful especially in the diagnosis of specific learning disabilities. Studies in India also reveal differences in eye movement pattern in children with specific learning disabilities especially in linguistic tasks as compared to non-linguistic tasks.

EYE AND THE VISUAL SYSTEM: A WINDOW TO THE BRAIN

The most primitive, immediate and involuntary behavior witnessed in infants is to look. This is a major route to the child's mind/brain functioning. Looking involves eye movement, when measured; provide insight into a child's spatial and temporal perception of his/her world. It is almost effortless and natural for humans to take the world through the eye. In fact, we live in a visual world perceiving almost everything through the eye and comprehending through the brain. Eye movements are considered to be the window to the brain hence a way to understand/ study cognitive abilities of an individual to perceive, recognize and comprehend the world around him/her. It is quite natural that we look at the most relevant and interesting part of an object/text/image necessary to recognize and comprehend and therefore move our eyes only to those selective areas. Furthermore, the pupil of the eye not only moves to extract information, decide where to see but also dilate rapidly to an array of cognitive and emotional stimuli thus revealing a great deal about processes like recognition, cognitive abilities, memory, thinking, feelings, learning, comprehension, socio-emotional and many other cognitive processes.

Therefore, studying eye movements may be a potential way to understand underlying cognitive abilities of an individual which is the neurobiological basis of developmental disabilities hence may be considered a very important tool for diagnostic procedures and health management systems. To understand eye movements, one has to know how the visual system works. The eye has to move in order to extract information from the stimuli. The visual angle is anywhere between 2 to 5 degrees; vision is accurate at the foveal region, that is, 2 ^{0} in the center of the retina where vision is sharpest and the information is extracted. The area around the foveal region, i.e. 5 ^{0} on either side of foveal region is the parafoveal region; partial information being extracted from the parafovea facilitates the reader. The area around the parafovea is said to be the peripheral vision where vision is very poor and extracting information is difficult to impossible (Lima & Inhoff, 1985; Rayner, Well, Pollatsek, & Bertera, 1982). Therefore, to bring the object into the foveal vision, one has to move the eye. When the information is extracted through the foveal vision, it is sent to specific centers of the brain through the optic nerve where the stimuli are recognized and comprehended. Especially, during the act of reading, the eye has to constantly and consistently move to bring the text to the foveal region.

Eye tracking as a tool for investigation becomes important because it is through the eye that individual gains information about the text being read or the stimuli being presented. Eye movements are involuntary, unconscious and automatic; it enables researchers to study the underlying processing strategies like attention, memory, comprehension, reasoning etc.

CURRENT ISSUES

Observational studies report children with learning disabilities often find difficulty in learning the skill of reading, writing or mathematical abilities, along with difficulty learning simple tasks like listening, attention, speaking, reasoning concentrating and organizing information; difficulty mastering social skills and motor coordination. When such difficulties are overlooked children with learning disabilities tend to either internalize or externalize their difficulties resulting in low confidence, low self-esteem (internalizing behavior) or frustration, aggression (externalizing behavior). Current issues in widely used psychometric tests are that they report difficulty in language and mathematical skills whereas there is much more to the diagnosis of specific learning disabilities.

Screening for specific learning disabilities has been a debated topic in diverse populations. Especially, in the Indian context, multilingualism, culturally diverse population, accessibility and expertise demand tailor-made batteries for screening children for specific learning disabilities. A common technique for diagnosing specific learning disabilities is the need of the hour and eye tracking may be the answer to overcome discrepancies owing to its accuracy and explicit data. The prevalence and patterns of dyslexia studied in the Indian context suggests:

- The incidence of children diagnosed with dyslexia increased with age attributed to the absence of screening procedures in schools.
- Order of birth has been reported as a reason for the incidence of dyslexia.
- Family type (nuclear family) for children affected with dyslexia 13%, 5-15% (Karande & Kulkarni, 2005), 15.75% (Moqasale, Paul, Patil, & Mogasale, 2012), 2-10% (Shah, Parwar, & Shah, 1998). The differences in results have been attributed to the different traditional scales used instead of one standard method. This may be highlighted as a limitation of psychometric tests and use of eye trackers as an aid for accurate results.
- It is noted that 5-10% of healthy looking children suffering from learning disability have been diagnosed only after they experienced academic problems in school and invariably failed.

The fundamental reason for lack of awareness in the diagnosis of learning disabilities is that many are unaware of the cognitive processes involved and the differences in learning a spoken language and learning the skill of reading. While spoken language is learnt almost naturally through observation, listening and differentiating sounds from infancy through childhood, reading and writing are skills that involve decoding and encoding phonemic structure indigenous to the language and therefore have to be explicitly taught. While reading is a skill of extracting meaning from written symbols, writing is phoneme encoded into an orthographic system. The ability to decode the encoded text and comprehend has to be skillfully learnt with consistent practice. Normally, children learn the skill that seems effortless for a typically growing child, conversely a few sets of children developing normally with their intellectual ability intact fail to pick up with the processes of decoding and encoding text. These children struggle with the different phonetic combinations in every word resulting in slowing down the whole process of learning the skill to read or write. As if conspiring intellectual ability with the skill to read thereby prevents the child from reaching his/her full potential. This group of children falls into the category of reading disability / specific learning disability/ dyslexia/ reading difficulty/disorder.

Hence, phonological knowledge becomes very important, that is, phonetic and acoustic features of a language; segmental knowledge like phonemes and suprasegmental knowledge like rhyme and prosody (Morais, 2003). Moreover, it is evident that phonological knowledge plays a critical role in learning the skill of reading. It is necessary to learn identification and manipulation of individual letters in a word which normal readers do effortlessly while children with dyslexia fall short in this area. This phonological deficit reported in children with dyslexia leads to poorer reading development (Bradley & Byrant, 1983).

Research in this field suggests that children with dyslexia have difficulty in the ability to generalize spelling-to-sound correspondence, that is, use of suprasegmental knowledge (Goswami, 1999). Other studies also report that children with dyslexia sparingly use rhyme analogy cues when compared to normal readers.

Furthermore, the phonological deficit hypothesis suggests the etiology of dyslexia may be due to impairment or difficulty in representing speech sounds resulting in low-level auditory processing seen in reading disabilities (Snowling, 1995; Shaywitz & Shaywitz, 2005). Studies in English (Rack, Snowling, & Olson, 1992) and German (Wimmer, 1996) reported dyslexic readers exhibited difficulty in suppressing/replacing initial/final phonemes. A cross-linguistic review of English, German, French and Spanish reported dyslexic readers experienced difficulty processing rhymes, syllables and phonemes, with respect to orthographic transparency, automatically.

Nevertheless, the phonemic complexity of a language is reflected in the ability to decipher individual phonemes in a written word which points out the linguistic origin (Vellutino, Fletcher, Snowling, & Scanlon, 2004; Granet, Castro, Gomi, 2006). Therefore, reading involves the integration of grapheme-phoneme-correspondence rules, phonological awareness, individual's experience, cognitive abilities and extent of neurological functioning.

With all the above intact, children with a neurological deficit may have difficulty in processing the sound structure of a given language in its written form. Research in this area has enough evidence proving the neurological basis of individuals experiencing processing difficulties as per the phonological coding deficit theory of reading disabilities (Shaywitz, Shaywitz, Pugh, Mencl, Fulbright, Skudlarski, …& Gore, 2002; Shaywitz, 1998).

Additionally, when compared to other cognitive abilities, dyslexia, stems from the processing difficulties of the written word in the brain. Studies in neuroimaging revealed the relationship between brain responses seen in infancy were good predictors of a reading problem later in life of an individual.

A study by Molfese (2000) confirmed that brain responses of speech sounds of an infant as early as 36 hours of birth could be used to discriminate dyslexia in later years with 81% accuracy in prediction. Also, neuroscientific research using fMRI and PET scans reported left hemisphere predominance for reading in general and inferior frontal, superior temporal, parieto-temporal, mid-temporal mid-occipital gyri, in particular, seemed to be involved in typical readers whereas children with dyslexia reported to demonstrate dysfunction in the left hemisphere and compensatory use of both hemispheres. However, these neurological abnormalities have found to have improved with phonological training and intervention over the years.

The issue of identifying and assessing children for specific learning disabilities is very difficult and crucial at the same time for the psychological, social, and personal well-being of a child growing into an adult. Furthermore, the manifestation of learning disabilities depends on varying settings, overtime, and environment making the task difficult to estimate the severity and specificity of the disorder. Diagnosis of specific learning disabilities needs comprehensive assessment. Hence, it is important to integrate other methods as tools for differential diagnosis, it is here that eye trackers come as an aid along with psychometric tests because differential diagnosis provides accurate distinguishing characteristics between and among other disorders.

In the Indian context, lack of awareness among parents and educators, policies and the gaps, socio-economic status, diverse cultures and environments, social beliefs, superstitions, faiths, multilingual-multi orthographic systems make the use of standardized tests questionable and a fundamental issue in the assessment of children with special needs (Ramaa, 2000).

A general consensus of assessment of any psychological disorder follows the standardized psychometric tests or criterion-referenced tests. These approaches are fairly well adapted and accepted for their reliability and validity for interpretation of results. What is overlooked in these approaches is that they often obscure the actual impairment of various skills. Especially in a country like India, these approaches lack revision, are not adept to the multilingual-multi orthographic society, less sensitive to reader's linguistic, cultural and economic background thereby limiting the interpretative capacity of the psychometric batteries and in the milieu labelling the child without much choice which later affects the child's personal growth and strategies for intervention. One needs to realize a method free of such limitations and more natural in assessing the child's abilities.

EYE TRACKING

Eye tracking as a tool for investigation becomes important because it is through the eye that an individual gains information about the surroundings. It enables researchers and psychologists to study and identify/point out the underlying processing strategies when information is being perceived from the surroundings. The fovea is a region of the eye where vision is sharpest and partial information is received from the parafovea facilitating the individual to comprehend the stimuli being perceived. Eye tracking as a tool, in reading research, has been successful in obtaining accurate, moment-to-moment, online, spatial and temporal record for every word irrespective and independent of a word being used in isolation or in context (Just & Carpenter, 1980; Rayner, 1998).

However, as the foveal region is limited, an individual has to make eye movements to access a particular part of the text while reading. This movement from one word or a part of the text to another is called a '*saccade*'. The duration of a saccade depends on its length and takes around 20-30ms hence no/

little information is extracted (Matin, 1974). After a saccade, the eye lands on an area of the text which is termed as a '*fixation*'. The duration of a fixation helps in extracting information from the text being read. The fixation duration can be short, long, skipped, or regressed according to the frequency, word length, linguistic features of a language, ease or difficulty of the text, visual acuity and the skill of the reader (Rayner, 1998).

It is understood that fixation duration measures reveal early and late processing stages. Extensive research in eye movement suggest lexical processing to be rapid (less than 50ms) (Rayner & Duffy, 1986), automatic and autonomous (Seidenberg, Tanenhaus, Leiman, & Beinkowski, 1982) while post-lexical effects to be slow (125-200ms) (Seidenberg et al., 1982). First fixation duration measure is said to be a window to early processing stage and Dwell time, which is the sum of total fixations and saccades on an area of interest irrespective of it is the only fixation or the first of multiple fixations, is considered a late processing measure. Eye movement studies suggest fixation duration lasts for about 200-250ms for English with 7-9 letter spaces saccades (Rayner & Bertera, 1979; Rayner, Inhoff, Morrison, Slowiaczek, & Bertera, 1981).

Eye tracking enables recording of different variables in a natural set up when other methods like the direct assessment of static or dynamic stimuli in accordance with the cognitive task demands become difficult. To understand eye movements, one has to know the different eye movement measures.

1. **Calibration:** The first step to use an eye tracker effectively to record eye movements is to calibrate. The eye has to be tuned to the eye tracker algorithm. The points of calibration ensure that the external stimulus is coordinated to the participants' eye and the eye tracker algorithm. The process of calibration cues the participants' attention to a series of locations and the eye tracking camera records these coordinates of the pupil center and the first Purkinge image (a small, bright reflection created on the cornea). To ensure the subjects attention on a particular area the eye tracking system marks the number of calibration points from 2-13. The more the number of points the better the spatial accuracy. The calibrated area has to correspond exactly to the location of the stimuli both the distance between the eye tracker and the eye; and the horizontal and vertical extensions of the scene. To ensure accuracy in calibration, the experimenter presents different cues on the area of the stimulus being presented so that the participant's eye movement matches the points marked on the location of stimulus. This is a very important step, only after successful calibrations can the eye tracker record data that is accurate and useful for analysis.
2. **Saccades:** The movement of the eye while viewing a visual scene or object is called a saccade. This movement of the eye helps in building a 'mental map' consisting the relevant parts of the scene/ object. The movement is involuntary, unconscious, and automatic. The reason for this is the small central region of the retina (fovea). Unless the image/scene does not come into the foveal region, it becomes difficult to perceive or comprehend the stimuli. To enable this eye makes the ballistic movement to bring the visual stimuli to the foveal region necessary for the cognitive ability of comprehension. The duration of the saccade depends on the angular distance the eye travels with an approximate velocity of 600^0 per second lasting form 10-100 milliseconds (Duchowski, 2007). The main measure of a saccade is duration, peak velocity, amplitude, gain (saccade amplitude/target amplitude) and latency. The initiation of a saccade lasts for about 30-120ms for amplitude up to 45 degrees; a peak velocity ranges from 200 to 400 degrees/second and it takes 180-250 milliseconds after stimulus onset for a saccade to initiate.

3. **Fixation:** The eye lands on an area of interest after a saccade. This landing of the eye is called a fixation. The time/duration of the eye stays in the area of interest is called a *fixation duration (FD)*. The first time the eye lands and stays on the area of interest are called the *first fixation duration (FFD)*. The total number of fixation duration on an area of interest between two saccades is the *gaze duration (GD)*. *Regressions* are another set of eye movements when the eye returns back to the previous area of interest after having crossed it, that is while reading a text when we return back to a word/sentence after having read it is a regression. First fixation duration is a measure that indicates the ease of processing a stimulus or the simple characteristics of the stimuli. For example, if the stimulus is a frequent object the FFD measure reflects ease of processing and if the stimulus is complex the FFD is not found to be significant. Hence FFD is considered to be an early processing measure of cognitive abilities.
4. **Fixation Duration (FD):** Is a measure that indicates the time taken by the subject to comprehend the stimuli. Gaze Duration (GD) measure is a late processing measure indicating difficulty in comprehending (a cognitive process) or the difficulty (complexity of the stimuli) of the stimuli and regression measure suggests the difficulty in comprehending the stimuli as the eye had to return back for a second look to understand the presented stimuli.
5. **Pursuit:** To track eye movement on small slow-moving objects, researchers use smooth pursuit. In comparison to saccades that are ballistic and involuntary, smooth pursuit eye movements are non-ballistic, voluntary and match gaze velocity to target velocity to keep the object in foveal vision. For example, when we see a moving car we tend to follow the moving car with slower velocity and longer duration. To assess smooth pursuit eye movement participants visually track small, slow-moving predictable velocity stimuli along a horizontal path. Low gain scores indicate difficulty in the functioning of the smooth pursuit eye movement.
6. **Eye Movements Through Scene Perception:** Typically growing individuals take 3-4 saccades/second and pause in between (fixate) for about 300-400ms at a time on a stimulus. During this time not only do we try to recognize and comprehend the stimuli but also decide where to fixate next? The most important eye movement measure to study scene/face perception are fixation location (where the eyes fixate), fixation duration (how long does the eye stay on the area of interest) and sequence (the pattern of the fixation on different areas of the stimuli and the distance between successful, subsequent and consecutive fixations. Location and sequencing measures infer attention and order/pattern. Fixation duration measure infers the speed of processing and distance between fixations signifies width of attentional spotlight. When a task is difficult and needs more fine-grained information, fixation duration increases and saccade amplitude decreases.

Data Coding and Analysis

1. The software tools provided in the eye tracker enables researchers to examine specific locations of the stimuli set.
2. The eye tracker comes with a built-in software to generate and control the stimuli and export the required data. In case of SMI eye trackers, software like Experiment center 3.6 is used to generate and control experiments and BGaze is used to collect and export data. The data thus exported can be analyzed as excel sheets, in SPSS or R statistical tools.
3. Programs like e-prime, Matlab, presentation software can also be used to generate stimuli, control the experiment, collect data, and export data for statistical analysis.

4. Therefore, the position of the eye initially fixates seem to have a strong influence on the ease/ difficulty with which a stimulus is recognized. The measures to understand ease in word recognition can be the overall time spent inspecting the word (O'Regan & Levy Schoen, 1987), word naming latencies (O'Regan & Jacobs, 1992), lexical decision latencies and errors (Nazir, O'Regan, & Jacobs, 1991) and perceptual identification errors (Nazir, Heller, & Sussmann, 1992).

Eye Tracking Paradigms

A few very common and useful paradigms using eye movement measures to understand foveal and parafoveal processing are discussed.

1. **Visual World Paradigm:** This paradigm was pioneered by Cooper initially and perfected by Tenenhaus and colleagues (Allopenna, Magnuson & Tenenhaus, 1998). It determines as to how linguistic and non-linguistic processes determine an individual understands of stimuli. The paradigm enables researchers to understand eye movement behavior while presenting the stimuli audio-visually. This paradigm helps researchers to study how the presence of a relevant visual stimulus along with an acoustic cue affects the underlying cognitive processes in time. In this paradigm, the participant hears an acoustic clue while looking at the target embedded in the experimental display. It equips researcher to study what happens before, during and after the presentation of the target and the time taken in milliseconds. It reflects the direction of visual attention, visual processing, recognition and comprehension and the ways in which visual and auditory information determines attention and gaze direction automatically and unconsciously.
2. **Moving Window or Gaze-Contingent Paradigm:** It is usually used in investigating perceptual span and parafoveal preview benefit during reading. This paradigm synchronizes the display of the target area in accordance with the fixation of the participant's eye movement with the rest of the stimuli being masked. In other words, the stimuli/text is displayed only when the participant fixates on a particular area of the text and as he/she moves the eye the text will be displayed accordingly obscuring the previous area and the forthcoming area of the stimuli. It helps researchers to understand cognitive processes involved in processing a stimulus from the parafovea and ease in comprehending it when the stimuli are fixated in the foveal region. The parafoveal processing is again unconscious where the participant doesn't even realize having seen the preview before fixating the target in the foveal region. The size of the text displayed at a time is called the moving window where the size of the moving window may be manipulated and controlled by the experimenter.
3. **Reading Paradigm:** It is a very simple paradigm in reading the research. The target word is embedded in sentences keeping the position of the target constant. The participant is instructed to simply read the sentence or paragraph with an occasional question to check comprehension. The area of interest is marked after data is collected and statistically analyzed.

Eye Tracking Systems

For experimental and diagnostic purposes, it is important that the eye tracking systems are affordable, portable, wearable, non-invasive and efficient in collecting data with high resolution. There are many different types of eye trackers available in the market and it is up to the institution or researcher to decide on which type of eye tracker would be tailor-made for their purpose. The commonly used eye trackers are discussed below.

1. **Video-Based Eye Trackers:** It is highly accurate and portable. It comes with a laptop and a head gear, or wearable glasses and a small pocket size processing and data storage unit.
2. **Electrooculography (EOG):** EOG is light weight wearable goggles capable of recording data for over 7 hours and analyze the same online with a 250Hz sampling resolution and 87% accuracy (Bulling, Roggen, & Röster, 2009). Other types offer signal acquisition with a customized iPhone application for data collection with a resolution rate of 2048Hz and data being transmitted through the Bluetooth device on to the iPhone. The data can be transferred on to the laptop for statistical analysis.
3. **Head-Mounted Eye Trackers:** It comes with a resolution of 1240Hz with built-in software for generating stimuli, controlling experiment and analyzing data.
4. **Screen-Based Eye Trackers:** It is best suited for outside the laboratory experimental research and tools for diagnosis. It is well designed to study visual attention.
5. **Optical Eye Trackers:** It reflects light from the eye to on an optical sensor. The data collected is then exported and statistically analyzed.

REVIEW OF LITERATURE

The period between 70's to 90's revolutionized the use of eye tracking as a tool to investigate cognitive processing by measuring an individual's eye movements to infer online, moment-to-moment cognitive processing and reported shorter fixations to be associated with better readability and ease of text presented while longer fixations indicated a processing load (Just, & Carpenter, 1980; Rello, Baeza-Yates, Dempere, & Saggion, 2013).

Research using eye tracking since then reported differences in eye movements in children with and without dyslexia and that reading ability of a child with dyslexia matched that of beginning readers with longer fixation duration, shorter saccades and increased regressions. Eye tracking research also ruled out the differences in eye movement in dyslexia as a cause of erratic eye movements (Pavlidis, 1981; 1983), instability during fixations and selective attention deficit (Farmer, & Klein, 1995). Nevertheless, the reading disability to be a reflection of underlying processes rather than oculomotor deficits. Hence differences in eye movement in children with dyslexia are not the cause of reading problems but a reflection of the difficulties in the underlying cognitive processes required to decode the presented stimuli.

Eye tracking has been extensively used in the past decade to study moment-to-moment online linguistic processing in different populations and languages. These studies have given insights on how linguistic features like grapheme-phoneme-correspondence, morphology, phonology, orthography, syntax and semantics play a crucial role in reading on one hand and the underlying cognitive processes like decoding, comprehension, attention, memory on the other play a role in an individual's skill of reading. Therefore, eye tracking measures enable researchers to understand linguistic features of a language through eye movement. The comparison of time taken in measures like FFD, FD, GD or saccadic amplitude between typically developing readers and dyslexic readers gives a clear understanding of the differences in reading patterns and reason out the divergent eye movement patterns reported in children with dyslexia.

Additionally, eye tracking measures provide enough proof on features like word length, word frequency, and orthographic depth in lexical processing. They also have report fixation to a target is delayed when a phonologically/morphologically related distracter is presented along with the target pointing out the effect of a related distracter to that of an unrelated one (Allopenna et al., 1998). Studies also reveal how the morphological structure of a language affects the recognition of words. A study by Azeez and Prakash (2016) using Urdu as a language of the investigation reveals that morphology plays a crucial role as compared to phonology during target recognition. A study by Benfatto et al. (2016) reports longer fixation durations and shorter saccadic movements for high risk than the low risk for dyslexia. A series of other studies also report differences in vergence and binocular coordination during saccades and fixations in dyslexic as compared to normal readers.

A comparative study in English-German report dyslexic readers took 5-6 times longer while reading English than the German dyslexic readers as compared to normal readers of the respective languages; similar results were reported in an Italian study (De Luca, Di Pace, Judica, Spinelli, & Zoccolotti, 1995). Furthermore, other eye movement studies report increased the percentage of regression in dyslexic readers during passage reading task; low-frequency words (Hyona & Olason, 1995); disproportionate and longer fixation duration and shorter saccades.

Eye tracking has been used by researchers as a means to identify children at risk for dyslexia as it allows online measurement in real time while reading in the most natural way, the difference in the role a language plays in comprehension and the subtle differences that could be recorded as compared to language-specific psychometric tests. Research using eye trackers suggests eye movements of dyslexic readers are different from those of normal readers. A study tracking eye movement for linguistic versus non-linguistic tasks reported altered eye movement pattern with more frequent and smaller rightward saccades and longer fixation duration for dyslexic children in a linguistic task while no such difference was observed for non-linguistic tasks. Pirozzolo and Rayner (1978) as well as Olson, Kliegl, and Davidson (1983) reported eye movements of dyslexic readers were similar to individual's eye movement when they were matched on reading age and contrastingly normal readers eye movements matched eye movements of dyslexic readers when the stimuli were difficult to read/comprehend.

Psycholinguistic research using eye movements report dyslexic readers exhibit longer FD, higher regressions, shorter saccades during a reading task reflecting impaired cognitive functioning (Rayner, 1998; Hutzler, Kronbichler, Jacobs, & Wimmer, 2006). Hyona & Olson (1995) concluded that differences in eye movement patterns in dyslexic readers were due to the linguistic features like word length and frequency of a language, the findings were further consistent with German text (Hutzler & Wimmer, 2004). Hristova, Gerganov, Todorova, and Georgieva (2010) reported young dyslexic readers were very slow in reading due to the effects of word length and word frequency which is a prerequisite of skilled reading. More interestingly they reported eye movements highlighted the specificity of reading difficulty without the confounding effect of different strategies that develop over time.

Abnormal eye movements in dyslexic readers have been well researched and reported longer fixation durations, shorter saccades, increased regressions and number of fixations as compared to normally developing chronologically aged matched children. Additionally, linguistic structure of a language, grapheme-phoneme-correspondence, frequency of a word, orthographic transparency, semantics etc. plays an important role in learning the skill to read. Eye movement studies explicitly bring about the differences in normal readers and dyslexic readers specific to the language structure or orthographic transparency.

Since dyslexia is a reading disorder, research findings report divergent eye movement patterns reflecting the difficulty in word recognition (Hyona & Olson, 1995) and suggest the presenting divergent eye movement patterns are due to the difficulty in psycholinguistic processing rather than oculomotor control or visual processing.

Nevertheless, it is also noted that impairment of visual-perceptual mechanisms and visual attentional processes in dyslexic readers could be the reason for atypical or divergent eye movement patterns again a link to difficulty in cognitive processing rather that oculomotor control typically seen in dyslexic children. The connectionistic multi-trace model postulate that the size of the visual attention window determines the global or analytic processing of the stimulus and a large visual attention window size is responsible for analytic processing. In case of the dyslexic reader, the visual attention span is reduced resulting in lesser number of letters being processed parallelly. Furthermore, Hawelka, and Wimmer (2005) reported low performance on an array of multi-element processing task in dyslexic readers.

The study by (Prado, Dubois, & Valdois, 2007) reported that visual span abilities impacted eye movement patterns and showed that dyslexic readers processed only a few letters at each fixation in a reading task as compared to the non-reading task. In other words, dyslexic readers had difficulty in processing a linguistic stimulus due to the small visual attention span hence affected reading efficiency as compared to the visual search which had a non-linguistic task and exhibited a high probability of analytic reading. Thus, confirming that visual attention span disorders in dyslexic children limit processing of many letters simultaneously limiting comprehension abilities in a linguistic task but the underlying cognitive processes seemed to be intact in the visual search that had a non-linguistic task pointing out the difficulties in reading and comprehension typical of individuals with dyslexia.

Hence, the authors concluded that the divergent eye movement patterns seen in dyslexic children were primarily due to a visual attention span disorder resulting in increased number of fixations signaling analytic reading while the age-matched controls showed the decreased number of fixations signaling global reading strategies.

In an interesting study by Desroches, Joanisse, and Robertson (2006) reported eye movement during auditory word recognition in isolation were similar in both dyslexic and normal readers. The dyslexic group showed no sensitivity to a phonological competitor while normal readers showed slower recognition rate suggesting that dyslexic readers could perceive segmental information and that they were less sensitive to perceive suprasegmental knowledge as compared to normal readers who can perceive both segmental and suprasegmental knowledge simultaneously, unconsciously and automatically. The finding reasons out the divergent eye movement patterns of dyslexic readers' deficit in phonological processing.

When the authors compared eye tracking data with traditional phonological awareness paper-pencil tests, revealed that while eye tracking measures showed abnormal rhyme processing in dyslexia, their performance on traditional phonological awareness paper-pencil test data was reported to be similar to that of controls especially in the overt rhyme judgment task. This finding suggests a clear strength of eye tracking as a tool for investigation for its ability to identify subtle processing deficits more explicitly as compared to traditional paper-pencil tests. Eye tracking measures reported difficulty in rhyme relationship that could not be detectable in traditional tests.

Another eye tracking study using RAN suggested dyslexic subjects suffered phonological and visual processing necessary for speed reading. A series of studies using visual-world paradigm to understand visual-auditory word recognition have reported that presence of rhyme competitor delayed the target recognition in typically developing children (Allopenna et al., 1998) while Desroches et al. (2006) reported dyslexic readers showed cohort competitor effect only while non-dyslexic readers were sensitive to both rhyme and cohort competitors. Furthermore, Tiadi et al. (2016) explain that healthy controls were sensitive to the rhyme and cohort competitors because they automatically encode the phonological relationship during visual-auditory word recognition processing whereas dyslexic readers were less sensitive to rhyme/cohort signaling phonological deficit in the same task.

Additionally, even recognition speed is slower in dyslexics than in non-dyslexics because dyslexics tend to spend significantly shorter time on targets due to their attentional deficits. This may be due to impairment in posterior parietal cortex and magnocellular path responsible for visual-spatial attention processing (Stein, 2001; Pugh, Mencl, Jenner, Katz, Frost, Lee... & Shaywitz, 2001). A longitudinal study reported a developmental trend in phonological awareness and its relationship with orthographic and morphological awareness improved with age (Berninger, Abbot, & Nagy Carlisle, 2010).

EYE MOVEMENT AND MENTAL DISORDERS

Any differences in the eye movement can reflect disorders or diseases in the functional areas of cerebral cortex, brain stem, cerebellum, and other areas of the brain. Thus, when we analyze the data from eye movement, we find that dysfunctional eye movements can reveal dysfunction in that area of the brain (Cogan, Chu, & Reingold, 1982). Analysis of smooth pursuit eye movements can reveal the extent of damage in the brain in patients with AIDS dementia complex, Alzheimer's disease (Kuskowski, 1988), Schizophrenia (Radant, & Hommer, 1992), and multiple sclerosis (Roche & King, 2010). Eye tracking research on attention deficit hyperactivity disorder (ADHD) with children and adolescents revealed increased premature saccades on a large number of saccades reflecting difficulty with inhibition and executive dysfunction- a characteristic of ADHD.

A case study on developmental dyscalculia prevalence 3-6% (Rotzer et al., 2009) have linked deficits in the spatial processing of numbers (Geary, Hoard, Nugent, & Bailey, 2012) may be due to impaired functioning of the intra-parietal sulcus (Rotzer, Loenneker, Kucian, Martin, Klaver, & Von Aster, 2009). An eye movement study by van Viersen, Slot, Kroesbergen, van't Noordende, and Leseman (2013) on children with developmental dyscalculia and typically developing children reported performance significantly differed both qualitatively and quantitatively. With regard to autism research using eye trackers, several studies have reported reduced looking time to people and faces and failure to orient to biological motion in young infants and toddlers with autism spectrum disorder (ASD). The studies have been able to discriminate reasonably between children with ASD and normal growing children at an individual level (Sasson & Touchstone, 2014) and characterize subgroups of ASD (Rice, Moriuchi, Jones, & Klin, 2012) useful to understand in detail the heterogeneity of ASD.

The easy access, accuracy and the possibility of integrating eye movement results with several other investigative methods have produced a high incidence of ASD between 2012-2016. The versatility of eye movement applications has also suggested for better identification, understanding of similarities and differences between ASD and other genetic syndromes (Crawford et al., 2016).

CONCLUSION

Eye acts as a window to the mind. The visuo-spatial orientation reveals how an individual perceives his/her surroundings. Any disturbance can reveal differences in one's cognitive abilities. Also, eye movements are autonomous and automatic hence not in the control of the individual. Studying eye movements can provide authentic data under controlled environmental variables. Eye tracking is a technique that tracks the eye movement in the most natural settings. The heat maps and scan paths provide qualitative data while first fixation duration, fixation duration, saccades, and regression provide quantitative data. The data thus obtained reveals the differential cognitive abilities on one hand and function of the stimuli on the other. For example, if one is studying cognitive abilities of the participant, the differences in the eye movement measures of the participant group versus the control group enables studying differential abilities; if stimuli are the research objective then the impact of the characteristic feature of the stimuli can be investigated. Hence, eye tracking may be seen as an effective tool for research and diagnosis may be suggestive for its precision in results.

The contemporary methods used in the psychological or neurological evaluation of developmental delays are painstakingly developed batteries which do provide precise reports under the experienced psychologist. The evaluation is time consuming, costly, need the experienced practitioner, take a lot of time for analysis on one hand and put the client, especially a child, under stress, anxiety and confusion which may affect performance blurring precision in the outcome on the other. Contrarily, eye tracking technique may be used to aid such apprehensions in the client, save time, cost and the like. Additionally, the data reveals moment-to-moment online measures in a conducive environment giving little clue to the client with regard to his/her skill in performing the tasks as seen in the assessment batteries. Eye movement patterns can be studied with precision in cases like specific learning disabilities and autism spectrum disorders using eye tracker as a diagnostic tool with linguistic and non-linguistic tasks as stimuli. With the ongoing research and the technological improvements, one can easily predict that eye tracking will soon be integrated as a potential tool in screening and diagnostic assessments.

REFERENCES

Allopenna, P. D., Magnuson, J. S., & Tanenhaus, M. K. (1998). Tracking the time course of spoken word recognition using eye movements: Evidence for continuous mapping models. *Journal of Memory and Language*, *38*(4), 419–439. doi:10.1006/jmla.1997.2558

Azeez, R., & Prakash, P. (2016). *Phonological and morphological processing in Urdu: An eye tracking investigation* (Unpublished Doctoral dissertation). University of Mysore, Mysore.

Benfatto, M. N., Seimyr, G. Ö., Ygge, J., Pansell, T., Rydberg, A., & Jacobson, C. (2016). Screening for dyslexia using eye tracking during reading. *PLoS One*, *11*(12), e0165508.

Berninger, V. W., Abbot, R. D., & Nagy Carlisle, J. (2010). Growth in phonological, orthographic and morphological awareness in grades 1 to 6. *Journal of Psycholinguistic Research*, *39*(2), 141–163. doi:10.100710936-009-9130-6 PMID:19826956

Bradley, L., & Bryant, P. E. (1983). Categorizing sounds and learning to read-A causal connection. *Nature*, *301*(3), 419–421. doi:10.1038/301419a0

Bulling, A., & Roggen, D., & Tröster, G. (2009). Wearable EOG goggles: Seamless sensing and context-awareness in everyday environments. *Journal of Ambient Intelligence and Smart Environments*, *1*, 157–171.

Cogan, D. G., Chu, F. C., & Reingold, D. B. (1982). Ocular signs of cerebellar disease. *Archives of Ophthalmology*, *100*(5), 755–760. doi:10.1001/archopht.1982.01030030759007 PMID:7082205

Crawford, H., Moss, J., Oliver, C., Elliot, N., Anderson, G. M., & McCleery, J. P. (2016). Visual preference for social stimuli in individuals with autism or neurodevelopmental disorders: An eye-tracking study. *Molecular Autism,* 7- 24. doi:10.118613229-016-0084-x

De Luca, M., Di Pace, E., Judica, A., Spinelli, D., & Zoccolotti, P. (1999). Eye movement patterns in linguistic and non-linguistic tasks in developmental surface dyslexia. *Neuropsychologia*, *37*(12), 1407–1420. doi:10.1016/S0028-3932(99)00038-X PMID:10606014

Desroches, A. S., Joanisse, M. F., & Robertson, E. K. (2006). Specific phonological impairments in dyslexia revealed by eye tracking. *Cognition*, *100*(3), B32–B42. doi:10.1016/j.cognition.2005.09.001 PMID:16288732

Duchowski, A. T. (2007). *Eye Tracking Methodology: Theory and Practice*. New York: Springer-Verlag Inc.

Farmer, M. E., & Klein, R. M. (1995). The evidence for a temporal processing deficit linked to dyslexia: A review. *Psychonomic Bulletin & Review*, *2*(4), 460–493. doi:10.3758/BF03210983 PMID:24203785

Geary, D. C., Hoard, M. K., Nugent, L., & Bailey, D. H. (2012). Mathematical cognitive deficits in children with learning disabilities and persistent low achievement: A five-year prospective study. *Journal of Educational Psychology*, *104*(1), 206–233. doi:10.1037/a0025398 PMID:27158154

Goswami, U. (1999). Causal connections in beginning reading: The importance of rhyme. *Journal of Research in Reading*, *22*(3), 217–240. doi:10.1111/1467-9817.00087

Granet, D. B., Castro, E. F., & Gomi, C. F. (2006). Reading: Do the eyes have it? *The American Orthoptic Journal*, *56*(1), 44–49. doi:10.3368/aoj.56.1.44

Grund, M., Naumann, C. L., & Haug, G. (2004). Diagnostischer Rechtschreibtest f¨ur 5. Klassen: DRT 5; *Manual. Deutsche Schultests*. Beltz Test, G¨ottingen, 2., aktual. aufl. in neuerrechtschreibung edition.

Hawelka, S., & Wimmer, H. (2005). Impaired visual processing of multielement arrays is associated with increased number of eye movements in dyslexic reading. *Vision Research*, *45*(7), 855–863. doi:10.1016/j.visres.2004.10.007 PMID:15644226

Hristova, E., Gerganov, A., Todorova, E., & Georgieva, S. (2010, January). Eye-Movements of Dyslexic Children Reading in Regular Orthography: Exploring word frequency and length effects. *Proceedings of the Annual Meeting of the Cognitive Science Society*, 32.

Hutzler, F., Kronbichler, M., Jacobs, A. M., & Wimmer, H. (2006). Perhaps correlational but not causal: No effect of dyslexic readers' magnocellular system on their eye movements during reading. *Neuropsychologia*, *44*(4), 637–648. doi:10.1016/j.neuropsychologia.2005.06.006 PMID:16115655

Hutzler, F., & Wimmer, H. (2004). Eye movements of dyslexic children when reading in a regular orthography. *Brain and Language*, *89*(1), 235–242. doi:10.1016/S0093-934X(03)00401-2 PMID:15010255

Hyönä, J., & Olson, R. K. (1995). Eye fixation patterns among dyslexic and normal readers: Effects of word length and word frequency. *Journal of Experimental Psychology. Learning, Memory, and Cognition*, *21*(6), 1430–1440. doi:10.1037/0278-7393.21.6.1430 PMID:7490575

Just, M. A., & Carpenter, P. A. (1980). A theory of reading: From eye fixations to comprehension. *Psychological Review*, *87*(4), 329–354. doi:10.1037/0033-295X.87.4.329 PMID:7413885

Kapur, M., John, A., Rozario, J., & Oommen, A. (2002). NIMHANS index of specific learning disabilities. In U. Hirisave, A. Oommen, & M. Kapur (Eds.), *Psychological Assessment of Children in the Clinical Setting* (pp. 88–126). Bangalore: Department of Clinical Psychology, National Institute of Mental Health and Neurosciences.

Karande, S., & Kulkarni, M. (2005). Poor school performance. *Indian Journal of Pediatrics*, *72*(11), 961–967. doi:10.1007/BF02731673 PMID:16391452

Kuskowski, M. A. (1988). Eye movements in progressive cerebral neurological disease. In C. W. Johnston & F. J. Pirozzolo (Eds.), *Neuropsychology of Eye Movements* (pp. 146–176). Hillsdale, NJ: Psychology Press.

Lima, S. D., & Inhoff, A. W. (1985). Lexical access during eye fixations in reading: Effects of word-initial letter sequence. *Journal of Experimental Psychology. Human Perception and Performance*, *11*(3), 272–285. doi:10.1037/0096-1523.11.3.272

Matin, E. (1974). Saccadic suppression: A review and an analysis. *Psychological Bulletin*, *81*(12), 899–917. doi:10.1037/h0037368

Molfese, M. L. (2000). Predicting dyslexia at 8 years of age using neonatal brain responses. *Brain and Language*, *72*(3), 238–245. doi:10.1006/brln.2000.2287 PMID:10764519

Moqasale, V., Paul, D. V., Patil, M. N., & Mogasale, V. (2012). Prevalence of specific learning disabili ties among primary school children in South Indian city. *Indian Journal of Pediatrics*, *79*(3), 432–347. PMID:21887581

Morais, J. (2003). Levels of phonological representation in skilled reading and learning to read. *Reading and Writing*, *16*(1/2), 123–151. doi:10.1023/A:1021702307703

Nazir, T. A., Heller, D., & Sussmann, C. (1992). Letter visibility and word recognition: The optimal viewing position in printed words. *Perception & Psychophysics*, *52*(3), 315–328. doi:10.3758/BF03209148 PMID:1408642

Nazir, T. A., O'regan, J. K., & Jacobs, A. M. (1991). On words and their letters. *Bulletin of the Psychonomic Society*, *29*(2), 171–174. doi:10.3758/BF03335227

O'Regan, J. K., & Jacobs, A. M. (1992). Optimal viewing position effect in word recognition: A challenge to current theory. *Journal of Experimental Psychology. Human Perception and Performance*, *18*(1), 185–197. doi:10.1037/0096-1523.18.1.185

O'Regan, J. K., & Lévy-Schoen, A. (1987). Eye-movement strategy and tactics in word recognition and reading. In M. Coltheart (Ed.), *Attention and performance 12: The psychology of reading* (pp. 363–383). Hillsdale, NJ: Lawrence Erlbaum Associates, Inc.

Olson, R. K., Kliegl, R., & Davidson, B. J. (1983). Dyslexic and normal readers' eye movements. *Journal of Experimental Psychology. Human Perception and Performance*, *9*(5), 816–825. doi:10.1037/0096-1523.9.5.816 PMID:6227691

Pavlidis, G. T. (1981). Do eye movements hold the key to dyslexia? *Neuropsychologia*, *19*(1), 57–64. doi:10.1016/0028-3932(81)90044-0 PMID:7231665

Pavlidis, G. T. (1983). The "dyslexia syndrome" and its objective diagnosis by erratic eye movements. In Eye movements in reading: Perceptual and language Processes (pp.441–466). Academic Press.

Pirozzolo, F. J., & Rayner, K. (1979). The neural control of eye movements in acquired and developmental reading disorders. In Studies in Neurolinguistics (vol. 4, pp. 97-123). Academic Press. doi:10.1016/B978-0-12-746304-9.50009-4

Prado, C., Dubois, M., & Valdois, S. (2007). The eye movement of dyslexic children during reading and visual search: Impact of the visual attention span. *Vision Research*, *47*(19), 2521–2530. doi:10.1016/j.visres.2007.06.001 PMID:17719073

Pugh, K. R., Mencl, W. E., Jenner, A. R., Katz, L., Frost, S. J., Lee, J. R., ... Shaywitz, B. A. (2001). Neurobiological studies of reading and reading disability. *Journal of Communication Disorders*, *34*(6), 479–492. doi:10.1016/S0021-9924(01)00060-0 PMID:11725860

Rack, J. P., Snowling, M., & Olson, R. (1992). The non-word reading deficit in developmental dyslexia: A review. *Reading Research Quarterly*, *27*(1), 29–53. doi:10.2307/747832

Radant, A. D., & Hommer, D. W. (1992). A quantitative analysis of saccades and smooth pursuit during visual pursuit tracking. A comparison of schizophrenics with normals and substance abusing controls. *Schizophrenia Research*, *6*(3), 225–235. doi:10.1016/0920-9964(92)90005-P PMID:1349241

Ramaa, S. (2000). Two decades of research on learning disabilities in India. *Dyslexia (Chichester, England)*, *6*(4), 268–283. doi:10.1002/1099-0909(200010/12)6:4<268::AID-DYS177>3.0.CO;2-A PMID:11129452

Rayner, K. (1998). Eye Movements in Reading and Information Processing: *20* Years of Research. *Psychological Bulletin*, *124*(3), 372–422. doi:10.1037/0033-2909.124.3.372 PMID:9849112

Rayner, K., & Duffy, S. A. (1986). Lexical complexity and fixation times in reading: Effects of word frequency, verb complexity, and lexical ambiguity. *Memory & Cognition*, *14*(3), 191–201.

Rayner, K., Inhoff, A. W., Morrison, R. E., Slowiaczek, M. L., & Bertera, J. H. (1981). Masking of foveal and parafoveal vision during eye fixations in reading. *Journal of Experimental Psychology. Human Perception and Performance*, *7*(1), 167–179. doi:10.1037/0096-1523.7.1.167

Rayner, K., Well, A. D., Pollatsek, A., & Bertera, J. H. (1982). The availability of useful information to the right of fixation in reading. *Perception & Psychophysics*, *31*(6), 537–550.

Rello, L., Baeza-Yates, R., Dempere, L., & Saggion, H. (2013). Frequent words improve readability and short words improve understandability for people with dyslexia. Proc. INTERACT '13. doi:10.1007/978-3-642-40498-6_15

Rice, K., Moriuchi, J. M., Jones, W., & Klin, A. (2012). Parsing heterogeneity in autism spectrum disorders: Visual scanning of dynamic social scenes in school aged children. *Journal of the American Academy of Child and Adolescent Psychiatry*, *51*(3), 238–248. doi:10.1016/j.jaac.2011.12.017 PMID:22365460

Roche, D. J. O., & King, A. C. (2010). Alcohol impairment of saccadic and smooth pursuit eye movements: Impact of risk factors for alcohol dependence. *Psychopharmacology*, *212*(1), 33–44. doi:10.100700213-010-1906-8 PMID:20635179

Rotzer, S., Loenneker, T., Kucian, K., Martin, E., Klaver, P., & Von Aster, M. (2009). Dysfunctional neural network of spatial working memory contributes to developmental dyscalculia. *Neuropsychologia, 47*(13), 2859-2865. doi:psychologia.2009.06.009 doi:10.1016/j.neuro

Sasson, N. J., & Touchstone, E. W. (2014). Visual attention to competing social and object images by preschool children with autism spectrum disorder. *Journal of Autism and Developmental Disorders, 44*(3), 584–592. doi:10.100710803-013-1910-z PMID:23918441

Seidenberg, M. S., Tanenhaus, M. K., Leiman, J. M., & Bienkowski, M. (1982). Automatic access of the meanings of ambiguous words in context: Some limitations of knowledge-based processing. *Cognitive Psychology, 14*(4), 489–537.

Shah, N., Parwar, A., & Shah, L. P. (1998). Specific learning disability. *Converse, 2*(2), 5–12.

Shaywitz, B. A., Shaywitz, S. E., Pugh, K. R., Mencl, W. E., Fulbright, R. K., Skudlarski, P., ... Gore, J. C. (2002). Disruption of posterior brain systems for reading in children with developmental dyslexia. *Biological Psychiatry, 52*(2), 101–110. doi:10.1016/S0006-3223(02)01365-3 PMID:12114001

Shaywitz, S. E. (1998). Dyslexia. *The New England Journal of Medicine, 338*(5), 307–312. doi:10.1056/NEJM199801293380507 PMID:9445412

Shaywitz, S. E., & Shaywitz, B. A. (2005). Dyslexia (Specific Reading Disability). *Biological Psychiatry, 57*(11), 1301–1309. doi:10.1016/j.biopsych.2005.01.043 PMID:15950002

Snowling, M. J. (1995). Phonological processing and developmental dyslexia. *Journal of Research in Reading, 18*(2), 132–138. doi:10.1111/j.1467-9817.1995.tb00079.x

Stein, J. (2001). The Magnocellular theory of developmental dyslexia. *Dyslexia (Chichester, England), 7*(1), 12–36. doi:10.1002/dys.186 PMID:11305228

Tiadi, A., Seassau, M., Gerard, C. L., & Bucci, M. P. (2016). Differences between dyslexic and non-dyslexic children in the performance of phonological visual-auditory recognition task: An eye tracking study. *PLoS One, 11*(7), e0159190. doi:10.1371/journal.pone.0159190 PMID:27438352

van Viersen, S., Slot, E. M., Kroesbergen, E. H., van't Noordende, J. E., & Leseman, P. P. (2013). The added value of eye-tracking in diagnosing dyscalculia: A case study. *Frontiers in Psychology, 4*, 679. doi:10.3389/fpsyg.2013.00679 PMID:24098294

Vellutino, F. R., Fletcher, J. M., Snowling, M. J., & Scanlon, D. M. (2004). Specific reading disability (dyslexia): What have we learned in the past four decades? *Journal of Child Psychology and Psychiatry, and Allied Disciplines, 45*(1), 2–40. doi:10.1046/j.0021-9630.2003.00305.x PMID:14959801

Wilkinson, G. S. (1993). *WRAT-3: Wide range achievement test administration manual.* Wide Range, Incorporated.

Wimmer, H. (1996). The nonword reading deficit in developmental dyslexia: Evidence from children learning to read German. *Journal of Experimental Psychology, 61*, 80–90. PMID:8812031

KEY TERMS AND DEFINITIONS

Calibration: It is a process whereby the participant's eye is synchronized to the eye tracker's camera. The participant is instructed to follow points displayed so as to estimate the geometric characteristics of the participant's eye. The accuracy of data collected depends on the exactness of the calibration.

Diagnosis: The process of identifying an illness, disorder or disability based on the presenting symptoms.

Eye Tracker: It is a tool that has built-in cameras and enables online recording of eye movements.

Fixation: The point where the eye lands on a stimulus after a saccade is a fixation. The time spent on the area of a fixation is said to be fixation duration.

Moving Window or Gaze-Contingent Paradigm: A paradigm in which the stimulus display changes depending on where the participant looks.

Reading Paradigm: It is simple sentence reading paradigm, wherein participants will have to read the sentences while eye movement measures are recorded online. The stimulus will be a sentence with a target word embedded in a destined position as per the research requirement.

Saccades: The movement of the eye from one area to another area of a stimulus to bring it to the foveal vision is said to be a saccade.

Specific Learning Disabilities: A disorder in more than one of any psychological processes with regard to learning to read, write or comprehend due to imperfection in cognitive ability.

Visual System: The ability of the eye and the central nervous system to process the visual world around us. It's the ability to detect, interpret and comprehend a given stimulus.

Visual World Paradigm: It is an experimental paradigm wherein participants hear utterances while looking at a visual display of target word along with competitors and distracters on the visual display. The task assigned to the participants is usually to look and listen.

Section 2

Neurodevelopmental Disorders:
Intervention and Certification

Chapter 9
Animal-Assisted Therapy as a Treatment for Autism Spectrum Disorder:
Encouraging Physician Participation in Research

Nicola Claire Pellew
Seton Hall University, USA

ABSTRACT

Research studies report that animal-assisted therapy (AAT) may be an effective alternative method for treating autism spectrum disorder (ASD). However, the presence of many methodological weaknesses and the limited replication of such studies have resulted in divided opinion on the actual effectiveness of AAT for treating ASD, and much hesitancy surrounding its use. Reliable clinically based studies must be conducted if this uncertainty is to be put to rest. Because these studies require the participation of physicians who are often hesitant to participate, it is suggested that leadership interventions be used as tools to encourage their participation in AAT research. This chapter aims to discuss the necessity for physician participation, the reasons for the lack of clinician participation in such research, and recommendations for encouraging physician and policymaker participation in specifically targeted research studies.

INTRODUCTION

Autism Spectrum Disorder (ASD) has received much attention over the past decade. During this time, research on the mystifying disorder has evolved significantly and has led to greater understanding of the condition and its underlying pathophysiology (Patel, Preedy, & Martin, 2014). Accordingly, the expansion of the *Diagnostic and Statistical Manual of Mental Disorders 4th Edition Text Revised* (DSM-IV TR) reflected this change in the broadened ASD diagnostic criteria now outlined in the DSM-V (American Psychiatric Association [APA], 2013). Treatments have followed suit, with new treatment combinations often greatly improving the condition and quality of life of many sufferers. However, these treatments

DOI: 10.4018/978-1-5225-7004-2.ch009

can be costly (Amendah, Grosse, Peacock, & Mandell, 2011; Lavelle, Weinstein, Newhouse, Munir, Kuhlthau, & Prosser, 2014; Patel, Preedy, & Martin, 2014). As such, obtaining treatment not only places financial strain on many individuals (Ganz, 2007; Kogan, Strickland, Blumberg, Singh, Perrin, & Van Dyck, 2008; Montes & Halterman, 2008; Shimabukuro, Grosse, & Rice, 2008); it creates a ripple effect on the U.S. healthcare system and economy as a whole (Amendah, Grosse, Peacock, & Mandell, 2011).

Animal-assisted therapy (AAT) has been suggested as an effective adjunct to many treatment types. However, a lack of robust clinical trials specifically targeting AAT for ASD has meant that most evidence is reflective of AAT as an alternative treatment for other mental and behavioral disorders such as depression, schizophrenia, and addictions (Kamioka, Okada, Tsutani, Park, Okuizumi, Handa, . . .Abe, 2014). Additionally, there are no randomized, double-blind case-controlled two-group experimental studies targeted at individuals with ASD (Kamioka, Okada, Tsutani, Park, Okuizumi, Handa, . . .Abe, 2014). Therefore, practitioners and policymakers are hesitant to fully endorse the method for treating ASD. Determining the efficacy and suitability of AAT for ASD requires the participation of physicians in specifically targeted case-controlled studies.

This review aims to discuss the necessity for physician participation in AAT for ASD research, explore AAT as a possible adjunct treatment for the disorder, discuss reasons for the lack of participation of clinicians in such research, and make recommendations for encouraging physicians and policymakers to participate in specifically targeted research studies. The chapter's objectives are to systematically identify, describe, and compare literature, in order to:

- Define and describe ASD and AAT;
- Explore current ASD treatment methods;
- Discuss the financial impact of ASD management;
- Discuss current AAT practices;
- Identify the benefits and challenges of using AAT to treat ASD;
- Suggest ways to encourage physician participation in AAT for ASD based research; and
- Provide recommendations for safely incorporating AAT into ASD treatments so that safe, high-quality case-control studies can be conducted.

Lastly, findings and future directions are discussed.

BACKGROUND

Autism Spectrum Disorder

ASD is a lifelong condition characterized by underdeveloped social interactions, poor communication skills, deficits in social-emotional reciprocity, limited ability to form and maintain relationships, and the display of restricted, repetitive, and stereotypical behaviors (APA, 2013). The symptoms of autism spectrum disorder are first recognizable in early childhood and often result in severe lifelong disability (Newschaffer, Croen, Daniels, Giarelli, Grether, Levy, . . . Windham, 2007). An ASD diagnosis is made if an individual has noticeable troubles in social relatedness, communication/play, and interests and activity (APA, 2013). Emotional dysregulation is also a common feature of ASD, and often considered evidence of a coexisting psychiatric disorder (Mazefsky, Pelphrey, & Dahl, 2012). Although intellectual disability is common among those affected by ASD, the disorder's presentation is broad and unique from person to person (Volkmar, Siegel, Woodbury-Smith, King, McCracken, & State, 2014).

ASD had been classified into subtypes (i.e., Autistic Disorder, Asperger's Disorder, Pervasive Developmental Disorder Not Otherwise Specified, Rett's Disorder, and Childhood Disintegrative Disorder) (APA, 2013). However, as a broad range of phenotypes became recognized, these subtypes were removed. As such, the progression, impact, and treatments of the conditions are select to an individual (Volkmar, Siegel, Woodbury-Smith, King, McCracken, & State, 2014). Current ASD diagnosis is based on clinical symptoms, and traditional therapies aim at reducing the manifestation of clinical symptoms (Eapen, Nicholls, Spagnol, & Mathew, 2017). These therapies often include pharmacotherapeutic agents such as antipsychotics, used in conjunction with tailored non-pharmacotherapeutic methods such as psychotherapy, speech therapy, and occupational therapy (Eapen, Nicholls, Spagnol, & Mathew, 2017).

ASD can be a challenge to diagnose and manage, and many individuals with ASD do not always obtain treatment upon initial presentation (Eapen, Nicholls, Spagnol, & Mathew, 2017). ASD is associated with several developmental and behavioral problems that may present simultaneously, making coordinated care as well as support for affected individuals and their families necessary (Eapen, Nicholls, Spagnol, & Mathew, 2017; Volkmar, Siegel, Woodbury-Smith, King, McCracken, & State, 2014). As such, Volkmar et al. (2014) recommend that ASD is managed early, using sustained multiple treatment interventions.

Financial Impact of ASD on the United States

The prevalence of ASD in North America is among the highest in the world and continues to increase (Baxter, Brugha, Erskine, Scheurer, Vos, & Scott, 2015; Centers for Disease Control and Prevention [CDC], 2017). According to the CDC (2016), ASD affects 1 in 68 school-aged children in the United States and is 4.5 times more common in males than in females (Baxter, Brugha, Erskine, Scheurer, Vos, & Scott, 2015). Baio (2012) reported that between 2002 and 2008, the prevalence of ASD increased by 78%. Additionally, the data from the National Survey of Children's Health has shown an increase in parent-reported ASD among children aged 6 to 17 years, from 1.2% in 2007 to 2.0% between 2011 and 2012 (Blumberg, Bramlett, Kogan, Schieve, Jones, & Lu, 2013).

The increasing prevalence of ASD indicates a growing need for resources and care, which has resulted in higher costs associated with the disorder (Amendah, Grosse, Peacock, & Mandell, 2011; Lavelle, Weinstein, Newhouse, Munir, Kuhlthau, & Prosser, 2014). According to Chiri and Warfield (2012), unmet healthcare needs are higher among those with ASD than those without the disorder. Additionally, studies have suggested that children with parent-reported ASD may have a higher risk of mortality (Hirvikoski, Mittendorfer-Rutz, Boman, Larsson, Lichtenstein, & Bolte, 2016; Jain, Spencer, Yang, Kelly, Newschaffer, Johnson,. . .Dennen, 2014; King, 2016; Van Heijst & Geurts, 2015), need more frequent healthcare office visits, and make greater use of prescription drugs (Hirvikoski, Mittendorfer-Rutz, Boman, Larsson, Lichtenstein, & Bolte, 2016). As such, out-of-pocket expenses for those affected with ASD and their families are high and continue to increase (Ganz, 2007; Kogan, Strickland, Blumberg, Singh, Perrin, & Van Dyck, 2008; Montes & Halterman, 2008; Shimabukuro, Grosse, & Rice, 2008). Moreover, in their review, Amendah et al. (2011) reported that the economic burden of ASD outside the healthcare system has also added to the overall economic burden of ASD in the United States.

Animal Assisted Therapy

AAT is a structured and goal-directed ASD treatment intervention that makes use of animals in health, education, and human services for therapeutic gains (O'Haire, 2013). The bond between animals and humans can be traced back centuries, and the earliest therapeutic use of animals has been traced back to Quaker England in 1792 (Connor & Miller, 2000). Animal-assisted therapy was first introduced to the United States in 1942, and in 1969 Boris Levinson established a therapeutic approach to AAT, which still forms the basis of AAT methods used today (Gammonley & Yates, 1991). Currently, AAT can be used as part of critical and acute care, physical rehabilitation, psychotherapy, and behavioral modification; however, this list is not exhaustive (Chandler, 2012). AAT can be beneficial due to the natural tendency for animals to easily form bonds with people and create calm and safe environments where patients are more open to therapy and the therapists' demands (Chandler, 2012; Kruger & Serpell, 2010; Martin & Farnum, 2002).

AAT is a fairly common practice in the United States health care facilities and is thought to be a more cost-effective alternative to currently used traditional ASD treatment methods (Lefebvre, Golab, Christensen, Castrodale, Aureden, Bialachowski,... Weese, 2008; O'Haire, 2013; Souter & Miller 2007). Currently, AAT is used in an assortment of healthcare settings, is applied to a number of clinical problems, and has proved a useful adjunct to traditional ASD treatments (Chandler 2012; Nimer & Lundahl, 2007). Currently, AAT is not uniform and can be adapted to the setting (e.g., inpatient, outpatient, group, individual, and short or long term) and type of animal used (e.g., dog, cat, and horse) (Bauman, 2010; Chandler, 2012).Patient homes, prisons, nursing homes, and hospitals are some examples of settings where AAT sessions are typically conducted (Chandler, 2012). AAT sessions are commonly conducted by certified handlers and/or certified mental and physical healthcare professionals (Chandler, 2012).

AAT is considered to be complementary and alternative medicine (CAM) and is thought to decrease the overall cost of ASD treatment when it is used in the long term (Lefebvre et al., 2008). According to the National Institutes of Health (2017), CAM consists of varied nonconventional medical and healthcare structures, practices, and products. Thus, in this sense, AAT would be used as an adjunct therapy incorporated either directly or indirectly into conventional therapeutic activities (Tielsch-Goddard & Gilmer, 2015). Comparably effective in its approach, this previously overlooked therapeutic method has become more popular over the past decade and has led to a surge in novel methodologies aimed at exploring CAM intervention (Tielsch-Goddard & Gilmer, 2015).

Although dogs and cats are the most commonly used animals in AAT, many kinds of animals have been used (Fine, 2015). For example, small animals such as fish, rabbits, and guinea pigs, and large animals such as horses, dolphins, and elephants have also been used (Fine, 2015). For the purpose of this review, dog therapy, equine therapy, rabbit therapy, and dolphin therapy will be discussed briefly.

- **Dog Therapy:** Dog therapy (DT) or canine therapy is a form of canine-assisted activity and therapy (CAAT) and refers to incorporating dogs into therapeutic activities so that interaction between the patient and the dog can occur (Fung, 2017). It has been suggested that dogs can improve social engagement in individuals with ASD due to the animal's simple, predictable, easy-to-interpret movements, demonstrated by activities such as fetch, play, walking, and giving commands (Redefer & Goodman, 1989; Sams, Fortney, & Willenbring, 2006; Silva, Correia, Magalhães, & de Sousa, 2011; Solomon, 2010). As a multisensory stimulus, interactions with a dog may target the low sensory and affective arousal levels of those with ASD (Redefer & Goodman, 1989). Dog-therapy sessions are not standardized and can run from 6 weeks to 15 weeks and may involve two to eighteen sessions of varying duration between 14 and 45 minutes (Fung, 2017).

- **Horse Therapy**: Horse therapy, equine therapy, or equine-assisted activity and therapy (EAAT) is an AAT intervention approach that involves interaction between patients and horses (Gabriels, Agnew, Holt, Shoffner, Zhaoxing, Ruzzano. . . Mesibov, 2012). EAAT in the form of therapeutic horseback riding (THR) is a method of AAT that has increased in popularity over the past four decades and is used to improve physical, psychosocial, and cognitive functioning in patients with a variety of conditions (Gabriels, Agnew, Holt, Shoffner, Zhaoxing, Ruzzano. . . Mesibov, 2012; Snider, Korner-Bitensky, Kammann, Warner, & Saleh, 2007). THR is the method often pursued by the ASD population and is suggested to arouse physiological, psychological, and social responses in both children and adolescents (Prothmann & Fine, 2011). A THR session is typically facilitated by a riding instructor qualified to teach riders with disabilities how to control the horse (Snider, Korner-Bitensky, Kammann, Warner, & Saleh, 2007). The number of sessions (9 to 12), the frequency of sessions (typically once a week), and the duration of each session (typically 60 minutes) of THR are standardized (Fung, 2017).
- **Rabbit Therapy:** Rabbit therapy is generally used when dog therapy is unavailable, typically due to lack of space (Samfira & Petroman, 2011). Additionally, being clean animals, rabbits may be the ideal choice for patients who have compromised immune systems or are allergic to dogs or other animals. Rabbit therapy is not standardized and has not been well researched (Samfira & Petroman, 2011).
- **Dolphin Therapy:** Dolphin-Assisted Therapy (DAT) involves swimming and interacting with captive dolphins (Marino & Lilienfeld, 2007; Samfira & Petroman, 2011). DAT is suggested to assist individuals with ASD and attention deficit hyperactivity disorder (ADHD) refine their motor skills and vocabulary by moving in the water with the dolphins (Marino & Lilienfeld, 2007). This movement is proposed to help them focus and be attentive for longer periods of time. Although DAT is suggested to stimulate communication, movement, and social interaction, these claims have not been scientifically substantiated (Samfira & Petroman, 2011).

Service Animals

There is often confusion between therapy animals and service animals, but they differ in many respects. Unlike therapy animals, service animals live with their owners permanently, assist them one-on-one with their activities of daily living, and are protected legally by the Americans with Disabilities Act (Chandler, 2012). In contrast, therapy animals work with professionals and with many of their clients (Chandler, 2012).

METHOD FOR LITERATURE SEARCH

Articles related to AAT and/or ASD were identified by conducting electronic searches using the Academic Search Complete, ERIC, EBSCO, Google Scholar, Proquest, PubMed, and Science Direct databases. The keywords searched were autism, autism spectrum disorder, pervasive developmental disorder, animal-assisted therapy, animal-assisted intervention, equine-assisted therapy, dog-assisted therapy, clinical research, and healthcare leadership. Criteria for inclusion in this review were as follows, published between 1985 and 2018, published in a peer-reviewed journal, in English, and focused on the social, emotional, and/or behavioral adjustment of individuals with ASD, and on AAT as a therapeutic intervention for ASD. Studies that were focused on the cost of ASD to the U.S. and studies based on physician participation in clinical trials were also included. Studies focused on the physiological effects of AAT or on the psychological disorders other than ASD were excluded. Additionally, the search was limited to peer-reviewed articles and books.

ANIMAL-ASSISTED THERAPY AS AN ADJUNCT ASD TREATMENT METHOD

Advantages of AAT for ASD

Therapeutic Benefits

Existing literature shows that the use of AAT for treating ASD may encourage positive emotions, improve mood, promote the development of empathy, improve social and communication skills, increase self-confidence, and reduce anxiety (Chandler, 2012; Kruger & Serpell, 2010; Martin & Farnum, 2002; Palley, O'Rourke, & Niemi, 2010). Additionally, AAT has been shown to reduce loneliness, insecurity, sadness, social isolation, and anger in ASD-affected individuals (Kruger & Serpell, 2010; Palley, O'Rourke, & Niemi, 2010). An AAT case example may involve petting or stroking the animal, gentle play with the animal, feeding the animal, riding the animal (equine therapy), and/or talking to the animal. These approaches aim to develop touch-related skills, a child's sense of connection to a living entity, and a variety of other skills (Chandler, 2012).

The benefits of classroom-based animal interactions were demonstrated in a study conducted by O'Haire, McKenzie, McCune, and Slaughter (2014). Using a multisite, control-to-intervention-based study, the social functioning of children diagnosed with ASD was assessed using a classroom-based animal-assisted activities (AAA) model. The study included 41 classrooms across 15 Australian schools. Sixty-four children aged 5-to-12 years and previously diagnosed with ASD (n = 25), Asperger's Disorder (n = 21), Pervasive Developmental Disorder Not Otherwise Specified (PDD-NOS)(n = 10), or Autistic Disorder (n = 8) were selected to participate in the study. An eight-week waitlist control group was included before starting the AAA program. Guinea pigs were introduced to the classroom setting and remained in the classroom during the school week (Monday to Friday) over an eight-week period. Participants were introduced to animal care and exposed to16-to-20-minute animal-interaction sessions per day. Teacher and parent-reported child behavior and social-functioning data were collected at three-time points using standardized instruments—i.e., upon study entry (T1), eight weeks prior to AAA program implementation (T2), and one week following the eight-week AAA program (T3). Results showed that there were significant improvements in social functioning, social approach behaviors, and social skills, as well as a decrease in social withdrawal behaviors in study participants exposed to the animal, an increased interest in attending school during the program was also reported (O'Haire, McKenzie, McCune, & Slaughter, 2014). The investigators concluded that results might demonstrate the cost-effectiveness and potential efficacy of the classroom-based AAA model (O'Haire, McKenzie, McCune, & Slaughter, 2014).

Bass, Duchowny, and Llabre (2009) evaluated the effects of therapeutic horseback riding on social functioning in children with autism. Their study included 34 children diagnosed with ASD who had no previous exposure to equine-assisted activity exposure. Participants were randomly assigned to the experimental or the control group. The experimental group consisted of girls (n=2) and boys (n=17) aged between 5 and 10 years (M = 6.95, SD = 1.67), and the wait-list control group consisted of girls (n=3) and boys (n=12) aged between 4 and10 years (M = 7.73, SD = 1.65). Results showed that after a 12-week horseback-riding intervention, children in the experimental group displayed improved sensory seeking, sensory sensitivity, and social motivation, and fewer inattention, distractibility, and sedentary behaviors. The investigators concluded that the results provided evidence of the possible viability of therapeutic horseback riding as a therapy option for treating children diagnosed with autism spectrum disorders.

Becker, Rogers, and Burrows (2017), aimed to evaluate the efficacy of an animal-assisted social skills training group for children diagnosed with ASD. Social skills groups with therapy dogs were compared to traditional social skills groups without a dog present. Students attending a therapeutic treatment-facility-based school who were diagnosed with ASD (n = 31; ages 8–14) were assigned to experimental or control groups and underwent 12 weeks of weekly treatment. A between-within repeated measures design was used in the study, and the severity of each participant's ASD symptoms (Childhood Autism Rating Scale-Second Edition [CARS-2]) was assessed; their depressive symptoms measured (Children's Depression Inventory-Second Edition [CDI-2]); theory of mind ability determined (Reading the Mind in the Eyes Test [RMET]); and level of social skill identified (Social Language Development Test [SLDT]), Making Inferences and Supporting Peers Subtests, Social Responsiveness Scale-Second Edition [SRS-2]). These assessments were conducted within the 2 weeks prior to and12 weeks following the intervention. The intervention involved the interaction of the experimental group participants with the dogs—for example, greeting the dog with "hello" and "goodbye," co-leading a dog by giving basic commands, and grooming the dog. The final review stage consisted of reviewing session goals by asking children to either verbalize or demonstrate the skill to the group. The control group session goals were closely aligned to those of the experimental group and attempted to introduce similar levels of movement and hands-on activity in the traditional groups. Results showed that theory of mind improved in both groups, and feelings of isolation and overall depressive symptoms were reduced. No significant differences were observed on the Social Language Development Test (SLDT). Based on study results, it was suggested that the animal-assisted social skills training model may be better at improving social skills and reducing the related affective symptoms in children with ASD than traditional training models (Bass, Duchowny, & Llabre, 2009). Currently, no evidence that refutes the benefits of AAT could be found.

Cost Benefits

Despite the resistance toward AAT, advocates have recognized it as an effective alternative ASD treatment option (Levy, Frasso, Colantonio, Reed, Stein, Barg, . . Fiks, 2016; Palley, O'Rourke, & Niemi, 2010). As such, the rising popularity and demonstrated effects of AAT have encouraged certain organizations to provide AAT free of charge (Palley, O'Rourke, & Niemi, 2010). For example, visits from therapy dogs may be provided as part of school programs, cost-free horseback riding may be subsidized by sponsorships and organizations, or instead of paying cash, time and energy may be accepted as payment for AAT services (Chandler, 2012). However, these services are not widespread and are only accessible to certain patients.

While it may seem that AAT is a more expensive childhood ASD treatment in the short term, should insurance companies accept the modality as a reimbursable cost the long-term savings will actually outweigh the short-term costs of treating childhood ASDs. Thus, if AAT improves patient outcomes in the long term, it potentially can also improve the patient's adherence to prescribed treatments, improve therapeutic outcomes, and reduce or shorten hospital stays (Chandler, 2012; Palley, O'Rourke, & Niemi, 2010). Increased application of AAT in childhood ASD treatment could also reduce the need for certain therapeutic interventions (Chandler, 2012). Thus, AAT ultimately could assist in reducing healthcare costs and become a more widely accepted reimbursable expense by third-party payers (Palley, O'Rourke, & Niemi, 2010). Should AAT be established as a credible, effective, safe, and cost-effective treatment, it could improve healthcare accessibility for many ASD-affected children and families (Palley, O'Rourke, & Niemi, 2010). Although these suggestions may sound reasonable, no studies have been conducted to substantiate this cost-saving claim.

DISADVANTAGES OF AAT FOR ASD

Not Suitable for All

AAT serves a diverse population and consists of clients of various ages, genders, and cultures (Chandler, 2012). Thus, for treatment to be effective, AAT practitioners must consider these differences (Chandler, 2012; Haubenhofer & Kirchengast, 2006). Since people may perceive animals differently, their beliefs and attitudes toward AAT may differ. Some clients may accept animals as pets, others may see them as sources of food, or be afraid of them due to past experiences (Matuszek, 2010). Clients who have had good experiences with animals and have felt the attachment to past animal companions are more likely to feel more comfortable with AAT. Those who have had negative experiences or have been taught to view animals in a certain way may feel uncomfortable, scared, or anxious during AAT sessions (Matuszek, 2010).

Concerns Over Hygiene and Safety

AAT may not be suitable for clients with animal allergies and other conditions that may result from the presence of certain animals (Morrison, 2007; Rossetti & King, 2010). Thus, to ensure that no possible contraindications of using the animal in therapy occur, clients must be individually assessed before introducing them to AAT-facilitated ASD therapy (Rossetti & King, 2010). Safety, sanitation, and hygiene are other factors that must be considered when bringing an animal into certain environments (Sillery, Hargreaves, Marin, Lerma, Kuznia, & Abbe, 2004). If AAT is to be implemented safely, both the animal and the therapist must receive proper annual check-ups to ensure that they are properly inoculated and remain up-to-date on all vaccines (Gagnon, Bouchard, Landry, Belles-Isles, Fortier, & Fillion, 2004). Additionally, behavioral assessments of both the therapist and animal should be carried out regularly to safeguard patients, handlers, and animals (Cullen, Titler, & Drahozal, 1999). If the utmost care is to be taken to protect the safety of all involved during the AAT process, stringent policies and protocols must be developed and implemented (Wu, Niedra, Pendergast, & McCrindle, 2002).

Ethical Issues and Animal Welfare

The debate surrounding the morality of integrating animals into AAT is ongoing (Zamir, 2006). According to Zamir (2006), integrating animals into therapeutic interventions violates their moral status by limiting their freedom and life purpose, violating the animal's well-being, removing their social connection, increasing their risk of injury, and causing the animal to be objectified. This notion has been partially supported by the results of studies conducted by Hatch (2007) and Heimlich (2001), who both reported inappropriate behaviors such as the teasing and mistreatment of therapy dogs displayed by some recipients and staff members in certain animal-based therapeutic environments. Heimlich's (2001) study to measure the effectiveness of AAT for children with multiple disabilities provides a classic example of an instance where animal welfare can be violated. During the study, the health of the therapy dog slowly declined due to stress, excessive panting, and tiredness (Heimlich, 2001), and the study was terminated early. Iannuzzi and Rowan (1991) reported concerns about resident animals regarding their need to be monitored closely for signs of poor health, their need for adequate rest, the availability of water that they can easily access and their comfort during sessions. Additionally, respondents suggested that AAT visits be kept to a maximum of three 60-minute sessions per week to ensure the health and well-being of the animal (Iannuzzi & Rowan, 1991).

Zamir (2006) suggested that if animal-assisted interventions (AAI) can support the animal's welfare while addressing human interests, the animal could benefit from the AAI process, thereby justifying its involvement as therapeutic. Zamir (2006) goes on to suggest that integrating dogs and horses into AAI programs may be more ethically justifiable than integrating smaller animals such as rodents, birds, and wild animals. Currently, there is a general agreement that AAIs could negatively affect the welfare of animals involved (Glenk, 2017). As such, the International Association of Human-Animal Interaction Organizations (IAHAIO) has developed guidelines aimed at increasing therapy animals' quality of life by reducing work-related strain (Fine, 2015). While many efforts have been made by IAHAIO, the European Union, and the Austrian Ministry of Labor, no standardized, universal criteria to protect the welfare of therapy animals has been developed, due to the broad spectrum of AAI activities (Glenk, 2017).

Limited Accessibility to Treatment

Although in the U.S Medicaid and certain corporate private insurance providers now offer AAT service reimbursement, this is only under certain circumstances and is only billable when it is incorporated into individualized treatment plans (Chandler, 2012). Conversely, AAT is not billable if it is used as routine care or is not thoroughly documented by a credentialed source (Chandler, 2012). Thus, despite the possibility of being more a cost-effective modality than conventional treatments, if AAT is not currently covered by health insurance, it may still be unaffordable for certain patients.

CHALLENGES FACING THE IMPLEMENTATION OF AAT AS AN ADJUNCT TREATMENT FOR ASD

Lack of Quantitative Research

The use of AAT for ASD is currently a popular topic for investigation and many studies are now making use of more meticulous methodology, randomized designs, and simple pre and post test strategies, and are investigating basic research questions. Although the findings of a number of peer-reviewed studies have reported positive results for the effects of AAT on ASD, the lack of quantitative research has kept divided opinions on the actual effectiveness of AAT for ASD. In her review, O'Haire (2013) described then current AAT research as "scattered" and cited scarce "high-quality studies, many methodological weaknesses, and limited replication" as the cause of much of the hesitancy in using AAT for treating ASD (p. 1619). Similarly, Nimer and Lundahl (2007) identified a lack of comparison and control groups in quantitative AAT studies as a common issue affecting the reliability of their outcomes.

Upon reviewing the literature, Morrison (2007) suggested that small sample size, inconsistent participant randomization, lack or inadequacy of control groups, selection bias, and poor generalizability were the main cause of resistance toward AAT in general. In addition, the author identified the validity of measurement tools and attrition rates as two other factors contributing to the hesitancy to use AAT. Friedmann, Son, and Saleem (2015) described the limitations of AAT-based research as focusing on the short term instead of over longer periods, and/or focused primarily on dogs as the therapy animal.

Kamioka et al. (2014) conducted a systematic review to summarize the results of randomized controlled trials (RCTs) that investigated the effects of animal-assisted therapy (AAT). The RCTs used in the review employed dogs, cats, dolphins, birds, cows, rabbits, ferrets, or guinea pigs as therapy animals. Although the authors were able to summarize the findings, they were unable to conduct a meta-analysis, because many of the studies were of poor quality and had high levels of heterogeneity. The authors concluded that AAT could be effective for treating certain mental and behavioral disorders. Additionally, they suggested an RCT methodology, reasons for nonparticipation, intervention dose, adverse effects, withdrawals, and cost should be assessed in future research (Kamioka, Okada,Tsutani, Park, Okuizumi, Handa,. . .Abe, 2014).

Lack of Physician Participation in Research

The spread of AAT and its benefits in published accounts has led to its increased implementation in ASD treatments. However, despite the reported effectiveness of the approach, AAT is still considered a CAM in many areas of health and, as such, is not viewed as a mainstream treatment method (Palley, O'Rourke, & Niemi, 2010). In their review of the literature, Palley et al. (2010) maintain that this was caused by physician resistance to using AAT in treatment. The authors claimed physician resistance was due to insufficient evidence of the clinical effectiveness of AAT and a lack of acceptable standard results.

In their study, Fayter, McDaid, Ritchie, Stirk, and Eastwood (2006) identified the barriers to physician participation in research as system, organization, research, and physician-related barriers. In their systematic review, Rahman et al. (2011) identified lack of time and resources, trial-specific issues, poor communication, clinician-scientist role conflicts, lack of physician training, lack of research-based experience, poor or no incentives or recognition, and a disinterest in the research topic as barriers preventing physicians from participating in AAT research. Clinical-trial recruitment, the trial process, and follow-ups require time, may result in an increased workload, and result in more physician responsibility (Foley & Moertel, 1991). Physicians may also be deterred from participating in research studies due to their perceived responsibility for their own clinical practice and patients. Furthermore, a lack of support staff to assist with the extra workload may be another contributing factor (Foley & Moertel, 1991; Smyth, Mossman, Hall, Hepburn, Pinkerton, Richards. . . Box, 1994; Yanagawa, Kishuku, Akaike, Azuma, & Irahara, 2010). Other reasons for physician reluctance toward clinical studies include their fear of altering the doctor-patient relationship and losing their rapport with patients (Levy, Frasso, Colantonio, Reed, Stein, Barg, . . .Fiks, 2016).

Even if physicians may be eager to become involved in clinical research studies, many are not familiar with the research-study process. Bylund et al. (2017) describe a clear example of how physician knowledge, attitudes, and beliefs can act as unnecessary barriers preventing physicians from participating in research. The study was conducted to assess the knowledge, attitudes, beliefs, experience, and interest of physicians regarding cancer clinical trials. Physicians (n=613) serving primarily minority ethnic and racial groups in the New York City area were emailed and encouraged to participate a 20-minute online survey about their patient population, and their knowledge of and attitudes toward clinical trials. Results showed that overall the 127 participants had little knowledge of and experience with cancer-based clinical trials. Despite this, it was noted that overall they felt positively toward clinical trials, 41.4% were eager to learn more about trials, and 35.7% indicated they might be interested in participating. Additionally, it was noted that Black and Latino physicians and those with positive views of clinical trials were more likely to partake in future training opportunities. The investigators suggested that methods of delivering education on clinical trials to interested providers should be explored.

SOLUTIONS AND RECOMMENDATIONS

Develop a Vision and Strategy

A possible way to increase the participation of physicians in clinical research could involve developing a vision and strategy that focus on encouraging physicians to participate. If the vision and strategy are to be strong, factors that possibly could influence the level of physician participation in clinical research must be considered (Ward, 1994). According to Croughan (2001), such factors include personal interest in the research topic are the clinical relevance of the research, a personal connection to the researchers, collective ownership of the project, costs associated with research participation, and little interference of research with patient care.

The participation of physicians in research studies on the suitability of AAT as an ASD treatment can greatly influence whether the treatment modality becomes mainstreamed or not. As such, physicians inadvertently hold the key to its possible therapeutic and cost-saving potential, since without the support of prescribing physicians, it is unlikely that the treatment modality will ever be accepted into mainstream medicine. Thus, to realize the vision of improving research on AAT as a treatment for ASD, the proposed goal of expanding physician participation in AAT research needs to be achieved (Smith, 2013). The implementation of a briefly proposed strategy to encourage physician participation in research involving AAT for treating ASD could focus on educating physicians, offering incentives, forming interdisciplinary teams, and implementing policy.

Educate

Encouraging physicians to participate in clinical studies focused on AAT as a treatment for ASD requires familiarizing them with the topic and the study process (Ganz, 2007). To become familiar with AAT concepts, physicians must become acquainted with study processes, receive up-to-date information, and be encouraged to participate in clinical studies (Lefebvre, Golab, Christensen, Castrodale, Aureden, Bialachowski, . . . Weese, 2008). Education that focuses on changing physician attitudes, knowledge, and beliefs is paramount if their participation in AAT research is to occur. In addition, countering the perceptions of skeptics calls for demonstrating the logicality and effectiveness of AAT as an ASD management tool. Therefore, we recommend development of interactive, applicable, and knowledge-based programs promoting the participation of physicians in AAT, and strategies such as incorporating training programs into undergraduate and graduate medical education courses, and reinforcing concepts through continuing medical education. These programs could include hands-on interactions during AAT sessions and knowledge-based workshops that could be offered online or in a class-based setting. Furthermore, educational programs could focus on fostering a culture of inquiry and research-based learning (Rahman, Majumder, Shaban, Rahman, Ahmed, Abdulrahman, & D'Souza, 2011). Collaborative efforts between ASD-based research organizations, healthcare organizations, and ASD advocate organizations could provide support for these programs. Rahman et al. (2011) also recommend that physicians with prior clinical research be selected as "physician ambassadors" who could share their experiences and positive perspectives.

Motivate

Motivation drives change and is an important factor that could influence a physician's willingness to participate in clinical research. To appeal to a physician's, intrinsic and extrinsic motivators must be identified (Herzer & Pronovost, 2015). Herzer's theory describes intrinsic motivation as the drive within an individual to make an effort due to interest in the work being performed and posits that it consists of a desire to achieve, have purpose, obtain autonomy, reach mastery, take responsibility, and grow and learn (Pink, 2011). Assigning responsibility for more difficult tasks, granting additional authority or autonomy, providing direct feedback on performance, cultivating a collegial rather than a competitive atmosphere, and inspiring a collective purpose and vision are all strategies that can foster intrinsic motivation (Pink, 2011). Since Herzberg's intrinsic motivation theory suggests that appealing to intrinsic motivation determinants could effectively improve performance, this could apply to improving participation in clinical research. An example of intrinsic motivation would be a physician's desire to improve patients' health, appealed to by encouraging research participation through programs, and providing collaborative environments that involve solving complex and interesting research-related issues.

Extrinsic motivators refer to motivating factors based on rewards or punishments (Herzer & Pronovost, 2015). Extrinsic motivators are outside influences that are not related to the nature of work itself and have no bearing on internal satisfaction (Herzer & Pronovost, 2015). Money is an example of an extrinsic motivator. Results of a study conducted by Donaldson et al. (1999) show that appealing to a physician's external motivation in the form of incentives can significantly improve physician participation in research. Thus, offering them appealing financial rewards could encourage physicians to participate in clinical research. These rewards could vary according to the complexity of the study, the level of physician participation, and the quality of their contribution to the study itself.

Make Participating in Research Convenient

The responsibility that physicians feel toward their patients may often mean that participating in research studies is not a priority for them (Hoffman, Benda, Fairbanks, & Auguste, 2017). Due to time constraints, many physicians may find participating in clinical research studies inconvenient. Developing flexible participation methods that provide the adequate freedom and autonomy might make participating in clinical research more appealing to physicians.

Form Interdisciplinary Healthcare Teams

Physicians may feel more open to participating in clinical studies if they feel supported. Since interdisciplinary healthcare teams bring expertise from a variety of healthcare areas, the support and a feeling of inclusion may improve the appeal of clinical studies to physicians. Thus, the development of specialized interdisciplinary healthcare teams could be beneficial, with teams comprised of physicians, AAT experts, ASD related therapists, and organizational leadership representatives. The interdisciplinary input may broaden physician and clinician insight, knowledge, and understanding of AAT (Wright, Sparks, & O'Hair, 2013). In addition, a team environment may be more conducive to open dialogue between physicians, clinicians, and AAT experts. This environment may then provide a comfortable platform for physicians and clinicians to voice their opinions and concerns and create an interactive learning environment.

Implement Policy

Development of suitable organizational and departmental guidelines and policies could successfully gain physician buy-in (Rugari, Hunter, & Carswell, 2017). These policies could cover both general program implementation and AAT health and safety. In order to implement a successful program, the policy should consider the setting in which AAT will be implemented (e.g., home, clinic, and school); the governing processes (e.g., laws and legislation protecting the treatment of animals and patient safety); and assessing the economic issues that could arise during its implementation (e.g., expense of running educational programs and loss of physician work hours due to participation in AAT related activities) (Collins, 2005).

General Program Policies

General program policies should provide physicians with necessary information to give them with the freedom to make informed decisions before consenting to study participation. Many of the physicians' concerns related to the development and implementation of an AAT program could also be addressed by clearly outlining animal and handler training and certifying standards (Rugari, Hunter, & Carswell, 2017), and specifying educational program standards and guidelines within the policy.

Infection-Control Policies

Developing and maintaining appropriate policies and procedures are vital to protecting patients and animals. Linder, Siebens, Mueller, Gibbs, and Freeman (2017) conducted a study to evaluate the animal-assisted intervention (AAI) policies and procedures of hospitals, eldercare facilities, and animal-therapy organizations. A United States national survey of 45 eldercare facilities, 45 hospitals, and 27 therapy-animal organizations were surveyed to evaluate their AAI healthcare and safety policies. Results showed great variation in AAI health and safety policies and procedures, and while some were adequate to maintain safety, others had the potential to harm both humans and animals (Linder, Siebens, Mueller, Gibbs, & Freeman, 2017). The study also revealed that hospitals generally had more stringent AAI requirements than eldercare facilities (Linder, Siebens, Mueller, Gibbs, & Freeman, 2017). Healthcare facilities with AAI programs should review their guidelines and update policy to ensure the safety of patients and animals (Linder, Siebens, Mueller, Gibbs, & Freeman, 2017).

Infection-control policies could specify training and certification requirements as well as infection-control standards for AAT animals and handlers. Consideration could also be given to animal and handler health screenings and vaccinations, staff training in animal management and patient-animal contact, patient suitability, and zoonotic infection prevention (Rugari, Hunter, & Carswell, 2017). Policies might also identify unsuitable AAT candidates who may have open wounds, infectious diseases, or are immune compromised. These teams could maintain open communication and make themselves available to the physician and the interdisciplinary teams whenever necessary.

Health Insurance Policies

Should physician participation in research lead to the acceptance of AAT as an ASD treatment, a "push" toward mainstreaming the treatment for ASDs may occur. Consequently, health-insurance providers may then be obliged to cover AAT as a "standard treatment." in this regard. Therefore, health insurance providers could develop affordable AAT inclusive coverage policies that could cover AAT as they would any other reimbursable condition. The ripple effect may significantly improve the accessibility of AAT for those who cannot afford the treatment. Over time, this spread could increase the affordability of ASD treatments for both the patient and the U.S. healthcare system, as the cost-saving potential of AAT for treating ASDs will be realized (Ganz, 2007).

FUTURE DIRECTIONS

Further scientific studies are needed to better understand the therapeutic actions of AAT on ASD and evaluate its potential long-term benefits. While no studies refuting the benefits of AAT as a treatment for psychological disorders (including ASD) could be found, the quality of "AAT-supportive" studies is questionable. Thus, any future trends in AAT as a treatment for ASD will strongly depend on whether evidence confirming its safety, efficacy, and reliability is brought forward. Developing a strong evidence base is vital if physicians are to begin considering AAT as an adjunct treatment for ASD. Nevertheless, providing a strong evidence base requires physician participation in AAT-based research. Thus, if physicians are not encouraged to participate in AAT-related research, true evidence and the possibility of obtaining the likely benefits of this modality could be lost.

Leadership strategies provide a tailor able framework that could guide the collaboration between physicians and other AAT research stakeholders. As healthcare continues to transform itself, the flexibility of relationships between healthcare service providers and health corporations are being pushed to follow suit. Strategies could provide direction, outline objective guidelines, and protect patients', physicians', and researchers' interests, leading to improved AAT research, and possibly to increased acceptance of

AAT for ASD. Furthermore, developing and refining collaboration-based strategic pathways require more leadership-focused research.

While increasing AAT-based research and implementing AAT as a treatment for ASD may come at a large initial expense, AAT improving patient outcomes could offset these expenses in the long term. Since AAT may have the potential to improve a patient's adherence to prescribed treatments, improve therapeutic outcomes, and reduce or shorten hospital stays (Chandler, 2012), a ripple effect may lead to reduced healthcare costs. Subsequently, AAT could become a reimbursable expense for third-party payers. This may then lead to a shift of AAT from a "niche" practice to a mainstream practice, thereby increasing the affordability of ASD treatment for patients, families, and ultimately the U.S. healthcare system as a whole. However, no reliable research has been conducted to substantiate these claims. Therefore, additional quantitative research would be required to more precisely identify, assign a value to, and quantify the expenses and savings.

CONCLUSION

This review summarized the key work related to AAT as a method to treat ASD, discussed possible reasons for low physician participation in this area of clinical research, and outlined a leadership method to improve AAT-related research as it applies to ASD. In the end, using leadership strategies that aim to encourage physicians to participate in clinical research is imperative for determining the safety, efficacy, and suitability of AAT as an adjunct treatment for ASD. Additionally, the potential cost savings of the treatment modality are an additional outcome to consider alongside other key variables, such as improved treatment outcomes and behaviors. Given that cost savings relate to important outcomes, comprehensive research should consider quantifying and identifying leadership strategies as essential factors in AAT and healthcare research.

REFERENCES

Amendah, D., Grosse, S. D., Peacock, G., & Mandell, D. S. (2011). The economic costs of autism: A review. In D. Amaral, D. Geschwind, & G. Dawson (Eds.), *Autism spectrum disorders* (pp. 1347–1360). New York, NY: Oxford University Press. doi:10.1093/med/9780195371826.003.0088

American Psychiatric Association. (2013). *Diagnostic and statistical manual of mental disorders* (5th ed.). Arlington, VA: American Psychiatric Association.

Baio, J. (2012). Prevalence of autism spectrum disorders: Autism and developmental disabilities monitoring network, 14 sites, United States, 2008. *MMWR. Surveillance Summaries*, *61*(3), 1–19. PMID:22456193

Bass, M. M., Duchowny, C. A., & Llabre, M. M. (2009). The effect of therapeutic horseback riding on social functioning in children with autism. *Journal of Autism and Developmental Disorders*, *39*(9), 1261–1267. doi:10.100710803-009-0734-3 PMID:19350376

Bauman, M. L. (2010). Medical comorbidities in autism: Challenges to diagnosis and treatment. *Neurotherapeutics; the Journal of the American Society for Experimental NeuroTherapeutics*, *7*(3), 320–327. doi:10.1016/j.nurt.2010.06.001 PMID:20643385

Baxter, A., Brugha, T., Erskine, H., Scheurer, R., Vos, T., & Scott, J. (2015). The epidemiology and global burden of autism spectrum disorders. *Psychological Medicine*, *45*(3), 601–613. doi:10.1017/S003329171400172X PMID:25108395

Becker, J. L., Rogers, E. C., & Burrows, B. (2017). Animal-assisted social skills training for children with autism spectrum disorders. *Anthrozoos*, *30*(2), 307–326. doi:10.1080/08927936.2017.1311055

Blumberg, S. J., Bramlett, M. D., Kogan, M. D., Schieve, L. A., Jones, J. R., & Lu, M. C. (2013). *Changes in prevalence of parent-reported autism spectrum disorder in school-aged U.S. children: 2007 to 2011-2012*. Hyattsville, MD: National Center for Health Statistics.

Bylund, C. L., Weiss, E. S., Michaels, M., Patel, S., D'Agostino, T. A., Peterson, E. B., ... McKee, M. D. (2017). Primary care physicians' attitudes and beliefs about cancer clinical trials. *Clinical Trials*, *14*(5), 518–525. doi:10.1177/1740774517717722 PMID:28693389

Centers for Disease Control and Prevention. (2016, March 31). *CDC estimates 1 in 68 school-aged children have autism: No change from previous estimate*. Retrieved from https://www.cdc.gov/media/releases/2016/p0331-children-autism.html

Centers for Disease Control and Prevention. (2017, March 10). Autism spectrum disorder (ASD). Retrieved from https://www.cdc.gov/ncbddd/autism/data.html

Chandler, C. K. (2012). *Animal-assisted therapy in counseling*. New York, NY: Taylor & Francis.

Chiri, G., & Warfield, M. (2012). Unmet need and problems accessing core health care services for children with autism spectrum disorder. *Maternal and Child Health Journal*, *16*(5), 1081–1091. doi:10.100710995-011-0833-6 PMID:21667201

Collins, T. (2005). Health policy analysis: A simple tool for policy makers. *Public Health*, *119*(3), 192–196. doi:10.1016/j.puhe.2004.03.006 PMID:15661129

Connor, K., & Miller, J. (2000). Animal-assisted therapy: An in-depth look. *Dimensions of Critical Care Nursing*, *19*(3), 20–26. doi:10.1097/00003465-200019030-00006 PMID:11998003

Croughan, M. (2001). Factors influencing physician participation in practice-based research network studies: A call for further research. [Commentary]. *The Journal of Family Practice*, *50*(11), 978. PMID:11711017

Cullen, L., Titler, M., & Drahozal, R. (1999). Family and pet visitation in the critical care unit. *Critical Care Nurse*, *19*(3), 84. PMID:10661096

Donaldson, G. W., Moinpour, C. M., Bush, N. E., Chapko, M., Jocom, J., Siadak, M., & Sullivan, K. M. (1999). Physician participation in research surveys: A randomized study of inducements to return mailed research questionnaires. *Evaluation & the Health Professions*, *22*(4), 427–441. doi:10.1177/01632789922034392 PMID:10623399

Eapen, V., Nicholls, L., Spagnol, V., & Mathew, N. E. (2017). Current status of biological treatment options in autism spectrum disorder. *Asian Journal of Psychiatry*, *30*, 1–10. doi:10.1016/j.ajp.2017.07.025 PMID:28704714

Fayter, D., McDaid, C., Ritchie, G., Stirk, L., & Eastwood, A. (2006). *Systematic review of barriers, modifiers and benefits involved in participation in cancer clinical trials. Research Report. CRD Report (31)*. University of York NHS Centre for Reviews & Dissemination.

Fine, A. H. (2015). *Handbook on Animal-Assisted Therapy: Foundations and Guidelines for Animal-Assisted Interventions*. New York, NY: Academic Press.

Foley, J. F., & Moertel, C. G. (1991). Improving accrual into cancer clinical trials. *Journal of Cancer Education*, *6*(3), 165–173. doi:10.1080/08858199109528114 PMID:1931596

Friedmann, E., Son, H., & Saleem, M. (2015). The animal–human bond: Health and wellness. In A. H. Fine (Ed.), *Handbook on Animal-Assisted Therapy: Foundations and Guidelines for Animal-Assisted Interventions* (4th ed., pp. 73–88). Burlington, MA: Academic Press. doi:10.1016/B978-0-12-801292-5.00007-9

Fung, S. C. (2017). An observational study on canine-assisted play therapy for children with autism: Move towards the phrase of manualization and protocol development. *Global Journal of Health Science*, *9*(7), 67. doi:10.5539/gjhs.v9n7p67

Gabriels, R. L., Agnew, J. A., Holt, K. D., Shoffner, A., Zhaoxing, P., Ruzzano, S., ... Mesibov, G. (2012). Pilot study measuring the effects of therapeutic horseback riding on school-age children and adolescents with autism spectrum disorders. *Research in Autism Spectrum Disorders*, *6*(2), 578–588. doi:10.1016/j.rasd.2011.09.007

Gagnon, J., Bouchard, F., Landry, M., Belles-Isles, M., Fortier, M., & Fillion, L. (2004). Implementing a hospital-based animal therapy program for children with cancer: A descriptive study. *Canadian Oncology Nursing Journal/Revue canadienne de soins infirmiers en oncologie, 14*(4), 217-222.

Gammonley, J., & Yates, J. (1991). Pet projects: Animal assisted therapy in nursing homes. *Journal of Gerontological Nursing*, *17*(1), 12–15. doi:10.3928/0098-9134-19910101-05 PMID:1899683

Ganz, M. L. (2007). The lifetime distribution of the incremental societal costs of autism. *Archives of Pediatrics & Adolescent Medicine*, *161*(4), 343–349. doi:10.1001/archpedi.161.4.343 PMID:17404130

Glenk, L. M. (2017). Current perspectives on therapy dog welfare in animal-assisted interventions. *Animals (Basel)*, *7*(2), 7. doi:10.3390/ani7020007 PMID:28157145

Hatch, A. (2007). The view from all fours: A look at an animal-assisted activity program from the animals' perspective. *Anthrozoos*, *20*(1), 37–50. doi:10.2752/089279307780216632

Haubenhofer, D. K., & Kirchengast, S. (2006). Austrian and American approaches to animal-based health care services. *Anthrozoos*, *19*(4), 365–373. doi:10.2752/089279306785415484

Heimlich, K. (2001). Animal-assisted therapy and the severely disabled child: A quantitative study. *Journal of Rehabilitation*, *67*(4), 48.

Herzer, K. R., & Pronovost, P. J. (2015). Physician motivation: Listening to what pay for performance programs and quality improvement collaboratives are telling us. *Joint Commission Journal on Quality and Patient Safety*, *41*(11), 522–528. doi:10.1016/S1553-7250(15)41069-4 PMID:26484685

Hirvikoski, T., Mittendorfer-Rutz, E., Boman, M., Larsson, H., Lichtenstein, P., & Bolte, S. (2016). Premature mortality in autism spectrum disorder. *The British Journal of Psychiatry*, *208*(3), 232–238. doi:10.1192/bjp.bp.114.160192 PMID:26541693

Hoffman, D. J., Benda, N. C., Fairbanks, R. J., & Auguste, T. C. (2017). Simulated motivations: Understanding influences on medical professionals' decision making to participate in human factors research studies. *Proceedings of the International Symposium on Human Factors and Ergonomics in Health Care*, *6*(1), 9-12. 10.1177/2327857917061003

Iannuzzi, D., & Rowan, A. N. (1991). Ethical issues in animal-assisted therapy programs. *Anthrozoos*, *4*(3), 154–163. doi:10.2752/089279391787057116

Jain, A., Spencer, D., Yang, W., Kelly, J. P., Newschaffer, C. J., Johnson, J., ... Dennen, T. (2014). Injuries among children with autism spectrum disorder. *Academic Pediatrics*, *14*(4), 390–397. doi:10.1016/j.acap.2014.03.012 PMID:24976351

Kamioka, H., Okada, S., Tsutani, K., Park, H., Okuizumi, H., Handa, S., ... Abe, T. (2014). Effectiveness of animal-assisted therapy: A systematic review of randomized controlled trials. *Complementary Therapies in Medicine*, *22*(2), 371–390. doi:10.1016/j.ctim.2013.12.016 PMID:24731910

King, B. H. (2016). Psychiatric comorbidities in neurodevelopmental disorders. *Current Opinion in Neurology*, *29*(2), 113–117. doi:10.1097/WCO.0000000000000299 PMID:26840045

Kogan, M. D., Strickland, B. B., Blumberg, S. J., Singh, G. K., Perrin, J. M., & Van Dyck, P. C. (2008). A national profile of the health care experiences and family impact of autism spectrum disorder among children in the United States, 2005-2006. *Pediatrics*, *122*(6), e1149–e1158. doi:10.1542/peds.2008-1057 PMID:19047216

Kruger, K. A., & Serpell, J. A. (2010). Animal-assisted interventions in mental health: Definitions and theoretical foundations. In A. H. Fine (Ed.), *Handbook on Animal-Assisted Therapy: Foundations And Guidelines For Animal-Assisted Interventions* (3rd ed.; pp. 33–48). Burlington, MA: Academic Press; doi:10.1016/B978-0-12-381453-1.10003-0

Lavelle, T. A., Weinstein, M. C., Newhouse, J. P., Munir, K., Kuhlthau, K. A., & Prosser, L. A. (2014). Economic burden of autism spectrum disorders. *Pediatrics*, *133*(3), e520–e529. doi:10.1542/peds.2013-0763 PMID:24515505

Lefebvre, S. L., Golab, G. C., Christensen, E., Castrodale, L., Aureden, K., Bialachowski, A., ... Weese, J. S. (2008). Writing panel of working group. Guidelines for animal-assisted interventions in health care facilities. *American Journal of Infection Control*, *36*(2), 78–85. doi:10.1016/j.ajic.2007.09.005 PMID:18313508

Levy, S. E., Frasso, R., Colantonio, S., Reed, H., Stein, G., Barg, F. K., ... Fiks, A. G. (2016). Shared decision making and treatment decisions for young children with autism spectrum disorder. *Academic Pediatrics*, *16*(6), 571–578. doi:10.1016/j.acap.2016.04.007 PMID:27132050

Linder, D. E., Siebens, H. C., Mueller, M. K., Gibbs, D. M., & Freeman, L. M. (2017). Animal-assisted interventions: A national survey of health and safety policies in hospitals, eldercare facilities, and therapy animal organizations. *American Journal of Infection Control*, *45*(8), 883–887. doi:10.1016/j.ajic.2017.04.287 PMID:28673680

Marino, L., & Lilienfeld, S. O. (2007). Dolphin-assisted therapy: More flawed data and more flawed conclusions. *Anthrozoos*, *20*(3), 239–249. doi:10.2752/089279307X224782

Martin, F., & Farnum, J. (2002). Animal-assisted therapy for children with pervasive developmental disorders. *Western Journal of Nursing Research*, *24*(6), 657–670. doi:10.1177/019394502320555403 PMID:12365766

Matuszek, S. (2010). Animal-facilitated therapy in various patient populations: Systematic literature review. *Holistic Nursing Practice*, *24*(4), 187–203. doi:10.1097/HNP.0b013e3181e90197 PMID:20588128

Mazefsky, C. A., Pelphrey, K. A., & Dahl, R. E. (2012). The need for a broader approach to emotion regulation research in autism. *Child Development Perspectives*, *6*(1), 92–97. doi:10.1111/j.1750-8606.2011.00229.x PMID:22639681

Montes, G., & Halterman, J. S. (2008). Association of autism spectrum disorders and loss of family income. *Pediatrics*, *121*(4), 1594. doi:10.1542/peds.2007-1594 PMID:18381511

Morrison, M. L. (2007). Health benefits of animal-assisted interventions. *Complementary Health Practice Review*, *12*(1), 51–62. doi:10.1177/1533210107302397

National Institutes of Health. (2017, September 24). Complementary, alternative, or integrative health: What's in a name? Retrieved from https://nccih.nih.gov/health/integrative-health

Newschaffer, C. J., Croen, L. A., Daniels, J., Giarelli, E., Grether, J. K., Levy, S. E., ... Windham, G. C. (2007). The epidemiology of autism spectrum disorders. *Annual Review of Public Health*, *28*(1), 235–258. doi:10.1146/annurev.publhealth.28.021406.144007 PMID:17367287

Nimer, J., & Lundahl, B. (2007). Animal-assisted therapy: A meta-analysis. *Anthrozoos*, *20*(3), 225–238. doi:10.2752/089279307X224773

O'Haire, M. E. (2013). Animal-assisted intervention for autism spectrum disorder: A systematic literature review. *Journal of Autism and Developmental Disorders*, *43*(7), 1606–1622. doi:10.100710803-012-1707-5 PMID:23124442

O'Haire, M. E., McKenzie, S. J., McCune, S., & Slaughter, V. (2014). Effects of classroom animal-assisted activities on social functioning in children with autism spectrum disorder. *Journal of Alternative and Complementary Medicine (New York, N.Y.)*, *20*(3), 162–168. doi:10.1089/acm.2013.0165 PMID:24156772

Palley, L. S., O'Rourke, P. P., & Niemi, S. M. (2010). Mainstreaming animal-assisted therapy. *ILAR Journal*, *51*(3), 199–207. doi:10.1093/ilar.51.3.199 PMID:21131720

Patel, V. B., Preedy, V. R., & Martin, C. R. (2014). *Comprehensive guide to autism*. New York, NY: Springer. doi:10.1007/978-1-4614-4788-7

Pink, D. H. (2011). *Drive: The surprising truth about what motivates us*. New York, NY: Penguin Group.

Prothmann, A., & Fine, A. H. (2011). Animal-assisted interventions in child psychiatry. In P. McCardle, S. McCune, J. A. Griffin, L. Esposito, & L. S. Freund (Eds.), *Animals in our lives: Human animal interaction in family, community and therapeutic settings* (pp. 143–162). Baltimore, MD: Paul H. Brooks Publishing.

Rahman, S., Majumder, M. A. A., Shaban, S. F., Rahman, N., Ahmed, M., Abdulrahman, K. B., & D'Souza, U. J. (2011). Physician participation in clinical research and trials: Issues and approaches. *Advances in Medical Education and Practice*, *2*, 85–93. doi:10.2147/AMEP.S14103 PMID:23745079

Redefer, L. A., & Goodman, J. F. (1989). Brief report: Pet-facilitated therapy with autistic children. *Journal of Autism and Developmental Disorders*, *19*(3), 461–467. doi:10.1007/BF02212943 PMID:2793790

Rossetti, J., & King, C. (2010). Use of animal-assisted therapy with psychiatric patients: A literature review. *Journal of Psychosocial Nursing and Mental Health Services*, *48*(11), 44–48. doi:10.3928/02793695-20100831-05 PMID:20873700

Rugari, S. M., Hunter, C. L., & Carswell, B. M. (2017). Animal-assisted therapy and activities in the critical care setting. *Nursing 2017. Critical Care (London, England)*, *12*(6), 32–40. Retrieved from http://journals.lww.com/nursingcriticalcare/Fulltext/2017/11000/Animal_assisted_therapy_and_activities_in_the.5.aspx

Samfira, M., & Petroman, I. (2011). Therapeutic value of the human being-animal relationship. *Lucrari Stiintifice. Zootehnie si Biotehnologii*, *44*(2), 512–515.

Sams, M. J., Fortney, E. V., & Willenbring, S. (2006). Occupational therapy incorporating animals for children with autism: A pilot investigation. *The American Journal of Occupational Therapy*, *60*(3), 268–274. doi:10.5014/ajot.60.3.268 PMID:16776394

Shimabukuro, T. T., Grosse, S. D., & Rice, C. (2008). Medical expenditures for children with an autism spectrum disorder in a privately insured population. *Journal of Autism and Developmental Disorders*, *38*(3), 546–552. doi:10.100710803-007-0424-y PMID:17690969

Sillery, J., Hargreaves, J., Marin, P., Lerma, E., Kuznia, C., & Abbe, C. (2004). Pasteurella multocida peritonitis another risk of animal-assisted therapy. *Infection Control and Hospital Epidemiology*, *25*(1), 5–6. doi:10.1086/503486 PMID:14756211

Silva, K., Correia, R., Lima, M., Magalhães, A., & de Sousa, L. (2011). Can dogs prime autistic children for therapy? Evidence from a single case study. *Journal of Alternative and Complementary Medicine (New York, N.Y.)*, *17*(7), 655–659. doi:10.1089/acm.2010.0436 PMID:21689015

Smith, K. (2013). Evidence-informed policy in public health. In K. Smith (Ed.), *Beyond evidence-based policy in public health: The interplay of ideas* (pp. 42–69). London: Palgrave Macmillan UK; doi:10.1057/9781137026583_2

Smyth, J. F., Mossman, J., Hall, R., Hepburn, S., Pinkerton, R., Richards, M., ... Box, J. (1994). Conducting clinical research in the new NHS: The model of cancer. *British Medical Journal, 309*(6952), 457–461. doi:10.1136/bmj.309.6952.457 PMID:7920132

Snider, L., Korner-Bitensky, N., Kammann, C., Warner, S., & Saleh, M. (2007). Horseback riding as therapy for children with cerebral palsy: Is there evidence of its effectiveness? *Physical & Occupational Therapy in Pediatrics*, *27*(2), 5–23. PMID:17442652

Solomon, O. (2010). What a dog can do: Children with autism and therapy dogs in social interaction. *ETHOS Journal of the Society of Psychological Anthropology*, *38*(1), 143–166.

Souter, M. A., & Miller, M. D. (2007). Do animal-assisted activities effectively treat depression? A meta-analysis. *Anthrozoos*, *20*(2), 167–180. doi:10.2752/175303707X207954

Tielsch-Goddard, A., & Gilmer, M. J. (2015). The role and impact of animals with patients. *Nursing*, *41*(2), 65–71. PMID:26292453

Van Heijst, B. F., & Geurts, H. M. (2015). Quality of life in autism across the lifespan: A meta-analysis. *Autism*, *19*(2), 158–160. doi:10.1177/1362361313517053 PMID:24443331

Volkmar, F., Siegel, M., Woodbury-Smith, M., King, B., McCracken, J., & State, M. (2014). Practice parameter for the assessment and treatment of children and adolescents with autism spectrum disorder. *Journal of the American Academy of Child and Adolescent Psychiatry*, *53*(2), 237–257. doi:10.1016/j.jaac.2013.10.013 PMID:24472258

Ward, J. (1994). General practitioners' experience of research. *Family Practice*, *11*(4), 418–423. doi:10.1093/fampra/11.4.418 PMID:7895971

Wright, K. B., Sparks, L., & O'Hair, H. D. (2013). *Health communication in the 21st century*. New York, NY: John Wiley & Sons.

Wu, A. S., Niedra, R., Pendergast, L., & McCrindle, B. W. (2002). Acceptability and impact of pet visitation on a cardiology inpatient unit. *Journal of Nursing*, *17*(5), 354–362. PMID:12395303

Yanagawa, H., Kishuku, M., Akaike, M., Azuma, H., & Irahara, M. (2010). View of physicians on and barriers to patient enrollment in a multicenter clinical trial: Experience in a Japanese rural area. *International Archives of Medicine*, *3*(7). doi:10.1186/1755-7682-3-7 PMID:20525325

Zamir, T. (2006). The moral basis of animal-assisted therapy. *Society & Animals*, *14*(2), 179–199. doi:10.1163/156853006776778770 PMID:16862727

KEY TERMS AND DEFINITIONS

Animal-Assisted Therapy: A therapeutic modality in which a certified animal forms an essential part of the treatment process.

Autism Spectrum Disorder: An incurable condition whereby an individual has poor social and communication skills and may display restricted and repetitive behaviors.

Clinical Study: Any research study that prospectively assigns human participants or groups of humans to one or more health-related interventions to evaluate the effects on health outcomes.

Complementary and Alternative Medicine: A group of various medical and health approaches that are used in place of or as an adjunct to allopathic approaches, but that is not considered to be allopathic in nature.

Conventional/Allopathic Medicine: Widely accepted treatment that is used by most healthcare professionals.

Double-Blind Study: A type of medical study characterized by the unawareness of both the study participants and researcher are unaware of whether the treatment or procedure has been administered. Double-blinded studies are frequently used if initial studies have demonstrated particular promise.

Extrinsic Motivation: The drive of an individual to make an effort based on rewards or punishments.

Health Policy: Decisions, plans, and actions that are outlined and followed to achieve specific healthcare goals.

Interdisciplinary Healthcare Teams: A group of healthcare professionals from various fields who work collaboratively to achieve a common goal for the patient.

Intrinsic Motivation: The drive within an individual to make an effort due to interest in the work being performed, consisting of a desire to achieve, have purpose, obtain autonomy, reach mastery, take responsibility, and grow and learn.

Leadership: The ability to motivate a group of people to work towards achieving a common goal.

Leadership Vision: A mental image that is used to guide an organization or group into the future. A leadership vision forms the basis upon which goals are set, plans are made, and problems are solved.

Randomized Control Trial: A study in which participants are selected at random to receive one of several clinical interventions. One of these interventions the control which, may be a standard practice, a placebo, or no intervention at all.

Strategic Leadership: A plan developed using well-considered tactics to communicate a vision, and the outline, the goals, and objectives to be met, in order to achieve it.

Chapter 10
Autism and Diet:
An Insight Approach

Komal Srivastava
Apollo Gleneagles Hospitals, India

ABSTRACT

The parents of children with autism spectrum disorder (ASD) often try alternative treatments to reduce their children's symptoms, and one of the alternatives is a specialized diet. This diet is called gluten-free casein-free or GFCF diet. The GFCF diet has grown popular over the years. These children may be sensitive to the taste, smell, color, and texture of foods. They may limit or totally avoid some foods and even whole food groups. They may have difficulty focusing on one task for an extended period of time. It may be hard for a child to sit down and eat a meal from start to finish. The chapter highlights the impact of maternal nutrition, nutritional deficiencies, and GFCF diet in ASD.

INTRODUCTION

Nutrition plays a very important role in growth and development of the brain. Nutrients present in different food are required in sufficient amount for its development. There are a certain group of nutrients which are supposed to have an important role and thus making it more crucial. Brain development and function are affected by the timing of nutrient supplement and deficiency. For proper brain development and functional homeostasis, there must be a constant flow of nutrients across the blood-brain barrier, which is ensured by a group of transporters and regulator. It functions in such a way that brain receives neither too much nor too little of each nutrient (Fuglestad, Rao, & Georgieff, 2008).

IMPORTANCE OF MATERNAL NUTRITION

Various biological, socio-economic and demographic factors which vary in different population influence the complex association between maternal nutrition and birth outcome thus proving that nutrition plays an important role in maternal and child health (Villar, Merialdi, Gulmezoglu, Abalos, Carroli,

DOI: 10.4018/978-1-5225-7004-2.ch010

Kulier, & de Onis, 2003). The significance of adequate nutrition during fetal life for long-term physical health is well documented (Barker, 1998; Harding, 2001). However, the relationship between maternal nutrition during pregnancy and child mental health is less established (Heindel & Vandenberg, 2015). The prenatal environment is crucial in relation to the cognitive development of the child, particularly during critical periods of brain development, which highlights that the fetus needs for optimal nutrition (Thapar, Cooper, Jefferies, & Stergiakouli, 2012). There are documented detrimental effects of severe maternal malnutrition during pregnancy (Roseboom, Painter, van Abeelen, Veenendaal, & de Rooij, 2011). Severe deficiencies of certain micronutrients, like iron and iodine (Prado & Dewey, 2014) has effects on child's neurodevelopment and general cognitive functions, as well as severe deficiencies of folate and choline on child neural tube defects but the impact of more subtle variations in maternal diet quality on child neurodevelopment has received little attention until recently (Zeisel, 2008).

ROLE OF NUTRITION IN BRAIN DEVELOPMENT

Intelligence is the global capacity of the individual to act purposefully, to think rationally and to deal effectively with his environment. Intelligence Quotient (IQ) refers to general cognitive ability, such as learning aptitude, reasoning, and problem-solving qualities. Development of brain begins in the very early period of conception i.e as early as 18 days after fertilisation and tends to continue even after birth. The fastest growth of brain occurs in utero, a vulnerable and important period. Suboptimal nutrition during brain development may affect cognitive development and behavioral performance over time (Anjos, Altmäe, Emmett, Tiemeier, Closa-Monasterolo, Luque, & Egan, 2013; Rees & Inder, 2005; Thompson & Nelson, 2001).

During pregnancy, important neurologic functions are developing in the fetus (Rees & Inder, 2005). Brain development in the last trimester of gestation is particularly vulnerable to inadequacy in the mother's diet (Anjos, Altmäe, Emmett, Tiemeier, Closa-Monasterolo, Luque, & Egan, 2013). Maternal diet has a long-term effect on their child's neurodevelopment. It includes cognitive, psychomotor and mental development, IQ scores (verbal, verbal-executive function, and performance) and its effects on behavioral status. (Anjos, Altmäe, Emmett, Tiemeier, Closa-Monasterolo, Luque, & Egan, 2013; Hibbeln, Davis, Steer, Emmett, Rogers, Williams, & Golding, 2007; Gil & Gil, 2015; Starling, Charlton, McMahon, & Lucas, 2015). Intakes of specific food items, such as fish, during pregnancy, have shown positive associations with neurodevelopmental outcomes in childhood (Anjos, Altmäe, Emmett, Tiemeier, Closa-Monasterolo, Luque, & Egan, 2013; Gil & Gil, 2015; Starling, Charlton, McMahon, & Lucas, 2015).

Various cross-sectional studies conducted has shown relation between dietary patterns and cognitive outcomes, in childhood, in adolescence, and in the elderly (Gale, Martyn, Marriott, Limond, Crozier, & Inskip, 2009; Kim, Yu, Choi, Nam, Kim, Oh, & Yang, 2015; Leventakou, Roumeliotaki, Sarri, Koutra, Kampouri, Kyriklaki, & Chatzi, 2016; Northstone, Joinson, Emmett, Ness, & Paus, 2012; Nyaradi, Foster, Hickling, Li, Ambrosini, Jacques, & Oddy, 2014). Optimum intake of healthy foods such as fruits, vegetables, and fish was measured in these stages of life, are linked with better cognitive outcomes, including higher childhood IQ. In addition, unhealthy dietary patterns were found to be associated with poorer cognitive outcomes in childhood and adolescence (Gale, Martyn, Marriott, Limond, Crozier, & Inskip, 2009; Kim, Yu, Choi, Nam, Kim, Oh, & Yang, 2015; Leventakou, Roumeliotaki, Sarri, Koutra, Kampouri, Kyriklaki, & Chatzi, 2016; Northstone, Joinson, Emmett, Ness, & Paus, 2012; Nyaradi, Foster, Hickling, Li, Ambrosini, Jacques, & Oddy, 2014; Smithers, Golley, Mittinty, Brazionis, Northstone, Emmett, & Lynch, 2012; Smithers, Golley, Mittinty, Brazionis, Northstone, Emmett, & Lynch, 2013).

COGNITION

Cognition represents a complex set of higher mental functions subserved by the brain and includes attention, memory, thinking, learning, and perception (Bhatnagar & Taneja, 2001). Apart from nutrition, cognitive development is influenced by many factors. The literature has suggested a strong connection between improved nutrition and optimal brain function. Nutrients present in food plays a vital role in cell proliferation, DNA synthesis, neurotransmitter and hormone metabolism. It also serves an important role in the enzyme systems of the brain (Bhatnagar & Taneja, 2001; Lozoff & Georgieff, 2006; Zeisel, 2009; De Souza, Fernandes, & Tavares do Carmo, 2011; Zimmermann, 2011). Brain development is more rapid in the early years of life compared to the rest of the body which may make it more susceptible to nutrient deficiencies (Benton, 2010).

Role of Nutrition in Cognition

The role of nutrition from the perspective of cognitive development is critical to appreciate. Likewise, adequate nutrient delivery alone does not ensure normal brain growth and development. The role of nutrition in cognitive development must be considered keeping in mind other biological and environmental factors. Optimum nutrition is essential for normal development. Environmental factors along with poor nutrition have its effects on development. Nutritional deficiencies (as measured by the mental development index of Bayley Scales) has effects on cognition which are more severe for children living in homes where there is less motivation compared to homes with higher levels of motivation (Grantham-McGregor, Lira, Ashworth, Morris, & Assunçao, 1998). Studies on the role of micronutrients such as omega-3 fatty acids, vitamin B12, folic acid, zinc, iron, and iodine has been carried out to isolate the importance on these nutrients in context to the relationship between nutrition and cognitive development. From observational studies carried out, it can be concluded that these micronutrients play an important role in the cognitive development of children.

AUTISM SPECTRUM DISORDER

The *diagnostic and statistical manual of mental disorders* (DSM-5; APA, 2013) has described Autism Spectrum disorder (ASD) along with Autism which is one of the complex neurodevelopmental conditions. ASD affects almost 1 in 100 children (Kogan, Blumberg, Schieve, Boyle, Perrin, Ghandour, & van Dyck, 2009) and is characterized, in varying degrees, by deficits in verbal and nonverbal communication, and is associated with repetitive behaviors (APA, 2013). Several forms of ASD have been described, such as Asperger syndrome or Kanner type autism (Kanner, 1949) revealing that ASD is a highly heterogeneous disorder, likely with multiple underlying causes. Intense scientific work has been performed in recent years to understand the potential origin of ASD, revealing that this disorder arises from both genetic and environmental factors, especially those influencing fetal and early-life development (Lai et al., 2013).

Various studies carried out on ASD children have suggested that it is highly heritable which is estimated to be 38 – 54%, thus resulting to investigate on its mechanism (Hallmayer, Cleveland, Torres, Phillips, Cohen, Torigoe, & Lotspeich, 2011). ASD cases (10%) are also in genetic etiology, such as fragile X syndrome, tuberous sclerosis, and Rett disorder. Supporting the idea of heterogeneity of ASD, single genetic mutations account for only 1-2% of ASD cases (Abrahams, & Geschwind, 2008) with the majority of cases remaining idiopathic. Mutations identified by genetic studies have revealed that some affected genes are involved in brain development from in utero through infancy. Frequent aberrations in brain cytoarchitectural organization and neuronal connectivity have been observed in the brains of ASD patients, leading to the concept that ASD is a synaptopathy (Won, Mah, & Kim, 2013). Genes involved in synapse formation or brain connectivity (e.g., fmr1, mecp2, shank3, tsc, neuroligin, and cntnap2) have been repeatedly linked to ASD (Oddi, Crusio, D'amato, & Pietropaolo, 2013; Shcheglovitov, Shcheglovitova, Yazawa, Portmann, Shu, Sebastiano, & Dolmetsch, 2013; Penagarikano, Abrahams, Herman, Winden, Gdalyahu, Dong, & Golshani, 2011).

ASD brain transcriptome studies identify molecular abnormalities in synaptic and immune/microglia markers gene expression, with the former being down-regulated and the latter upregulated (Voineagu, Wang, Johnston, Lowe, Tian, Horvath, & Geschwind, 2011). Other genes related to inflammation (e.g., il-1raplp1, il-1r2, c4b, met, mch2, par2, mtor1, and µpar) have been reported to be differentially expressed in ASD as well (Warren, Singh, Cole, Odell, Pingree, Warren, & White, 1991; Odell, Maciulis, Cutler, Warren, McMahon, Coon, ... & Torres, 2005). This is of particular interest as the prenatal environment generating chronic neuroinflammatory processes lead to the rapid development of ASD in susceptible children (Estes, Zwaigenbaum, Gu, John, Paterson, Elison, & Kostopoulos, 2015). Indeed, maternal inflammation linked to infection, autoimmunity, obesity, or gestational diabetes during pregnancy is associated with a higher risk of neurodevelopmental disorders, particularly in ASD. Many experimental studies have linked maternal immune activation (MIA) in the pathogenesis of ASD with neuro - inflammatory events in the developing brain as an important component of brain malformation (Smith, Li, Garbett, Mirnics, & Patterson, 2007; Patterson, 2011). Experimental studies also revealed that MIA induces long-lasting changes in immune system activity and microbiota, which are believed to be involved in behavioral alterations in offspring (Cryan & Dinan, 2015; Hsiao, McBride, Hsien, Sharon, Hyde, McCue, & Patterson, 2013). Interestingly, the host microbiota has been shown to modulate local immune responses in the brain (Erny, de Angelis, Jaitin, Wieghofer, Staszewski, David, & Schwierzeck, 2015) and conversely neuro inflammation can influence the microbiota composition (Cryan, & Dinan, 2015). In addition to the microbiota, nutrition is an important component of inflammatory regulation and the nutritional deficiency could also be an important risk factor for ASD (Bazinet & Layé, 2014). Recent animal studies have revealed that maternal nutritional statuses in n-3 polyunsaturated fatty acids (PUFAs), essential fatty acids with anti-inflammatory properties that are present in the brain (Calder, 2013; Delpech, Thomazeau, Madore, Bosch-Bouju, Larrieu, Lacabanne, & Layé, 2015), regulate microglia activity in the developing brain (Madore, Nadjar, Delpech, Sere, Aubert, Portal,... & Layé, 2014) and influence ASD-like behavioural disorders (Pietropaolo, Goubran, Joffre, Aubert, Lemaire-Mayo, Crusio, & Laye, 2014).

Impact of Maternal Nutrition on ASD

Nutritional deficiencies are particularly common during pregnancy due to increased metabolic demands imposed by a growing placenta, fetus and maternal tissues, and have been shown to influence brain development in terms of structure and function. There is strong biological plausibility, therefore, that maternal nutrition might influence ASD risk as well (Picciano, 2003). In a large population-based case-control study, consumption of prenatal vitamin supplements near the time of conception was associated with about 40% reduction in risk for ASD (Schmidt, Hansen, Hartiala, Allayee, Schmidt, Tancredi, & Hertz-Picciotto, 2011). Impaired methylation capacity and altered DNA methylation have been implicated in ASD etiology (Schanen, 2006). The current research suggests that autism spectrum disorders (ASD) occur as a result of events that take place during pregnancy. Apart from genetic factors, non-heritable risk factors contribute to a substantial proportion of ASD cases. Focus on maternal nutrition has been an area of interest as a factor which may influence risk for ASD. Various population-based studies carried out in this context have yielded conflicting results.

Different studies on maternal nutritional status were been carried out in which two studies-one an American case-control study, CHARGE (Childhood Autism Risks from Genetics and Environment) and, the other, a Norwegian cohort study (Norwegian Mother and Child Cohort Study (MoBa)) has strong results. It focused on folic acid intake during the peri-conceptual period and early pregnancy with a reduction in risk for of ASD. In the CHARGE study, maternal iron intake and multivitamin use were also associated with a reduced risk of ASD.

ASD and Feeding Difficulties

Multiple eating and nutritional challenges which serve as a core feature of ASD. Children are observed where they are unable to recognize and address such problems. These children are found to have feeding problems and difficulties 5 times higher than those of non-ASD peers (Sharp, Berry, McCracken, Nuhu, Marvel, Saulnier, & Jaquess, 2013). ASD children are picky eaters. They are highly selective while choosing foods for themselves and only eating a narrow variety of foods–is the most prominent feeding concerns among children with autism". It typically involves strong preferences for starchy and processed foods and snack foods, along with a bias against fruits and vegetables (Berry, Novak, Withrow, Schmidt, Rarback, Feucht, & Sharp, 2015).

Nutritional deficiencies and medical complications are seen as a consequence of eating issues in children with ASD, thus resulting in serious health risks. Children with ASD have been found to have lower vitamin D and calcium intake from food compared with that of their typically developing peers and children with and without autism generally do not consume sufficient amounts of those nutrients or vitamin E, potassium, and choline. A cross-sectional study published in 2015 in the *Journal of the Academy of Nutrition and Dietetics* investigated micronutrient intake and the use of supplements in 288 children aged 2–11 with ASD. The results show that while 56% of the sample was taking nutritional supplements, there remained deficits in vitamin D, calcium, potassium, pantothenic acid, and choline. Nearly one-third of participants were deficient in vitamin D, for example, and up to 54% were calcium-deficient (Stewart, Hyman, Schmidt, Macklin, Reynolds, Johnson, & Manning-Courtney, 2015).

Concentration on detail, perseveration, impulsivity, fear of novelty, sensory impairments, deficits in social compliance, and biological food intolerance are the few feeding problems which are found in ASD children (Cumine, Leach, & Stevenson, 2000). Parental anxiety, reinforcement of negative feeding patterns, and communication difficulties have been suggested as additional social reinforcers that contribute to the maintenance of maladaptive feeding behaviors in this population (Shaw, Garcia, Thorn, Farley, & Flanagan, 2003). Ahearn, Castine, Nault, and Green (2001) suggested that selective feeding in children with ASD was a manifestation of their restricted interests and activities.

Mealtime behavior and eating problems are usually not assessed unless a child exhibits failure to thrive (Hutchinson, 1999), which might explain the lack of research on problem feeding behavior in children with ASD. When nutritional rehabilitation is delayed until after a child is 8 years of age, however, growth rates fall below average (Schwarz, 2003). Thus, some evidence has indicated that even when failure to thrive is not evident and health is not immediately at risk, assessment and treatment of aberrant feeding behaviors in this population should be a priority.

Feeding problems are often seen in children with ASD wherein its prevalence has been reported to be as high as 90% (Kodak & Piazza, 2008), with close to 70% of children described as selective eaters (Twachtman-Reilly, Amaral, & Zebrowski, 2008). In fact, some authors have suggested that the presence of feeding difficulties in infancy may be an early sign of autism (Keen, 2008; Laud, Girolami, Boscoe, & Gulotta, 2009).

Repeated behaviors in children with ASD have narrow and fanatical interests which lead to selective food choices and eating habits. This can lead to the following health concerns.

- **Food Selection or Food Dislikes:** The attributes of food like the taste, smell, color and texture are found to be one of the difficult accept in consuming meals by these children as they are sensitive towards it. This limits or total avoidance of some foods and even whole food groups. Common dislikes include fruits, vegetables and slippery, soft foods.
- **Inadequate Intake:** Children with autism may have difficulty focusing on one task for an extended period of time. It may be hard for a child to sit down and eat a meal from start to finish.
- **Constipation:** Due to selective food choice and avoidance of food groups from diet children with ASD are more prone to constipation. The problem can be remedied by incorporating plenty of fluids and fiber-rich foods along with physical activity.
- **Food and Drug Interactions:** Certain drugs used in the treatment of ASD have a side effect thus, reducing the appetite of the child. This can reduce the amount of food a child eats, which can affect growth. Other medications may increase appetite or affect the absorption of certain vitamins and minerals.

Nutritional Deficiencies in ASD

Restricted diets and inadequate nutrient intake of children with ASD have been reported. A study carried out by Liu et al. (2016), the study examined the nutritional statuses of children with ASD and the relationships between their behaviors and nutritional intake. 154 diagnosed children with ASD and 73 typically-developing (TD) children from Chongqing, China, were enrolled. The serum ferritin, folate, vitamin B12, 25(OH) vitamin D, and vitamin A concentrations in the children with ASD were determined. All participants underwent anthropometric examinations, dietary assessments, and questionnaire assessments about their feeding behaviors, and gastrointestinal symptoms. The Z_{HA}, Z_{WA}, and Z_{BMIA} were found to be significantly lower in the children with ASD compared with those without ASD. A higher percentage of picky eaters, resistances to new foods as well as severe eating problems and constipation were reported in ASD children. These children consumed significantly fewer macronutrients compared with the children without ASD. In addition, the children with ASD had the highest rate of vitamin A deficiency, followed by iron deficiency. From the study, it was concluded that children with ASD had reduced macronutrient intake, severe feeding issues, constipation and vitamin A deficiency. A low serum vitamin A level may be a risk factor for symptoms of ASD. Similarly a study carried by Srivastava, Raman, and Bhattacharya (2016), with ASD children and normal children (2 – 6 years) in a tertiary care hospitals of Kolkata showed that ASD children showed deviation in anthropometrics in terms of height, weight and head circumference when compared to normal children at 5 percent level of significance.

Gluten-Free Casein-Free (GFCF) Diet in ASD

Various approaches have been adopted to improve the quality of life of ASD children, wherein diet and nutrition are considered to be very important. Parents of children with ASD have reported that there has been an improvement in the behavior of their children after adopting a special diet that is free from gluten and casein. Gluten is proteins of wheat and casein of milk. Exclusion of gluten and casein from the diet of these children is based on the theory that these children may have an allergic reaction or high sensitivity to foods containing gluten or casein. Children with autism, according to the theory, process, peptides, and proteins in foods containing gluten and casein differently. Hypothetically, this difference in processing may exacerbate autistic symptoms. The brain treats this protein like false opiate chemicals which in turn leads the child to behave in a certain way. The reason behind the use of this diet is to reduce symptoms and improve social and cognitive behaviors and speech (Table 1).

Studies conducted on ASD children have found the abnormal level of peptides in body fluids. There may be some scientific merit to the reasoning behind a gluten-free/casein-free diet. The efficacy of a GFCF diet for autism has not been supported by medical research as a review conducted on recent and past studies concluded that there is a lack of scientific evidence to suggest whether this diet can be helpful or not. Gluten and casein are found in the majority of the food that is usually consumed on a daily base, it has become difficult to conduct randomized clinical trials in ASD. The protein of cereals i.e, gluten is found in the seeds of several grains such as barley, rye, and wheat. It is found in maximum cereals. This protein in cereals helps in binding or gives structure to bakery products. It's difficult to avoid gluten. Nowadays stores have separate counters named as "Gluten – Free" foods, but still, it is important to read the nutritional levels to check if there are additives containing gluten.

A gluten-free diet, forbidden most bread and cereal products. Thus, the diet should be planned in such a way that contains adequate fiber, vitamins, and minerals. Nutritional Supplementation can be done to bridge the gap thus overcoming the nutritional deficiencies. Lactose is the carbohydrate and casein is the protein which is found in milk and all dairy products. It's important to read the nutritional information and ingredients present in packed food as it might happen that products proclaiming lactose-free might contain casein.

INTERVENTION

Parent Education

Family involvement and engagement along with the professional is important and essential in the treatment of ASD (Angell, 2010). If the child is still young, one would anticipate that the child will become more food selective around the age of two or three years, as seen in typical development, and that this stage will be more challenging for a child with ASD. When parents first learn of the child's diagnosis, it may be wise to show them a number of coping strategies, in order to prepare them for the developmental food refusals or to prevent some problems from getting worse. Particular attention must be paid

Table 1. Foods to be included and excluded in Gluten-Free Casein-Free (GFCF)

	Foods to be Included in GFCF Diet	Foods to be Excluded in GFCF Diet
1.	Cereal Grains and Products: Ragi, Bajra, Jowar, Flaxseed, Maize Flour, Rice, Rice flakes, Rice Flour, Puffed rice, Sanwa millet, Sorghum, Rice Noodles, Corn Flakes	Wheat and Wheat Products: Bread, Pastries, Chocolates, Cookies, Biscuits, Muffins, Pizza, Chapatis, Oats, Barley, Noodles, Pasta, Maggi
2.	Pulses and Legumes: All	Milk and Milk Products: Chocolates, Ice Cream, Butter, Curd,
3.	Vegetables: All	
4.	Fish, Chicken, Eggs	
5.	Fruits: All	
6.	Milk and its products (check for additives), Almond Milk	

to prevent intrusive feeding and to assure the child is regularly exposed to variation in the menu and presentation of foods (Levine, Bachar, Tsangen, Mizrachi, Levy, Dalal,... & Boaz, 2011; Schreck & Williams, 2006). Parents' actions and their relationship with their child influence the course of mealtimes. Eating is not only about food. At the table members of the family enjoy each other's company, the meal, exchange feelings an family/cultural values. Unpleasurable mealtimes affect the relationship and some members do not feel respected with regard to their needs and choices. When the strategies chosen by the parent affect the relationship and contribute to the maintenance of a feeding problem, alternatives may be suggested and modelling used, to demonstrate different actions and attitudes in response to the child's behaviours. Regardless which treatment approach is chosen, parents must learn it and the transfer to different social environments must be carefully planned. It is hoped that regular follow-up with the family can be established, so that parent support is ensured and that changes can be made when needed (Nadon, Feldman, & Gisel, 2013).

Nutritional Supplementation

Feeding problems may be long-term problems. This is one reason why nutritional supplements may be useful to ensure that the child's health is not compromised (Williams & Foxx, 2007). This will require a nutritionist's evaluation, to determine whether supplementation or modification of the existing diet is indicated. A routine follows up is mandatory and changes to be made carefully to ensure that they don't suppress the child's appetite or interfere with digestion. Another option is to introduce supplements in small quantities after each meal, or before bedtime. Introduction of nutritional supplementation in the diet of children and modification of diet is may present to be a major challenge and considerable risk. The changes to be done in the diet of children should be under strict guidance and supervision of the profession because, if done wrong, children may eliminate another food from their already limited repertoire. To increase the chance of success, it will be best not to change the sensory properties of preferred foods and to present modifications as similar as possible to the taste and texture of preferred foods (Fraker, Fishbein, Cox, & Walbert, 2009). Fading and desensitizing techniques are usually best for introducing food supplements (Williams & Foxx, 2007).

Behavioral Treatment Approaches

The functional analysis must be carried out before implementing behavioral treatments as it determines to which behaviors contribute to the maintenance of feeding problems and what function these behaviors serve (avoidance, attention seeking, pleasure-seeking, obtaining a reward). Qualified professionals must supervise interventions so that no undesirable behaviors are reinforced (Kodak & Piazza, 2008). A number of studies have shown the effectiveness of behavioral interventions for increasing acceptance of new foods (Williams & Seiverling, 2010; Matson & Fodstad, 2009). However, there are only a few studies demonstrating that acceptance of new foods generalizes to other foods or other environments and that preference of the child has been taken into account (Kozlowski, Matson, Fodstad, & Moree, 2011; Koegel, Bharoocha, Ribnick, Ribnick, Bucio, Fredeen, & Koegel, 2012). Different types of behavioural interventions are often used in varying combinations (Sharp, Jaquess, Morton, & Herzinger, 2010; Kozlowski, Matson, Fodstad, & Moree, 2011). Positive reinforcement, for example, consists of rewarding the child when he shows the desired response. A sequential presentation is a form of positive reinforcement. This type of interventions helps in acceptance of a non-preferred food immediately followed by a preferred food. Along with the preferred the new, non-preferred food is also presented. Although not mentioned in the literature, clinical practice requires great care with this approach. If parents report that their child can detect the slightest change to a familiar recipe, or reacts negatively to different commercial brands when they look exactly alike, the child may be hypersensitive to flavors. When new foods are hidden in what is familiar to the child, they are often detected by the child. The danger of this approach is, that if the child has limited communication abilities, he may not understand what happened to his food and thus, may refuse to ever eat it again for fear that this problem will repeat itself. It is best not to use this method without the knowledge of the child.

FUTURE RESEARCH DIRECTIONS

Recent increases in ASD prevalence estimates suggest the pressing need to translate these gains into access to effective interventions for all individuals with ASD. Future research includes:

- Awareness among the population;
- Early identification and intervention of these children;
- Proper channelizing of ASD children through various programmes in order to make their life comfortable;
- Behavioral changes;
- Need for an interdisciplinary approach to managing atypical eating patterns in children with ASD;
- Considering several factors when implementing GFCF diet for individuals with ASD, and;
- Evaluating the nutritional adequacy of children with ASD.

CONCLUSION

Optimum nutrition is the cornerstone of proper growth and development of children. For better birth outcome, maternal nutritional status is very important, thus resulting in low post-partum complication for both mother and infant. Good nutrition of mother prior to conception results in better birth outcomes. The role of nutrition in cognitive development is crucial, keeping in mind other factors such as biological and environmental factors. Children with ASD have feeding problems as they are "picky eaters" with highly restricted food choices. This behavior of selective food choices results in many nutritional deficiencies among these children, thus affecting their anthropometrics. Among various treatment plan followed by parents/ caregivers of these children, "elimination diet" is one important intervention. This diet results in the elimination of dairy and wheat completely from their daily menu. The exclusion of major food groups is also one of the reasons of developing nutritional deficiencies among ASD children. By giving education to the parents and creating awareness in terms of nutritional intervention, behavioral changes can bring help these children to embrace much better thus improving their quality of life and making the more acceptable and cooperative in the society.

REFERENCES

Abrahams, B. S., & Geschwind, D. H. (2008). Advances in autism genetics: On the threshold of a new neurobiology. *Nature Reviews. Genetics*, *9*(5), 341–355. doi:10.1038/nrg2346 PMID:18414403

Ahearn, W. H., Castine, T., Nault, K., & Green, G. (2001). An assessment of food acceptance in children with autism or pervasive developmental disorder-not otherwise specified. *Journal of Autism and Developmental Disorders*, *31*(5), 505–511. doi:10.1023/A:1012221026124 PMID:11794415

American Psychiatric Association. (2013). *Diagnostic and statistical manual of mental disorders (DSM-5®)*. American Psychiatric Pub.

Angell, A. (2010). Selective eaters and tactile sensitivity: A review of classification and treatment methods that address anxiety and support a child's need for a sense of control. *ICAN: Infant, Child, &. Adolescent Nutrition*, *2*(5), 299–303.

Anjos, T., Altmäe, S., Emmett, P., Tiemeier, H., Closa-Monasterolo, R., Luque, V., & Egan, B. (2013). Nutrition and neurodevelopment in children: Focus on NUTRIMENTHE project. *European Journal of Nutrition*, *52*(8), 1825–1842. doi:10.100700394-013-0560-4 PMID:23884402

Barker, D. J. P. (1998). *Mothers, babies and health in later life* (2nd ed.). Edinburgh, UK: Churchill Livingstone.

Bazinet, R. P., & Layé, S. (2014). Polyunsaturated fatty acids and their metabolites in brain function and disease. *Nature Reviews. Neuroscience*, *15*(12), 771–785. doi:10.1038/nrn3820 PMID:25387473

Benton, D. (2010). The influence of dietary status on the cognitive performance of children. *Molecular Nutrition & Food Research*, *54*(4), 457–470. doi:10.1002/mnfr.200900158 PMID:20077417

Berry, R. C., Novak, P., Withrow, N., Schmidt, B., Rarback, S., Feucht, S., & Sharp, W. G. (2015). Nutrition management of gastrointestinal symptoms in children with autism spectrum disorder: Guideline from an expert panel. *Journal of the Academy of Nutrition and Dietetics, 115*(12), 1919–1927. doi:10.1016/j.jand.2015.05.016 PMID:26164551

Bhatnagar, S., & Taneja, S. (2001). Zinc and cognitive development. *British Journal of Nutrition, 85*(S2), S139–S145. doi:10.1079/BJN2000306 PMID:11509102

Calder, P. C. (2013). Omega-3 polyunsaturated fatty acids and inflammatory processes: Nutrition or pharmacology? *British Journal of Clinical Pharmacology, 75*(3), 645–662. doi:10.1111/j.1365-2125.2012.04374.x PMID:22765297

Cryan, J. F., & Dinan, T. G. (2015). More than a gut feeling: The microbiota regulates neurodevelopment and behavior. *Neuropsychopharmacology, 40*(1), 241–242. doi:10.1038/npp.2014.224 PMID:25482171

Cumine, V., Leach, J., & Stevenson, G. (2000). *Autism in the early years: A practical guide*. London: David Fulton.

De Souza, A. S., Fernandes, F. S., & Tavares do Carmo, M. D. G. (2011). Effects of maternal malnutrition and postnatal nutritional rehabilitation on brain fatty acids, learning, and memory. *Nutrition Reviews, 69*(3), 132–144. doi:10.1111/j.1753-4887.2011.00374.x PMID:21348877

Delpech, J. C., Thomazeau, A., Madore, C., Bosch-Bouju, C., Larrieu, T., Lacabanne, C., & Layé, S. (2015). Dietary n-3 PUFAs deficiency increases vulnerability to inflammation-induced spatial memory impairment. *Neuropsychopharmacology, 40*(12), 2774–2787. doi:10.1038/npp.2015.127 PMID:25948102

Erny, D., de Angelis, A. L. H., Jaitin, D., Wieghofer, P., Staszewski, O., David, E., & Schwierzeck, V. (2015). Host microbiota constantly control maturation and function of microglia in the CNS. *Nature Neuroscience, 18*(7), 965–977. doi:10.1038/nn.4030 PMID:26030851

Estes, A., Zwaigenbaum, L., Gu, H., John, T. S., Paterson, S., Elison, J. T., & Kostopoulos, P. (2015). Behavioral, cognitive, and adaptive development in infants with autism spectrum disorder in the first 2 years of life. *Journal of Neurodevelopmental Disorders, 7*(1), 24. doi:10.118611689-015-9117-6 PMID:26203305

Fraker, C., Fishbein, M., Cox, S., & Walbert, L. (2009). *Food chaining: The proven 6-step plan to stop picky eating, solve feeding problems, and expand your child's diet.* Da Capo Lifelong Books.

Fuglestad, A. J., Rao, R., & Georgieff, M. K. (2008). The role of nutrition in cognitive development. In C. A. Nelson & M. Luciana (Eds.), *Handbook in Developmental Cognitive Neuroscience* (2nd ed.; pp. 623–641). Cambridge, MA: MIT Press.

Gale, C. R., Martyn, C. N., Marriott, L. D., Limond, J., Crozier, S., Inskip, H. M., ... Robinson, S. M. (2009). Dietary patterns in infancy and cognitive and neuropsychological function in childhood. *Journal of Child Psychology and Psychiatry, and Allied Disciplines, 50*(7), 816–823. doi:10.1111/j.1469-7610.2008.02029.x PMID:19236526

Gil, A., & Gil, F. (2015). Fish, a Mediterranean source of n-3 PUFA: Benefits do not justify limiting consumption. *British Journal of Nutrition, 113*(S2), S58–S67. doi:10.1017/S0007114514003742 PMID:26148923

Grantham-McGregor, S. M., Lira, P. I., Ashworth, A., Morris, S. S., & Assunçao, A. M. (1998). The development of low birth weight term infants and the effects of the environment in northeast Brazil. *The Journal of Pediatrics*, *132*(4), 661–666. doi:10.1016/S0022-3476(98)70357-9 PMID:9580767

Hallmayer, J., Cleveland, S., Torres, A., Phillips, J., Cohen, B., Torigoe, T., & Lotspeich, L. (2011). Genetic heritability and shared environmental factors among twin pairs with autism. *Archives of General Psychiatry*, *68*(11), 1095–1102. doi:10.1001/archgenpsychiatry.2011.76 PMID:21727249

Harding, J. E. (2001). The nutritional basis of the fetal origins of adult disease. *International Journal of Epidemiology*, *30*(1), 15–23. doi:10.1093/ije/30.1.15 PMID:11171842

Heindel, J. J., & Vandenberg, L. N. (2015). Developmental origins of health and disease: A paradigm for understanding disease etiology and prevention. *Current Opinion in Pediatrics*, *27*(2), 248–253. doi:10.1097/MOP.0000000000000191 PMID:25635586

Hibbeln, J. R., Davis, J. M., Steer, C., Emmett, P., Rogers, I., Williams, C., & Golding, J. (2007). Maternal seafood consumption in pregnancy and neurodevelopmental outcomes in childhood (ALSPAC study): An observational cohort study. *Lancet*, *369*(9561), 578–585. doi:10.1016/S0140-6736(07)60277-3 PMID:17307104

Hsiao, E. Y., McBride, S. W., Hsien, S., Sharon, G., Hyde, E. R., McCue, T., & Patterson, P. H. (2013). Microbiota modulate behavioral and physiological abnormalities associated with neurodevelopmental disorders. *Cell*, *155*(7), 1451–1463. doi:10.1016/j.cell.2013.11.024 PMID:24315484

Hutchinson, H. (1999). Feeding problems in young children: Report of three cases and review of the literature. *Journal of Human Nutrition and Dietetics*, *12*(4), 337–343. doi:10.1046/j.1365-277x.1999.00171.x

Kanner, L. (1949). Problems of nosology and psychodynamics of early infantile autism. *The American Journal of Orthopsychiatry*, *19*(3), 416–426. doi:10.1111/j.1939-0025.1949.tb05441.x PMID:18146742

Keen, D. V. (2008). Childhood autism, feeding problems and failure to thrive in early infancy. *European Child & Adolescent Psychiatry*, *17*(4), 209–216. doi:10.100700787-007-0655-7 PMID:17876499

Kim, J., Yu, A., Choi, B. Y., Nam, J. H., Kim, M. K., Oh, D. H., & Yang, Y. J. (2015). Dietary patterns derived by cluster analysis are associated with cognitive function among Korean older adults. *Nutrients*, *7*(6), 4154–4169. doi:10.3390/nu7064154 PMID:26035243

Kodak, T., & Piazza, C. C. (2008). Assessment and behavioral treatment of feeding and sleeping disorders in children with autism spectrum disorders. *Child and Adolescent Psychiatric Clinics*, *17*(4), 887–905. doi:10.1016/j.chc.2008.06.005 PMID:18775376

Koegel, R. L., Bharoocha, A. A., Ribnick, C. B., Ribnick, R. C., Bucio, M. O., Fredeen, R. M., & Koegel, L. K. (2012). Using individualized reinforcers and hierarchical exposure to increase food flexibility in children with autism spectrum disorders. *Journal of Autism and Developmental Disorders*, *42*(8), 1574–1581. doi:10.100710803-011-1392-9 PMID:22042309

Kogan, M. D., Blumberg, S. J., Schieve, L. A., Boyle, C. A., Perrin, J. M., Ghandour, R. M., & van Dyck, P. C. (2009). Prevalence of parent-reported diagnosis of autism spectrum disorder among children in the US, 2007. *Pediatrics*, *124*(5), 1395–1403. doi:10.1542/peds.2009-1522 PMID:19805460

Kozlowski, A. M., Matson, J. L., Fodstad, J. C., & Moree, B. N. (2011). Feeding therapy in a child with autistic disorder: Sequential food presentation. *Clinical Case Studies*, *10*(3), 236–246. doi:10.1177/1534650111405189

Lai, M. C., Lombardo, M. V., Suckling, J., Ruigrok, A. N. V., Chakrabarti, B., Ecker, C., ... Baron-Cohen, S. (2013). Biological sex affects the neurobiology of autism. *Brain*, *136*(9), 2799–2815. doi:10.1093/brain/awt216 PMID:23935125

Laud, R. B., Girolami, P. A., Boscoe, J. H., & Gulotta, C. S. (2009). Treatment outcomes for severe feeding problems in children with autism spectrum disorder. *Behavior Modification*, *33*(5), 520–536. doi:10.1177/0145445509346729 PMID:19748900

Leventakou, V., Roumeliotaki, T., Sarri, K., Koutra, K., Kampouri, M., Kyriklaki, A., & Chatzi, L. (2016). Dietary patterns in early childhood and child cognitive and psychomotor development: The Rhea mother–child cohort study in Crete. *British Journal of Nutrition*, *115*(8), 1431–1437. doi:10.1017/S0007114516000246 PMID:26887648

Levine, A., Bachar, L., Tsangen, Z., Mizrachi, A., Levy, A., Dalal, I., ... Boaz, M. (2011). Screening criteria for diagnosis of infantile feeding disorders as a cause of poor feeding or food refusal. *Journal of Pediatric Gastroenterology and Nutrition*, *52*(5), 563–568. doi:10.1097/MPG.0b013e3181ff72d2 PMID:21464761

Liu, X., Liu, J., Xiong, X., Yang, T., Hou, N., Liang, X., ... Li, T. (2016). Correlation between nutrition and symptoms: Nutritional survey of children with autism spectrum disorder in Chongqing, China. *Nutrients*, *8*(5), 294. doi:10.3390/nu8050294 PMID:27187463

Lozoff, B., & Georgieff, M. K. (2006). Iron deficiency and brain development. *Seminars in Pediatric Neurology*, *13*(3), 158–165. doi:10.1016/j.spen.2006.08.004 PMID:17101454

Madore, C., Nadjar, A., Delpech, J. C., Sere, A., Aubert, A., Portal, C., ... Layé, S. (2014). Nutritional n-3 PUFAs deficiency during perinatal periods alters brain innate immune system and neuronal plasticity-associated genes. *Brain, Behavior, and Immunity*, *41*, 22–31. doi:10.1016/j.bbi.2014.03.021 PMID:24735929

Matson, J. L., & Fodstad, J. C. (2009). Issues in identifying the etiology of food refusal in young children. *Journal of Pediatric Gastroenterology and Nutrition*, *48*(3), 274–275. doi:10.1097/MPG.0b013e31818af6b6 PMID:19242285

Nadon, G., Feldman, D., & Gisel, E. (2013). Feeding issues associated with the autism spectrum disorders. In *Recent Advances in Autism Spectrum Disorders* (Vol. 1, pp. 614–616). IntechOpen Publications; doi:10.5772/53644

Northstone, K., Joinson, C., Emmett, P., Ness, A., & Paus, T. (2012). Are dietary patterns in childhood associated with IQ at 8 years of age? A population-based cohort study. *Journal of Epidemiology and Community Health*, *66*(7), 624–628. doi:10.1136/jech.2010.111955 PMID:21300993

Nyaradi, A., Foster, J. K., Hickling, S., Li, J., Ambrosini, G. L., Jacques, A., & Oddy, W. H. (2014). Prospective associations between dietary patterns and cognitive performance during adolescence. *Journal of Child Psychology and Psychiatry, and Allied Disciplines*, *55*(9), 1017–1024. doi:10.1111/jcpp.12209 PMID:24673485

Nyaradi, A., Li, J., Hickling, S., Foster, J., & Oddy, W. H. (2013). The role of nutrition in children's neurocognitive development, from pregnancy through childhood. *Frontiers in Human Neuroscience*, *7*, 97. doi:10.3389/fnhum.2013.00097 PMID:23532379

Oddi, D., Crusio, W. E., D'amato, F. R., & Pietropaolo, S. (2013). Monogenic mouse models of social dysfunction: Implications for autism. *Behavioural Brain Research*, *251*, 75–84. doi:10.1016/j.bbr.2013.01.002 PMID:23327738

Odell, D., Maciulis, A., Cutler, A., Warren, L., McMahon, W. M., Coon, H., ... Torres, A. (2005). Confirmation of the association of the C4B null allelle in autism. *Human Immunology*, *66*(2), 140–145. doi:10.1016/j.humimm.2004.11.002 PMID:15694999

Patterson, P. H. (2011). Maternal infection and immune involvement in autism. *Trends in Molecular Medicine*, *17*(7), 389–394. doi:10.1016/j.molmed.2011.03.001 PMID:21482187

Penagarikano, O., Abrahams, B. S., Herman, E. I., Winden, K. D., Gdalyahu, A., Dong, H., & Golshani, P. (2011). Absence of CNTNAP2 leads to epilepsy, neuronal migration abnormalities, and core autism-related deficits. *Cell*, *147*(1), 235–246. doi:10.1016/j.cell.2011.08.040 PMID:21962519

Picciano, M. F. (2003). Pregnancy and lactation: Physiological adjustments, nutritional requirements and the role of dietary supplements. *The Journal of Nutrition*, *133*(6), 1997S–2002S. doi:10.1093/jn/133.6.1997S PMID:12771353

Pietropaolo, S., Goubran, M., Joffre, C., Aubert, A., Lemaire-Mayo, V., Crusio, W. E., & Laye, S. (2014). Dietary supplementation of omega-3 fatty acids rescues fragile X phenotypes in Fmr1-Ko mice. *Psychoneuroendocrinology*, *49*, 119–129. doi:10.1016/j.psyneuen.2014.07.002 PMID:25080404

Prado, E. L., & Dewey, K. G. (2014). Nutrition and brain development in early life. *Nutrition Reviews*, *72*(4), 267–284. doi:10.1111/nure.12102 PMID:24684384

Rees, S., & Inder, T. (2005). Fetal and neonatal origins of altered brain development. *Early Human Development*, *81*(9), 753–761. doi:10.1016/j.earlhumdev.2005.07.004 PMID:16107304

Roseboom, T. J., Painter, R. C., van Abeelen, A. F., Veenendaal, M. V., & de Rooij, S. R. (2011). Hungry in the womb: What are the consequences? Lessons from the Dutch famine. *Maturitas*, *70*(2), 141–145. doi:10.1016/j.maturitas.2011.06.017 PMID:21802226

Schanen, N. C. (2006). Epigenetics of autism spectrum disorders. *Human Molecular Genetics*, *15*(2), R138–R150. doi:10.1093/hmg/ddl213 PMID:16987877

Schmidt, R. J., Hansen, R. L., Hartiala, J., Allayee, H., Schmidt, L. C., Tancredi, D. J., & Hertz-Picciotto, I. (2011). Prenatal vitamins, one-carbon metabolism gene variants, and risk for autism. *Epidemiology (Cambridge, Mass.)*, *22*(4), 476–485. doi:10.1097/EDE.0b013e31821d0e30 PMID:21610500

Schreck, K. A., & Williams, K. (2006). Food preferences and factors influencing food selectivity for children with autism spectrum disorders. *Research in Developmental Disabilities*, *27*(4), 353–363. doi:10.1016/j.ridd.2005.03.005 PMID:16043324

Schwarz, S. M. (2003). Feeding disorders in children with developmental disabilities. *Infants and Young Children*, *16*(4), 317–330. doi:10.1097/00001163-200310000-00005

Sharp, W. G., Berry, R. C., McCracken, C., Nuhu, N. N., Marvel, E., Saulnier, C. A., & Jaquess, D. L. (2013). Feeding problems and nutrient intake in children with autism spectrum disorders: A meta-analysis and comprehensive review of the literature. *Journal of Autism and Developmental Disorders*, *43*(9), 2159–2173. doi:10.100710803-013-1771-5 PMID:23371510

Sharp, W. G., Jaquess, D. L., Morton, J. F., & Herzinger, C. V. (2010). Pediatric feeding disorders: A quantitative synthesis of treatment outcomes. *Clinical Child and Family Psychology Review*, *13*(4), 348–365. doi:10.100710567-010-0079-7 PMID:20844951

Shaw, R. J., Garcia, M., Thorn, M., Farley, C. A., & Flanagan, G. (2003). Treatment of feeding disorders in children with Down syndrome. *Clinical Child Psychology and Psychiatry*, *8*(1), 105–117. doi:10.1177/1359104503008001010

Shcheglovitov, A., Shcheglovitova, O., Yazawa, M., Portmann, T., Shu, R., Sebastiano, V., & Dolmetsch, R. E. (2013). SHANK3 and IGF1 restore synaptic deficits in neurons from 22q13 deletion syndrome patients. *Nature*, *503*(7475), 267–271. doi:10.1038/nature12618 PMID:24132240

Smith, S. E., Li, J., Garbett, K., Mirnics, K., & Patterson, P. H. (2007). Maternal immune activation alters fetal brain development through interleukin-6. *The Journal of Neuroscience*, *27*(40), 10695–10702. doi:10.1523/JNEUROSCI.2178-07.2007 PMID:17913903

Smithers, L. G., Golley, R. K., Mittinty, M. N., Brazionis, L., Northstone, K., Emmett, P., & Lynch, J. W. (2012). Dietary patterns at 6, 15 and 24 months of age are associated with IQ at 8 years of age. *European Journal of Epidemiology*, *27*(7), 525–535. doi:10.100710654-012-9715-5 PMID:22810299

Smithers, L. G., Golley, R. K., Mittinty, M. N., Brazionis, L., Northstone, K., Emmett, P., & Lynch, J. W. (2013). Do dietary trajectories between infancy and toddlerhood influence IQ in childhood and adolescence? Results from a prospective birth cohort study. *PLoS One*, *8*(3), e58904. doi:10.1371/journal.pone.0058904 PMID:23516574

Srivastava, K., Raman, M., & Bhattacharya, A. (2016). A study on comparison of anthropometrics of autism spectrum disorder children with normal children. *International Journal of Innovative Research and Development*, *5*(6), 484–487.

Starling, P., Charlton, K., McMahon, A. T., & Lucas, C. (2015). Fish intake during pregnancy and fetal neurodevelopment: A systematic review of the evidence. *Nutrients*, *7*(3), 2001–2014. doi:10.3390/nu7032001 PMID:25793632

Stewart, P. A., Hyman, S. L., Schmidt, B. L., Macklin, E. A., Reynolds, A., Johnson, C. R., & Manning-Courtney, P. (2015). Dietary supplementation in children with autism spectrum disorders: Common, insufficient, and excessive. *Journal of the Academy of Nutrition and Dietetics*, *115*(8), 1237–1248. doi:10.1016/j.jand.2015.03.026 PMID:26052041

Thapar, A., Cooper, M., Jefferies, R., & Stergiakouli, E. (2012). What causes attention deficit hyperactivity disorder? *Archives of Disease in Childhood, 97*(3), 260–265. doi:10.1136/archdischild-2011-300482 PMID:21903599

Thompson, R. A., & Nelson, C. A. (2001). Developmental science and the media: Early brain development. *The American Psychologist, 56*(1), 5–15. doi:10.1037/0003-066X.56.1.5 PMID:11242988

Twachtman-Reilly, J., Amaral, S. C., & Zebrowski, P. P. (2008). Addressing feeding disorders in children on the autism spectrum in school-based settings: Physiological and behavioral issues. *Language, Speech, and Hearing Services in Schools, 39*(2), 261–272. doi:10.1044/0161-1461(2008/025) PMID:18420528

Villar, J., Merialdi, M., Gulmezoglu, A. M., Abalos, E., Carroli, G., Kulier, R., & de Onis, M. (2003). Nutritional interventions during pregnancy for the prevention or treatment of maternal morbidity and preterm delivery: An overview of randomized controlled trials. *The Journal of Nutrition, 133*(5), 1606S–1625S. doi:10.1093/jn/133.5.1606S PMID:12730475

Voineagu, I., Wang, X., Johnston, P., Lowe, J. K., Tian, Y., Horvath, S., & Geschwind, D. H. (2011). Transcriptomic analysis of autistic brain reveals convergent molecular pathology. *Nature, 474*(7351), 380–384. doi:10.1038/nature10110 PMID:21614001

Warren, R. P., Singh, V. K., Cole, P., Odell, J. D., Pingree, C. B., Warren, W. L., & White, E. (1991). Increased frequency of the null allele at the complement C4b locus in autism. *Clinical and Experimental Immunology, 83*(3), 438–440. doi:10.1111/j.1365-2249.1991.tb05657.x PMID:2004485

Williams, K. E., & Foxx, R. M. (2007). *Treating eating problems of children with autism spectrum disorders and developmental disabilities: Interventions for professionals and parents*. Pro-ed.

Williams, K. E., & Seiverling, L. (2010). Eating problems in children with autism spectrum disorders. *Topics in Clinical Nutrition, 25*(1), 27–37. doi:10.1097/TIN.0b013e3181d10958

Won, H., Mah, W., & Kim, E. (2013). Autism spectrum disorder causes, mechanisms, and treatments: Focus on neuronal synapses. *Frontiers in Molecular Neuroscience, 6*, 19. doi:10.3389/fnmol.2013.00019 PMID:23935565

Zeisel, S. H. (2008). Is maternal diet supplementation beneficial? Optimal development of infant depends on mother's diet. *The American Journal of Clinical Nutrition, 89*(2), 685S–687S. doi:10.3945/ajcn.2008.26811F PMID:19116319

Zeisel, S. H. (2009). Importance of methyl donors during reproduction. *The American Journal of Clinical Nutrition, 89*(2), 673S–677S. doi:10.3945/ajcn.2008.26811D PMID:19116320

Zimmermann, M. B. (2011). The role of iodine in human growth and development. *Seminars in Cell & Developmental Biology, 22*(6), 645–652. doi:10.1016/j.semcdb.2011.07.009 PMID:21802524

KEY TERMS AND DEFINITIONS

Autism Spectrum Disorder: It is a neurodevelopmental disorder that begins in early childhood and affects the communication, social interaction, cognition and behavior in children.

Casein Free: A casein-free diet in which milk protein (casein) is eliminated by removing all dairy products from the diet.

Cognition: Cognition is a term referring to the mental processes involved in gaining knowledge and comprehension. These processes include thinking, knowing, remembering, judging and problem-solving. These are higher-level functions of the brain and encompass language, imagination, perception, and planning.

Diet: It is a sum of nutritious food that is eaten by an individual.

Digestion: Digestion is the breakdown of large insoluble food molecules into small water-soluble food molecules so that they can be absorbed into the watery blood plasma. In certain organisms, these smaller substances are absorbed through the small intestine into the bloodstream.

Gluten-Free: A gluten-free diet is a diet that strictly excludes gluten, a mixture of proteins found in wheat and related grains, including barley, rye, oat, and all their species and hybrids (such as Spelt, Kamut, and Triticale).

Nutrition: Nutrition is the process of taking food into the body and absorbing the nutrients in those foods.

Chapter 11
Application of Bio-Feedback in Neurodevelopmental Disorders

Srinivasan Venkatesan
All India Institute of Speech and Hearing, India

Hariharan Venkataraman
All India Institute of Speech and Hearing, India

ABSTRACT

Biofeedback is a non-invasive process to electronically monitor normal automatic bodily function to acquire its voluntary control. Traditional medical models place the onus on the physician to "cure" the illness. Biofeedback places responsibility on the patient to gain self-control. Its application as evidence-based practice in neurodevelopmental disorders is a nascent, unexplored, and debated area of study. This chapter outlines the meaning, nature, types, protocols, procedure, practices, challenges, benefits, and limitations in its use. Its history is traced for efficacy vis-à-vis other treatments, and other issues like cost-effectiveness, certification of professionals, gadget-enabled, and computer-assisted variants. Studies have attempted, albeit with methodological limitations, to validate its utility for neurodevelopmental disorders without any definitive or conclusive evidence for or against its use given the inability to replicate results, control or exclude confounding factors, placebo effects, and/or bias. An agenda for prospective research is given.

INTRODUCTION

Biofeedback (BF) uses electrical signals to monitor and amplify body functions that are too subtle for body awareness. Electronic instruments sense bioelectrical signals emitted by subliminal body behavior. They then deliver information back to the subject (feedback) via sensory modalities-usually auditory, visual, tactile, or a combination of all. When the internal visceral cues are made explicit, through practice, the client can gain control over specific body functions. Traditional medical models place the onus on the physician to 'cure' the illness. BF places responsibility on the patient to gain self-control. Thus, individuals can gain control over Sympathetic Nervous System, and later, on own without the help of instrumentation (Frank, Khorshid, Kiffer, Moravec, & McKee, 2010).

DOI: 10.4018/978-1-5225-7004-2.ch011

BF help gain greater awareness of many physiological functions by primarily using instruments that provide information on the activity of those same systems, with the goal of being able to manipulate them at will (Durand & Barlow, 2009; p. 331). There are two models of BF training: operant conditioning and psycho-physiological psychotherapy. The former is based on consequences to modify the behavior. The principles of operant conditioning, schedules of reinforcement, shaping, discrimination, generalization, extinction, and habituation apply to these procedures too. For BF, the reinforcement of the signal displays prompt for the patients to change their physiology. The latter model views the patient as an individual to combine the use of BF with stress management and other psychotherapeutic interventions. BF is training and not a treatment. Much like being taught how to ride a bicycle or a new language, individuals undergoing BF training must take an active role and practice in order to develop the skill. Rather than passively receiving a treatment by swallowing pills, the patient is an active learner. Treatment is what insurance reimbursement is traditionally designed to reimburse. An insured would not want to cover a course on BF training in as much they would not cover courses on personal development or read self-help books.

BF is an education. As sensors are placed on the patient's skin, the therapist explains what each sensor will be measuring. The patient is assured that the sensors do not cause any pain or shock. Rather, they simply record signals from the body and display them on the screen. The therapist chooses specific signal displays and explains it to the individual. This may be as simple as 'the green line is muscle tension, the blue line is temperature'. Patients are then taught how the signals being displayed relate to their physiology. For example, the therapist may say, 'Raise your shoulders' or 'Scrunch your face,' using the muscle tension signal on the screen to point out the patient's physiological responses (Schwartz & Andrasik, 2006). How much ever sophisticated they might be, BF instruments are the only aides to the training. They are not the end of it. They are meant to monitor a physiological process, measure what is monitored, and to present what is monitored or measured as meaningful information. The common methods of BF drawn from various classical texts on the theme are listed below (Schwartz & Andrasik, 2016; Khazan, 2013; Basmajian, 1989; Rickles, Sandweiss, Jacobs, Grove, & Criswell, 1983; Beatty & Legewie, 1977; Brown, 1977):

- Electromyography (EMG-BF) measures muscle tension as it changes over time.
- Skin conductance is a correlate of sweat gland activity. Also called Galvanic Skin Response (GSR) or Electro-dermal Activity (EDA), thermal or temperature BF, it measures body temperature changes over time by Skin Conductance Activity (SCA) by measuring Skin Conductance Level (SCL) or Skin Conductance Response (SCR). This is an indirect measure of sympathetic outflow. It measures changes in the amount of heat given off by the skin, a measurement that indicates any changes in blood flow.
- Electroencephalography (EEG) or Neurofeedback Electroencephalography (NF-EEG)-measures brain wave activity over time. This is an electrophysiological monitoring method to record the electrical activity of the brain. Based on electrode placements on the scalp, it measures the brain's spontaneous electrical activity over a period of time.
- Galvanic Skin Response (GSR) training or thermal feedback measures the amount of sweat on your body over time. Skin temperature is a correlate of peripheral vasoconstriction and is an indirect measure of sympathetic outflow.
- Heart variability BF measures pulse and heart rate as beats per minute through sensors.
- Respiration is measured in breaths per minute typically by a strain gauge worn around the chest or abdomen.

- Electropalatography (EPG) is used to monitor contacts between the tongue and hard palate, particularly during articulation and speech.
- Audio-visual feedback involves conveying messages through hearing and/or sight modalities.
- Ultrasound imaging or visual feedback makes use of high frequency sounds one cannot hear but can be emitted and detected by special machines.

BF training has been used on a variety of clinical and non-clinical condition, such as, asthma (Lehrer, Vaschilio, Lu, Shou-En., Eckberg Vaschillo, Scardellaa, & Habib, 2006), pain (Turk, Meichenbaum, & Berman, 1979), stroke (Nelson, 2007), migraine and tension headache (Nestoriuc, Martin, Rief, & Andrasik, 2008), disordered defecation, fecal incontinence and constipation (Enck, Van Der Voort, & Klosterhalfen, 2009; Erick, 1993), substance use disorders (Sokhadze, Cannon, & Trudeau, 2008), cardiovascular diseases (Kranitz & Lehrer, 2004), hemiplegia (Armagan, Tascioglu, & Oner, 2003), balance and mobility in older populations (Zijlstra, Mancini, Chiari, & Zijlstra, 2010), neuro-motor rehabilitation (Huang, Wolf, & He, 2006), sports, exercise and rehabilitation medicine (Prinsloo, Raunch, & Derman, 2014).

Ancient records testify that the yogis in Indian sub-continent have consciously mastered controlling their autonomic nervous system (slowing down their heart rate, increasing body temperature, decreasing oxygen consumption and so on) for thousands of years. The act of self-regulation of the autonomic nervous system was not believed as possible in the west till the late 1950s. Among their early proponents of BF was Edmund Jacobson, who developed progressive relaxation technique in the 1930s and Johann Schultz who developed autogenic training. Both these self-regulatory techniques have become the basis for research and discovery of BF. Hence, BF is nicknamed as 'Yoga of the West' or 'Zen Technology' (Kuruvilla, 2010; Peper & Shaffer, 2010).

The general consensus is that the technique is effective in reducing the frequency and severity of migraine and tension headaches often allowing patients to decrease their dependence on medication. It is found to be effective in patients with acute and intense panic attacks than those with chronic, long-standing and generalized anxiety. It has been used with limited success as a conservative choice of treatment in depression and post-traumatic stress disorder. Its gadgetry has helped controlling mild sleep bruxism although it has not been proved effective in severe cases. Moreover, long-term efficacy on maintenance of initial symptomatic improvement during follow up after 12-64 months in constipation and incontinence has been disappointing. It is also reported to lower and ameliorate short-term pain, improving heart health, reduce hyper-arousal and ameliorate troubled sleeping. Nonetheless, there are also criticisms about its absence of standardized protocols, limited empirical support, or that the mechanism of its action is still not fully understood, or that statistical significance between pre and post treatments need not be necessarily equal to clinical significance, or that laboratory settings are not equal to clinical settings. A schematic depiction of the principles of BF application is given in figure one (Source: https://www.thinglink.com/scene/712052688614850562).

NEURODEVELOPMENTAL DISORDERS

Neurodevelopmental disorders (NDD) are a group of conditions in which the development of the central nervous system is disturbed. Cognitive-related disorders involving functions of the brain due to genetic causes and that present from early childhood are known as NDD. There is no single agreed-upon defi-

Figure 1. Schematic representation of the BF technique

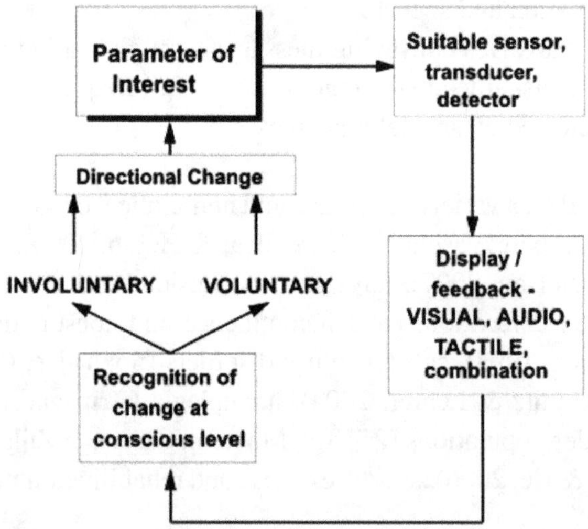

nition or classified listing on the types of NDD. Although these conditions are recognized on the basis of molecular substrates like genes, CNS malformations, obstetric complications before, during or after birth, congenital anomalies, intrauterine insults, and what are called as biomarkers; in clinical practice, the various NDD are documented and classified on the basis of observable, behavioral, phenomenological, and/or morphological features. The origins and history of development of the concept of NDD are credited to recent or ongoing discoveries in clinical genetics despite the fact that the technology of dissecting complex diseases is not as easy as decoding single gene disorders.

The two major diagnostic classification systems that are used for this classification are: Diagnostic and Statistical Manual, 5th Revision (American Psychiatric Association, 2016; 2013) and International Classification of Diseases and Related Health Problems, 10th Revision (World Health Organization, 2008). The official list under DSM-5 includes: intellectual developmental disorder or disability, global developmental delay, language disorder, speech sound disorder, childhood onset fluency disorder (stuttering), social (pragmatic) communication disorder, ASD, ADHD, specific learning disability (SLD), developmental coordination disorder, stereotypic movement disorder, Tourette's disorder, persistent (chronic) motor or vocal tic disorder, and provisional tic disorder. ICD-10 describes a distinct axis of NDD as a group of conditions with three main criteria: onset in infancy or childhood, impairments related to central nervous system maturation; and expressed steadily without remissions or relapse (World Health Organization, 2008).

From a psychological perspective, NDD is defined as a condition of abnormal brain dysfunction that adversely affects a child's emotional and social functioning as well as cognitive and learning capabilities over time across developmental stages (Farran & Karmiloff-Smith, 2012). The developmental brain dysfunction can manifest as an impaired motor function, emotion, self-control, learning, memory, language or non-verbal communication. A characteristic feature in the study of NDD is the adherence to a developmental perspective. They are different from acquired disorders in which their cause and onset can happen during any time of a person's lifespan. Even as the heterogeneity and variability of children with NDD are acknowledged, there are unanswered questions on whether the stated boundaries between these disorders really do exist. Are they overlapping, do they co-exist, or whether many of them are comorbid conditions is a matter of perennial debate. The term NDD has gained popularity in the past two decades (Bishop & Rutter, 2009).

The diagnosis of NDD is not completely stable since there is constant movement in and out of it over time (Woolfendon, Sarkozy, Ridley, & Williams, 2012). Moreover, it is alleged that many of them share the same genetic factors, specific environmental or risk factors, neural substrates, biomarkers, temperamental antecedents, abnormalities of cognitive and emotional processing, symptom similarity, the course of illness and treatment response. When this is so, it becomes pertinent to ask whether there is any empirical validation in having so many different names and types of NDD (Farran, Riby, & Herwegen, 2014; Clegg, Gillott, & Jones, 2013; Andrews, Pine, Hobbs, Anderson, & Sunderland, 2009).

Other conditions considered as NDD include motor developmental disorders, dyspraxia, traumatic brain injury, cerebral palsy, genetic disorders like schizophrenia, Down syndrome, disorders of behavior and conduct. Apart from these, some authors have also added eating, feeding and elimination disorders, separation anxiety disorders, and selective/elective mutism under the list.

Although considered as multi-factorial, NDD is typically understood as caused by language, social or emotional deprivation on the developing brain. Further, they may be also genetically determined by a chromosomal disturbance (as also in Fragile X Syndrome, Prader-Willi Syndrome or Angelman Syndrome), or by physical trauma, poor nutrition, metabolic disturbances, systemic infections and immune reactions during pregnancy (De Felice, Ricceri, Venerosi, Chiarotti, & Calamandrei, 2015; Vargo, 2012). The notion that some substances in the environment can damage the nervous system has an ancient history. The neurotoxicity of lead, mercury, manganese and certain pesticides in use are the most commonly implicated agents (Szpir, 2006). The role of hippocampus dysfunction in some of these disorders is recently being implicated (Prehn-Kristensen, Cooke, Baving, & Schumann, 2012).

Bibliographic searches were conducted to identify publications between 1985 and 2009 concerned with 35 NDD show that a bulk of studies have focused only on ADHD and ASD (Bishop, 2010). It is assumed that the symptoms and behaviors of NDD often change and evolve as a child grows older. In some cases, the disabilities are permanent (United States Environmental Protective Agency, 2015). A lifespan approach to NDD is a wanting area of inquiry. Although the condition in children, adolescents, and young adults have attracted clinical and research attention, the question of their ageing, its affect on their cognition, evidence on gene hunting, search for biomarkers, histopathological, imaging, neuropharmacological and other key brain abnormalities have not yielded conclusive results till date (Mukaetova-Ladinska, Perry, Baron, & Povey, 2012; Piven & Rabins, 2011).

Studies have shown that there is a higher incidence of medical problems related to neurodegeneration, gastrointestinal functioning, obesity, and hypertension in elderly persons with Fragile X Syndrome (Utari, Adams, Berry-Kravis, Chavez, Scaggs, Ngotran, ... & Tartaglia, 2010). Many studies have targeted children with ASD with great promise but to no avail in converging towards either understanding its etiology or helping in their treatment (Ben-Ari, 2016; Berg & Dobyns, 2015; Geschwind & State, 2015; Ecker, Bookheimer, & Murphy, 2015). Can there be or is there a late-life ASD is a question that has been unconvincingly raised. Through case history, corroborated or supplemented by information from a close relative is considered to be the most important diagnostic tool to identify such conditions (van Niekerk, Groen, Vissers, & van-Driel-de Jong, 2011). Older patients with undiagnosed Asperger's Syndrome have been illustrated through case studies (James, Mukaetova-Ladinska, Reichelt, Briel, & Scully, 2006). Studies on aging in autism are needed to plan appropriate services and shed light on the full course, development and prognosis of this neurodevelopmental condition. It is shown that 'neurotypical' aging in core domains of autistic impairments: social cognition, executive function, cognitive style and memory, reserve, compensation, quality of life, loneliness, and physical health are areas of concern even during their old age (Happe & Charlton, 2012).

The persistence of ADHD symptoms to old age was reported in a population-based sample of >1500 persons aged 65-80 years (Guldberg-Kjar, Sehlin, & Johansson, 2013). While the life expectancy of persons with mild intellectual disability is reported as similar to the general population, those in severe-profound grades over 40 years are less than 20% (Patja, Livanainen, Vesala, Oksanen, & Ruoppila, 2000; Janicki, Dalton, Henderson, & Davidson, 1999). It is shown that adults with intellectual disability are at risk of developing dementia in old age (Strydom, Hassiotis, King, & Livingston, 2009; Strydom, Livingston, King, & Hassiotis, 2007). Psychiatric morbidity also appears to be high for older people with SLD (Cooper, 1997; Patel, Goldberg, & Moss, 1993). Diagnosis and treatment of these disorders can be difficult; treatment often involves a combination of applied behavior analysis, drugs as well as home- and school-based programs. Wherein genomics, neuroimaging, and brain development are the cornerstones for NDD, its treatment must expectedly target neurobiological mechanisms (Hamilton, 2015). A variety of drugs, although lacking in the specificity of action, are currently prescribed to treat this condition for acting on neurotransmitter and physiological systems (Homberg, Kyzar, Stewart, Nguyen, Poudel, Echevarria, ... & Pittman, 2016).

BIOFEEDBACK AND NEURODEVELOPMENTAL DISORDERS: LITERATURE REVIEW

Available literature on the application of BF in NDD is scattered. The tapestry of BF history has been woven from many independent threads. Some have blossomed and disappeared. Others have continued to nurture the field. The technique of BF itself evolved out of laboratory research in 1940's. In the 1950s and 1960s, researchers from different fields studied various applications of BF to modify physiological functions in animals and humans. In an early study, changes in consciousness were observed to be accompanied by variations in EEG alpha rhythm of human subjects (Kamiya, 1968). Dicara and Miller (1968) observed that curarized rats could learn to avoid a shock by lowering their heart rate. Later, visceral conditioning, through the use of feedback techniques was demonstrated in human beings (Miller & Dworkin, 1974). At that time, operant conditioning models were used to further BF research (Kimmel, 1981; Birbaumer & Kimmel, 1979). Kimmel (1974) found that subjects' GSR could be conditioned using pleasant odors. Kimmel (1974) summarized the research up to 1967, including 16 studies of GSR, five of heart rate, and three of the vasomotor response. Most of these studies supported the contention that the ANS could be modified through operant conditioning. The first clinical application of thermal feedback training was attempted along with 'Autogenic Training' in the treatment of migraine (Green & Green, 1977; Luthe & Schultz, 1969). Around the same time, EMG training was being used to reduce tension headache by means of a 16-week program (Budzynski, Stoyva, & Adler, 1970). Even earlier, Marinacci (1955) demonstrated that EMG feedback could be applied to improve neuromuscular functioning in several disorders. Available bibliographies on BF covering over 1000 un-annotated titles are available (Butler, 1978; Butler & Stoyva, 1973) although not specific to NDD.

With growing recognition for the biological basis of NDD, earlier conceptualizations focused on a psychogenic etiology stemming from disruptions in parent-child relationships are now relegated to the background (Bettelheim, 1967; p. 484). The role of electrophysiological, protein, pupillary light reflex, eye-blink conditioning or eye-tracking, mirror neuron network dysfunction, cognitive task performance, brain oscillations and/or immune cell biomarkers of genetic risks in diagnosis, treatment and outcome in NDD is gaining recognition (McPartland, 2016; Jeste, Frohlich, & Loo, 2015; Tye, McLoughlin, Kuntsi, & Asherson, 2011; Tye, Rijsdijk, Greven, Kuntsi, Asherson, & McLoughlin, 2012). There is no single or straight-forward list of biomarkers that is offered as a template for these conditions. Genetic, metabolic, inflammatory brain sites as well as mitochondrial dysfunction and oxidative stress, are the commonly investigated biomarkers for NDD. The identification of brain-based biomarkers could potentially assist in objective diagnosis, monitoring of treatment response and prediction of outcomes for children with NDD. At present, the field is yet to identify reliable and reproducible biomarkers for these disorders. It is still grappling to address issues related to clinical heterogeneity, methodological standardization, and cross-site validation before further progress can be achieved. It is like the proverbial search for a needle in the haystack, wherein the quest for identifying or listing specific, sensitive, reliable and valid biomarkers based on the measure of brain function is going on (Gnanavel, 2017).

Owing to the preceding, a '*terroir* model' of neurodevelopment is proposed. In this five-tier model illustrated in another chapter, BF training paradigms is considered as an intervention at level four for NDD. It targets below overt 'symptoms' but above or closer to cognitions emanating from brain structure or functions. It would be worthwhile to review and take stock of the available but scattered technical literature on the application of BF on NDD. Such an attempt would clarify many research questions: What is the nature, extent, intensity, depth or diversity of research that has already gone into this theme? What are the salient findings in the already accumulated body of research on this problem area? What has been the identified historical course and trends in BF research vis-à-vis persons with NDD? Have all types of these disorders been addressed by researchers and practitioners of BF? Are all the types of clinical populations affected by such conditions amenable to effective use of BF techniques? Are there or can there be any qualifiers to be taken into account at intake levels or during sample recruitment to justify such a gadget-driven, expensive, time-consuming and labor-intensive activity as trying out the BF training? Could certain forms or types of BF than the others may be more appropriate for certain conditions of such disorders? What might be the returns on such investments in the long run as generalization effect to real-life behaviors for children with NDD? Undeterred by this long list of research questions and challenged by the paucity of answers in this area, the present inquiry attempts to undertake a comprehensive qualitative and quantitative analysis of bibliographic listing of references and citations on BF and NDD. An attempt is also being undertaken to study broad trends in the distribution of the publications in relation to specific variables such as timeline or years, type, themes or are of research. A historical and cross-sectional empirical and systematic bibliographic survey design was adopted for this study.

METHOD

Apart from perusing available bibliographies on the subject (Hammond, 2008), key-word searches were carried out in open access databases, internet-based resources and search engines like Google Scholar, Scopus, Refseek, MEDLINE via PubMed, CINHAL, Web of Science, Ichushi Web, GHL, WPRIM, JSTOR, ProQuest, PsycINFO, WOK, EMBASE, searches in Applied Psychophysiology and Biofeedback, and Journal of Neurotherapy. Wherever available cross-references were checked for author credentials and before they were added. The key-words used in the internet searches were: 'biofeedback', 'neurodevelopmental disorders', or along with their specific subtypes.

Procedure

Data collection involved approaching every known or available source of information and documentation for procuring old issues of journals, visiting online archives, validating cross-references, and listing citations by names of authors, year of publication, the title of book, article, and journal, recording their volume, issue and page numbers. Additional information on DOI, ISSN/ISBN, Impact Factor (if available) and periodicity of the journal, place of origin, internet source, and year of commencement of the journal was also collected. A schematic representation of the procedure used in the study is given in figure two. The inclusion/exclusion criteria for collection of the bibliographic database are given below:

Inclusion

Only indexed journal articles with complete details on author/s, their affiliation, year of publication, the title of the journal, volume, issue and page numbers were taken;

Any or all authored, co-authored, written or published research articles mentioning BF or its equivalent terms obtained from national and/or international journals having print and/or electronic ISSN to date;

Only the most typical categories of NDD as given under DSM-5, such as intellectual disability, global developmental delays, language disorder, speech sound disorder, childhood onset fluency disorder (stuttering), social communication disorder, ASD, ADHD, and SLD were targeted for bibliographic search on BF in this study;

Published original research articles, review articles, and case reports were included; Manuscripts addressing the select list of childhood-onset NDD as included under official lists of disease classifications were alone included;

Exclusion

Research titles by authors on BF or its equivalent terms appearing in periodicals, newsletters, magazines, proceedings of seminars, webinars, or conferences, mimeographs, video or audio materials, and unpublished pre-doctoral doctoral or post-doctoral dissertations;

Entries on books, monographs, mimeographs, lecture notes, although related to the topic were excluded;

Incomplete, misleading, repeated, and unverified cross-references from available full- text articles and books were excluded;

Editorials, letters to editor, notes and news about seminars or conferences, short communications, book reviews, and blogs were excluded;

Other categories of NDD, such as developmental coordination disorder, Tourette's disorder, persistent or chronic motor or vocal tic disorder, although included under DSM-5, were excluded for bibliographic search on BF in this study.

Certain acquired or adulthood onset related NDD like schizophrenia, depressive disorders, obsessive-compulsive disorders, substance abuse conditions were excluded from the purview of this study;

Data Analysis

The collected list of references was compiled in Microsoft Excel spreadsheet under appropriate headings along with distinct codes to enable their categorization and classification. Based on titles, readings of their abstract and text, clinical populations addressed, the articles were classified into seven diagnostic categories of NDD: (1) Learning Disability; (2) Stuttering; (3) Autism Spectrum Disorder; (4) Attention Deficit (Hyperactivity) Disorder; (5) Speech, Language and Hearing Disorders; (6) Voice Disorders, and; (7) Intellectual Disability. Another 5-tier sorting was carried out in terms of their 10-year term timelines beginning 1970s to date to verify how many research articles were published under different themes for every decade. To facilitate a thematic analysis, the text of the articles were studied for types of NDD targeted, research design used, sampling, interventions, and outcome measures respectively.

The codification, categorization, and classification of the themes reflected by the titles included in the study were subjected to inter-observer reliability checks by involving three mutually blinded independent coders for at least 50 entries each out of the overall sample of research articles. The tripartite inter-reviewer agreement as measured by Fleiss Kappa for multiple coders (contrasting Cohen's Kappa applicable only for two raters) (Fleiss 1981; Fleiss & Cohen, 1973) was 0.91 which is interpreted as 'almost perfect agreement' (Landis & Koch, 1977). Face validity is found to be high for the classification of the thematic categories covered by the research papers. The tone and tenor of ethical issues pertaining to bio-behavioral research as enshrined in the official mandate within the investigating institution were scrupulously adhered to (Venkatesan, 2009). A descriptive and interpretative statistical analysis was carried out by applying measures of non-parametric statistics using SPSS/PC (Carver & Nash, 2009).

Figure 2. Schematic representation of the steps used in the study

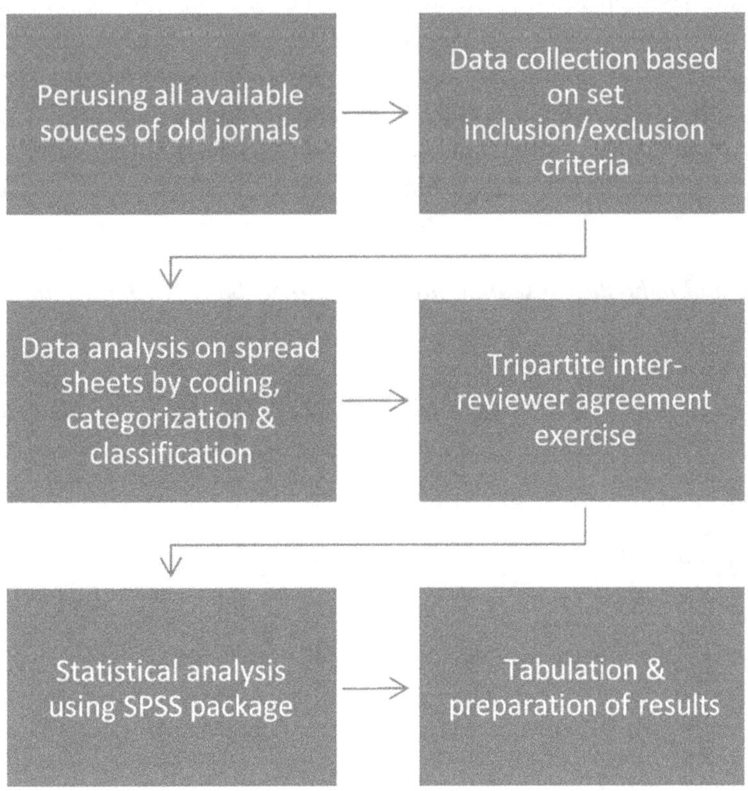

RESULTS

The findings of this study on published research papers about BF techniques vis-à-vis NDD are divided as: (a) Overall & Conditions against Type of BF Used; (b) Timelines; and; (c) Thematic Analysis.

Overall and Conditions Against Type of BF Used

For the *overall* 107 research articles sourced on the theme of BF techniques in NDD, the bibliographic search yielded a major share of work related to ADD/ADHD (N: 45; 42.06%), followed by ASD (N: 14; 13.08%) and SLHD (N: 14; 13.08%). SLHD covers an assortment of conditions including aphasia, apraxia, dysarthria, and disorders of phonation. While the reported use of BF on voice disorders (N: 9; 8.41%) and intellectual disability (N: 9; 8.41%) is low, its use on stammering or stuttering has been minimal (N: 5; 4.67%). NF-EEG appears to be the most preferred BF procedure by researchers on NDD (N: 72; 67.29%). This is followed by a preference for use of EMG (N: 19; 17.76%). The use of GSR or thermal feedback on NDD is nil. Studies based on the use of other forms of BF such as audio-visual, ultrasound, galvanic skin response and electropalatography are less. There are multiple NF-BF training protocols. More specifically, there is a paucity of BF research with NDD using qEEG, P300 and ERP abnormalities, or those based on the Peniston Protocol (Alpha-Theta Feedback), its Scott-Kaiser Modification (Table 1).

Timelines

The analysis of results based on decade wise stratification of *timelines* shows that the 1970s are marked with beginnings of BF research work undertaken on NDD. In this compilation, the oldest and earliest entry is a report on the use of 'contingent feedback to improve digital performance in a functionally deaf cerebral palsied child and another normal child (Sachs, Martin, & Fitch, 1972). The results were discussed in terms of the effects of contingent sensory feedback on motor functioning. Two other early case-reports using 'visual feedback in establishing normal vocal intensity in two mildly retarded adults'

Table 1. Distribution of published research papers on biofeedback techniques in neurodevelopmental disorders

Code	Heading	NF-EEG	EMG	BF	EPG	AV	US	TOTAL
A	Learning Disability	11						11
B	Stuttering		4	1				5
C	ASD	14						14
D	ADD/ADHD	41	4					45
E	SLH Disorders		4	3	1	3	3	14
F	Voice Disorders		6	2		1		9
G	Intellectual Disability	6	1			2		9
	Total	72	19	6	1	6	3	107

[NF-EEG: Neurofeedback-Electroencephalography; EMG: Electromyography; BF: Biofeedback; EPG: Electropalatography; AV: Audio-Visual Feedback; US: Ultrasound Feedback]

(Brody, Nelon, & Brody, 1975) and another on the use of EMG-BF for 11 sessions to control the hyperactivity of a 6 ½-year old boy. The child was instructed to turn off a tone which signaled the presence of muscular tension. A follow-up session after a 7-month interval indicated the improvements were continued to be maintained both in school as well as home settings (Braud, Lupin, & Braud, 1975). Other early studies of the 1970s have also been case reports on using 'analogue EMG feedback' (Guitar, 1975) or 'auditory EMG feedback' (Hanna, Wilfling, & McNeill, 1975) to reduce frequency of stuttering, treatment of hyper-functional voice disorders (Prosek, Montgomery, Walden, & Schwartz, 1978) and spastic dysphonia (Henschen & Burton, 1978). A study undertaken in this period has also attempted to follow up and replicate preliminary findings that suggested EEG-BF combined with the drug (Ritalin) showed better improvements than each of them used alone on children with ADD/ADHD (Shouse & Lubar, 1979).

The 1980s witnessed an onset of interest in trying BF training on children with SLD while continuing the saga of single case studies. There was interest on whether these children showed unique brain-wave signatures (Tansey, 1985), whether the application of BF training brought about improvements in their verbal, visuospatial, and creative skills (Cunningham & Murphy, 1981), or it facilitated their performance on arithmetic tasks (Jackson & Eberly, 1982). During the 1990s, there is a dip in the research interests as reflected by the fewer publications across the board, which has picked up in the post-millennium period. Since then, the focus is markedly turning toward attempting BF on NDD especially, ADD/ADHD and ASD (Table 2).

THEMATIC ANALYSIS

A thematic analysis of the compiled papers against specific, combined or comparative types of NDD is presented below in relation to their adopted research design, sampling, interventions, and outcome measures respectively.

The overall blueprint or strategy that is chosen to integrate the different components of the study in a coherent and logical manner thereby ensuring that the problem is answered for collection, measurement and analysis of data is the essence of research design. There are exploratory (Fernándezm, Harmony,

Table 2. Decade wise distribution of published research papers on biofeedback techniques in neurodevelopmental disorders

Condition	1970-79	1980-89	1990-99	2000-2009	2010+	TOTAL
SLD		5	1	5		11
Stammering/Stuttering	3	2				5
ASD		1	1	8	4	14
ADD/ADHD	3	1	7	25	9	45
SLHD	2	5	2	2	3	14
Voice	2	3	2	1	1	9
ID	1	1	1	3	3	9
TOTAL	11	18	14	44	20	107

[SLD: Specific Learning Disability; ASD: Autism Spectrum Disorder; ADD/ADHD: Attention Deficit (Hyperactivity) Disorder; SLHD: Speech, Language & Hearing Disorders; ID: Intellectual Disability]

Fernández-Bouzas, Díaz-Comas, Prado-Alcalá, Valdés-Sosa... García-Martínez, 2007), descriptive, cross-sectional, longitudinal-follow up (Becerra, Fernández, Harmony, Caballero, García, Fernández-Bouzas, Santiago-Rodríguez, & Prado-Alcalá, 2006; Ayers, 1995; Manschreck, Kalotkin, & Jacobson, 1980), meta-analytic (Tan, Thornby, Hammond, Strehl, Canady, Arnemann, & Kaiser, 2009), and mixed designs seen in the compiled bibliography of research publications on NDD. Instances of true experimental designs involving post-test only and pre-test post-test only involving random assignments to treatment groups and/or placebo-control groups (Kouijzer, van Schie, Gerrits, Buitelaar, & de Moor, 2013), and rarely a Solomon four-group design are seen. However, studies using factorial and crossover designs are minimal if not absent. A few papers have used quasi-experimental research designs involving the manipulation of the independent variable to observe the effect on the dependent variable (Moghanloo, Vafaie, Rostami, & Farahani, 2014). There is also use of pre-experimental research design involving one-shot case design and/or one group pretest-posttest design. Studies based on single case reports cover the use of NF treatment for dysarthria (Goldstein, Ziegler, Vogel, & Hoole, 1994), puberphonia (Franca & Bass-Ringdahi, 2015) and developmental disability (Fleischman & Othmer, 2005). A few studies have used single-subject ABCD baseline design with an ABABAB reversal design within the treatment others have tried a randomized pretest-posttest control group design with blinded active comparison and six-month follow-up by waitlisting the control group (Craig & Cleary, 1982). Some review papers have covered history or rationale for research and theory of BF with or without illustrative case studies (Nagai & Matsuura, 2011; Monastra, 2008; Maryn, De Bodt, & Van Cauwenberge, 2006; Monastra, Lynn, Linden, Lubar, Gruzelier, & LaVaque, 2006; Vernon, Frick, & Gruzelier, 2004; Lubar, 1991). Position papers provide the current evidence supporting the use of NF (Sherlin, Arns, Lubar, & Sokhadze, 2010), while a few are avowedly replication studies (Rossiter, 2004). Some theory-driven papers have examined whether a symptom or assessment/connectivity guided based approach was more effective in understanding BF against specific NDD (Coben & Myers, 2010).

There are wide differences with regard to the constitution of experimental and control groups since some researchers in the review have used IQ, type of disorder, their severity, sample characteristics like race, ethnicity, gender and age matching, while others have used criteria like handedness, low versus high functioning subjects to prepare their control groups. For cases of intellectual disability, the dilemma is seen between mental and/or chronological age matching across the research papers. Some have controlled the administration of medication, while others are silent on this issue. A few others have made two separate groups: drug and non-drug respectively. All these differences are bound to act as confounding variables. The role of artifacts or whether rest or pause periods are given, if so, for how long is seldom highlighted under procedure or discussion in most of the studies covered under this review.

The gold standard of research design (Misra, 2012; Sullivan, 2011), although dubbed as unobtainable (Bondemark & Ruf, 2015), is evidently single (or still better 'double-blind') multi-group randomized placebo case-controlled study is rarely seen in the field of BF on NDD (Geladé, Bink, Janssen, Van Mourik, Maras, & Oosterlaan, 2017; Bakhshayesh, Hansch, Wschkon, Rezai, & Esser, 2011; Perreau-Linck, Lessard, Levesque, & Beauregard, 2010; Leins, Goth, Hinterberger, Klinger, Rumpf, & Strehl, 2007). Going by the preceding, it is seen that BF and NF provide the kind of evidence-based practice that the healthcare establishment is demanding. Levels of evidence range from case report to observational studies to randomized clinical trials. BF has always emerged and remained a laboratory-based research combining neurophysiology and behavior therapy. 'Efficacy' is to do with determining how BF training works in controlled clinical laboratory settings. 'Effectiveness' assesses how well the treatment works in actual clinical settings.

There are five levels of efficacy, according to the professional associations in the area. They range from the lowest level ('not empirically supported') to the highest level ('efficacious and specific') as per the Guidelines for Evaluation of Clinical Efficacy of Psycho-physiological Interventions (LaVaque, Hammond, Trudeau, Monastra, Perry, & Lehrer, 2002). While the application of BF has been shown to be 'efficacious and specific' (highest level) for some clinical conditions, it has been also shown to 'not empirically supported' (lowest level) for some other clinical conditions. There are inherent difficulties in creating the so-called gold standard of double-blind randomized control trials at least for BF training, practice, and research which is founded on enhancing self-awareness of body-mind. Wherein 'placebos' or 'sham-biofeedback' is used as control condition by giving feedback that does not reflect the subject's physiological state, it raises ethical issues. Double- Research Society (renamed the Association for Applied Psychophysiology and Biofeedback) was founded in 1969 (Andrasik & Lords, 2008).

Irrespective of the history and the varied focus of BF on different clinical conditions, at least with respect to NDD, it has been shown that there are substantial variations in the findings. To begin with, there is no consensus on what constitutes NDD itself. A common criticism has been that the studies are based on a small sample size, or that they lack control group/placebo condition and follow the open-label approach. Despite the availability of efficacy guidelines established by the Association for Applied Psychophysiology and Biofeedback and the International Society for Neuronal Regulation, many papers are found not to apply them in actual research practice. Meticulously controlled large-scale group based clinical studies, additional randomized, double-blinded trials or those using correlation designs are needed to provide a better estimate of the robustness of this treatment and reached them to 'probably efficacious' level. Even wherein RCT is used, there are issues such as the efficacy and specificity of effects, treatment fidelity and problems inherent in placebo-controlled trials of NF-BF on NDD. Noting on the methodological flaws in double-blind placebo-controlled studies on ADHD, for example, a few reviews have not found any systematic beneficial effect of EEG-neurofeedback on their neurocognitive functioning (Vollebregt, van Dongen-Boomama, Bultelaar, & Slaats-Willemse, 2014a). However, it is also accepted that absence of evidence does not equate with evidence of absence. Future research needs to overcome these methodological limitations to provide conclusive evidence on this matter (Vollebregt, van Dongen-Boomama, Slaats-Willemse, & Bultelaar, 2014b).

It is argued that there is a long way to go before BF is recognized as a legitimate, scientific, and evidence-based intervention for the treatment of NDD. There are allegations on studies, particularly those presenting series of single cases that they might well have been based on spurious findings. On one side, research has repeatedly shown that a high proportion of children with NDD exhibit a dysfunctional BF profile relative to age-matched peers, and hence provides a rationale or justification for its use as an intervention on such cases. On the other side, there are also questions whether children with NDD are able to demonstrate learning of cortical self-regulation if treatment by BF can indeed lead to an improvement in cognition and behavior. Poor self-regulation is one of the major characteristic features of most children with NDD. Under such circumstances, it is both a challenge and limitation to use BF on them. Finally, the long-term effects of NF-BF and the potential negative side effects are still unclear. The small sample sizes in most studies and other confounding factors, such as motivation or expectations, might be also contributing to the outcome.

Operational definitions of NDD and/or its diagnostic sub-categories are missing in most of the reviewed research articles. Earlier publications have used DSM-IV criteria for the diagnosis of childhood psychiatric conditions, which have changed drastically in the later years. Some research papers mention how they address children who are ADD/ADHD, who were also intellectually or learning disabled. Such diagnostic heterogeneity takes away the basis for making any comparison between the findings of these studies. Although behavioral symptoms of inattention, impulsivity, and hyperactivity serve as a foundation for accurate diagnosis of ADD/ADHD, for example, the low inter-rater reliability and specificity of behavioral rating scales and the absence of comprehensive screening for associated or independent medical conditions that mimic these conditions have created a barrier for their effective identification, diagnosis and treatment.

Ideally, the use of BF mandates certified practitioners who have themselves undergone training in the handling of the instruments. It may also require that subjects are brought to the BF laboratory unless a portable device is being used. Subjects residing in far-flung geographical areas are likely to have limited access to this treatment modality. Contemporary efforts are on to provide these needed services via a telehealth modality. Such capability significantly improves access to care, particularly for subjects located at considerable distance from the provider. As the telecommunications infrastructure in rural and remote areas is often quite basic, such a system must be capable of operating within these limited parameters. The system provides real-time video and audio interactivity and allows the therapist to monitor and control BF equipment located at the remote site (Folen, James, Earles, & Andrasik, 2001).

Another mobile health application solution with BF based on body sensors, such as electrocardiogram, electromyography, blood pressure, electrodermal activity, and temperature, for remote monitoring of patients against falls and/or for use during knee rehabilitation in the elderly population is gathering momentum (Weber-Spickschen, Colcuc, Hanke, Clausen, James, & Horstmann, 2017). Breathwalk is a science of combining specific patterns of footsteps synchronized with breathing. Multimedia assisted breathwalk awareness systems to detect the user's walking and breathing conditions to provide appropriate multimedia guidance on the Smartphone is now available. It gives feedback to synchronize footstep with breathing to aid stress reduction (Dillon, Kelly, Robertson, & Robertson, 2016). Accordingly, they can effectively assist beginners in slowing down the walking speed and decreasing incorrect footsteps (Meng-Chieh, Huan, & Ming-Sui, 2012). Efforts are also being made to rope in the use of robotics for online affect detection and adaptation by BF mechanisms for rehabilitation of children with autism (Liu, Conn, Sarkar, & Stone, 2008). Most studies on clinical applications of robotics in the diagnosis and treatment of autism fall under four broad categories: (a) their response to robots or robot-like behavior in comparison to human behavior; (b) use of robots to elicit behaviors; (c) use of robots to model, teach, and/or practice a skill, and; (d) use of robots to provide feedback on performance. A critical review of the literature shows that most of the findings are exploratory and have methodological limitations that make it difficult to draw firm conclusions about the clinical utility of robots (Diehl, Schmitt, Villano, & Crowell, 2012).

Conditions that raise caution concerning the use of BF are patient age, intellectual disability, psychotic disorders, the presence of life-threatening disorders, medical conditions and personality disorders. Breath retraining, for example, may set off an asthma attack in vulnerable patients. Major losses, family conflicts, and stressful environments will distract from BF learning to block generalization of its benefits to daily life. There are no absolute contraindications for BF. However, one needs to tailor the BF training to the levels, the degree of insight and motivation, and level of cooperation of the subjects. Unauthorized use or modification of BF devices may be hazardous. It should not be used if the subject has a pacemaker, or those with symptomatic epilepsy, electrical hyperreactivity, have irritated, inflamed or broken skin, on pregnant women, children under age three, those under influence of drugs or alcohol. Rarely, transient complaints of brain fog (impaired concentration), chattering teeth, fatigue, depersonalization, dizziness, headaches, social anxiety, are mentioned. These symptoms do not linger for long.

The steadily growing brain-computer interface during use of BF in NDD is impacting not only on individuals but also on society as a whole. Ethical standards that govern human research as derived from Nuremberg Code and the revised Helsinki Declaration-2013 mandate informed consent of the patient or a legally authorized representative for using an unproven intervention (World Medical Association, 2015). Medical ethics question the use of no-treatment (placebo and sham procedure) controlled studies of new therapies when safe and effective standard therapies are available for use as an active or "equivalence" control. Withholding or denying the best proven diagnostic and therapeutic treatment to any participant in a clinical study, including those subjects who consent for randomization into a control group is best avoided.

LIMITATIONS AND FUTURE RESEARCH DIRECTIONS

Even though the study has attempted a pioneering effort to compile as many empirical research articles as a bibliography on BF as related to NDD, no claim can be or is made that the collection is exhaustive. Further, the categories of NDD addressed during this data gathering are along the lines, but not exactly fitting into a DSM-5 system of official classification.

Extending beyond the concerns within this chapter, the contemporary technology on BF must itself needs to undertake more extensive longitudinal studies, amass and utilize health monitoring data in real time, develop distinct protocols that can replicated, accredit its practitioners based on periodic competency-based certification, explore the possibility of using telemetry and ambulatory monitoring, and ameliorate its reliability or validity through double-blind randomized case-controlled studies using sham treatments.

SUMMARY

In sum, BF has been explained in this chapter as a strong possibility and promise for application in the field of NDD. Evidence-based practices and procedures are on the momentum. There is still a long way to go before its efficacy is convincingly proved beyond a practice as art or above prevalent systems of alternative medicine.

REFERENCES

American Psychiatric Association. (2013). Neuro-cognitive disorders. In The American Psychiatric Textbook of Psychiatry (5th ed.). Washington, DC: Author. doi:10.1176/appi.books.9781585625031.rh24

American Psychiatric Association. (2016). *Neuro-developmental disorders: DSM-5 selections*. Washington, DC: Author.

Andrasik, F., & Lords, A. O. (2008). Biofeedback. In L. Freeman (Ed.), *Mosby's Complementary and Alternative Medicine: A research-based approach* (pp. 189–214). St. Louis, MO: Mosby Elsevier.

Andrews, G., Pine, D. S., Hobbs, M. J., Anderson, T. M., & Sunderland, M. (2009). Neurodevelopmental disorders: Cluster 2 of the proposed meta-structure for DSM-V and ICD-11. *Psychological Medicine*, *39*(2), 2013–2023. doi:10.1017/S0033291709990274 PMID:19796427

Armagan, O., Tascioglu, F., & Oner, C. (2003). Electromyographic biofeedback in the treatment of the hemiplegic hand: A placebo-controlled study. *American Journal of Physical Medicine & Rehabilitation*, *82*(11), 856–861. doi:10.1097/01.PHM.0000091984.72486.E0 PMID:14566153

Ayers, M. E. (1995). Long-term follow up of EEG neurofeedback with absence seizures. *Biofeedback and Self-Regulation*, *20*(3), 309–310.

Bakhshayesh, A. R., Hansch, S., Wschkon, A., Rezai, M. J., & Esser, G. (2011). Neurofeedback in ADHD: A single-blind randomized controlled trial. *European Child & Adolescent Psychiatry*, *20*(9), 481–491. doi:10.100700787-011-0208-y PMID:21842168

Basmajian, J. V. (1989). *Biofeedback: Principles and practice for clinicians*. Philadelphia: Williams & Wilkins.

Beatty, J., & Legewie, H. (1977). *Biofeedback and behavior*. London: Plenum Press. doi:10.1007/978-1-4684-2526-0

Becerra, J., Fernández, T., Harmony, T., Caballero, M. I., García, F., Fernández-Bouzas, A., ... Prado-Alcalá, R. A. (2006). Follow-up study of learning-disabled children treated with neurofeedback or placebo. *Clinical EEG and Neuroscience*, *37*(3), 198–203. doi:10.1177/155005940603700307 PMID:16929704

Ben-Ari, Y. (2016). Progress in autism research and post-genomic studies. *Lancet Neurology*, *15*(2), 136. doi:10.1016/S1474-4422(15)00402-0 PMID:28463118

Berg, A. T., & Dobyns, W. B. (2015). Progress in autism and related disorders of brain development. *Lancet Neurology*, *14*(11), 1169–1170. doi:10.1016/S1474-4422(15)00048-4 PMID:25891008

Bettelheim, B. (1967). *The empty fortress: Infantile autism and the birth of the self*. New York: Free Press.

Birbaumer, N., & Kimmel, H. D. (Eds.). (1979). *Biofeedback and self regulation*. Hillsdale, NJ: Erlbaum.

Bishop, D., & Rutter, M. (2008). Neurodevelopmental disorders: conceptual issues. Rutter's child and adolescent psychiatry, 32-41.

Bishop, D. V. M. (2010). Which neurodevelopmental disorders get researched and why? *PLoS One*, *5*(11), e15112. doi:10.1371/journal.pone.0015112 PMID:21152085

Bondemark, L., & Ruf, S. (2015). Randomized controlled trial: The gold standard or unobtainable fallacy. *European Journal of Orthodontics*, *37*(5), 457–461. doi:10.1093/ejo/cjv046 PMID:26136438

Braud, L. W., Lupin, M. N., & Braud, W. G. (1975). The use of electromyographic biofeedback in the control of hyperactivity. *Journal of Learning Disabilities*, *8*(7), 420–452. doi:10.1177/002221947500800704

Brody, D. M., Nelon, B. A., & Brody, J. F. (1975). The use of visual feedback in establishing normal vocal intensity in two mildly retarded adults. *The Journal of Speech and Hearing Disorders*, *40*(4), 602–507. doi:10.1044/jshd.4004.502 PMID:1234966

Brown, B. B. (1977). *Stress and the art of biofeedback.* New York: Harper & Row.

Budzynski, T., Stoyva, J., & Adler, C. (1970). Feedback induced relaxation: Application to tension headache. *Journal of Behavior Therapy and Experimental Psychiatry*, *1*(3), 205–211. doi:10.1016/0005-7916(70)90004-2

Butler, F. (1978). *Biofeedback: A survey of literature*. New York: Plenum Publishing Corporation.

Butler, F., & Stoyva, J. (1973). *Biofeedback and self-regulation: A bibliography*. Colorado: Biofeedback Research Society.

Carver, R. H., & Nash, J. G. (2009). *Doing data analysis with SPSS: Version 20*. Belmont, CA: Brooks/Cole Cengage Learning.

Clegg, J., Gillott, A., & Jones, J. (2013). Conceptual issues in neurodevelopmental disorders: Lives out of synch. *Current Opinion in Psychiatry*, *28*, 1–3. doi:10.1097/ YCO.ObO13e32835f6771 PMID:23519204

Coben, R., & Myers, T. E. (2010). The relative efficacy of connectivity guided and symptom-based EEG biofeedback for autistic disorders. *Applied Psycho-physiological Biofeedback*, *35*(1), 13–23. doi:10.100710484-009-9102-5 PMID:19649702

Cooper, S. A. (1997). Deficient health and social services for elderly people with learning disabilities. *Journal of Intellectual Disability Research*, *41*(4), 331–338. doi:10.1111/j.1365-2788.1997.tb00717.x PMID:9297611

Craig, A. R., & Cleary, P. J. (1982). Reduction of stuttering by young male stutterers using EMG feedback. *Biofeedback and Self-Regulation*, *7*(3), 241–255. doi:10.1007/BF00998918 PMID:7171633

Cunningham, M., & Murphy, P. (1981). The effects of bilateral EEG biofeedback on verbal, visuospatial and creative skills in LD male adolescents. *Journal of Learning Disabilities*, *14*(4), 204–208. doi:10.1177/002221948101400406 PMID:7229554

De Felice, A., Ricceri, L., Venerosi, A., Chiarotti, F., & Calamandrei, G. (2015). Multifactorial origin of neurodevelopmental disorders: Approaches to understanding complex aetiologies. *Toxics*, *3*(1), 89–129. doi:10.3390/toxics3010089 PMID:29056653

Dicara, L. V., & Miller, N. E. (1968). Instrumental learning of vasomotor responses by rats: Learning to respond differentially in the two ears. *Science*, *159*(3822), 1485–1486. doi:10.1126cience.159.3822.1485 PMID:5732491

Diehl, J. J., Schmitt, L. M., Villano, M., & Crowell, C. R. (2012). The clinical use of robots for individuals with Autism Spectrum Disorders: A critical review. *Research in Autism Spectrum Disorders*, *6*(1), 249–262. doi:10.1016/j.rasd.2011.05.006 PMID:22125579

Dillon, A., Kelly, M., Robertson, I. H., & Robertson, D. A. (2016). Smartphone applications utilizing biofeedback can aid stress reduction. *Frontiers in Psychology*, *7*, 832. doi:10.3389/fpsyg.2016.00832 PMID:27378963

Durand, V. M., & Barlow, D. (2009). *Abnormal psychology: An integrative approach.* Belmont, CA: Wadsworth Cengage Learning.

Ecker, C., Bookheimer, S. Y., & Murphy, D. G. M. (2015). Neuroimaging in autism spectrum disorder: Brain structure and function across life span. *Lancet Neurology*, *14*(11), 1121–1134. doi:10.1016/S1474-4422(15)00050-2 PMID:25891007

Enck, P., Van Der Voort, I. R., & Klosterhalfen, S. (2009). Biofeedback therapy for fecal incontinence and constipation. *Neurogastroenterology and Motility*, *21*(11), 1133–1141. doi:10.1111/j.1365-2982.2009.01345.x PMID:19566591

Erick, P. (1993). Biofeedback training in disordered defecation: A critical review. *Digestive Diseases and Sciences*, *38*(11), 1953–1960. doi:10.1007/BF01297069 PMID:8223066

Farran, E. K., & Karmiloff-Smith, A. (2012). *Neurodevelopmental disorders across the lifespan: A neuro-constructive approach*. Oxford, UK: Oxford University Press.

Farran, E. K., Riby, D., & Herwegen, J. V. (2014). Neurodevelopmental disorders: Definitions and issues. In J. V. Herwegen & D. Riby (Eds.), *Neurodevelopmental disorders: Research challenges and solutions*. London: Psychology Press.

Fernándezm, T., Harmony, T., Fernández-Bouzas, A., Díaz-Comas, L., Prado-Alcalá, R. A., Valdés-Sosa, P., ... García-Martínez, F. (2007). Changes in EEG current sources induced by neurofeedback in learning disabled children: An exploratory study. *Applied Psychophysiology and Biofeedback*, *32*(3-4), 169–183. doi:10.100710484-007-9044-8 PMID:17978869

Fleischman, M. J., & Othmer, S. (2005). Case study: Improvements in IQ score and maintenance of gains following EEG biofeedback with mildly developmentally delayed twins. *Journal of Neurotherapy*, *9*(4), 35–46. doi:10.1300/J184v09n04_03

Fleiss, J. L. (1981). *Statistical methods for rates and proportions*. New York: John Wiley.

Fleiss, J. L., & Cohen, J. (1973). The equivalence of weighted kappa and the intra-class correlation coefficient as measures of reliability. *Educational and Psychological Measurement*, *33*(1), 613–619. doi:10.1177/001316447303300309

Folen, R. A., James, L. C., Earles, J. E., & Andrasik, F. (2001). Biofeedback via telehealth: A new frontier for applied psychophysiology. *Applied Psychophysiology and Biofeedback*, *26*(3), 195–204. doi:10.1023/A:1011346103638 PMID:11680283

Franca, M. C., & Bass-Ringdahi, S. (2015). A clinical demonstration of the application of audiovisual biofeedback in the treatment of puberphonia. *International Journal of Pediatric Otorhinolaryngology*, *79*(6), 912–920. doi:10.1016/j.ijporl.2015.04.013 PMID:25912681

Frank, D. L., Khorshid, L., Kiffer, J. F., Moravec, C. S., & McKee, M. G. (2010). Biofeedback in medicine: Who, when, why and how? *Mental Health in Family Medicine*, *7*(2), 85–91. PMID:22477926

Geladé, K., Bink, M., Janssen, T. W., Van Mourik, R., Maras, A., & Oosterlaan, J. (2017). An RCT into the effects of neurofeedback on neurocognitive functioning compared to stimulant medication and physical activity in children with ADHD. *European Child & Adolescent Psychiatry*, *26*(4), 457–468. doi:10.100700787-016-0902-x PMID:27665293

Geschwind, D. H., & State, M. W. (2015). Gene hunting in autism spectrum disorder: On the path to precision medicine. *Lancet Neurology*, *14*(11), 1109–1120. doi:10.1016/S1474-4422(15)00044-7 PMID:25891009

Gnanavel, S. (2017). Biomarkers in autism spectrum disorders: An illusion or promising reality. *Indian Journal of Psychological Medicine*, *39*(5), 714–715. doi:10.4103/IJPSYM.IJPSYM_122_17 PMID:29200579

Goldstein, P., Ziegler, W., Vogel, M., & Hoole, P. (1994). Combined palatal-lift and EPG-feedback therapy in dysarthria: A case study. *Clinical Linguistics & Phonetics*, *8*(3), 201–218. doi:10.3109/02699209408985307

Green, E., & Green, A. (1977). *Beyond biofeedback*. New York: Delacorte Press/Seymour.

Guitar, B. (1975). Reduction of stuttering frequency using analog electromyographic feedback. *Journal of Speech and Hearing Research*, *18*(4), 672–685. doi:10.1044/jshr.1804.672 PMID:1207099

Guldberg-Kjar, T., Sehlin, S., & Johansson, B. (2013). ADHD symptoms across life span in population-based Swedish sample aged 65-80. *International Psychogeriatrics*, *29*(4), 667–675. doi:10.1017/S1041610212002050 PMID:23237190

Hamilton, D. R. (2015). Treatment of neurodevelopmental disorders: Targeting neurobiological mechanisms. *Journal of Developmental and Behavioral Pediatrics*, *36*(6), 425. doi:10.1097/DBP.0000000000000183

Hammond, D. C. (2008). Comprehensive Neuro-feedback Bibliography: 2007 Update. *Journal of Neurotherapy*, *11*(3), 45–60. doi:10.1080/10874200802126241

Hanna, R., Wilfling, F., & McNeill, B. (1975). A biofeedback treatment for stuttering. *The Journal of Speech and Hearing Disorders*, *40*(2), 270–273. doi:10.1044/jshd.4002.270 PMID:1234938

Happe, F., & Charlton, R. A. (2012). Aging in autism spectrum disorders: A mini review. *Gerontology*, *58*(1), 70–78. doi:10.1159/000329720 PMID:21865667

Henschen, T. L., & Burton, N. G. (1978). Treatment of spastic dysphonia by EMG biofeedback. *Biofeedback and Self-Regulation*, *3*(1), 91–96. doi:10.1007/BF00998566 PMID:667194

Homberg, J. R., Kyzar, E. J., Stewart, A. M., Nguyen, M., Poudel, M. K., Echevarria, D. J., ... Pittman, J. (2016). Improving treatment of neurodevelopmental disorders: Recommendations based on preclinical studies. *Expert Opinion on Drug Discovery*, *11*(1), 11–25. doi:10.1517/17460441.2016.1115834 PMID:26558752

Huang, H., Wolf, S. L., & He, J. (2006). Recent developments in biofeedback of neuro-motor rehabilitation. *Journal of Neuroengineering and Rehabilitation*, *3*(1), 11. doi:10.1186/1743-0003-3-11 PMID:16790060

Jackson, G. M., & Eberly, D. A. (1982). Facilitation of performance on an arithmetic task as a result of the application of a biofeedback procedure to suppress alpha wave activity. *Biofeedback and Self-Regulation*, *7*(2), 211–221. doi:10.1007/BF00998784 PMID:7138953

James, I. A., Mukaetova-Ladinska, E., Reichelt, F. K., Briel, R., & Scully, A. (2006). Diagnosing Asperger's syndrome in the elderly: A series of case presentations. *International Journal of Geriatric Psychiatry*, *21*(10), 951–960. doi:10.1002/gps.1588 PMID:16927399

Janicki, M. P., Dalton, A. J., Henderson, C. M., & Davidson, P. W. (1999). Mortality and morbidity among older adults with intellectual disability: Health services considerations. *Disability and Rehabilitation, 21*(5-6), 284–294. doi:10.1080/096382899297710 PMID:10381241

Jeste, S. S., Frohlich, J., & Loo, S. K. (2015). Electrophysiological biomarkers of diagnosis and outcome in neurodevelopmental disorders. *Current Opinion in Neurology, 28*(2), 110–116. doi:10.1097/WCO.0000000000000181 PMID:25710286

Kamiya, J. (1968). Conscious control of brain waves. *Psychology Today, 1*, 56–60.

Khazan, I. Z. (2013). *The clinical handbook of biofeedback: A step-by-step guide for training and practice with mindfulness*. Sussex, UK: Wiley-Blackwell. doi:10.1002/9781118485309

Kimmel, H. D. (1974). Instrumental conditioning of autonomically mediated responses in human beings. *The American Psychologist, 29*(5), 325–335. doi:10.1037/h0037621 PMID:4847492

Kimmel, H. D. (1981). The relevance of experimental studies to clinical applications of biofeedback. *Biofeedback and Self-Regulation, 6*(2), 263–271. doi:10.1007/BF00998874 PMID:7260190

Kouijzer, M. E., van Schie, H. T., Gerrits, B. J., Buitelaar, J. K., & de Moor, J. M. (2013). Is EEG-biofeedback an effective treatment in autism spectrum disorders? A randomized controlled trial. *Applied Psychophysiology and Biofeedback, 38*(1), 17–28. doi:10.100710484-012-9204-3 PMID:22903518

Kranitz, L., & Lehrer, P. (2004). *Biofeedback applications in the treatment of cardiovascular diseases*. Academic Press. doi:10.1097/01.crd.0000107893.17799.95

Kuruvilla, K. (2010). India contribution to behavior therapy. *Indian Journal of Psychiatry, 52*(7S1), S371–S377. doi:10.4103/0019-5545.69271 PMID:21836708

Landis, J. R., & Koch, G. G. (1977). The measurement of observer agreement for categorical data. *Biometrics, 33*(1), 159-174.

LaVaque, T. J., Hammond, D. C., Trudeau, D., Monastra, V. J., Perry, J., Lehrer, P., ... Sherman, R. (2002). Template for developing guidelines for the evaluation of the clinical efficacy of psycho-physiological interventions. *Applied Psychophysiology and Biofeedback, 27*(4), 273–281. doi:10.1023/A:1021061318355 PMID:12557455

Lehrer, P., & Vaschilio, E. (2006). Heart rate variability biofeedback: Effects on age of heart rate variability, baroreflex gain, and asthma. *Chest Journal, 129*(2), 278–384. doi:10.1378/chest.129.2.278 PMID:16478842

Leins, U., Goth, G., Hinterberger, T., Klinger, C., Rumpf, N., & Strehl, U. (2007). EEG biofeedback for children with ADHD: A comparison of SCP and theta/beta protocols. *Applied Psychophysiology and Biofeedback, 32*(2), 73–88. doi:10.100710484-007-9031-0 PMID:17356905

Liu, C., Conn, K., Sarkar, N., & Stone, W. (2008). Online affect detection and robot behavior adaptation for intervention in children with autism. *IEEE Transactions on Robotics, 24*(4), 883–896. doi:10.1109/TRO.2008.2001362

Lubar, J. F. (1991). Discourse on the development of EEG diagnostics and biofeedback for attention-deficit/hyperactivity disorders. *Biofeedback and Self-Regulation*, *16*(3), 201–225. doi:10.1007/BF01000016 PMID:1932259

Luthe, W., & Schultz, J. H. (1969). *Autogenic therapy: Applications in psychotherapy*. New York: Grune & Stratton.

Manschreck, T. C., Kalotkin, M., & Jacobson, A. M. (1980). Utility of electro-myographic biological feedback in chronic stuttering: A clinical study with follow-up. *Perceptual and Motor Skills*, *51*(2), 535–540. doi:10.2466/pms.1980.51.2.535 PMID:7443374

Marinacci, A. A. (1955). *Clinical electromyography: A brief review of the electrophysiology of the motor unit and its application to the diagnosis of lower motor neuron diseases, peripheral neuropathy and the myopathies*. Los Angeles, CA: San Lucas Press.

Maryn, Y., De Bodt, M., & Van Cauwenberge, P. (2006). Effects of biofeedback in phonatory disorders and phonatory performance: A systematic literature. *Applied Psychophysiology and Biofeedback*, *31*(1), 65–83. doi:10.100710484-006-9005-7 PMID:16514557

McPartland, J. C. (2016). Considerations in biolmarker development for neurodevelopmental disorders. *Current Opinion in Neurology*, *29*(2), 118–122. doi:10.1097/WCO.0000000000000300 PMID:26844621

Meng-Chieh, Y., Huan, W., & Ming-Sui, L. (2012). Multimedia assisted breath walk aware system. *IEEE Transactions on Biomedical Engineering*, *59*(12), 3276–3282. doi:10.1109/TBME.2012.2208747 PMID:23203771

Miller, N. E., & Dworkin, B. (1974). Visceral learning: Recent difficulties with curarized rats and significant problems for human research. In P. A. Obrist, A. H. Black, J. Brener, & L. V. DiCara (Eds.), *Cardiovascular psychophysiology* (pp. 312–331). New York: Aldine.

Misra, S. (2012). Randomized double-blind placebo control studies, the 'Gold Standard' in intervention-based studies. *Indian Journal of Sexually Transmitted Diseases*, *33*(2), 131–134. doi:10.4103/0253-7184.102130 PMID:23188942

Moghanloo, M., Vafaie, M. E. A., Rostami, R., & Farahani, H. (2014). Determination of the effects of neurofeedback training in the neuropsychological rehabilitation in inattentive and combined subtypes of attention-deficit/hyperactivity disorder. *NeuroRegulaton*, *1*(2), 131–150. doi:10.15540/nr.1.2.131

Monastra, V. J. (2008). Quantitative electroencephalography and attention-deficit/hyperactivity disorder: Implications for clinical practice. *Current Psychiatry Reports*, *10*(5), 432–438. doi:10.100711920-008-0069-3 PMID:18803918

Monastra, V. J., Lynn, S., Linden, M., Lubar, J. F., Gruzelier, J., & LaVaque, T. J. (2006). Electroencephalographic biofeedback in the treatment of attention-deficit/ hyperactivity disorder. *Journal of Neurotherapy*, *9*(4), 5–34. doi:10.1300/J184v09n04_02

Mukaetova-Ladinska, E. B., Perry, E., Baron, M., & Povey, C. (2012). Ageing in people with autism spectrum disorder. *International Journal of Geriatric Psychiatry*, *27*(2), 109–118. doi:10.1002/gps.2711 PMID:21538534

Nagai, Y., & Matsuura, M. (2011). Biofeedback treatment for epilepsy. *Brain and Nerve*, *63*(4), 385–392. PMID:21441642

Nelson, L. A. (2007). The role of biofeedback in stroke rehabilitation: Past and future directions. *Topics in Stroke Rehabilitation*, *14*(4), 59–66. doi:10.1310/tsr1404-59 PMID:17698458

Nestoriuc, Y., Martin, A., Rief, W., & Andrasik, F. (2008). Biofeedback treatment for headache disorders: A comprehensive efficacy review. *Applied Psychophysiology and Biofeedback*, *33*(3), 125–140. doi:10.100710484-008-9060-3 PMID:18726688

Patel, P., Goldberg, D., & Moss, S. (1993). Psychiatric morbidity in older people with moderate and severe learning disability. II: The prevalence study. *The British Journal of Psychiatry*, *163*(4), 481–491. doi:10.1192/bjp.163.4.481 PMID:8252287

Patja, K., Livanainen, M., Vesala, H., Oksanen, H., & Ruoppila, I. (2000). Life expectancy of people with intellectual disability: A 35-year old follow-up study. *Journal of Intellectual Disability Research*, *44*(5), 591–599. doi:10.1046/j.1365-2788.2000.00280.x PMID:11079356

Peper, E., & Shaffer, F. (2010). Biofeedback history: An alternative view. *Biofeedback*, *38*(4), 142–147. doi:10.5298/1081-5937-38.4.03

Perreau-Linck, E., Lessard, N., Levesque, J., & Beauregard, M. (2010). Effects of neurofeedback training on inhibitory capacities in ADHD children: A single-blind, randomized, placebo-controlled study. *Journal of Neurotherapy*, *14*(3), 229–242. doi:10.1080/10874208.2010.501514

Piven, J., & Rabins, P. (2011). Autism spectrum disorders in older adults: Toward defining a research agenda. *Journal of the American Geriatrics Society*, *59*(11), 2151–2155. doi:10.1111/j.1532-5415.2011.03632.x PMID:22091837

Prehn-Kristensen, A., Cooke, R., Baving, L., & Schumann, C. (2012). Neurodevelopmental disorders. In T. Bartsch (Ed.), The clinical neurobiology of the hippocampus: An integrated view. Oxford, UK: Oxford Scholarship Online/Oxford University Press. doi:10.1093/acprof:oso/9780199592388.003.0010

Prinsloo, G. E., Raunch, H. G. L., & Derman, W. E. (2014). A brief review and clinical applications of heart rate variability biofeedback in sports, exercise and rehabilitation medicine. *The Physician and Sportsmedicine*, *42*(2), 88–99. doi:10.3810/psm.2014.05.2061 PMID:24875976

Prosek, R. A., Montgomery, A. A., Walden, B. E., & Schwartz, D. M. (1978). EMG biofeedback in the treatment of hyperfunctional voice disorders. *The Journal of Speech and Hearing Disorders*, *43*(3), 282–294. doi:10.1044/jshd.4303.282 PMID:692095

Rickles, W. H., Sandweiss, J. H., Jacobs, D. W., Grove, R. N., & Criswell, E. (Eds.). (1983). *Biofeedback and family practice medicine*. London: Plenum Press. doi:10.1007/978-1-4684-1173-7

Rossiter, T. (2004). The effectiveness of EEG biofeedback and stimulant drugs in treating AD/HD: Part II. Replication. *Applied Psychophysiology and Biofeedback*, *29*(4), 233–243. doi:10.100710484-004-0383-4 PMID:15707253

Sachs, D. A., Martin, J. E., & Fitch, J. L. (1972). The effect of visual feedback on a digital exercise in a functionally deaf cerebral palsied child. *Journal of Behavior Therapy and Experimental Psychiatry*, *3*(3), 217–222. doi:10.1016/0005-7916(72)90078-X

Schwartz, M., & Andrasik, F. (2016). *Biofeedback: A practitioner's guide* (4th ed.). New York: Guilford Publications.

Sherlin, L., Arns, M., Lubar, J., & Sokhadze, E. (2010). A position paper on neurofeedback for the treatment of ADHD. *Journal of Neurotherapy*, *14*(2), 66–78. doi:10.1080/10874201003773880

Shouse, M. N., & Lubar, J. F. (1979). Operant conditioning of EEG rhythms and Ritalin in the treatment of hyper-kinesis. *Biofeedback and Self-Regulation*, *4*(4), 299–312. doi:10.1007/BF00998960 PMID:526475

Sokhadze, T. M., Cannon, R. L., & Trudeau, D. L. (2008). EEG biofeedback as a treatment for substance use disorders: Review, a rating of efficiency, and recommendations for further research. *Applied Psychophysiology and Biofeedback*, *33*(1), 1–28. doi:10.100710484-007-9047-5 PMID:18214670

Strydom, A., Hassiotis, A., King, M., & Livingston, G. (2009). The relationship of dementia prevalence in older adults with intellectual disability (ID) to age and severity of ID. *Psychological Medicine*, *39*(1), 13–21. doi:10.1017/S0033291708003334 PMID:18410700

Strydom, A., Livingston, G., King, M., & Hassiotis, A. (2007). Prevalence of dementia in intellectual disability using different diagnostic criteria. *The British Journal of Psychiatry*, *191*(2), 150–157. doi:10.1192/bjp.bp.106.028845 PMID:17666500

Sullivan, G. M. (2011). Getting off the 'Gold Standard': Randomized controlled trials and education research. *Journal of Graduate Medical Education*, *3*(3), 285–289. doi:10.4300/JGME-D-11-00147.1 PMID:22942950

Szpir, M. (2006). New thinking on neurodevelopment. *Environmental Health Perspectives*, *114*(2), A100–A107. doi:10.1289/ehp.114-a100 PMID:16451834

Tan, G., Thornby, J., Hammond, C., Strehl, U., Canady, B., Arnemann, K., & Kaiser, D. A. (2009). Meta-analysis of EEG biofeedback in treating epilepsy. *Clinical EEG and Neuroscience*, *40*(3), 180–189. doi:10.1177/155005940904000310 PMID:19715180

Tansey, M. (1985). Brain wave signatures: An index reflexive of the brain's functional neuroanatomy: Further findings on the effect of EEG sensorimotor rhythm biofeedback training on the neurological precursors of learning disabilities. *International Journal of Psychophysiology*, *3*(2), 85–99. doi:10.1016/0167-8760(85)90030-3 PMID:4077617

Turk, D., Meichenbaum, D. H., & Berman, W. H. (1979). Application of biofeedback for the regulation of pain: A critical review. *Psychological Bulletin*, *86*(6), 1322–1338. doi:10.1037/0033-2909.86.6.1322 PMID:515286

Tye, C., McLoughlin, G., Kuntsi, J., & Asherson, P. (2011). Electrophysiological markers of genetic risk for attention deficit hyperactivity disorder. *Expert Reviews in Molecular Medicine*, *13*, e9. doi:10.1017/S1462399411001797 PMID:21426626

Tye, C., Rijsdijk, F., Greven, C. U., Kuntsi, J., Asherson, P., & McLoughlin, G. (2012). Shared genetic influences on ADHD symptoms and very low-frequency EEG activity: A twin study. *Journal of Child Psychology and Psychiatry, and Allied Disciplines*, *53*(6), 706–715. doi:10.1111/j.1469-7610.2011.02501.x PMID:22118296

United States Environmental Protective Agency. (2015). America's children and the environment: Neurodevelopmental Disorders (excerpt from the. In C. Croft (Ed.), *Environmental hazards and neurodevelopment: Where ecology and well being connect* (3rd ed.; pp. 3–40). Oakville, ON: Apple Academic Press.

Utari, A., Adams, E., Berry-Kravis, E., Chavez, A., Scaggs, F., Ngotran, L., ... Tartaglia, N. (2010). Aging in fragile X syndrome. *Journal of Neurodevelopmental Disorders*, *2*(2), 70–76. doi:10.100711689-010-9047-2 PMID:20585378

van Niekerk, M. E. H., Groen, W., Vissers, C. T. W. M., van-Driel-de Jong, D., Kan, C. C., & Oude Voshaar, R. C. (2011). Diagnosing autism spectrum disorders in elderly people. *International Psychogeriatrics*, *23*(5), 700–710. doi:10.1017/S1041610210002152 PMID:21110908

Vargo, F. E. (2012). *Neurodevelopmental disorders: A definitive guide for educators*. New York, NY: W. W. Norton & Company.

Venkatesan, S. (2009b). *Ethical guidelines for biobehavioral research*. Mysore: All India Institute of Speech and Hearing.

Vernon, D., Frick, A., & Gruzelier, J. (2004). Neurofeedback as a treatment for ADHD: A methodological review with implications for future research. *Journal of Neurotherapy*, *8*(2), 53–82. doi:10.1300/J184v08n02_04

Vollebregt, M. A., van Dongen-Boomama, M., Bultelaar, J. K., & Slaats-Willemse, D. (2014a). Does EEG-neurofeedback improve neurocognitive functioning in children with attention-deficit/hyperactivity disorder? A systematic review and a double-blind placebo-controlled study. *Journal of Clinical Psychology and Psychiatry*, *55*(5), 460–472. doi:10.1111/jcpp.12143 PMID:24168522

Vollebregt, M. A., van Dongen-Boomama, M., Slaats-Willemse, D., & Bultelaar, J. K. (2014b). What future research should bring to help resolving the debate about the efficacy of EEG-neurofeedback in children with ADHD. *Frontiers in Human Neuroscience*, *8*, 321. doi:10.3389/fnhum.2014.00321 PMID:24860487

Weber-Spickschen, T. S., Colcuc, C., Hanke, A., Clausen, J. D., James, P. A., & Horstmann, H. (2017). Fun during knee rehabilitation: Feasibility and acceptability testing of a new Android-based training device. *The Open Medical Informatics Journal*, *11*(1), 29–36. doi:10.2174/1874431101711010029 PMID:29081870

Woolfendon, S., Sarkozy, V., Ridley, G., & Williams, K. (2012). A systematic review of the diagnostic stability of autism spectrum disorder. *Research in Autism Spectrum Disorders*, *6*(1), 345–354. doi:10.1016/j.rasd.2011.06.008

World Health Organization. (2008). *The ICD-10 classification of mental and behavioral disorders descriptions and diagnostic guidelines*. Geneva: Author.

World Medical Association. (2015). *WMA Declaration of Helsinki-Ethical principles for medical research involving human subjects*. Author.

Zijlstra, A., Mancini, M., Chiari, L., & Zijlstra, W. (2010). Biofeedback for training balance and mobility in older populations: A systematic review. *Journal of Neuroengineering and Rehabilitation*, *7*(1), 58. doi:10.1186/1743-0003-7-58 PMID:21143921

KEY TERMS AND DEFINITIONS

Adaptive Behavior: A type of behavior that is used to adjust to another type of behavior or situation.

Biomarker: Biological markers are substances used as an objective indicator of a biological state.

Classical Conditioning: Also called Pavlovian or respondent conditioning it refers to learning procedure in which a biologically potent stimulus like food is paired with a previously neutral stimulus.

Developmental Motor Coordination Disorder: A childhood developmental disorder marked by clumsiness in otherwise healthy children.

Discrimination: The ability to perceive and respond to differences among stimuli.

Disorders of Behavior and Conduct: A repetitive and persistent pattern of behavior in which the basic rights of others or major age-appropriate norms are violated.

Dyspraxia: A developmental disorder of the brain in childhood causing difficulty in activities requiring coordination and movement.

Generalization: The tendency to respond in the same way to different but similar stimuli.

Intellectual Developmental Disorder or Disability: Also known by its earlier term "mental retardation," is a condition characterized by limitations in both intellectual functioning and in adaptive behavior which covers many everyday social and practical skills. The disability originates before the age of eighteen.

Operant Conditioning: Also called instrumental conditioning is a method of learning that occurs through rewards and punishments for behavior.

Shaping: It is the process of reinforcing successively closer and closer approximations to a desired terminal behavior.

Stereotypic Movement Disorders: A motor disorder with onset in childhood involving repetitive non-functional motor behaviors like hand waving, head banging that markedly interfere with normal activities or results in bodily injury.

Sympathetic Nervous System: A part of the autonomic nervous system which activates what is often called the fight or flight response.

Traumatic Brain Injury: A brain dysfunction caused by an outside force, usually a violent blow to the head.

Chapter 12
LearnEasy–Android Application as a Technological Intervention for Children With Dyslexia

Ganta Sandeep V. Padmakar
Dr. B. R. Ambedkar National Institute of Technology, India

Arun Khosla
Dr. B. R. Ambedkar National Institute of Technology, India

Kulbhushan Chand
Dr. B. R. Ambedkar National Institute of Technology, India

ABSTRACT

The recent studies show that the children with learning disabilities numbers have been gradually increased in India. Though the main reason for the cause of this disorder is unknown, the authors strongly believe that this neurological disorder is explained as a genetic disorder passed from elder hierarchy to the next generation. With the available resources, the awareness programs are limited to urban areas only on account of using current technology in diagnosing disorders. In developed countries, it is seen that new technologies taking birth every day for the treatment of these disorders. This includes LCD 3D display, Kinect games, computer games (psychotherapeutic) in therapy sessions, etc. These kinds of games make children more attentive towards the intervention bringing new changes in the day-to-day lives of the children. In this chapter, a new algorithm has been highlighted for the intervention of children with dyslexia by using the Android application as a source to increase the level of perception and sound-symbol association of the respective alphabets used and studied.

DOI: 10.4018/978-1-5225-7004-2.ch012

INTRODUCTION

Dyslexia is often specified as a learning disability where the children have trouble with reading and spelling despite having the ability to learn. It is often termed as a brain-based difference termed as one of the neurological disorders, which can be different from person to person. There is no cure as neuro-pathological studies have revealed an abnormal anatomy of the Corpus Callosum (CC) in dyslexic brains (Elnakib, Casanova, Gimelrfarb, Switala, & El-Baz, 2012).

Children with dyslexia are not much different from others but their inability to learn something makes them different. They need different techniques unlike ordinary methods implemented for normal children to learn something new. Because of this disorder, they cannot easily understand what has been taught to them in a regular manner. They often get confused with the letters like 'p' for 'q' and 'b' for 'd' and also similar in the case with the other alphabets and numbers (Vellutino & Scanlon, 1987; Sklar, Hanley, & Simmons, 1973). The problem of perception in dyslexia seemingly results from an inability to retrieve correct verbal labels for phonemes (Vellutino & Scanlon, 1987).

The mode of teaching should be different for children with learning disabilities like an entertaining game at the same time also the learning process. Gaming is the best method as it attracts the child's attention and can make an impact to remember for long periods of time (Cuschieri, Khaled, Farrugia, Martinez, & Yannakakis, 2014). It serves the purpose of creating enthusiasm in children to learn as well as make them enjoy learning also e.g. word shark a game developed to build words using alphabets (Singleton, & Simmons, 2001; Rello, Bayarri, & Gorriz, 2012).

Technology has opened the door to a new set of scalable tools that can address this challenge and help people with dyslexia live the most productive and learning lives as possible. When deciding on technology options, we must consider the individual needs of the child (including sensory, physical, social and communicative issues) characteristics and needs, and the environmental demands (Tanner, Dixon, & Verenikina, 2010).

The investigators identified one of the problems with the children with dyslexia as sound-symbol association and perception (Vellutino & Scanlon, 1987; Sklar, Hanley, & Simmons, 1973). As discussed perception in this regard is nothing but misinterpretation or misjudging the alphabets and writing them in a different manner. Coming to sound-symbol association children with the disability were unable to identify the sounds associated with the respective letters and their pronunciation (Rello, 2014). Thus, given the unique learning needs of individuals with dyslexia, the purpose was to design an android application based game in order to make them learn and understand the respective difficulty associated with their disability. The investigators have considered different subjects with dyslexia for intervention. This game enabled the subjects to understand the meaning of perception. The score comparison with the normal children, their performance and also accuracy helped the trainers to study the improvement of the children with dyslexia. The sound-symbol association technique helped them to identify the pronunciation of different words used in the game with respect to alphabets.

MODERN DAY TECHNOLOGY

Recent studies have indicated that children with dyslexia have responded dramatically to intervention and supports employed to improve their skills through gaming (Cuschieri, Khaled, Farrugia, Martinez, & Yannakakis, 2014). Their learning ability has shown a marked improvement when gadgets like an iPad and tablets were employed. A range of data is available to support this claim. Digital display boards, electronic tutors and even Power Point presentations have proved to be highly effective aids (Ismail & Jaafar, 2011). The core technical group believes that it can deliver solutions based on gaming, smart-phones and Haptic technologies that can go a long way in helping the caregivers, therapists and parents who work with children with dyslexia.

There are a lot of technological innovations growing in the field of health sciences for children with autism spectrum disorders, intellectual disabilities, attention deficit hyperactivity disorder, and also children with specific learning disability in which dyslexia is one. Specifically, about dyslexia, the global countries outside India are a step ahead in technological innovations in the field of neurology as they use projectors, virtual reality etc in the teaching methods. New methodologies with technology included in the teaching make the intervention process innovative as well as effective.

Considering the situation in India, awareness and understanding the level of disorder is important. Many social organizations and NGO's came forward to deal with these types of disorders. These organizations mostly follow traditional teaching methodologies rather than using technology in it. Now the point is beside the usage of traditional methodologies, have to start using the available technological interventions like projectors, LED display, smart phones etc (Ismail & Jaafar, 2011). Smart phones are now a revolution in the modern day technology as they become a handy device.

Assistive technology which offers a way for dyslexics to save time and overcome some of the issues like slow note taking and unreadable handwriting came to limelight (Madeira, Silva, Marcelino, & Ferreira, 2015). The authors specify two important technologies that facilitate this process namely Livescribe Smartpen and Dragon Naturally Speaking (Madeira, Silva, Marcelino, & Ferreira, 2015). Livescribe smartpen brings words and ideas into the digital world. It captures everything we write and everything that is spoken. Dragon Naturally Speaking for PC users and Dragon Dictate for Mac users is another technological tool that facilitates the learning process for the students with dyslexia and creates efficiency at the workplace. For those who have word-retrieval difficulties, grapho-motor weakness or problems committing ideas to paper in a timely fashion, Dragon may be the tool needed in order to improve writing skills. Dragon is a speech-recognition program, a technology which allows the computer to understand and also identify the words spoken by the user with the help of a microphone.

In addition to the above technology, there is different applications based program which helps the children with dyslexia (Tanner, Dixon, & Verenikina, 2010). Changes to the design and development methodologies can lead to better results.

PROPOSED WORK METHODOLOGY

In this section, the authors' describes the methodology implemented for the intervention of dyslexic children. The work is on dyslexia, sound-symbol association and perception. The problem of perception is to misjudge the letters and writing them in the wrong format. Similarly, the sound symbol association, where the recognition of correct pronunciation for the letters specified is difficult. For this purpose, the investigators used an Android application (Skiada, Soroniati, Gardeli, & Zissis, 2014) to overcome the problem of perception and phonology (sound-symbol association).

Motivation

Reading disability (RD) and language impairment (LI) are common learning issues that make developing a skill and utilization of reading and verbal language skills, respectively, complicated for affected individuals (Powers, Eicher, Butter, Kong, Miller, Ring, Mann, & Gruen, 2013). There are many successful people in their respective fields despite being dyslexic like Albert Einstein, Tom Cruise etc. There is a new teaching methodology for them to learn that can bring out the hidden talents lying in the dyslexics.

Algorithm

The algorithm to be followed for the intervention process for the children with dyslexia is shown in the below Figure 1 such that it makes the intervention easy and also to understand the subject will be simplified. The algorithm has the design of the intervention followed by application development. Intervention procedure begins and training of the children starts with and without the supervision of the parents and trainers. Final conclusions are drawn based on the performance of the children with dyslexia.

Application Development

Smart phones have become handy and in addition to that Android devices are very much affordable. Gaming is one of the processes implemented for creative techniques in order to make someone learn in an easy manner (Cuschieri, Khaled, Farrugia, Martinez, & Yannakakis, 2014; Skiada, Soroniati, Gardeli, & Zissis, 2014). There will be different levels in the gaming process which can be increased or decreased in order to test one's capability. Gaming is one of the easiest methods implemented in today's teaching methods. For the intervention purpose, an Android application has been designed and developed which will help the children with dyslexia to understand the alphabets and words and also the sound pronunciation associated with the alphabets respectively. The screenshots of the application are shown respectively in Figure 2.

Figure 1. The designed algorithm for dyslexia intervention

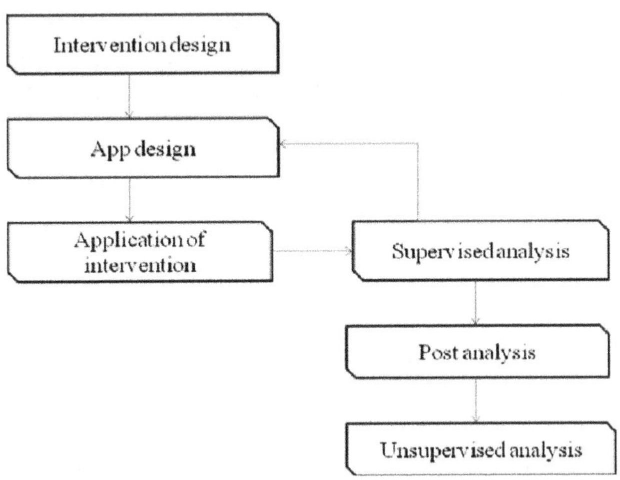

Figure 2. Screenshots of the application

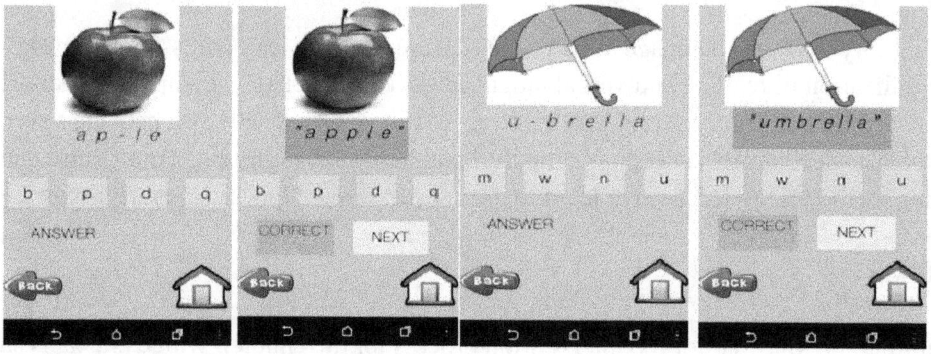

Firstly a layout is prepared i.e. the design and its logos on the application where images have to be placed for the children to identify. This is the pre-analysis before starting the development of an application. A complete application is developed based on the layout and the requirements and intervention procedure is initiated.

INTERVENTION PROCEDURE

Children with dyslexia having the problems of perception and sound-symbol association are identified of age 5-12 years old are made ready to start the intervention program. All the participants were chosen for the study from a special school for children with learning disabilities. The investigators explain the trainers and parents about the application i.e. for example if you see the figure 4, the objects in the screenshots are nothing but buttons. If you press the buttons the name of the object will be played. In the next label, a question will be asked to fill the missing letter from the given options. Now for the one particular question asked the kid with dyslexia has to choose the correct answer from the given four options. Once the answer was correct the question label will be displayed with complete word and next question option will be displayed. If a mistake was committed the next option won't be displayed and the child has to choose the answer in the successive attempts.

Next, the analysis of their performance is monitored day by day with the supervision of either with their parents or with the help of the trainers. The authors' continued this intervention for 2-3 weeks and once the children with the disability are familiar with how to start and understand the game, the unsupervised analysis is initiated.

Post Intervention

The children with dyslexia have to use the application without any supervision and the score obtained in each attempt they make will be noted by trainers or parents. If the performances of the children with dyslexia are able to identify the letters and the respective sounds of alphabets, leads to a conclusion that this intervention program helped them to understand and improve their sensing of sound and learning of words. By observing their performance the trainers can understand where they are lacking in using the application. Based on this certain modifications are made in that aspect for a better design and development to improve their performance.

RESULTS AND DISCUSSION

The investigators considered three subjects for studying the intervention procedure where they were analyzed in the following areas with respect to their disability level:

Attention: Their level of grasping and understanding the application.
Memory: Their level of memorizing the letters of the words.
Motivation: Whether they are interested to use the application or not.

The participants were under constant supervision for a period of approximately 14 weeks during their training and performing sessions.

Results

The rating was given by the trainers to each subject on a performance scale of 10 by analyzing and observing the performance.

Subject 1. (Male, 7 Years)

The below figure 3 shows the performance analysis of subject 1. The training and observation were held in three different phases each for a period of 3 weeks. During the first phase, the dyslexic child was observed on the basic part of the knowledge the participant has. The required data is collected from the trainers as they are dealing with the participant for the past 5 years. In this phase instructions regarding the usage of the application are well explained to the child, trainers and also for the parents. During the second phase, the child was asked to use the application. Based on the performance rating was given on a scale of 10. Similarly in the last phase during the post-intervention period, the child was asked to use the application without providing any help and based on the performance, the rating was given on a scale of 10 in front of the trainers. This also includes the concentration level of the sound symbol association of the subject. Below graph shows the subject's performance level in three different phases of intervention respectively.

Figure 3. Performance analysis graph of subject 1 during baseline, intervention and post-intervention

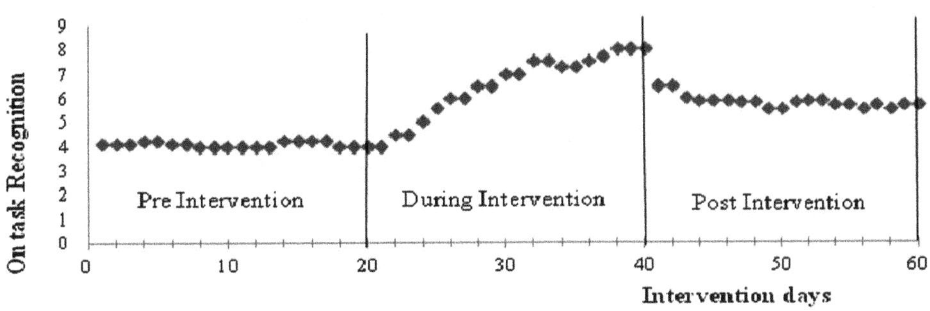

Subject 2. (Male, 10 Years)

The below figure 4 shows the performance analysis of Subject 2 who is severely dyslexic. The participant underwent all the training and intervention phases. The performance was rated on a scale of 10 in all the three phases. The graph below shows the subject's performance level in three different phases of intervention respectively.

Subject 3. (Female, 9 Years)

Figure 5 shows the performance analysis of Subject 3. The similar process of training and teaching methods was adopted with the subject 3 for the intervention phases. The performance graph was plotted with their results with respect to the total intervention days. The graph below shows the subject's performance level in three different phases of intervention respectively.

Analysis

The success of the intervention differed across the students, but Subjects 1 and 3 showed a good improvement. For Subject 1 the proposed application usage was 46.3% effective, as after intervention it was observed that the participant 1 started identifying the letters from the mirror image letters and for participant 3 it was 42% effective. However for participant 2 as mentioned earlier this intervention process helped him better than the traditional teaching methods but the performance is less compared with

Figure 4. Performance analysis graph of subject 2 during baseline, intervention and post-intervention

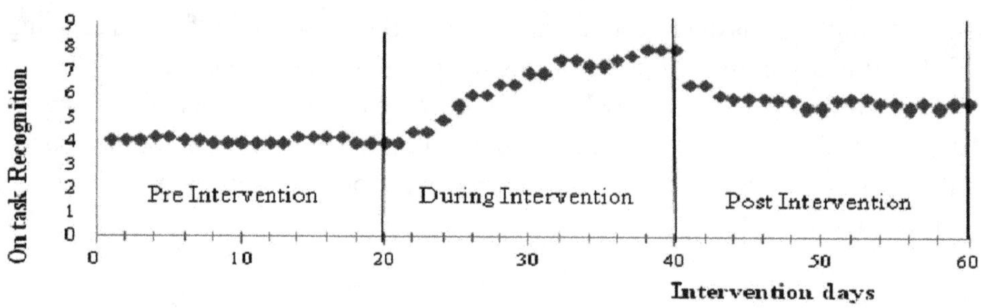

Figure 5. Performance analysis graph of subject 3 during baseline, intervention and post-intervention

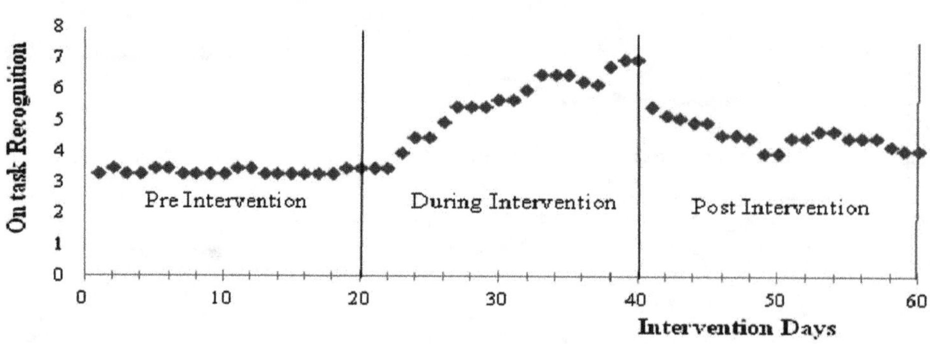

the other two subjects as the intervention process helped him to improve slowly as he took more no of intervention days and it was 36% effective. The authors gave the comparison with respect to traditional teaching methods adopted in the training center to the technological intervention. The record of each and every participant in the training center is studied carefully and analyzed with the help of a psychologist. Based on this, the performance of each participant using technological intervention showed the difference. Table 1, 2 and 3 present the analysis using this application for Subjects 1, 2 and 3 respectively. A comparison of graphed data between the baseline and intervention phases indicates a movement in improving the analysis of observed data.

Improvement Rate Difference

Improvement rate difference (IRD) is a special effect for single case research data (Parker, Vannest, & Brown, 2009). It expresses the difference in successful performance between baseline (pre-intervention) and Intervention phases. IRD can be calculated from visual analysis of non-overlapping data and is easily explained to most educators. The investigators calculated the mean of each phase and compared the performance in all the three sessions conducted and then finally calculated the efficiency and the progress of the children with dyslexia.

IRD was calculated in two ways:

1. Finding the mean of each phase for all the three phases respectively.
2. Finding the mean of all the values in all the phases collectively.

Mean IRD for each phase is: $$\frac{Sum\,of\,scores\,in\,that\,phase}{Total\,number\,of\,scores}. \tag{1}$$

Mean IRD for all phases collectively is: $$\frac{Sum\,of\,60\,all\,scores}{Total\,number\,of\,scores}. \tag{2}$$

Improvement rate Percentage is:

$$\frac{Difference\,of\,mean\,IRD\,values\,of\,phase\,3\,and\,1}{Mean\,IRD\,value\,of\,phase\,1}. \times 100 \tag{3}$$

The overall mean IRD for the three phases in consideration for Subject 1 was 6.32, suggesting that the subject had a 46% improvement rate from baseline to intervention phases of the strategy adopted to teach the letters as well as to recognize them from mirror-image letters and also synchronized sound symbols for respective alphabets.

The overall mean IRD for the three phases in consideration for Subject 2 was 4.5, suggesting that the subject had a 36% improvement rate from baseline to intervention phases of the strategy adopted to teach the subject respective sound symbols and also alphabets from their mirror images.

Table 1. Analysis of Subject 1's Graphed Data across Phases

Phase	Analysis
Baseline	Stable, slightly downward trend
	No variability
	Mean IRD – 5.05
During Intervention	Upward trend
	Relatively large variability
	Mean IRD – 7.5
Post Intervention	Stable trend
	Smaller variability
	Mean IRD – 7.39

Table 2. Analysis of Subject 2's Graphed Data across Phases

Phase	Analysis
Baseline	Stable, slightly downward trend
	Relatively low variability
	Mean IRD – 3.3
During Intervention	Upward trend
	Large variability
	Mean IRD – 5.5
Post Intervention	Stable downward trend
	Relatively large variability
	Mean IRD – 4.5

Table 3. Analysis of Subject 3's Graphed Data across Phases

Phase	Analysis
Baseline	Stable trend
	Relatively low variability
	Mean IRD – 4
During Intervention	Upward trend
	Large variability
	Mean IRD – 6.5
Post Intervention	Stable trend
	Relatively large variability
	Mean IRD - 5.82

The overall mean IRD for the three phases in consideration for Subject 3 was 5.49, suggesting that the subject had a 42% improvement rate from baseline to intervention phases of the strategy adopted to teach the subject respective sound symbols and also alphabets from their mirror images.

Discussion

As smart phones and tablets have become a handy device, it will be innovative if we start using them for the children with specific learning disabilities for the intervention purpose. With this motivation, an Android application was used by the investigators for the technological intervention of the children with dyslexia and started using them for their improvement in learning the alphabets and their respective sounds with the help of the trainers and their parents.

During the investigator's observation, in all the intervention phases the subjects responded well in using the application. Subject's 1 and 3 had an improvement from the baseline to pre-intervention phases compared to subject 2 where the participant needs more practice every day. Comparisons between the performance of using traditional methods and technological intervention as well as by observing the participants performance in presence of a psychologist helped the investigators to conclude that there is an improvement in their performance of overcoming the disability.

With the improvement rate difference percentage was on a good scale, the investigators specify that this application usage helped a lot for them to understand identifying alphabets and respective sounds. There are traditional teaching methodologies besides this technological intervention but this showed a good improvement in specific time. This is because of the keen interest was shown by the children with dyslexia playing with smart phones, tablets etc. as always they love to spend time on smart phones playing games. For all the three subjects besides the trainers, their mothers also had a good time teaching their children at home about the specifications of the application.

The application was used daily twice by the subjects at the training centers. The authors took care in observing the performance of each and every subject in all the three phases for all the different periods of time. The authors solved the difficulties if any faced by the children while using the application and took feedback from the trainers as well as from the mothers as if there are any necessary changes to be made for the application.

Analysis of data collected over 20 weeks indicated that this strategy proved to be successful. As hypothesized, the results revealed that the intervention was effective in changing the perspective of the subject and also increasing rate of attention in understanding the alphabets and recognizing the correct letters from their respective mirror images and also sound-symbol association.

In every field, technology plays a key role in designing and developing new things to meet objectives, likewise in the field of health and personality development. There are different methods developed day to day in which gaming is one of them. We can develop a new application-oriented gaming or can make changes to the already existing one which improves the learning process of dyslexic children. Recent advancements in mobile or handheld devices are assisting children with neurological disorders in different areas of impairment (Bogdanowiez, 2006; Crie, 2005; Dickinson, Gregor, & Newell, 2002). The electronic devices can be used to enhance communication, improve social imagination, participation, and enhancing independence. A number of applications have been developed to enhance different skills of children. The advantage of using electronic devices in technological interventions such as an iPad, or any Android tablet gives specific results because of its ease of operation. The availability of Multi-touch tabletop or floor wall projectors has emerged as a relatively new model in human-computer interaction that provides a shared interface to support interaction among co-located users supporting natural interactions.

These available technological tools are very promising that carry the immense potential to augment, enhance and extend the reach of existing dyslexia services for the benefits of families and individuals with dyslexia (Singleton & Simmons, 2001; Rello, Bayarri, & Gorriz, 2012).

CONCLUSION AND FUTURE DIRECTIONS

Technological intervention procedures for children with learning disabilities have been used globally. With the same motto, an initiation was taken in a locality to bring a change in the lives of specially disabled children to not make them separate from others to live a happy life. This initiative might bring a lot of change in the future which may help to come up with new applications with the help of technology for the children with dyslexia.

The authors show that with this application usage there is some improvement in learning the alphabets and their respective sounds from the baseline intervention stage to post-intervention stage. However for time being even if they show less improvement, regular practice with the help of their trainers and parents there might be some long-term responses. We can also see that some children are skilled with hidden special talents which can be unique from others in performances like math, reciting, art or music or it might be sport etc. The parents should recognize what their child is capable of and have to give proper training and guidance to improve their skills as we have the history in the past like Einstein, Tom Cruise etc who were also dyslexics but overcame their disability to reach greater heights in their respective fields. Dyslexia as well as other specific learning disorders might be lifelong but can be overcome through regular practice and starting the intervention as early as possible. The parents must understand the situation and should act according to it. There are other interventions like speech therapy and behavioral therapy which can be used for serving the purpose of children with dyslexia and other learning difficulties.

More research has to be done on the behavioral analysis of the children with dyslexia. Future work includes: a) to carry out more changes in the design of the application module according to the dyslexic child convenience and hence to proceed with the intervention and; b) the implementation of application services to integrate the intervention work for different modules.

ACKNOWLEDGMENT

The authors would like to thank Dr Pallavi Khanna, Psychologist and Child Specialist, Jalandhar and Ekalavya School for our collaboration and for the support during the whole process.

REFERENCES

Bogdanowiez, K. (2006). *A short introduction to dyslexia.* Available: http://www.jezykangielski.org/teacher6

Crie, M. (2005). *Teaching today: Helping dyslexic students succeed.* Available: http://www.glencoe.com/sec/teachingtoday/educationupclose.phtml/46

Cuschieri, T., Khaled, R., Farrugia, V. E., Martinez, H. P., & Yannakakis, G. N. (2014 September). The iLearnRW Game: Support for Students with Dyslexia in Class and at Home. In *Games and Virtual Worlds for Serious Applications (VS-GAMES), 2014 6th International Conference on* (pp. 1-2). IEEE.

Dickinson, A., Gregor, P., & Newell, A. F. (2002, July). Ongoing investigation of the ways in which some of the problems encountered by some dyslexics can be alleviated using computer techniques. In *Proceedings of the fifth international ACM conference on Assistive technologies* (pp. 97-103). ACM. 10.1145/638249.638268

Elnakib, A., Casanova, M. F., Gimelrfarb, G., Switala, A. E., & El-Baz, A. (2012). Dyslexia diagnostics by 3-D shape analysis of the corpus callosum. *IEEE Transactions on Information Technology in Biomedicine, 16*(4), 700–708. doi:10.1109/TITB.2012.2187302 PMID:22334032

Ismail, R., & Jaafar, A. (2011, November). Interactive Screen-Based design for dyslexic Children. In *User Science and Engineering (i-USEr), 2011 International Conference on* (pp. 168-171). IEEE. 10.1109/iUSEr.2011.6150559

Madeira, J., Silva, C., Marcelino, L., & Ferreira, P. (2015). Assistive Mobile Applications for Dyslexia. *Procedia Computer Science, 64*, 417–424. doi:10.1016/j.procs.2015.08.535

Parker, R. I., Vannest, K. J., & Brown, L. (2009). The improvement rate difference for single-case research. *Exceptional Children, 75*(2), 135–150. doi:10.1177/001440290907500201

Powers, N. R., Eicher, J. D., Butter, F., Kong, Y., Miller, L. L., Ring, S. M., ... Gruen, J. R. (2013). Alleles of a polymorphic ETV6 binding site in DCDC2 confer risk of reading and language impairment. *American Journal of Human Genetics, 93*(1), 19–28. doi:10.1016/j.ajhg.2013.05.008 PMID:23746548

Rello, L. (2014). Design of Word Exercises for children with dyslexia. *Procedia Computer Science, 27*, 74–83. doi:10.1016/j.procs.2014.02.010

Rello, L., Bayarri, C., & Gorriz, A. (2012, October). What is wrong with this word? Dyseggxia: A game for children with dyslexia. In *Proceedings of the 14th international ACM SIGACCESS conference on Computers and accessibility* (pp. 219-220). ACM. 10.1145/2384916.2384962

Singleton, C., & Simmons, F. (2001). An evaluation of Wordshark in the classroom. *British Journal of Educational Technology, 32*(3), 317–330. doi:10.1111/1467-8535.00201

Skiada, R., Soroniati, E., Gardeli, A., & Zissis, D. (2014). EasyLexia: A mobile application for children with learning difficulties. *Procedia Computer Science, 27*, 218–228. doi:10.1016/j.procs.2014.02.025

Sklar, B., Hanley, J., & Simmons, W. W. (1973). A Computer Analysis of EEG Spectral Signatures from Normal and Dyslexic Children. *IEEE Transactions on Biomedical Engineering*, *1*(1), 20–26. doi:10.1109/TBME.1973.324247 PMID:4681806

Tanner, K., Dixon, R., & Verenikina, I. (2010, June). The digital technology in the learning of students with autism spectrum disorders (ASD) in applied classroom settings. In *EdMedia: World Conference on Educational Media and Technology* (pp. 2586-2591). Association for the Advancement of Computing in Education (AACE).

Vellutino, F. R., & Scanlon, D. M. (1987). Phonological coding, phonological awareness, and reading ability: Evidence from a longitudinal and experimental study. *Merrill-Palmer Quarterly*, 321–363.

KEY TERMS AND DEFINITIONS

Assistive Technology: It refers to any item, piece of equipment or product system, whether acquired commercially off the shelf, modified, or customized, that is used to increase, maintain, or improve the functional capabilities of children with disabilities.

Dyslexia: It is also called as reading disability where the children have trouble with reading and spelling despite having the ability to learn.

LearnEasy-Android Application: It is a software application running on the Android platform.

Livescribe Smartpen: It refers to the smartpen, a ballpoint pen with an embedded computer and digital audio recorder. When used with Anoto digital paper, it records what it writes for later uploading to a computer, and synchronizes those notes with any audio it has recorded.

Perception: It is the ability to see, hear, or become aware of something through the senses.

Phonics: It is a method for teaching reading and writing of the English language to the children.

Technological Intervention: It refers to the use of latest devices in the intervention of children with disabilities.

Chapter 13
Yogic Care for Neurodevelopmental Rehabilitation:
Bringing Life Into Treatment, Management, and Prevention

Arun Pratap Singh
Mahatma Gandhi Antarrashtriya Hindi Vishwavidyalaya, India

ABSTRACT

Recent biological and behavioral studies indicate that several unhealthy alterations in ways of living (i.e., consumption-pattern, leisure activities, sleep routine, postures, breathing, stress-level, and use of high-tech gadgets) may be related with aggravation and augmentation of neurodevelopmental disorders. In this backdrop, it is important to recognize that yoga offers holistic knowledge for correction in lifestyle to not only prevent but also manage and alleviate neurodevelopmental disorders. Unfortunately, clinicians have been relying in their practice rather heavily on intrusive and pharmacological interventions and avoiding the use of sustainable techniques. Therefore, in order to increase awareness and promote its use in clinical settings, present work is ventured on the understanding effectiveness of and challenges in utilizing yogic practices for neurodevelopmental rehabilitation. It also identifies priorities for future research and action to amplify applicability of yogic lifestyle in hospitals, clinics, and other public health centers.

INTRODUCTION

In last few decades, Neurodevelopmental Disorders (NDD) has emerged as one of the greatest threats to public health. Persons with developmental deficits in speech, use of language, scholastic progress, social skills, communication and intellectual ability, constitute a substantial chunk of human population throughout the world. In a study, only among children of 4000 families in six regions of India, the prevalence rate for NDD ranged between 10-18 percent (Silberberg, Arora, Bhutani, Durkin, Gulati,

DOI: 10.4018/978-1-5225-7004-2.ch013

Nair, & Pinto-Martin, 2014). Autism Spectrum Disorder-which is only one specific disorder under the NDD- has been globally estimated to occur in one person in every 160 persons (Elsabbagh, Divan, Koh, Kim, Kauchali, Marcín,... & Yasamy, 2012); while prevalence rate for many other NDDs in many low-income countries remains unexplored (Hossain, Ahmed, Uddin, Chowdhury, Iqbal, Kabir,... & Hossain, 2017). Additionally, if we take full life course perspective into our account, then incidences of developmental deficits in the central nervous system and their consequent malady for human life, would present a much grim scenario.

In many countries, traditionally, persons lacking developmentally relevant capacities are socially ostracized and face inhumane stigma. While some peoples suffering from NDD have normal abilities to live independently but many others need life-long care and support. As a result, many families and communities have to carry a substantial degree of emotional and financial burden (Dykens, 2015). Due to lack of skilled health professionals, infrastructure, and financial constraints, a majority of developing and lower-income countries are not capable to provide appropriate health and education services to those, who are afflicted with these disorders and caregivers. In this context, with support from more than 60 nations, World Health Organization has sought to promote sharing of sustainable and cost-effective strategies to strengthen and expand integrated healthcare services for mental health and disability (Grupp-Phelan, Harman, & Kelleher, 2007).

Furthermore, although, we lack clear picture about causes of NDD, a number of pre-natal and environmental risk factors have been recognized. For long, previous studies have noted that childhood, in the modern age, has become susceptible to much vulnerability due to the unhealthy lifestyle of parents before and after conception (Dykens, 2015; Sampson, Streissguth, Bookstein, Little, Clarren, Dehaene, ... & Graham, 1997; Talge, Neal, & Glover, 2007). Also, many unhealthy alterations in lifestyle have been found to be major contributors in the development of social, behavioral and communicative disorders (Mattson, Allison, Fontana, Harvie, Longo, Malaisse, ... & Seyfried, 2014; Mattson, 2015; Singh & Misra, 2012, 2015, 2016). In this context, several agencies have articulated the urgent need to outline relevant cost-effective strategies.

We can also easily interpret following multiple aspects which denote for suitability of yoga in the care of persons suffering from developmental disabilities.

- First, it harmonizes multiple aspects of mind-body functioning (Singh, 2017).
- Second, being convenient to learn and practice, both for patients and healthcare providers, it can be adopted in any rehabilitation settings, comparably easily than any other therapy for management and treatment of NDD.
- Thirdly, yogic care involves little financial investment because it does not require a huge financial expenditure for purchasing equipment and training yoga therapists. It can be easily used in resource-deprived countries also (Chuang, Soares, Tilbrook, Cox, Hewitt, Aplin, ... & Torgerson, 2012; Hartfiel, Clarke, Havenhand, Phillips, & Edwards, 2017).
- Fourth, as evidenced in several studies for supplementing role, yoga can be integrated with any other therapy (Desikachar, 1999; Kalyani, Venkatasubramanian, Arasappa, Rao, Kalmady, Behere,... & Gangadhar, 2011).
- Fifth, because of holistic effects, it can resolve multiple concerns related to physical, mental, social and occupational domains (Jeter, Slutsky, Singh, & Khalsa, 2015).
- Sixth, being substantially free from any potential side effect, yogic care can be used for neurodevelopmental rehabilitation without minding much about negative repercussions of rehabilitation.

As observed, in view of several limitations of psychiatric, developmental, psychological and community interventions, the efficacy of yogic care for preventing, managing and providing cure from NDD, yogic techniques can be particularly relevant for neurodevelopmental rehabilitation (Dykens, 2015). Against this backdrop, this chapter discusses several dimensions of yogic care for facilitating neurodevelopmental rehabilitation.

In the first section, it orients towards an understanding of major challenges and issues of prevailing primary, secondary and tertiary rehabilitation services to address developmental deficits. Then, in next section, it provides a layout of opportunities found in potentials of yogic techniques as envisioned by popular experts of yoga and also summarizes major reviews on the effectiveness of yogic wisdom to address disorders related with the nervous system. In the third section, challenges of using yogic knowledge for rehabilitation of persons afflicted with NDD have been elaborated. In the following section, the author describes directions for research and actions for imbuing yogic care. Lastly, the author concludes with major highlights of this chapter.

CURRENT SCENARIO OF NEURODEVELOPMENTAL REHABILITATION: CHALLENGES AND ISSUES

Traditionally, resource-demanding interventions (i.e., drugs, psycho-educational, developmental and behavioral) are being utilized to address developmental deficits in communication, speech, language and scholastic performance. Some recommendations for systemic changes in the environment, to assuage disability, are also in focus. But, their delivery in any setting is marred by several challenges. A majority of these reside in financial, biological, systemic, environmental, cultural and contextual repertoire of dominating perspectives.

Most of the psycho-educational, developmental and behavioral interventions have been experienced to be resource and labor-intensive. Large randomized controlled studies have highlighted financial complications of behavioral rehabilitation (Rappley, 2005). In consequence, the paucity of healthcare professionals, and lack of resources for effective service management impede access to rehabilitative care in different countries. In vast parts of the world, mental health experts, psychologists, and psychiatrists are variably placed in rural and urban areas, with greater density in capital or metro regions.

The biomedical model had remained occupied in tracing specific etiology, underlying pathological processes, and their particular effects. Although, this model has held center stage it paid limited attention to the relevance of individual actions, the role of environment and individual perceptions in accounting for their developmental traces of mental health (Bury, 2004; Foucault, 1973). Initially, confined to morbidity and mortality, it had reduced all causes of developmental deficits to the biological territory. Recently, ill-effects of such conceptions have been widely recognized. Many negative side-effects of drugs in the prevention, management, and treatment are being substantially noticed. For instance, it has been found that treatment of ADHD by using drugs induces a decrease in appetite, headache, problems falling asleep, irritability and abdominal discomfort (Elia, Ambrosini, & Rapoport, 1999; Greydanus, 2005).

Freud's insistence on explaining any disability through unconscious conflicts is beginning to lose its credibility (Palombo, Bendicsen, & Koch, 2009). Psychological overemphasis on only individualistic view of disability and disorders is being challenged by the contrasting emergence of evidence of the effect of parent's lifestyle and environment on the shaping of the development of the child. Realizing the limitations of existing popular perspectives, the biopsychosocial model had broadened its ambit of understanding of disease and disability by dynamically adding the influence of psychological, social and behavioral factors to the biological factors. Currently, lay notions of disease and disorders, as explored and recognized in several scholarly studies, have emerged to challenge mainstream views of rehabilitation with their notion of 'reserve stock' to be invested in by adopting health behavior, or diminished by self-neglect or unhealthy behaviors (Blaxter, 1990).

Henceforth, many mechanical, artificial and materialistic changes in contemporary life have begun to be noticed to explain spurt in the prevalence of developmental disabilities. These changes are altering not only the pattern of everyday life but also shaping the micro-level contexts such as home, school, and work setting. A plethora of living choices (i.e., fast foods, cold drinks, alcohol, pornography etc.) offered by persuasive media and market is interfering with the mind-body functioning of a majority of the world population. Cut-throat competition glamorized by globalization and disturbances in traditional customs of leisure, consumption and daily life are creating constraints in multiple spheres of development. Prominently, inappropriate living choices (e.g. unhealthy dietary habits, intake of fast food, irregular sleep, less physical activity etc.) have been realized to contribute to developmental delay but unfortunately, these issues are not getting space in neurodevelopmental rehabilitation settings.

A majority of neurodevelopmental rehabilitation services and networks, in developing and low-income countries, are based on service-delivery models originated from research evidence of developed countries. Consequently, they are less affordable and ensuring their applicability becomes a huge challenge in any other setting. Furthermore, the genesis of NDD in childhood had received greater attention but a full-life course perspective has been ignored.

While the prevalence of NDD is higher in developing countries but most of the rehabilitation strategies have been derived from studies in developed countries and thus operate with cultural incongruence. Therefore, development of culturally-sensitive and socially-contextualized knowledge, for addressing these conditions, is becoming important. Recently, several healthcare agencies have realized the need for locally relevant knowledge.

It has been noted that non-specialist service providers and parent-mediated interventions are more effective in dealing issues of developmental disability. It has also been realized that there is a need to ensure greater participation of persons with developmental disorders and their families. In short, we find that in the process of neurodevelopmental rehabilitation role of ingredients of life have been avoided. Despite several pieces of evidence indicating the role of consumption patterns, sleep-related habits, daily routine habits, spiritual practices, their use in neurodevelopmental rehabilitation remains rather minimized.

POTENTIAL OF YOGIC CARE

Traditionally, yoga has been viewed as a set of practices which not only pacifies physical and psychological turmoil and confusion but also induces calmness, harmony and balance in the body (Saraswati, 1996). Maharshi Patanjali, who is believed to be the first person to summarize theory and practice of yoga in his most famous treatise-yoga sutra, outlines controlling and transformation of mind as the goal of yoga (Iyengar, 1993). Although in modern times, physiological aspects of yoga have been over-emphasized, if we try to explore rather deeply then we find that yoga had evolved with a variety of contours. It included not only postures, deep breathing practices, cleansing techniques, daily routine instructions, dietary restrictions, and habits for the spiritual uplift, but it evolved also as a set of cognitive and affective techniques to deal with problems in many other spheres of life (Acharya, 2008; Cornelissen, 2004). While doing so, it does not view the existence of individual as confined in one's physical realm but mutually dependent on the societal and environmental contexts (Aurobindo, 1917).

Several studies, in last few decades, have indicated towards multiple routes for the utility of yoga to prevent the occurrence of risk factors responsible for delay or defects in the central nervous system. According to a review of independent prospective studies, by reducing the stress level in pregnant mothers, the risk for attention-deficit/hyperactivity, anxiety, and language delay in the offspring can be substantially prevented (Talge, Neal, & Glover, 2007). Yoga-based practices can be useful as an add-on treatment for socio-occupational functioning (Behere, Arasappa, Jagannathan, Varambally, Venkatasubramanian, Thirthalli,... & Gangadhar, 2011), caregivers relationship with patients (Harrison, Manocha, & Rubia, 2004), improving mood-disturbance, anger, resilience, fatigue, negative stress-response behaviours and concentration on the task in children (Herbert & Esparaham, 2017; Jeter, Slutsky, Singh, & Khalsa, 2015).

Based on the yogic perspective of life and evidence-based knowledge, following techniques are being elaborated as follows:

Regulating Dietary Habits

Dietary regulations occupy major space in yogic life. Food items have been categorized into three types according to notions of their effects on the human mind (Aurobindo, 1917). Sattvic category, which quietens the mind, consists of organically grown sweet potato, cow milk and other milk products, wheat, barley, gram, dates, fruits, coconut, pumpkin and maize. Rajsic food items induce egoism, aggressiveness and excess of activity. It includes salt, pepper, tea, coffee, garlic, sugar, cold drinks, chocolates and other spicy, dry and bitter food preparations. In a third category called-Tamsic, different types of liquor, chips, meat, pickles and preserved food items have been experienced to result into dullness. In yoga, the act of eating food is required to be preceded by devotional actions and mood so as to induce calmness to facilitate proper digestion. In addition, appropriate chewing of each morsel, not to eat anything in between two meals during a day, eating only when feeling intense hunger, eating regularly and drinking enough amount of water are some important habits. Over-indulgence in eating and not eating at all during the period of intense hunger - both were suggested to result in serious health problems. Regarding the quantity of food, yogic instructions to fill half of the stomach with food, one fourth with water and remaining one fourth to be left for aeration are relevant for better digestion. In order to facilitate appropriate growth during different developmental trajectories, Yoga also emphasizes on the practice of rational fasting to promote vigor, vigilance, and well-being.

Recently, yogic notions of diet have been supported by psycho-biological studies. In modern studies, intake of protein-rich food has been found to be associated with an increase in awareness while of carbohydrate to lack of fatigue and vitamins to experience vigor (Benton & Donohoe, 1999). In neurological studies, intermittent fasting and intake of vegetables and fruits have been found to increase resistance to neuro-generative disorders (Mattson, Allison, Fontana, Harvie, Longo, Malaisse, ... & Seyfried, 2014; Mattson, 2015). In particular, fasting has been noted to be of great importance for the prevention of developmental problems in old age because it reduces intake of free radicals and increases production of neurotrophic factors and protein chaperons. Several yoga therapists have been reporting anecdotal evidence for the effectiveness of yogic dietary habits for ameliorating developmental delays in the nervous system. In one such article, fasting was reported to treat several neuro-generative disorders such as palsy, mental retardation and the age-dependent emergence of concerns of anxiety, depression, and loneliness. In another article, intake of tea or coffee was reported to be related to the developmental lagging of nervous system. However, it remains to be seen that whether these anecdotal findings may stand to empirical scrutiny.

Synchronising Sleep

Sleep is considered as one of three important foundations of health in equivalence with diet and sexual restrictions (Charak Samhita, 11/35). The period of sleep was recommended to be regulated in synchrony with daily natural events (e.g., sunrise, the appearance of stars). Particularly, 'Ayurveda' recommends sleep during early hours of the second quarter of the night till the onset of the fourth quarter of the night. Regular sleep during this period of the night is said to improve fitness, stamina, digestibility and self-esteem and serve several restorative functions of the body (Rigveda, 10/127; Charaka Sutra, 21/38). Remaining awake during the night was stated to increase physical illnesses. The second important suggestion was about getting up early in the morning. Early rising was conceived to have medicinal value for many diseases. Multiple effects of morning rise such as in enhancing gaiety, optimism, positive body image were especially emphasized (Ashtanga Hridaya, Sutrasthana, 2/3).

Some recent biological studies have validated Ayurvedic realizations about sleep. Positive changes in the biochemical constitution such as increased secretion of health-enhancing neuro-peptides (i.e., corticosteroids and hormones (i.e., melatonin) have been demonstrated to be associated with the timing of sleep in synchrony with sun-rise and sunset (Buschkens, Graham, & Cottrell, 2010; Roeser, Obergfell, Meule, Vögele, Schlarb, & Kübler, 2012). However, in the modern age, urbanization and technological predominance seem to have badly affected the practice of appropriate sleep habits resulting in several developmental complications.

Daily Routine and Positive Leisure

Regular pursuance of daily routine activities (i.e., bathing, massaging, physical exercises), positive leisure and religious behaviors (i.e., prayer, chanting religious mantras) have been widely mentioned in different yogic texts. Bathing was recommended to be performed daily for overcoming fatigue and sweat and promoting physical stamina (Ashtanga Hridaya Sutra, 2/16-18). Positive effects of oil massaging of children to prevent excessive sweating, fatigue, and increase flexibility, strength and fitness were eloquently recognized. Physical exercises were considered of great value for their positive contribution to improving digestion, physical fitness and strength (C.S., Sutrasthana, 7/ 31-32). Engagement in violent, addictive and sexual activities was suggested to be highly harmful during adolescence (C.S. 7/29). The sexual restriction was greatly recommended for gaining multiple positive effects of Yoga (Kathopanishada, 11/5). Chanting of mantras is a major religious behavior recommended in yogic tradition. Particularly, 'Om' is of major importance considered as 'syllable' of the God in different religions. In a study, chanting of 'Om' has been found to be correlated with deactivation of the limbic system and stimulation of vagus nerve and thus indicating for the potential to treat emotional reactivity and stress (Kalyani, Venkatasubramanian, Arasappa, Rao, Kalmady, Behere, ... & Gangadhar, 2011).

Postures

We find an astounding variety of structured postures in several spiritual texts of India (Desikachar, 1999). The effect of postures in the calming restlessness of mind was of special significance for spiritual seekers

(Yoga Sutra, 1.2). The postures (Asana) were particularly meant for effortless, relaxed and poised sitting in meditation (Yoga Sutra, 2/46-48). Yoga Sutra did not provide any more description of categorization and classification of postures (Iyengar,1993). But some other texts indicate about manifold forms of postures developed from minute observation of different creatures and their species-specific concomitant physical or mental capacities (Dhayanbindupanishad, 42). During later ages, multiple forms and series of postures were invented to alleviate psycho-physiological imbalances in body and mind. Effects of yogic postures operate through internal massaging of specific muscles, neural ganglions and organs of the body and in turn results into the improved functioning of the human nervous system, muscular system and circulatory system (C.S., Sutrasthana, 28/7, Acharya, 2008).

Postures play a facilitative role in ensuring proper absorption and distribution of nutrients to the different organs of the body. Rao (2002) contends that by attention to coordinated breathe and body movements, awareness of emotional blockages goes on to increase. In a study among children aged 5-16, diagnosed with ADHD, the practice of loosening kriya, postures, kapalbhati, Ujjayee, anuloma-villoma, and nadanusandhan resulted into a significant reduction in severity of symptoms (Hariprasad, Arasappa, Varambally, Srinath, & Gangadhar, 2013).

Breath Regulation (Pranayama)

Next to postures (Asanas), regulation of breath (Pranayama) is considered of crucial significance for increasing mental acumen. It was intuitively realized by yogic sages that particular forms of conscious breathing are related subsequently to specific kinds of mental experiences, cognitive abilities and states of human wellness. It came also to their experience that alleviation of many negative effects and reestablishment of harmony between human body and mind can be possible through breath-regulation (Y.S., 2/52; Prasnopanishad, 2/10-11). The spine and spinal muscles are a source of action and lungs are receiving instruments of breathing technique. There are three components of all breathing practices: inhalation, exhalation and retention (Iyengar, 1993, p., 30). In some types, deep breathing is practiced through both nostrils; in some others forceful expulsion of breath is undertaken and in other types, alternate breathing from nostrils is carried out. In some other techniques, certain divine syllables are mentally repeated in consonance with inhalation, retention or exhalation of breath. There are also some highly advanced practices in which there is no actual breathing but merely conscious visualization of receiving vital energy. These breath taking practices increase muscular strength of lungs. Increased availability of oxygen enhances functional capacity of different internal organs of the body. Especially, the positive effect of deep breathing (Pranayama) on purification of the nervous system, increasing concentration and mental vigor was considered of special importance (Shvetashvaropanishad, 2/9).

In congruence with yogic realizations, several recent clinical studies have identified less utilization of lungs and consequently reduced intake of oxygen as a major source of multiple ailments (Gupta, Gupta, Sood, & Arkham, 2014). The practice of alternate nostrils breathing (Anuloma-Viloma Pranayama) and Kapalbhati pranayama are viewed as special value during initiation of deep breathing practice (Saraswati, 1996).

Yognidra

Yoga Nidra, a classical yogic technique prescribed for psychophysical relaxation (Hatha Pradipika, 1.32; Gherand Samhita, 2.4; 2.19), is a state between sleep and awakening. In this state, relaxation is induced in simultaneity with mental alertness and experiential journey of different parts of the body (Desikachar, 1999). This technique is practiced by inculcating imagery, awareness of breathing and abdominal movements. It has a revitalizing impact on human existence (Brihadarakyopanishad, 4/3/18). It's regular practice develops self-control, attention and concentration and helps in overcoming stresses of life and gaining composure (Y. S., 2.54-56). As a result of widening recognition of Yognidra, its' different offshoots i.e. iRest, divine sleep have become popular in western countries.

Through its' practice, autonomic nervous system and the endocrine system gets harmonized resulting in greater energy, relaxation and strength. Many previous studies have noticed significant changes in the sympathetic activity in practitioners of Yognidra. It stabilizes glucose level (Amita, Prabhakar, Manoj, Harminder, & Pawan, 2009), blood pressure, heart-rate (Monica, Singh, Ghildiyal, Kala, & Srivastava, 2012) neural activity, and functioning of the hypothalamus and thus indicates for its potential benefit in anxiety, depression and different types of disabilities (Kim, 2017) (Vempati & Telles, 2002). Other concomitant changes such as increase in ATP and frequency of alpha and delta brain waves during Yoganidra may be linked positively with the nourishment of several parts of the human body (Dusek, Otu, Wohlhueter, Bhasin, Zerbini, Joseph,... & Libermann, 2008). Research evidences have corroborated for its great effect in reducing negative thought patterns and unhealthy habits (Pence, Katz, Huffman, & Cojucar, 2014). In patients of combat-related post-traumatic stress disorder, use of Yognidra only for eight weeks has shown promising potential to reduce rage, anxiety, emotional reactivity and increase relaxation, peace, self-awareness despite the intrusive memories in veterans (Stankovic, 2011).

Meditation

There are a variety of meditation techniques. These include focusing fixed attention on present moment or a fixed stimulus such as one's breathe, use some imagery or observing one's own thoughts rather than suppressing or engaging with them. Meditation has found to yield a positive contribution to well-being among a wide range of healthy people and persons with mental problems (Murphy & Donovan, 1999; Shapiro, Schwartz, & Santerre, 2002). In short term, it leads to a reduction in arousal by inducing changes in heart rate, respiration, skin conductance, cortisol levels, and by increasing alpha waves. In long term, it has been found to lead to increased health, cognitive functioning, creativity, empathy, and in the management of conditions such as hypertension, chronic pain, anxiety, and depression. Merely, 20 minutes a day of guided meditation for few weeks has been found to produce favourable changes in inflammation, ageing, and energy production (Bhasin, Dusek, Chang, Joseph, Denninger, Fricchione, ... & Libermann, 2013).

CHALLENGES AND ISSUES IN RESEARCH AND PRACTICE OF YOGIC CARE IN NEURODEVELOPMENTAL REHABILITATION

In mainstream research and practice of neurodevelopmental rehabilitation, pharmacological and to some extent behavioral approaches are highly emphasized. But, there is minimal availability of evidence-based knowledge on content and process-oriented aspects of yogic care (Salmon, Lush, Jablonski, & Sephton, 2009). As a result, although persons are utilizing yoga on their own to overcome several developmental disabilities and anecdotally reporting their effects but yogic approach for neurodevelopmental rehabilitation is largely invisible in hospitals and clinics. Taking into account existing scenario, this section recapitulates challenges in research and practice of yogic neurodevelopmental rehabilitation. In particular, it provides a snap of methodological limitations and practical constraints.

In last few decades, many studies have been conducted to explore and evaluate the promising possibility of yogic practices for neuro-developmental rehabilitation (Behere, Arasappa, Jagannathan, Varambally, Venkatasubramanian, Thirthalli,... & Gangadhar, 2011; Hariprasad, Arasappa, Varambally, Srinath, & Gangadhar, 2013; Harrison, Manocha, & Rubia, 2004; Hartfiel, Clarke, Havenhand, Phillips, & Edwards, 2017; Jeter, Slutsky, Singh, & Khalsa, 2015). Some attempts for randomized control trials have also been made (Chuang, Soares, Tilbrook, Cox, Hewitt, Aplin, ... & Torgerson, 2012; Jeter, Slutsky, Singh, & Khalsa, 2015). In popular academic view, RCTs are considered as 'perfect' scientific approach to validating effects of yoga. But, due to the impossibility of double-blind trials mental health associated effects are difficult to evaluate in an absolute sense (Mason, Tovey, & Long, 2002; Cornelissen, 2004). This is because any yogic practice has its own ontological and epistemological premises and also there is a gap in basic paradigmatic assumptions between science and yoga as a method. Moreover, yoga involves a variety of practices. Recently, different versions of Yoga, claiming for their supremacy have evolved. Across these different styles, there is the lack in uniformity in content and procedure and thus complicating any endeavour for the comparative assessment for standardization and replication (Mason, Tovey, & Long, 2002). Also, in any intervention, there may be plausibility of abundance of participatory bias that can influence the outcome either in positive or negative manner for or against its practitioners. Further, the settings in which the published studies are conducted, vary from laboratory, residence, clinics, yoga studios, to university campus. Outcome measures also vary considerably across studies.

Moreover, in any experimental study, a researcher faces an arduous task of separating effect of yoga from physical exercise. According to yogic philosophy, if any action is performed with awareness and particular intention then and only then it becomes Yoga; otherwise it remains merely an exercise (Saraswati, 1996). In such a scenario, a researcher is likely to be perplexed with the task of invoking a particular type of attitude in practitioners participating in a research.

Yoga consists of immense variety. It is like a vast sea of practices which can subsume almost any practice blended with an attitude of intention, awareness, and relaxation (Iyengar, 1993). Now the question before us is how can we empirically evaluate the effect of Yoga? Should we use it as a whole system or stand-alone practices? Yoga emphasizes on the experience of self by one-self (Aurobindo, 1917). Then, to what extent, neutral observation of the effect of yogic practices can actually provide real glimpse of yoga for mental health? Yoga is based on the basic idea of holism and continuity of existence but not on the broken idea of a dichotomy between body and mind (Aurobindo, 1917). But, existing research findings are based on reductionist notions and explanations. Conventional studies have mostly been merely limited to capturing of certain biochemical alterations and self-report of subjective experiences. Lack of detail in specifics of yogic intervention is frequently noticeable in different empirical studies (Salmon, Lush, Jablonski, & Sephton, 2009).

According to the yogic theory of human mind, these subjective experiences constitute a lower level of human existence and the effect of Yoga operates through qualitative alterations in different sheaths of consciousness and transgressing ordinary states of the mind (Cornelissen, 2004). As espoused in yogic tradition, the mind is of four layers. The deepest layer is Chitta, the transformation of which is related to experiences of divinity, mystical union, beauty, and space and time transcendence (Iyengar, 1993). Scientific studies are often caught in the puzzle of measurements of subtle changes at uppermost level-body; While, effects of Yoga are conceptualized to operate through body's undetectable nadis or energy vortices (Desikachar, 1999). Due to paradigmatic fixation to ritualistic to the Newtonian scientific inquiry, experiences at other levels of being are either rejected or sometimes believed in ambiguity (Cornelissen, 2004).

To gain benefits of yoga, a person needs to be motivated to practice. According to yogic theory, with an increase in motivation, benefits of yoga are maximized (Iyengar, 1993). Now the problem for researchers is related to increase motivation among subjects for participation in yoga to measure effects. If researchers get involved in motivating subjects then how will they be able to avoid intrusion of biases due to direct engagement of experimenter? And if not, then how to overcome effect of drop-out rate in any experimental research on yoga. Also, in view of the individual variation in motivation for participating in yoga, researchers remain perplexed about the relevance of generalized statements for the outcome of engagement in yoga.

A researcher does not act in oblivion but in the midst of contextual influences and pressures. The act of interpreting particular forms of yoga is often given varied orientation by socio-political debates and controversies (Saraswati, 1996). In such a backdrop, a researcher often gets baffled with the task of what to research and what not to research. The researcher himself/herself may be preoccupied with a certain type of perception due to his training in the particular type of research and disciplinary tradition; which may further prevent from unearthing culturally sensitive mechanisms underlying practice of Yoga. Therefore, we need to have a re-look towards our priorities of research in future.

FUTURE RESEARCH DIRECTIONS

There is need to strengthen research endeavors to address several issues and challenges of rehabilitation efforts through yogic interventions. In order to advance evidence-based knowledge, effective methodology for research on the effectiveness of yogic care needs to be undertaken. In view of holistic effects of yoga, research endeavors also need to undertake mixed-method approach. In view of Yoga being a set of multiple practices, effectiveness of isolated practices needs to be investigated. In addition, holistic modules of yogic lifestyle also need to be assessed for managing and treating individual disorders. In any such research endeavor, the collaboration would be needed in between yoga experts, psychologists, psychiatrists, and anthropologists.

Since, Yoga was developed in a particular historical and social context, several sociological issues related to the application of yoga in different types of settings need to be properly understood. Although Yoga as a term was developed in India, there can be multiple practices in different religions which can be clubbed under yogic care but any such endeavor needs to pay appropriate attention also to several issues related with faith. Also, we will need to work upon effective models for delivery of yogic care in different therapeutic settings.

For long, scientific method has been used to assess the effectiveness of Yoga. In this pursuance, whatever aspects of Yoga would have been scrutinized objectively has been accepted and denial mode has been adopted for all other aspects. As a result 'half-baked' truths are commonly noticeable (Carnelissen, 2004). But, if try to fathom deep into process and content of Yoga by using it's own method, then it can provide much more relevant knowledge.

CONCLUSION

This chapter has highlighted multiple issues and challenges for neurodevelopmental rehabilitation and effectiveness of yogic care for the same. It has also underlined challenges involved in yogic neurodevelopmental rehabilitation. In view of several lifestyle changes, yogic lifestyle and practices offer promising possibility to reduce the cost of services for prevention, management, and rehabilitation. Since, the practice of any particular component of Yoga also requires enough attention to balancing life style, daily routine affairs of living related to diet, sleep, daily routine habits cannot be segregated apart. In view of racial and communal perceptions for yoga, any such effort involves careful scrutiny and consideration of relevant yogic practices in different religions and countries.

REFERENCES

Acharya, P. S. R. S. (2008). *Yam, Niyam, Asana and Pranayam*. Mathura: Akhand Jyoti Sansthan.

Amita, S., Prabhakar, S., Manoj, I., Harminder, S., & Pawan, T. (2009). Effect of yoga-nidra on blood glucose level in diabetic patients. *Indian Journal of Physiology and Pharmacology*, *53*(1), 97–101. PMID:19810584

Aurobindo, S. (1917). *The synthesis of Yoga*. Pondicherry: Sri Aurobindo Ashram.

Behere, R. V., Arasappa, R., Jagannathan, A., Varambally, S., Venkatasubramanian, G., Thirthalli, J., ... Gangadhar, B. N. (2011). Effect of yoga therapy on facial emotion recognition deficits, symptoms and functioning in patients with schizophrenia. *Acta Psychiatrica Scandinavica*, *123*(2), 147–153. doi:10.1111/j.1600-0447.2010.01605.x PMID:20846271

Benton, D., & Donohoe, R. T. (1999). The effects of nutrients on mood. *Public Health Nutrition*, *2*(3a), 403–409. doi:10.1017/S1368980099000555 PMID:10610080

Bhasin, M. K., Dusek, J. A., Chang, B. H., Joseph, M. G., Denninger, J. W., Fricchione, G. L., ... Libermann, T. A. (2013). Relaxation response induces temporal transcriptome changes in energy metabolism, insulin secretion and inflammatory pathways. *PLoS One*, *8*(5), e62817. doi:10.1371/journal.pone.0062817 PMID:23650531

Blaxter, M. (1990). *Health and lifestyles*. London: Routledge. doi:10.4324/9780203393000

Bury, M. (2004). Researching patient/professional interactions. *Journal of Health Services Research & Policy*, *9*(1), 48–54. doi:10.1258/135581904322724130 PMID:15006228

Buschkens, J., Graham, D., & Cottrell, D. (2010). Well-being Under chronic stress: Is morningness an advantage? *Stress and Health*, *26*(4), 330–340. doi:10.1002mi.1300

Chuang, L. H., Soares, M. O., Tilbrook, H., Cox, H., Hewitt, C. E., Aplin, J., ... Torgerson, D. J. (2012). A pragmatic multicentered randomized controlled trial of yoga for chronic low back pain: Economic evaluation. *Spine*, *37*(18), 1593–1601. doi:10.1097/BRS.0b013e3182545937 PMID:22433499

Cornelissen, R. M. M. (2004). The evolution of consciousness in Sri Aurobindo's cosmo-psychology. In H. Wautischer (Ed.), *Ontology of consciousness: Percipient action* (pp. 1–29). Boston: The MIT Press.

Desikachar, T. K. V. (1999). *The heart of Yoga: Developing a personal practice*. Rochester, VT: Inner Traditions International.

Dusek, J. A., Otu, H. H., Wohlhueter, A. L., Bhasin, M., Zerbini, L. F., Joseph, M. G., ... Libermann, T. A. (2008). Genomic counter-stress changes induced by the relaxation response. *PLoS One*, *3*(7), e2576. doi:10.1371/journal.pone.0002576 PMID:18596974

Dykens, E. M. (2015). Family adjustment and interventions in neurodevelopmental disorders. *Current Opinion in Psychiatry*, *28*(2), 121–126. doi:10.1097/YCO.0000000000000129 PMID:25594421

Elia, J., Ambrosini, P. J., & Rapoport, J. L. (1999). Treatment of attention-deficit-hyperactivity disorder. *The New England Journal of Medicine*, *340*(10), 780–788. doi:10.1056/NEJM199903113401007 PMID:10072414

Elsabbagh, M., Divan, G., Koh, Y. J., Kim, Y. S., Kauchali, S., Marcín, C., ... Yasamy, M. T. (2012). Global prevalence of autism and other pervasive developmental disorders. *Autism Research*, *5*(3), 160–179. doi:10.1002/aur.239 PMID:22495912

Foucault, M. (1973). *The birth of clinic*. London: Tavistock.

Greydanus, D. E. (2005). Pharmacologic treatment of attention-deficit hyperactivity disorder. *Indian Journal of Pediatrics*, *72*(11), 953–960. doi:10.1007/BF02731672 PMID:16391451

Grupp-Phelan, J., Harman, J. S., & Kelleher, K. J. (2007). Trends in mental health and chronic condition visits by children presenting for care at U.S. emergency departments. *Public Health Reports*, *122*(1), 55–61. doi:10.1177/003335490712200108 PMID:17236609

Gupta, A., Gupta, R., Sood, S., & Arkham, M. (2014). Pranayam for treatment of chronic obstructive pulmonary disease: Results from a randomized controlled trial. *Integrative Medicine: A Clinician's Journal, 13*(1), 26-31.

Hariprasad, V. R., Arasappa, R., Varambally, S., Srinath, S., & Gangadhar, B. N. (2013). Feasibility and efficacy of yoga as an add-on intervention in attention deficit-hyperactivity disorder: An exploratory study. *Indian Journal of Psychiatry*, *55*(7S3), S379–S384. doi:10.4103/0019-5545.116317 PMID:24049203

Harrison, L. J., Manocha, R., & Rubia, K. (2004). Sahaja yoga meditation as a family treatment programme for children with attention deficit-hyperactivity disorder. *Clinical Child Psychology and Psychiatry*, *9*(4), 479–497. doi:10.1177/1359104504046155

Hartfiel, N., Clarke, G., Havenhand, J., Phillips, C., & Edwards, R. (2017). Cost-effectiveness of yoga for managing musculoskeletal conditions in the workplace. *Occupational Medicine*, *67*(9), 1–9. doi:10.1093/occmed/kqx161 PMID:29202204

Herbert, A., & Esparham, A. (2017). Mind–Body Therapy for children with attention deficit hyperactivity disorder. *Children*, *4*(5), 31. doi:10.3390/children4050031 PMID:28441363

Hossain, M. D., Ahmed, H. U., Uddin, M. J., Chowdhury, W. A., Iqbal, M. S., Kabir, R. I., ... Hossain, S. W. (2017). Autism Spectrum disorders (ASD) in South Asia: A systematic review. *BMC Psychiatry*, *17*(1), 281. doi:10.118612888-017-1440-x PMID:28826398

Iyengar, B. K. S. (1993). *Light on the Yogasutras of Patanjali*. New Delhi: Harper Collins.

Jeter, P., Slutsky, J., Singh, N., & Khalsa, S. B. (2015). Yoga as a therapeutic intervention: A bibliometric analysis of published research studies from 1967 to 2013. *Journal of Alternative and Complementary Medicine (New York, N.Y.)*, *21*(10), 586–592. doi:10.1089/acm.2015.0057 PMID:26196166

Kalyani, B. G., Venkatasubramanian, G., Arasappa, R., Rao, N. P., Kalmady, S. V., Behere, R. V., ... Gangadhar, B. N. (2011). Neurohemodynamic correlates of 'OM'chanting: A pilot functional magnetic resonance imaging study. *International Journal of Yoga*, *4*(1), 3–6. doi:10.4103/0973-6131.78171 PMID:21654968

Kim, S. D. (2017). Psychological effects of yoga nidra in women with menstrual disorders: A systematic review of randomized controlled trials. *Complementary Therapies in Clinical Practice*, *28*, 4–8. doi:10.1016/j.ctcp.2017.04.001 PMID:28779936

Mason, S., Tovey, P., & Long, A. F. (2002). Evaluating complementary medicine: Methodological challenges of randomised controlled trials. *British Medical Journal*, *325*(7368), 832–834. doi:10.1136/bmj.325.7368.832 PMID:12376448

Mattson, M. P. (2015). What doesn't kill you? *Scientific American*, *313*(1), 40–45. doi:10.1038cientifi camerican0715-40 PMID:26204714

Mattson, M. P., Allison, D. B., Fontana, L., Harvie, M., Longo, V. D., Malaisse, W. J., ... Seyfried, T. N. (2014). Meal frequency and timing in health and disease. *Proceedings of the National Academy of Sciences of the United States of America*, *111*(47), 16647–16653. doi:10.1073/pnas.1413965111 PMID:25404320

Monika, S. U., Ghildiyal, A., Kala, S., & Srivastava, N. (2012). Effect of Yoga Nidra on physiological variables in patients of menstrual disturbances of reproductive age group. *Indian Journal of Physiology and Pharmacology*, *56*(2), 161–167. PMID:23387245

Murphy, M., & Donovan, S. (1999). *The physical and psychological effects of meditation: A review of contemporary research with a comprehensive bibliography 1931-1996 (2nd ed.)*. Sausalito, CA: Institute of Noetic Sciences.

Palombo, J., Bendicsen, H. K., & Koch, B. J. (2009). *Guide to psychoanalytic developmental theories*. New York: Springer.

Pence, P. G., Katz, L. S., Huffman, C., & Cojucar, G. (2014). Delivering Integrative Restoration-Yoga Nidra Meditation (iRest®) to women with sexual trauma at a Veteran's Medical Center: A pilot study. *International Journal of Yoga Therapy*, *24*, 53–62. PMID:25858651

Rao, K. (2002). Stress and its management. In P. Jose (Ed.), *Indian health –A reference document* (pp. 433–435). Kerala: Deepika Publishers.

Rappley, M. D. (2005). Clinical practice: Attention deficit-hyperactivity disorder. *The New England Journal of Medicine*, *352*(2), 165–173. doi:10.1056/NEJMcp032387 PMID:15647579

Roeser, K., Obergfell, F., Meule, A., Vögele, C., Schlarb, A. A., & Kübler, A. (2012). Of larks and hearts—morningness/eveningness, heart rate variability and cardiovascular stress response at different times of day. *Physiology & Behavior*, *106*(2), 151–157. doi:10.1016/j.physbeh.2012.01.023 PMID:22330324

Salmon, P., Lush, E., Jablonski, M., & Sephton, S. E. (2009). Yoga and mindfulness: Clinical aspects of an ancient mind/body practice. *Cognitive and Behavioral Practice*, *16*(1), 59–72. doi:10.1016/j.cbpra.2008.07.002

Sampson, P. D., Streissguth, A. P., Bookstein, F. L., Little, R. E., Clarren, S. K., Dehaene, P., ... Graham, J. M. (1997). Incidence of fetal alcohol syndrome and prevalence of alcohol-related neurodevelopmental disorder. *Teratology*, *56*(5), 317–326. doi:10.1002/(SICI)1096-9926(199711)56:5<317::AID-TERA5>3.0.CO;2-U PMID:9451756

Saraswati, S. S. (1996). *Asana, Panayama, Mudra Bandh*. Munger: Yog Publications Trust.

Shapiro, S., Schwartz, G., & Santerre, C. (2002). Meditation and positive psychology. In C. R. Snyder & S. J. Lopez (Eds.), *Handbook of positive psychology* (pp. 632–645). New York: Oxford University Press.

Silberberg, D., Arora, N., Bhutani, V., Durkin, M., Gulati, S., Nair, M., & Pinto-Martin, J. (2014). Neuro-Developmental Disorders in India - From Epidemiology to Public Policy (I10-1.006). *Neurology*, *82*(S10), I10–I11.

Singh, A. P. (2017). Effectiveness of yogic lifestyle for promoting mental health and well-being: Implications for therapeutic value and school health-care policy. In A. Dubey & A. Shukla (Eds.), Mental health: Psychosocial perspectives (vol. 4). New Delhi: Concept.

Singh, A. P., & Misra, G. (2012). Adolescent lifestyle in India: Prevalence of risk and health-promotive factors. *Psychology and Developing Societies*, *24*(2), 145–160. doi:10.1177/097133361202400203

Singh, A. P., & Misra, G. (2015). Pattern of leisure-lifestyles in Indian school adolescents: Contextual influences and implications for health concerns. *Cognitive Psychology*, *2*(1), 1–11. doi:10.1080/23311908.2015.1050779

Singh, A. P., & Misra, G. (2016). Gender difference in life Style: Results of a survey among Indian school adolescents. *Social Change*, *46*(3), 1–16. doi:10.1177/0049085716654816

Stankovic, L. (2011). Transforming trauma: A qualitative feasibility study of integrative restoration (iRest) yoga Nidra on combat-related post-traumatic stress disorder. *International Journal of Yoga Therapy*, *21*, 23–37. PMID:22398342

Talge, N. M., Neal, C., & Glover, V. (2007). Early Stress, translational research and prevention science network: Fetal and neonatal experience on child and adolescent mental health. Antenatal maternal stress and long-term effects on child neurodevelopment: How and why? *Journal of Child Psychology and Psychiatry, and Allied Disciplines*, *48*(3-4), 245–261. doi:10.1111/j.1469-7610.2006.01714.x PMID:17355398

Vempati, R. P., & Telles, S. (2002). Yoga-based guided relaxation reduces sympathetic activity judged from baseline levels. *Psychological Reports*, *90*(2), 487–494. doi:10.2466/pr0.2002.90.2.487 PMID:12061588

KEY TERMS AND DEFINITIONS

Daily Routine and Positive Leisure: This term denotes ordinary activities of life in the transaction with daytime and seasonal variation.

Dietary Habits: It refers to habits related to ingestion.

Meditation: This term is defined as concentration towards any object/situation with full awareness and relaxation.

Neurodevelopment Disorders: These disorders indicate developmental deficits in the development of the central nervous system.

Posture: It denotes a particular bodily position influencing physical and mental aspects of health.

Pranayama: Ordinarily, this word is used for breath-regulation but in actual yogic terminology, this term means for controlling and harmonizing vital force of the body.

Yoga: This term refers to a perspective of life/therapy/a cluster of spiritual practices as ingrained in Indian traditional systems of knowledge.

Yognidra: In order to maintain harmony in the body, this practice involves loosening of each part of the body with full awareness and successively relaxes the body.

Chapter 14
Play Therapy for Children With Neurodevelopmental Disorders

Gaurav Thapliyal
Sweekar Academy of Rehabilitation Sciences, India

Sushma Kotnala
Pyare Foundation, India

ABSTRACT

A play is referred to the language of children through which they express and communicate their feelings, thoughts, and behavior in a playful way. Play therapy enables children to gain an understanding of themselves and the world around them and helps them to overcome behavioral, emotional, social, and various other issues through play activities. The chapter majorly focuses on the effectiveness of play therapy in different neurodevelopmental disorders. Recent trends and studies suggested that play therapy is one of the most favored therapeutic approaches used in the children with various neurodevelopmental disorders.

INTRODUCTION

Human life begins from childhood to adulthood. From the first day of life, everyone has their own temperament, perception and meaning to strive for survival which we call as "individual differences". Childhood is the initial stage of the circle of development. It is the utmost factor to be followed appropriately for achieving all the developmental milestones successfully. If this stage of childhood does not function properly, it may lead to the psychological, social, emotional and behavioral issues.

Presently, increased numbers of children have been diagnosed with neurodevelopmental disorders such as intellectual disability, autism spectrum disorder, attention deficit hyperactivity disorder (ADHD), and specific learning disorders. There are many therapeutic practices that help in the management of these disorders; one of them is play therapy. The most prominent activity, in which children mostly involve, is playing. Through playing children are availed with valuable cognitive, emotional, and interpersonal learning opportunities. For children playing is the way to express their significant emotions, feelings and behavioral pattern of life. By the process of play therapy, children work on their own emotional and

DOI: 10.4018/978-1-5225-7004-2.ch014

psychological problems in their own way. It is a natural expression of play where the therapist provides a secure and comfortable environment for children to express their feelings, thoughts, and behaviors within the acceptable limits. The present chapter focuses the use of play therapy and its effective application among children with neurodevelopmental disorders.

DEFINITIONS OF PLAY AND PLAY THERAPY

Play provides a developmentally responsive means for expressing thoughts and feelings, exploring relationships, make sense of experiences, disclosing wishes, and developing coping strategies. (Landreth, 2002)

"For children, play is the natural, spontaneous, and comfortable medium through which children express themselves" (Axline, 1947).

Play therapy is a developmentally-sensitive intervention to help the children with significant emotional problems. It:

is a well thought-out, philosophically conceived, developmentally-based, and research-supported method of helping children cope with and overcome the problems they experience in the process of living their lives. (Landreth, 1996)

Play Therapy is defined as:

the systematic use of a theoretical model to establish an interpersonal process wherein trained play therapists use the therapeutic powers of play to help clients prevent or resolve psychosocial difficulties and achieve optimal growth and development. (Association for Play Therapy, 2011)

HISTORICAL DEVELOPMENT

The famous Greek philosopher Plato (429-347 B.C) stated that "You can discover more about a person in an hour of play than in a year of conservation". The effective use of play as an intervention with childhood problems was initiated by Freud (1909) who published his work with the classical case of "Little Hans," a five-year-old boy with phobia. During his treatment, it was based on the father's notes about Hans' play that Freud advised the father to resolve his son's underlying conflicts and fear. It was the first recorded case of "Little Hans" in which a child's difficulty was understood in the terms of emotional problems. Hug-Hellmuth (1921) was the pioneer therapist who provided play materials in the therapy with children to promote their self-expression. Hug-Hellmuth discouraged psychoanalysis of children below six years of age and opined it to be potentially dangerous. Hug-Hellmuth introduced play as an intervention in child therapy. Klein (1955) started using play to analyses children under the age of six years. Klein believed that a child's play was served same as that of free association used among adults for their underlying conflicts. Freud (1946) applied the basic principles of psychoanalysis to children in therapy. Freud described that the children's play may be a conscious repetition of their day-to-day life activities. On the other hand, Klein used play as a medium for the verbalized free association to work with children. Levy (1938) developed a structured play approach known as "release therapy". It helped children in recreating their feelings and thoughts or any other experiences towards a specific traumatic situation through play. Levy described that when a child feels comfortable, gets support, and security, along with appropriate play materials then the child may be able to play out a previous traumatic event over and over until the child will be able to let go of his/her fear, anxiety and other emotions related to those traumatic situations or events.

Axline (1947) was the most well-known personality in the field of play therapy. Axline developed a concept of non-directive play therapy to work with children and also revealed the value of the relationship between the therapist and the child via play, which allows the child to feel safe so that the process of growth may occur. Through establishing the rapport with the child in play therapy, the therapist will be able to balance his/her emotional maturity and could easily develop varied emotional expression and exploration of the various levels of the emotional process. Axline (1969) created eight basic principles as a help to guide the child-centered play therapist: (1) the therapist should develop a trusting and affectionate relationship with the child; (2) the therapist must accept the child the way he or she is; (3) the therapist should be lenient enough for the child to experience freedom in expressing his or her emotions completely; (4) the therapist should recognize the feelings and reflect them back to the child in a genuine manner; (5) the therapist must truly believe that the child is able to solve his or her own problems; (6) the therapist must refrain from directing any actions, speech, or play for the child; (7) the therapist should have patience throughout the gradual therapeutic process, and; (8) the therapist should be the one to create limitations necessary to anchor the relationship in the world of reality.

Rogers (1951) developed "client-centered therapy". Basically, it was the foundation for "child-centered play therapy". Carl Rogers emphasized deeply the relationships between the child and the play therapist based on trust and acceptance. It was a new perspective on emotional and psychological difficulties and the altered process within the therapy. Solomon (1938) developed an "active play therapy" in which a procedure was used with acting out and making children impulsive. It is a technique of abreaction that may occur through the safe play and also a supportive relationship. A child can play out difficult feelings and experiences, and thereby avoid acting them out through socially inappropriate behaviors.

In the year of 1982, Schaefer and O'Connor established the Association for Play Therapy (APT) who showed a major advancement in the field of play therapy. Later, the concepts of play therapy were applied and extended into many other various situations and ways such as in different clinical settings and among a diverse population. According to Landreth (1991), the different objectives of child-centered play therapy were to help children with various problems:

- To develop the positive self-concept.
- Become more self-directing.
- Become more self-accepting.
- Become more self-reliant.
- Experience a feeling of control.
- Become sensitive to the process of coping.
- Become more trustworthy.
- Develop an internal source of evaluation.

RATIONALE FOR PLAY THERAPY

The rationale of play therapy is to act as the symbolic language of self-expression in the children with maladjustment. Normally, adults communicate their emotions and thought process through verbal language. It is a process which transforms personal experiences into abstract skills. Children do not have that specific skill to perform complex operations until eleven years of age (Piaget, 1962). Children express their emotions and experiences through play (Ginott, 1960). Jernberg (1979) suggested the technique of touch to reconnect and provide a secure relationship between parents and the child. The parents were taught to respond empathically and to understand the nonverbal communication of the child through a playful approach.

Packman and Bratton (2003) found an activity-based intervention for children with learning disability. They described this specialized treatment to be very effective on those children who exhibited problem behavior at home and school. These kinds of interventions often involve the use of the symbolic expression which helps adolescents to develop their expression and exploration. It also allows children to have a safe distance between themselves and reality (Bratton & Ferebee 1999; Malchiodi, 2005). Harvey (2006) has developed a concept of "dynamic family play therapy". Basically, it is an action-oriented therapeutic process in which family members are involved in therapy sessions. Parents are instructed to display their creativity and help them adapt to traumatic situations. There are various techniques used to rely on the strength of the parent-child relationships as a significant factor in the healing process. Schaefer (2003) promoted and suggested play therapy for adolescents to encourage the use of language and benefits of play across the lifetime. The major goal of play therapy with adolescents was to help them feel more secure, comfortable and talk willingly about their feelings and experiences (Gallo-Lopez & Rubin, 2012).

GOALS OF PLAY THERAPY

Though there are various types of psychotherapies, the basic goals of play therapy are to decrease and modify maladaptive behaviors and also to help improve the adaptive ones. Some major goals of play therapy include:

- Improving communication pattern with verbal expression.
- Enhancing problem-solving and coping skills.
- Improving mood and affect.
- Improving impulse control.
- Developing underlying conflict.
- Developing self-awareness.
- Improving self-confidence.
- Developing greater self-esteem.
- Developing the more positive self-concept.
- Improving social skills.

FORMS OF PLAY THERAPY

In different types of play therapies, some basic concepts were originated from the past and several most influential forms of therapies that are existing in the current scenario.

Psychoanalytic Play Therapy

Freud (1928) published comprehensively about how they incorporated play as a therapy into the psychoanalytic approach. As free association technique was used in adult clients, they substituted the natural tendency of the children to play together with free association. They described that the process of play uncovered the underlying problems or conflicts of children. In support to the therapy, the study done by Clausen, Ruff, Wiederhold, and Heineman (2012) applied the treatment for foster children who received psychodynamic play therapy over three years. Researchers found significant improvements with regard to reduction in anxiety, aggressive behavior, depression, interpersonal issues and problems related to school.

Structured Play Therapy

Structured play therapy is the exact opposite of non-structured approaches because the functions of play therapy is considered to be within the confined limits which are organized by various play materials provided in various play situations. Levy (1938) described structured therapy as a directive approach where the therapist provides security, support and other materials required to recreate stressfully or deal with any traumatic events of the child so that the child may cognitively understand the negative emotions and feelings associated with those adverse situations.

Adlerian Play Therapy

Adlerian play therapy is the most flexible approach which is based on the human needs regarding feeling the sense of "belongingness". The goal of the therapy is to meet the individual needs of the child as well as to give a sense of control and mastery to the participant. Taylor and Bratton (2014) applied Adlerian play therapy in their study with a four-year-old boy who was experiencing bereavement after the loss of his mother. After the treatment sessions, the authors found significant changes, as well as, an increased in his feelings of belonging.

The responsibility of the therapist is not only to explore children's lifestyle but also to gain knowledge about their emotions, behavior, relationships and perceptions towards self and others. The therapist should also conceptualize the thought pattern, behavior and feelings of the child's parents because it will be beneficial for him to understand the underlying factors of parents with regard to their in the relationship with children (Schaefer, 2003). Many play therapists include even parents or caregivers to train them on the methods to communicate with the child in a constructive way.

Client-Centered Play Therapy

Axline (1947) discussed that client-centered play therapy emphasizes the therapist's role including the qualities of genuineness, unconditional positive regard and empathic understanding towards the children. In the therapy, the therapist provides an acceptance, support and secure feeling instead of focusing on the problems of children. Axline indicated that therapist ought not to be in hurry of the problems of the child. The primary goal of client-centered play therapy is self-directed growth and change in the child. Moustakas (1959) indicated that this process develops the exploration of feelings and culminates in the child's an increased sense of self-worth. Ray, Armstrong, Balkin, and Jayne (2015) conducted a systematic review and meta-analytical study on 23 children who received child-centered play therapy in school. The conclusion of the study revealed that play therapy generated statistically significant outcomes in the children with internalizing problems, disruptive behavior, and academic problems.

Cognitive Behavioral Play Therapy (CBPT)

Knell (1993) developed the concept of cognitive behavioral play therapy in which cognitive and behavioral interventions are incorporated into a play therapy paradigm. Knell described six steps of CBPT:

- CBPT focuses on all the children through play in therapy.
- It incorporates children's imaginations, thinking, fantasies and environment in therapy sessions.
- It provides various techniques to improve appropriate behavior and positive thinking.
- It is a directive and goal-directed approach and not open-ended.
- It involves demonstrated techniques into therapy such as modeling.
- It involves an empirical examination of treatment into therapy.

Hall, Kaduson, and Schaefer (2002) used 15 techniques of cognitive behavioral play therapy with the children of age range between 4 to 12 years diagnosed with ADHD. After the completion of the therapy, children showed the significant reduction in the symptoms of hyperactivity and attentional problems.

Filial Play Therapy

Guerney (1964) developed filial therapy. It became the most popular therapy in the field of play therapy. This technique was unique as it allowed parents to implement play therapy sessions at home. The basic concept of this therapy was to make the parents and caregivers get involved in play therapy sessions. In the sessions, parents were the primary participants so that the lack of family intimacy, knowledge and the emotional conditions of the child can be eliminated. Furthermore, Schaefer (2003) described that if the parents understand the problem and psychological state of the child, they need not seek any psychological help from any professional play therapist. They will involve in the therapy sessions on their own as a primary play therapist with the child.

TECHNIQUES OF PLAY THERAPY

The Feeling Word Game

The Feeling Word Game allows children to express and connect their emotions and feelings in a non-fearful and non-threatening way. It is very difficult for children to express their emotions verbally because sometimes they do not connect themselves with emotion-provoking situations. When they are involved in play activities, they talk and express their feelings via play.

The therapist narrates a story regarding himself including both positive and negative feelings. At the end of the story, therapist place poker chips in front of the child for every appropriate feeling. It shows that everyone can have more than one feeling at the same time. Then therapist tells another story which is completely non-threatening to the child including both positive and negative feelings. Now, the child receives a tin of feelings and is instructed to put down what he may feel under those situations. After that, child narrates another story to the therapist to put down his feelings in the tin of feelings. It continues until major issues are discussed.

Application

The specific technique is effective to the children with conduct problems, ADHD and anxiety issues.

The Pick-Up-Sticks Game

The Pick-Up-Sticks Game was developed by Barbara McDowell (see Kaduson & Schaefer, 1997, pp. 145–149) for the purpose of improving affective expression in children. It is a technique designed for the children to express their emotions and pair various affective states related to the environmental conditions. To use the technique, children must know color-feeling pairs which mean Color- Your- Life.

Therapist starts with reviewing color-feelings pairs by playing Color-Your-Life. It may be discussed verbally also. Then the therapist describes the use of Pick-Up-Sticks in therapy sessions. Now, either the therapist or the child holds sticks in his fist and drop it on the table. Basically, they have to remove one stick without moving any other sticks. The game ends up when one of the players move other sticks accidently. Every time the stick is removed, the child must tell about a time when he had a feeling associated with the color of the stick. Once the therapist gets his turn, the therapist gives the response, tailored to the particular need of the child. This technique evaluates and interprets the color of the sticks chosen and avoided by the children and the overall affect during the play session.

Application

This technique is used among children individually or by making them into or in a small group. The child must have adequate verbal skills and knowledge about color-feeling pairs. This therapeutic strategy is more successful with children who are competitive because they have a particular desire to win that force them to choose the particular Pick-Up-Sticks which they normally avoid.

The Mad Game

The Mad Game is designed by Patricia Davidson (see Kaduson & Schaefer, 1997, pp. 224–225) to provide awareness to the children with anger suggesting that anger is a primary emotion which is easily acceptable. During the session, therapist divides blocks between himself and the child. Then, he instructs the child to put each block on the top of the previous one once the turn comes. Every time they have to express any incidence which makes them angry. All events are acceptable either it is silly or serious. Once all blocks are stacked then the child would be instructed to mention one last event which made him seriously angry. At last, the child has to make a mad face and knock down all the blocks.

Application

This technique can be used to show the slightly altered emotions rather than anger such as fear, anxiety and sadness.

Relaxation Training: Bubble Breaths

Bubble breaths technique is a very effective relaxation technique which involves teaching children deep and controlled breathing to make them aware regarding their body and mind connections. The therapist will take the child into a specific room where the child blows bubbles. The child and the therapist can pop those bubbles before they fall. After that, the therapist instructs the child to blow only one big bubble. Now, the therapist tells the child to take a deep breath from the stomach and exhale in very slow manner. Here, the therapist discusses with the child that whenever he gets angry, his brain demands more air and lungs cannot provide it. When they breathe slowly then the brain will not demand more air and heart and lungs will work slowly in a far better way. If they get angry and take a deep bubble breath they can prevent their anger easily.

Application

It is very simple, non-expansive and non-threatening technique, especially for those children with anger and anxiety.

Using a Puppet to Create a Symbolic Client

The use of puppets has a precious role in play therapy. All children attribute their emotions onto puppets. There are various children who are extremely anxious, fearful and withdrawn towards involving in therapies. But puppet is very useful as a symbolic technique so as to engage these kinds of children into therapy. The therapist observes anxiety and fear of the child and shows him a puppet. Then he remarks the puppet as anxious and fearful. Therapist discuss with the child to make the puppet comfortable. Actually, the therapist is achieving three major goals:

- Show empathy to child's emotions.
- Involving in the child's participation in the therapy.
- Establishing rapport with the child.

Application

The age range of children to adopt this technique is, between 4 and 8 years and is especially applicable to those children who are anxious and withdrawn regarding the therapy.

The Spy and the Sneak

The Spy and the sneak technique were developed to change the adverse and the negative interactions among family members in a positives way. Once it is transformed, it increases the enjoyment among each other. Parents start observing positive and adaptive qualities of their children and give positive reinforcement towards their adaptive behavior. It gives an insight to the children as well, that they are getting more attention from the parents in an adaptive manner.

The therapist discusses with the child about a sneaky positive behavior that makes the parents surprised. The therapist guides the child to be a "sneak" and the parents are the "spy" who will find out what the sneak has done. He has to do brainstorming for the child to do at least three to four behavior related to the treatment goals. In the further sessions, parents will be informed about the role of the spy and will be invited to the session. They have to jot down all the good behaviors of their child for a week at home. Both the parents and the child are instructed not to discuss the findings with each other. Finally, the therapist will set a discussion regarding how the parents and the child feel about the child's engagement in positive activities. The child also gets pleasure to receive the positive attention followed by surprising the parents more.

Application

It is an excellent technique to be used among families experiencing negative interactions. After few therapeutic sessions, therapist switches the roles of parents and the child with each the sneak.

PLAY THERAPY IN NEURODEVELOPMENTAL DISORDERS

Various evidence-based studies have assessed the effectiveness of play therapy among different populations. Only very few experimentally designed studies were done. Some of them were in the form of case studies while others were anecdotal reports. Gall et al. (1996) described that case studies are the weakest method to measure the outcome of the treatment due to its lack of internal and external validity. All the experimental studies have been mostly preferred with various case studies since it has increased the validity of the studies that controlled their effects by confounding variables. In this section, controlled studies showed the effectiveness of play therapy, especially, all those studies that investigated the effectiveness of play therapy with children.

Intellectual Developmental Disorder

Morrison and Newcomer (1975) did a study to measure the effectiveness of directive and non-directive play therapy for children with mental retardation. The study concluded that no evidence revealed more effectiveness regarding directive and non-directive play therapy. Swan and Ray (2014) did a study related to CCPT on the children with intellectual disabilities who were showing the symptoms of irritable behavior and hyperactivity. The study showed the reduction in irritable behavior and hyperactivity after following the treatment. After three weeks, despite the treatment sessions, all the improvements were maintained by the children with intellectual disability.

Kachalaki and Faghirpour (2015) conducted a study on "The effect of play therapy in the development of cognitive skills, social and motor educable mentally retarded students". The research findings suggested that play therapy indicated improvements in the concept of mental development such as "length, weight, volume, appropriate eye-hand coordination, social development, academic achievement and motor developmental skills among educable children who were already diagnosed with intellectual developmental disorder. Jacob and Brinda (2017) did a study on "The effect of non-directive play therapy on development among mentally challenged children in selected institutions of Coimbatore". The major findings of the study showed that non-directive play therapy has a significant effect on the development of mentally challenged children.

Autism Spectrum Disorder

Kenny and Winick (2000) utilized the techniques of directive play therapy in the treatment of children with autism. The treatment showed significant changes in the children with Autism. Josefi and Ryan (2009) took 16 sessions of non-directed play therapy with 6 years old boy who was diagnosed with severe autism. After receiving all the sessions, he developed the ability to engage in pretend play, increased autonomy and showed improvement regarding the level of empathy. Parker and O'Brien (2011) discussed regarding a 7 years old boy diagnosed with ASD and showed a significant improvement after receiving sand play activity as part of play therapy in his/her school. Ware (2014) did a single case design study on play therapy for children with ASD. The study was to find out the impact of non-directive play therapy on social competence, empathy and self-regulation with the children who diagnosed with ASD. The results supported play therapy as an intervention that helps children to develop all these areas.

Attention Deficit Hyperactivity Disorder

Naderi et al (2010) conducted a study on "efficacy of play therapy on ADHD, Anxiety and Social Maturity in 8 to 12 years aged clientele of Ahwaz metropolitan counseling clinics". The results revealed that play therapy is an effective intervention for children who experience various problems such as ADHD, and anxiety. Barzegary and Zamini (2011) did a study to examine the effect of play therapy of 14 male participants with ADHD. The results found that play therapy was an effective method of treating children with ADHD. Robinson et al. (2017) conducted a study on "The effects of child-centered play therapy on the behavioral performance of three first grade students with ADHD". The findings suggested that CCPT was an effective intervention for the first-grade students with ADHD in school settings.

Learning Disorders

Blanco and Ray (2011) revealed in their study that children who received Client Centered Play Therapy (CCPT) as an experimental group showed significant improvement in their academic performances as compared to the children with the control group. Khaledi et al. (2014) did a study on "The positive impact of play therapy on writing performance of students with dysgraphia". Results revealed that play therapy had a positive impact on the students with dysgraphia who had spelling difficulties. Sarpoulaki and Kolahi (2016) did a study to evaluate the efficacy of play therapy on children with spelling disorders and aggressive behavior. The result found that after using play therapy there was a significant reduction in aggressive behavior. They also noted an improvement in spelling disorder among the subjects. Esmaili, Shafaroodi, and Zardkhaneh (2017) conducted a study on:

Effect of play-based therapy on the meta-cognitive and behavioral aspect of executive functions, a randomized, controlled, clinical trial on the students with learning disabilities.

The result concluded that play-based therapy is highly effective on meta-cognitive and behavioral aspects of executive functioning among the subjects.

PLAY THERAPY IN OTHER CHILDHOOD DISORDERS

Play therapy is the best therapeutic technique which provides opportunities to the children to express their underlying conflicts or various other problems in a better way. In India, the prevalence rate of substance abuse is very high which lead to domestic violence, family crises, conflicts in interpersonal relationships and major psychiatric illnesses. Substance abuse or multiple addictions cause violence at home. Mostly, parents are the primary suspects in children with physical abuse. Once it is cleared, the child has to be removed from his home for security and safety. There are thousands of children who can get benefits from the long-term treatment of play therapy. It includes all kind of children such as children with sexual abuse (Hill, 2006), violent abuse (Chazan & Cohen, 2010), traumatic events (Webb, 2011), and children who lost their loved ones (Rakesh & Srinath, 2010).

Most of the time in an extreme case, children and adolescents experience unresolved anxiety, fear and sudden traumatic events that may not exhibit any negative behavioral changes; however, they develop aggressive, rebellious and withdrawn behavior which may lead to severe psychological problems in their life (Schaefer, 2010). In addition, children with grief reaction experience differently than an adult individual. They display their pain and the reaction of grief in "short bursts" which is opposite to prolonged period of time due to their short attention span (Landreth, 1996). It may affect their temperament, family dynamics as well as other resources even more if they do not receive any psychological help or treatment. (Collins & Collins, 2005). Schaefer (2003) described that children who experience grief must participate in filial therapy until they bereaved both the parents. However, it is a must for the parents or caregivers to observe initial sessions of play therapy and then to receive specific training for further treatment process (Schafer, 2010).

Various research studies have shown that after receiving play therapy, children who have been abused in any way such as sexually, emotionally, physically and neglectfully has come up with stability and positive effects in their lives (White & Allers, 1994). These studies also found a strong correlation between faster and effective healing progress from the use of play as a therapy either by a trained play therapist or parents. A research study conducted on 26 children with sexual abused showed improvement in their coping skills and behavior after receiving 10 sessions of play therapy (Blankenship & Lawver, 2008). Although, 10 sessions were not well enough to generate the appropriate outcome of the study. Due to that researcher monitored the study for a longer period of time. After that, approximately one-third of all the children showed significant improvement with regard to the reception of play therapy.

Flahive and Ray (2007) discussed that those samples, who received sand tray/play therapy in their study, showed significant differences in the problem of externalizing & internalizing disorders as compared with a control group. Ray, Schottelkorb, and Tsai (2007) conducted a study on the children, exhibiting symptoms of ADHD. After receiving play therapy, there was a positive impact on the overall symptoms such as internalizing and externalizing problems, depression, anxiety, self-concept, and treatment compliance.

IMPLICATIONS OF PLAY THERAPY

Play therapy is a non-threatening and effective treatment for the children with emotional and behavioral problems. Basically, it is an issue for the adults who use their energies to change the maladaptive behavior of their children and deal with their emotional problems. Therefore, play therapy is a very effective intervention to provide help to those children with various problems.

Play therapy is also very effective across all settings, age, race, gender as well as clinical and non-clinical populations. It is extremely useful in a school setting with all age groups. There is an implication in Indian scenario where it applies for different children belonging to diverse socio-economic backgrounds. Even the involvement of the parents is very common in both Indian as well as western studies. It is also found that the role of the parents in therapy sessions showed a significant treatment outcome. To give proper training to parents regarding how to help the child while play at home is worthwhile.

Various research studies suggested that play therapy may take approximately 30 sessions to indicate the improvement and overall functioning of the children. The understanding views of all trained play therapists are crucial towards their small and young clients who receive therapy sessions with its full effects. This approach prevents all the future problems which may develop in children across their life-span.

INDICATIONS OF PLAY THERAPY

Play therapy has been used as a major psychotherapeutic technique to treat disorders among children with:

- Specific phobia
- Panic disorders
- Generalized anxiety disorders
- Obsessive-compulsive disorder
- Depression
- Post-traumatic stress disorder
- Separation anxiety disorder
- Selective mutism
- Autism spectrum disorders
- ADHD
- Enuresis
- Sleep problems
- Learning disorders
- Conduct disorders

CONTRAINDICATIONS OF PLAY THERAPY

There are very few disorders to which play therapy cannot be applied. They include:

- Chronic illnesses
- Burn victims

- Children with deaf
- Children with physically challenged
- Dissociation
- Schizophrenia

FUTURE RESEARCH DIRECTIONS

In the field of play therapy, the future research needs to take into consideration the following factors:

- Play therapy still works on the small number of participants which cannot be generalized to a normal population. Sample size must be large for future studies.
- Mostly, studies do not report work experience of the therapist in this field. Various studies also do not show any standardized protocol, even though all the procedures of play therapy provide clear guidelines and clarity.
- There are significant research studies which reveal the design of therapy versus absence of treatment but still, researchers are not able to provide clarity about play therapy being the most effective intervention. It must be compared with other therapeutic treatment with children.
- Different studies focused on specific play therapy treatment among specific populations. The most important question is that whether the interventions facilitate play and it ought to be empirically researched. There are few research guidelines regarding how to facilitate play but of those only very few are based on empirical works.

CONCLUSION

Play therapy is a universal, dynamic and upcoming field in the ground of psychotherapy. From the earlier period, play therapy has been used as a most effective psychotherapeutic treatment for different psychiatric disorders. The present chapter mainly focused on the efficacy of play therapy as an intervention in the children with neurodevelopmental disorders. Through various evidence-based research studies, it is found that play therapy is an intervention which may be significant to reduce symptoms of disorders and improve adaptive behavior. The conclusion of the chapter revealed the effectiveness of play therapy in various neurodevelopmental disorders.

REFERENCES

Association for Play Therapy. (n.d.). Retrieved November 30, 2011, from http://www.a4pt.org/index.html

Axline, V. M. (1969). *Play therapy*. New York, NY: Ballenti.

Axline, V. M. (1947). *Play therapy: The inner dynamics of childhood*. Boston: Houghton Mifflin.

Barzegary, L., & Zamini, S. (2011). The effect of play therapy on children with ADHD. *Procedia: Social and Behavioral Sciences*, *30*, 2216–2218. doi:10.1016/j.sbspro.2011.10.432

Blanco, P., & Ray, D. (2011). Play therapy in the schools: A best practice for improving academic achievement. *Journal of Counseling and Development*, *89*(2), 235–242. doi:10.1002/j.1556-6678.2011.tb00083.x

Blankenship, K., & Lawver, T. (2008). Play therapy: A case-based example of a nondirective approach. *Psychiatry (Edgmont)*, *5*(10), 24–28. PMID:19724720

Bratton, S. C., & Ferebee, K. W. (1999). The use of structured expressive art activities in group activity therapy with preadolescents. In D. S. Sweeny & L. E. Homeyer (Eds.), *The handbook of group play therapy: How to do it, how it works, whom it's best for* (pp. 192–214). San Francisco, CA: Jossey-Bass.

Chazan, S., & Cohen, E. (2010). Adaptive and defensive strategies in post-traumatic play of young children exposed to violent attacks. *Journal of Child Psychotherapy*, *36*(2), 133–151. doi:10.1080/0075417X.2010.495024

Clausen, J. M., Ruff, S. C., Wiederhold, W. V., & Heineman, T. V. (2012). For as long as it takes: Relationship-based play therapy for children in foster care. *Psychoanalytic Social Work*, *19*(1-2), 43–53. doi:10.1080/15228878.2012.666481

Collins, B. C., & Collins, T. M. (2005). *Crisis and trauma: Developmental-ecological intervention*. Boston: Houghton Mifflin.

Esmaili, S. K., Shafaroodi, N., & Zardkhaneh, S. A. (2017). Effect of play based therapy on meta-cognitive and behavioral aspects of executive functions: A randomised, controlled, clinical trial on the students with learning disabilities. *Basic and Clinical Neuroscience*, *8*(3), 2003–2012.

Flahive, M., & Ray, D. (2007). Effect of group sand tray therapy with preadolescents in a school setting. *Journal for Specialists in Group Work*, *32*(4), 362–382. doi:10.1080/01933920701476706

Freud, A. (1928). *Introduction to the technique of Child Analysis* (L. P. Clark, Trans.). New York: Nervous and Mental Disease Publishing.

Freud, A. (1946). *The psycho-analytical treatment of children*. New York: International Universities.

Freud, S. (1909). Analysis of a Phobia in a Five-Year-Old Boy. *The Standard Edition of the Complete Psychological Works of Sigmund Freud*, *X*, 3–149.

Gall, M. D., Borg, W. R., & Gall, J. P. (1996). *Educational Research*. White Plains.

Gallo-Lopez, L., & Rubin, L. C. (2012). *Play-Based Interventions for Children and Adolescents with Autism Spectrum Disorders*. New York: Routledge.

Ginott, H. (1960). A rationale for selecting toys in play therapy. *Journal of Consulting Psychology*, *24*(3), 243–246. doi:10.1037/h0043980 PMID:13850211

Guerney, B. Jr. (1964). Filial therapy: Description and rationale. *Journal of Consulting Psychology*, *28*(4), 304–310. doi:10.1037/h0041340 PMID:14198792

Hall, T. M., Kaduson, H. G., & Schaefer, C. E. (2002). Fifteen effective play therapy techniques. *Professional Psychology, Research and Practice*, *33*(6), 515–522. doi:10.1037/0735-7028.33.6.515

Harvey, S. (2006). Dynamic play therapy. In C. E. Schaefer & H. G. Kaduson (Eds.), *Contemporary play therapy: Theory* (pp. 55–81). Research, and Practice.

Hill, A. (2006). Play therapy with sexually abused children: Including parents in therapeutic play. *Child & Family Social Work, 11*(4), 316–324. doi:10.1111/j.1365-2206.2006.00411.x

Hug-Hellmuth, H. V. (1921). On the technique of Child-Analysis. *The International Journal of Psycho-Analysis, 2*, 287–305.

Jacob, S., & Brinda, V. (2017). The effect of non-directive play therapy on development among mentally challenged children in selected institutions of Coimbatore. *Asian Journal of Nursing Education and Research, 7*(4), 482–490. doi:10.5958/2349-2996.2017.00094.5

Jernberg, A. M. (1979). *Theraplay: A new treatment using structured play for problem children and their families.* Academic Press.

Josefi, O., & Ryan, V. (2009). Non-directive play therapy for young children with autism: A case study. *Clinical Child Psychology and Psychiatry, 9*(4), 533–551. doi:10.1177/1359104504046158

Kachalaki, S. M., & Faghirpour, M. (2015). The effect of play therapy in the development of cognitive skills, social and motor educable mentally retarded students. *Journal UMP Social Sciences and Technology Management, 3*, 3.

Kaduson, H., & Schaefer, C. (Eds.). (1997). *101 favorite play therapy techniques.* Northvale, NJ: Jason Aronson.

Kenny, M. C., & Winick, C. B. (2000). An integrative approach to play therapy with an autistic girl. *International Journal of Play Therapy, 9*(1), 11–33. doi:10.1037/h0089438

Khaledi, S., Pak, A. V., Mirkhan, I., & Atai, M. (2014). The positive impact of play therapy on writing performance of students with dysgraphia. *International Journal of School Health, 1*(2), e22655. doi:10.17795/intjsh-22655

Klein, M. (1955). The psychoanalytic play technique. *The American Journal of Orthopsychiatry, 25*(2), 223–227. doi:10.1111/j.1939-0025.1955.tb00131.x PMID:14376493

Knell, S. (1993). *Cognitive-behavioral play therapy.* Northvale, NJ: Aronson.

Landreth, G. L. (1991). Play therapy: The art of the relationship. Accelerated Development.

Landreth, G. L. (1996). *Play therapy interventions with children's problems.* Northvale, NJ: Aronson.

Landreth, G. L. (2002). *Play therapy: The art of the relationship.* New York: Routledge.

Levy, D. M. (1938). Release therapy in young children. *Psychiatry, 1*(3), 387–389. doi:10.1080/00332747.1938.11022205

Malchiodi, C. A. (Ed.). (2005). *Expressive Therapies.* Guilford Publications.

Morrison, T. L., & Newcomer, B. L. (1975). Effects of directive vs. nondirective play therapy with institutionalized mentally retarded children. *American Journal of Mental Deficiency, 79*, 666–669. PMID:1146857

Moustakas, C. E. (1959). *Psychotherapy with children: The living relationship*. New York: Harper & Brothers.

Naderi, F., Heidarie, L. B., & Asgari, P. (2010). The efficacy of play therapy on ADHD, anxiety and social maturity in 8 to 12 years aged clientele children of Ahwaz metropolitan counseling clinics. *Journal of Applied Sciences (Faisalabad)*, *10*(3), 189–195. doi:10.3923/jas.2010.189.195

Packman, J., & Bratton, S. C. (2003). A school-based group play/activity therapy intervention with learning disabled preadolescents exhibiting behavior problems. *International Journal of Play Therapy*, *12*(2), 7–29. doi:10.1037/h0088876

Parker, N., & O' Brien, P. (2011). A play therapy reaching the child with autism. *International Journal of Special Education*, *26*(1), 80–87.

Piaget, J. (1962). *Play, dreams, and imitation in childhood*. New York: Norton.

Rakesh, A., & Srinath, S. (2010). Play therapy: Voice of a silent scream. *Journal of Indian Association for Child and Adolescent Mental Health*, *6*(1), 13–18.

Ray, D. C., Armstrong, S., Balkin, R., & Jayne, K. (2015). Child centered play therapy in the schools: Review and meta-analysis. *Psychology in the Schools*, *52*(2), 107–123. doi:10.1002/pits.21798

Ray, D. C., Schottelkorb, A., & Tsai, M. H. (2007). Play therapy with children exhibiting symptoms of ADHD. *International Journal of Play Therapy*, *16*(2), 95–111. doi:10.1037/1555-6824.16.2.95

Robinson, A., Simpson, C., & Hott, B. L. (2017). The effects of child centered play therapy on the behavioral performance of three first grade students with ADHD. *International Journal of Play Therapy*, *26*(2), 73–83. doi:10.1037/pla0000047

Rogers, C. (1951). *Client-centered therapy*. Boston: Houghton Mifflin Co.

Sarpoulaki, B., & Kolahi, P. (2016). Role of play therapy on aggression and learning disabilities in students: A Quasi-experimental design. *International Journal of Indian Psychology*, *3*(4), 57.

Schaefer, C. E. (2003). *Foundations of play therapy*. Hoboken, NJ: John Wiley & Sons.

Schaefer, C. E. (2010). *Play therapy for preschool children*. Washington, DC: American Psychological Association. doi:10.1037/12060-000

Schaefer, C. E., & O'Connor, J. K. (1982). *Handbook of Play Therapy* (Vol. 1). Somerset, NJ: John Wiley & Sons, Inc.

Solomon, J. C. (1938). Active play therapy. *The American Journal of Orthopsychiatry*, *8*(3), 479–498. doi:10.1111/j.1939-0025.1938.tb06398.x

Swan, K., & Ray, D. (2014). Effects of child-centered play therapy on irritability and hyperactivity behaviors of children with intellectual disabilities. *Journal of Humanistic Counseling*, *53*(2), 120–133. doi:10.1002/j.2161-1939.2014.00053.x

Taylor, D. D., & Bratton, S. C. (2014). Developmentally appropriate practice: Adlerian play therapy with preschool children. *Journal of Individual Psychology*, *70*(3), 205–219. doi:10.1353/jip.2014.0019

Ware, J. N. (2014). *Play Therapy for Children with Autism Spectrum Disorder: A Single-Case Design (Doctor of Philosophy)*. Counseling.

Webb, N. (2011). Play therapy for bereaved children: Adapting strategies to community, school, and home settings. *School Psychology International*, *32*(2), 132–143. doi:10.1177/0143034311400832

White, J., & Allers, C. T. (1994). Play therapy with abused children: A review of the literature. *Journal of Counseling and Development*, *72*(4), 390–394. doi:10.1002/j.1556-6676.1994.tb00955.x

KEY TERMS AND DEFINITIONS

Bubble Breaths: It is a technique of relaxation which involves teaching children deep and controlled breathing to make them aware regarding their body and mind connections.

Feeling Word Game: It allows children to express and connect their emotions and feelings in a non-fearful and non-threatening way.

Mad Game: It is designed to provide awareness to the children with anger suggesting that anger is a primary emotion which is easily acceptable.

Neurodevelopmental Disorders: It is a group of disorders that occur during the developmental period and affects all the developmental aspects of the child such as communication, cognition, social, etc.

Non-Directive Play Therapy: It is a psychological intervention method used to help children communicate their inner experiences through the use of toys and play.

Play: It is a physical or mental activity that engages the individual either for enjoyment or recreation.

Play Therapy: It is a form of psychological intervention where the play is used as a medium to help children to express or communicate their feelings.

Chapter 15
Certification and Medico-Legal Aspects of Neurodevelopmental Disorders in India

Srinivasan Venkatesan
All India Institute of Speech and Hearing, India

G. Y. Yashodharakumar
All India Institute of Speech and Hearing, India

ABSTRACT

With the emerging fields of medical jurisprudence and forensic medicine, cases of neurodevelopmental disorders in engagement or conflict with law are on the rise. Affected persons as alibi, victims, or perpetrators of crime are dotting as civil or criminal proceedings in contemporary courts. Rehabilitation specialists must be conversant with the medico-legal process, their duties, and responsibilities as subject experts to witness given their role in the certification of these cases. They must be aware of the problems and issues in certification during clinical practice. This chapter outlines the concerns related to estimation, measurement, and disability certification. Case vignettes are used to illustrate sample court proceedings during deposition before the attorney and at the time of cross-examination. Empirical research is reviewed before concluding this narrative with an agenda for future action to move away from traditional medical models toward understanding these disorders from human rights and person-in-environment perspectives.

INTRODUCTION

Psychiatrists are continued to be viewed as the mainstay in matters of certification for affected persons with mental ill-health conditions. The adjuvant role of clinical psychologists and psychiatric social workers (deemed as paraprofessionals) becomes important only as we move away from the traditional medical toward the contemporary human rights model (Goswami, Venkatesan, & Mathew, 2015; Morris, 2001). During legal proceedings, the courts are interested in a numerical quantification of the degree or extent of impairment, disability or handicap affecting such persons. The disability estimation, although

DOI: 10.4018/978-1-5225-7004-2.ch015

a simplistic derivative for referring to a complex behavioral phenomenon is required for grant of various benefits, concessions and/or compensations. To do so, issuing certificates has become an integral part of professional work.

The dictionary meaning of certificate is straightforward. It is 'an official document stating the result of a satisfactory examination'. It is meant to 'attest a fact in particular'. It is a 'written testimony of status, privileges or the truth of something'. In the context of disability, the certificate is not merely a document for the affected person. It is also a documentary proof of the condition for availing facilities, rights, or entitlements provided by the respective state or government of which one is the citizen. Certification involves and ensures a variety of functions. It gives a diagnostic label or nomenclature based on some official system of classification. It suggests treatment recommendation. Unlike a medical certificate of illness and/or fitness, whose validity is temporary, a certificate of disability has a longer shelf life or is sometimes issued for permanent use by the affected individual. There are usually similar or different guidelines for application, issue or receipt of disability certificates. There are authorities that are typically empowered or earmarked to issue them, a term or period until which they are deemed valid, prescribed formats in which they are issued, or some stated purposes for which they are given, and certain laws under which they are safeguarded (Perry & Drogin, 2007).

MEDICO-LEGAL CASE

Irrespective of their nature, type, purpose, or content, all disability reports and certificates have the potential of becoming an instrument of a Medico-Legal Case (MLC). For example, a psychological report stating below average level of intellectual functioning in a student can turn into a medico-legal document following a complaint of any discriminatory practice at school. MLCs involve both medical and legal aspects. They require investigation by law enforcing agencies in order to essentially fix the responsibility regarding causation of some harm, offense or that which explains the present state of the individual (Meera, 2016; Raveesh, Nayak, & Kumbar, 2016; Aggrawal, 2015).

Encounters with judicial system for persons with Neurodevelopmental Disorders (NDD) can occur through civil or criminal proceedings. Civil proceedings occur wherein one party sues another for personal injuries. Criminal proceedings take place where the law is broken and charges are made by police as a result of an assault. In either case, it involves procedures and practices of questioning, production of records, swearing by a document called affidavit including case sheet, interview reports, audio-video samples, written samples, test protocols, etc. The questioning happens wherein the lawyer representing plaintiff (complainant or petitioner) has the opportunity to question the defendant (accused) under oath (Carter, 2011). Some examples of medico-legal cases related to NDD are assault or battery including domestic violence and child abuse, road traffic accidents or sports injuries, cases of physical or mental trauma with suspicion of foul play, electrical injuries, poisoning, drug overuse or alcohol intoxication, burns and chemical injuries, sexual offences, attempted suicide, cases of asphyxia, hanging, strangulation, drowning, suffocation, unnatural deaths, or firearm injuries.

The medicolegal process begins with marking or labeling a file as 'MLC'. Registration of medicolegal cases is a must under Section 39 of the Code of Criminal Procedure. The medical profession is duty bound by contract under the law to serve and not to refuse. Failure to do so will attract legal penalty and prosecution. Referrals as MLCs are likely to come from the police, fellow professionals or institutions, from the courts or by relatives of the affected cases with some ulterior motive. The case record must have a separate identity or record number. The obtaining of 'consent' is an important prerequisite for all these cases. Consent happens between two or more persons who agree upon the same thing in the same sense. For clinical examination, diagnosis and treatment, any person who is conscious, mentally sound and 18+ years of age are entitled to give consent. The consent is invalid if given or extracted by intimidation, under fear, fraud, duress, or by misrepresentation of facts or from persons below adult age. There are three types of consent: (a) Implied Consent; (b) Expressed Verbal or Written Consent, and; (c) Informed Consent. The informed consent formats prescribed for use in clinical studies, for assent from children or minors during research are different from those used in medical-legal context.

Once registered, the medicolegal case record or document must be carefully maintained and attended on priority. The attending specialist is liable to be summoned as an expert witness to give evidence for or on behalf of the case. The expert is one whom either through education or experience has developed skill or knowledge in a particular subject enabling them to form an opinion that will assist the fact-finder. It may include doctors, paramedics, statisticians, or anyone whose proficiency or opinion matters for a given case. In the Indian context, medical practitioners are expected to be registered with the Medical Council, and rehabilitation professionals must have a registration number from Rehabilitation Council of India.

Witness in a court can come in many forms. A lay witness is different from a professional witness who has given treatment for the case. An eyewitness is a person who has seen the event occur firsthand through the senses of seeing, hearing, smelling and touching. An expert witness is asked to furnish a considered opinion owing to superior knowledge of an art or profession about a case. They are deemed to have special skills since they are trained in that given science, technique, language, or foreign law. They are experienced by practice and observation in that trade or science. They may not be required to have witnessed the event when it occurred. The expert witness is permitted to refer textbooks, check archives or standard references, consult seniors or colleagues to substantiate their claims. The expert may be summoned by the prosecution, defense, judge or a tribunal. A distinction is made between a testifying expert who appears under oath in front of the judge to speak the truth and nothing but the truth in the name of God; and, non-testifying expert, who may be hired by a contesting party to evaluate the facts of the case. Such an expert helps the attorney to prepare a case without testifying in the court of law (Brodsky, 2013; Kapardis, 2010). All expressions of statements made by the expert in court must be carried out only after a professional examination of the parties involved. A 30-day time frame is typically given to experts for submission of their technical report. The fee for experts and the charges for the medical-legal report are fixed by the court. An opportunity for rebuttal of expert opinion is allowed. Attendance of the expert upon summon from the court is mandatory. Summons may be issued by the Registrar or the Prothonotary of the court to appear in a particular court, on a given day, and at a stated time for a given case. The recipient must acknowledge summons by affixing a signature and seal. If the time is unsuitable or too short a notice, mention must be made on the summons before seeking a fresh date in writing or through personal appearance. Summons may not be honored only under exceptional circumstances like personal preoccupation, indisposition, or professional priorities. Whatever the reason for non-appearance, it must be conveyed to the court in proper time and permission must be sought thereof without delay (Blau, 2001).

Every medico-legal case must have a unique identification number along with the personal and socio-demographic details of the client, such as name, date of birth, age, gender, education, occupation, religion, residential address (permanent and temporary), AADHAR (it is a 12-digit unique identity number and can be obtained by residents of India) details, and cell-phone or email contacts. It is vital to record their date and time of visit, details of the accompanying escorts (police and/or relatives), their duration of acquaintance, as well as a mention about the professional colleague in whose presence all the transactions have taken place. Where possible, a written transcript or audio-video recording of the professional-patient transactions must be retained. Lady examiners must opt for cases involving gender sensitive issues. Cutting, over-writing, use of abbreviations must be avoided in the notes. Preservation of records in sealed envelopes in safe custody is a must. Their alteration, loss or destruction is a punishable offense (Sharma, 2008).

Medico-legal expert testimony in cases involving NDD is different from the clinical skills needed for their diagnosis or treatment planning. There are many ethical, legal, and business stipulations that come with such undertakings. This is quite different from standard clinical practice. The assessment and diagnostic formulation must meet contemporary practices called in the medico-legal parlance as 'Daubert Standard'. This provides a rule of evidence regarding the admissibility of expert witness testimony during legal proceedings. The examiners are expected to understand and use medico-legal terminology. The report should incorporate all details related to developmental, academic, family, and past history. Complicated cases must be discussed with seniors or colleagues (Gutheil & Drogin, 2013). Last, but not the least, the court demeanour and etiquette must be respected. Dress and appearance are important. Wearing of mutilated clothing, night dress, bathroom slippers, and transparent clothing is punishable. Standing up when the judge enters or leaves the court or when one's name is called is expected. One must speak aloud and address the judge with respect. All answers must be given briefly, to the point, and not uttered unless asked to explain. Use of mobile phones, ringtones, honking, or shouting is banned in court premises. Admitting that one does not know is appreciated by the court rather than making exaggerations talking excessively or pretentiously without knowing a subject. One must be cautious while answering hypothetical questions involving 'suppose', compounded or multiple questions, or queries under duress or when they are based on false assumptions even when posed during the cross-examination (Stevens, 2008).

Persons with NDD in engagement with judicial system or those in conflict with law may appear either as victims or accused during the medico-legal proceedings at court. In these circumstances, the expert witness is expected to professionally examine and testify by explaining the clinical condition of the patient in objective, accurate, observable and measurable terms. The retained written or audio-visual records are deemed as evidence in a court of law. The expert is obligated to explain their contents to the satisfaction of the court. One cannot or must not rely simply on one's memory. The reports must be preferably prepared in duplicate and supported with photographs, identification marks, consent forms, and/or biometrics. There are various sections under the Indian Penal Code stipulating sanctions and punishments even to the expert witness for infringements like fabricating or giving false evidence, causing their disappearance, intentional omission of information, destruction of record to prevent its use as evidence, etc. The recommended time duration for the preservation of records is at least ten years in case of adults and twelve years for minors. The court has right to take over any or all original documents or records at any time. Parties lose their right to get a copy of the records or test protocols while the investigations are going on or when the case is under judgment.

PRESENT SITUATION IN INDIA

Medical boards have been constituted at State Level, District Level, and Taluk Level to assess the percentage of disability in a given individual and then issue disability certificates for those who have 40 percent or more of the problem. An online portal is beginning to get into shape for the issue of identity cards and certificate of disability for net savvy seekers. The composition of a Medical Board is as follows: (a) Medical Superintendent/Principal/Director/Head of the institution or his nominee as Chairperson; (b) Psychiatrist-Member, and; (c) Physician-Member. At least two of them, including Chairperson of the board, must be present and sign the disability certificate. The certificate would be valid for a period of five years for those whose disability is 'temporary' and are below the age of 18 years. It is deemed 'permanent' for the older persons (Srivastava & Kumar, 2015; Nizamie, Prakash, Praharaj, & Akhtar, 2009). The working team of medical-rehabilitation professions earmarked in the Indian scenario for different disability conditions is as follows. The neurologist, neurophysician, neurosurgeon, and orthopaedic specialty group along with physiatrist and physiotherapists work for screening and certifying conditions like cerebral palsy, physical, or locomotion handicap and dwarfism. The psychiatrist and clinical psychologist dyad address certification issues of chronic mental illness as mental disability and/or intellectual disability. Clinical psychologists are earmarked to certify autism and specific learning disability. The neurologist-clinical neuropsychologist combines jointly to address organically brain damaged conditions with a cognitive-behavioral sequel. The audiologist, speech, and language specialist work with ENT specialists to measure and certify persons with hearing loss and/or speech-language impairments. The ophthalmologist-refractionist-oculist combine help certify persons with visual impairments. Depending on the nature, location or type of multiple disabilities, respective specialists are involved in the combined calculation of the percentage of handicap using a specified formula. There is a growing plea and momentum towards moving away from the medical models of disability certification towards the rights-based person-in environment positive and functional approaches by roping in the services of trained or licensed paraprofessionals in the field of rehabilitation (Goswami, Venkatesan, & Mathew, 2015).

The assessment of disability in mental illness is carried out by using a brief and simple instrument called 'Indian Disability Evaluation Assessment Scale' (IDEAS; 2002) developed by a Rehabilitation Committee or Disability Task Force of the Indian Psychiatric Society. This is used by a practitioner after receiving training for use only on out-patients living in the community. A watered-down adaptation of WHO-Disability Assessment Schedule-II (WHO-DAS-II; Ustun, Kostanjsek, Chatterji, & Rehm, 2010), the IDEAS cannot be used on in-patients during their short or long stay in the hospital. The ratings are carried out based on interviews of the primary caregivers although information from case records and patient interviews may be supplemented. The scale addresses only three diagnostic conditions-all deemed as NDD: Schizophrenia, Bipolar Disorder, and Obsessive Compulsive Disorder. The total duration of illness must have been for at least two years. The disability must be re-assessed and re-certified at least once in two years. The domains covered by this tool include self-care, interpersonal activities (or social relationships), communication and understanding and work-related either to employment, housework or education. Scoring ranges from zero (no disability), 1 (mild disability), 2 (moderate disability), 3 (severe disability) and 4 (profound disability) respectively. The maximum score is 20. It must be noted that many psychological, lifestyle and social issues can inflate or deflate the scores on this tool to give a false impression (Kumar, 2017; Mohan, Tandon, Kalra, & Trivedi, 2005; Thara, 2005). The most commonly found patients with disability among mental illness by this scale are those with schizophrenia and affective disorder (Kasthuri, Sharan, Chandrashekar, & Kumar, 2016).

A disability resulting from neurological illness is more than the diagnosis of a neurological condition. It is a measurement of the clinical manifestations of disability, impairment or handicap resulting from that condition. Moving away from medical domain, this borders on to legal aspects. For example, a rule states that no person who has acquired a neurological disability or has become permanently incapacitated while in government service can be dispensed with, reduced in rank or denied promotion on the ground of the disability. Despite all this, neurological disability has not been taken as a separate entity. It is grouped under orthopedic or locomotor disability under the Rights of Persons with Disabilities Act, 2016 (Radhakrishna, 2008).

The criteria for measurement of clinical manifestations of neurological disorders take into account clinical features like speech impairment (moderate dysarthria as 25% and severe dysarthria as 50%), motor nerve involvement (20% for each), sensory nerve involvement (10% for each), hemiparesis (mild as 25%, moderate as 50%, and severe degree as 75%), anaesthesia (of each limb as 10%), bladder problems (mild hesitancy or frequency as 25%, moderate as 50%, severe recurrent incontinence as 75%, and very severe or total incontinence as 100%). Similar yardsticks are given for post head injury fits and epileptic convulsions of moderate degree (1-5 episodes per month as 26%), severe degree (6-10 attacks per month as 50%) and very severe degree (more than 10 events per month as 75%). Ataxia of moderate degree is scored 50%, severe nature is rated as 75%, and the very severe condition is taken as 100% respectively. The measurements depend upon a given examination or evaluation of a neurologically affected patient by the specialist, which can be dubbed as not being entirely objective. The evaluation of disability for neurological conditions against these many parameters could be tedious and time-consuming. Further, other important parameters especially those related to neuropsychological deficits in attention-concentration, thinking, memory, judgment, problem-solving, or cognition, as well as those related to swallowing dysfunction, spasticity, dystonia, rigidity, tremors and muscular fatigue, are not addressed at all (Murali, 2006).

All disabilities are expectedly expressed as percentages. Therefore, it is expected that intellectual disability is also expressed in terms of a percentage. In this process, Intelligence Quotient (IQ) range will be the fundamental criteria to derive the disability percentage. One should remember IQ itself cannot be interpreted as disability percentage. A common misunderstanding is that IQ is direct equivalent of its percentage. An IQ of 70 is NOT equal to 70% intellectual disability just as another IQ of 25 is NOT to be mistaken for 25% intellectual disability. The percentage equivalents along with their International Classification for Disease (ICD) codes for the different range of IQs are as follows (Table 1):

There are other drawbacks in disability estimation of neurological disorders. The maximum percentage allowed for severe dysarthria as speech impairment is 50 only. The use of Mini-Mental Status Examination (MMSE; Upton, 2013; Jain & Passi, 2005; Folstein, Folstein, & McHugh, 1975) is insufficient to certify disability. Ideally, a comprehensive neuropsychological testing and profiling of cognitive assets-deficits along with the involvement of lobe functions would be required to estimate disability quotient. Epilepsy

Table 1. IQ range and degree/level of mental retardation

IQ Range	Degree/Level of Mental Retardation	ICD Code	Percentage
70-90	Below Average Intelligence (Slow Learner)	R41.83	25
50-69	Mild Intellectual Disability	F70	50
35-49	Moderate Intellectual Disability	F71	75
20-34	Severe Intellectual Disability	F72	90
<20	Profound Intellectual Disability	F73	100

(Source: 7.3 Table II: Intellectual Impairment to be assessed by a clinical psychologist; Office of the Chief Commissioner of Persons with Disabilities, Ministry of Social Justice and Empowerment, Government of India; No. 16-18/98-NI.

is graded only by its frequency irrespective of whether or not the patient is on anti-epileptic medication. A challenge for disability certification in neurological conditions is prediction and prognostication based on an individual's current status or functioning based on the age of onset, severity, quality of life, leisure participation, lifestyle, available social supports and other apparently invisible factors (Dahan-Oliel, Shikako-Thomas, & Majnemer, 2012).

CASE VIGNETTES

Given below are illustrative case vignettes to highlight the common themes of persons with NDD in contact or conflict with the law and judicial system. A perusal of these sketches will reveal that they cover a wide range of life areas covering different real-life problems or issues (Table 2).

Case Vignette #1

Reference is hereby made to MS Gill vs. the State of Punjab on 11 January 2001, in Punjab-Haryana High Court. The case pertains to a petition seeking admission to MBBS Course in the reserve category for persons with disability on account of hearing impairment. It was appealed that he was called for counseling but not admitted into the course despite being fully eligible in every respect on account of the arbitrary, discriminatory and illegal action of the respondents at the time of counseling. Eligibility criteria for a candidate seeking admission under the category were 40%, and it was claimed that the petitioner had a 50db hearing loss in right ear along with atresia of external and canal lobule. It was contended by the respondents that a final decision on the extent of disability was taken by a Medical

Table 2. Common themes and problems of conflict with the law and judicial system in persons with NDD

Sl No.	Common Themes	Problems of Conflict with the Law and Judicial System
1.	Work, Employment and Labor	Loss of job; retention in sinecure positions; compensations for voluntary retirement, absenteeism, under-performance…
2.	Marriage & Family	Separation or divorce, pre-marriage non-disclosure, payment of alimony, custody of a child, dowry harassment, domestic violence…
3.	Succession and Inheritance	Hereditary positions, bequeath of property, guardianship …
4.	Education	Concessions and benefits related to inclusion, amanuensis, and allotment of extra time during examinations, providing calculators, word processors or choice of alternative subjects
5.	Health	Euthanasia, organ donation or transplant, consent for treatment …
6.	Community Participation	Voting, driver license, accessible visitations, non-discrimination …
7.	Insurance Cover/Compensation	Proportional to life expectancy, opportunity cost, based on age, education, social status …
8.	Guardianship	Proxy decision making, reconciling to alternate therapies or low-cost therapeutic management…
9.	Legality to witness	Validity, competence to testify in the court of law, or give informed consent …

Board with overriding effect on the findings of a single doctor. Moreover, it was noted that the defect of the petitioner is surgically treatable for giving good hearing thereafter. It was recommended that the audiology testing would have to be carried out in the sound-treated room to get accurate results. During repeat testing, it was observed that the petitioner's hearing responses were inconsistent and that he was malingering. In the left ear, his conversation was within normal limits. Going by the facts of the case, the honorable court dismissed the writ petition leaving the parties to bear their own costs (Anand, 2001).

Case Vignette #2

Reference is hereby made to appellants Rama s/o Late Muniyellappa and Muniraju s/o Thyagarajappa vs. State of Karnataka represented by Anekal Police, Bangalore Rural, on 16 December 2013, in High Court of Karnataka, Bangalore. The case pertains to section 374 Cr. P. C. (Unlawful compulsory labour liable for punishment with imprisonment for a term of one year or with fine, or with both) against the judgment passed by lower court under section 376 (g) of IPC (commits gang rape is punishable with rigorous imprisonment not less than ten years or for life along with fine).

The appellants were tried and convicted of an offense punishable under 376(g) IPC to undergo rigorous imprisonment for ten years and pay a fine of Rs. 12000/- each. The victim of the offense was referred by the court as 'mentally retarded girl'. She was aged about 16 years as in the year 2002. The accused and the victim belong to the same vicinity. The reports state that when the victim was playing with other children near tank bund in the village, the two accused took her in a two-wheeler to a nearby eucalyptus grove, and committed rape on her one after the other. A police complaint was lodged the next day. The honorable high court sought to determine whether the prosecution has proved the occurrence of the incident on the said date at the designated location, and whether the learned trial judge has properly appreciated evidence on record and to what order.

A reading of the judgment shows that the victim has deposed before the honorable court under oath, and during cross-examination has narrated the sequence of events with 'certain variations and discrepancies'. She denied the suggestion that she was tutored by her father. The mental age of the victim as inferred by the court was about 10-12 years. With no other direct witness at the scene of crime and the father's evidence only relating to 'post occurrence events', 'medical evidence adduced by prosecution not being sufficient to hold that there was a complete act of rape' by the accused, 'from the evidence of the investigating officer and other documents relied thereupon by the prosecution' not being established as belonging to the accused, and eventually, the 'victim not consenting for examination of her genitals', and giving a 'consistent, cogent' evidence that can be 'corroborated from other circumstantial evidence', as well as the learned counsel for the two accused submitting 'that a lenient view may be taken in the matter of sentence', an order was passed that the accused are acquitted of an offence punishable under section 376 (g) IPC. Instead, they are convicted of an offense punishable under sections 376 r/w 511 IPC, which amounts to only an attempt and not the consummation of rape (Swamy, 2014a, 2014b).

Case Vignette #3

Reference is hereby made to appellants Suchitha Srivastava and Anr and to Chandigarh administration as respondent on 28 August 2009, in Supreme Court of India. A division bench of the High Court of Punjab and Haryana ruled that it was in the best interests of a mentally retarded orphaned woman to undergo an abortion. The victim had become pregnant as a result of alleged rape that took place while she was an inmate at a government-run welfare institution located in Chandigarh. Based on the set of questions answered by an Expert Body constituted by it, the High Court directed the termination of pregnancy even though the victim had expressed her willingness to bear the child. Based on an appeal for hearing on an urgent basis, since the woman was already pregnant for 19 weeks, a list of the following key questions was posed: whether it was correct on part of the High Court to direct the termination of pregnancy without the consent of the woman in question? Even if the woman was assumed to be mentally incapable of making an informed decision, what are the appropriate standards for a Court to exercise `Parens Patriae' (the doctrine that grants inherent power and authority to the state to protect persons who are legally unable to act on their own)? What if she is incapable of making the distinction between a child born before or after marriage or outside the wedlock and is unable to understand the social connotations attached thereto? What about her mental and physical capacity to bear and raise a child? Is she able to understand she has been impregnated through unvolunteered sex? The final verdict was based on a consideration that termination of pregnancy cannot be permitted without the consent of the victim in this case. Based on results of an ossification test it is revealed that the physical age of the victim is around 19-20 years and therefore conclusively it is shown that she is not a minor (Balakrishnan, Sathasivam, & Chauhan, 2009).

Case Vignette #4

Reference is hereby made to petitioner G. Nithyanandam and to respondents Tmt. Saritha & Sri. G. Jeevanandam on 16 April 2013, in the High Court of Judicature at Madras. The original petition filed under section 3, 7-10, and 29 of Guardians and Wards Act, 1890, praying for the appointment of the petitioner (brother) as guardian of the person and property of Kum. G. Prabhavathy, mentally retarded person. The other two respondents are also siblings of the mentally retarded person. The further plea was that the father had already expired and the mother's whereabouts were unknown since 1995. Going by the circumstances of the case, a doubt arose as to how the provisions of Guardians and Wards Act, 1890, would apply in a case of appointment of a guardian to a 31-year old person with mental retardation. Therefore, an advocate with experience in handling similar issues was appointed as Amicus Curiae (someone who is not a party to a case and is not solicited by a party, but who assists a court by offering information that bears on the case). Based on the submissions made by Amicus Curiae, distinctions were clarified between mental retardation and mental illness, or that the provisions of the Mental Health Act (1987) do not apply in this case, and that sections under National Trust for Welfare of Persons with Autism, Cerebral Palsy, Mental Retardation, and Multiple Disabilities Act (1999) would be relevant. The said Act provides for constitution of Local Level Committee which as empowered for the appointment of guardian upon application in prescribed forms in such cases. In the result, the petitioner was directed to approach the District Collector, Chennai, Chairperson, Local Level Committee for claims of nomination as guardian (Nithyanandam, 2013).

Note that the role of Local Level Committee was reiterated in petitioner Sri. Narayan Kutty Menon s/o Govinda vs. Respondent in State of Kerala represented by Chief on 17 February 2009, in High Court of Kerala, Ernakulam.

Case Vignette #5

There are continuing confusions between 'mental retardation' and 'mental illness' within the walls of many courts is testified in the judgment of Petitioner Jagjit Singh and Anr vs. Respondent in Delhi Developmental Authority on 26 November 2012 in the High Court of Delhi, New Delhi, wherein 'one of the sellers of premises is Mukesh s/o Late Narain Singh who is suffering from severe degree of mental retardation'. It excludes the applicability of the Mental Health Act (1987) as the definition of 'mentally ill person'. It is a case wherein the learned counsel for petitioners makes it clear that the two terms are 'two different ailments of same species but are governed by two different enactments' (Gaur, 2012).

Case Vignette #6

In the Petitioner Tarun Chatterjee and Anr vs. Respondent as Union of India and Ors on 4 September, 2017, in Calcutta High Court, Calcutta, eight persons, who are all employees of Tea Board, an autonomous body under Government of India, since their entry into service, were transferred to different zones and regional offices. The petitioners contended that the transfers were illegal, arbitrary and mala fide. The wife of the first appellant is working under Integrated Child Development Scheme and is posted in the district of North 24-Parganas and his son is also suffering from attention deficit hyperactivity disorder (ADHD). Despite all this, the court dismissed the application (Mukherjee & Sadhu, 2014).

Case Vignette #7

Reference is hereby made to petitioner Shubang Sharma s/o Shridhar Sharma vs. Chairman, Bar Council of India, Vice Chancellor, Hidayathullah National Law University, and Registrar and Examination Controller, Hidayathullah National Law University, as respondents on 28 April 2017, in the High Court of Chattisgarh, Bilaspur. The honorable court order directed the Bar Council of India to take a decision regarding allowing one-hour extra time to the petitioner for writing the examination and awarding 20 grace marks in view of his learning disability. In addition, the petitioner was permitted to write in margins (header and footer) and was exempted from writing those papers which are not taught in law colleges under the five-year integrated law course (Khanna & Misra, 2011).

While there are or could be many more instances of children, juveniles or adults with NDD seeking justice at the honorable courts, most reported cases are on persons with intellectual disabilities. Cases of individuals affected by other NDD like ADHD, autism spectrum disorders (ASD), speech-language disabilities, and others are seldom reported. A few public interest litigations floated by enterprising and enthusiastic non-government organizations have sought court interventions for implementation of the mandated reservations in jobs under public service and/or school admissions under the 'disadvantaged' or 'under-privileged' quota for students with a disability having special needs. Although there are regular media reports on the use of corporal punishment against known or unknown children with disabilities, they seldom amble their way to eventually reach the corridors of the courts (Venkatesan, 2015). Even wherein laws undergo periodic change, it is unlikely that people at the helm of affairs do undergo knowledge and attitudinal change at the same pace (Box #2). Until then, children continue to be blamed, coerced, stripped of their opportunities, denied the exercise of their rights and subjected to various ignominies or insults at home and school (Venkatesan, 2014; 2011). There is the likelihood that sizeable numbers of these affected children may get recognized or adjudged as juvenile delinquents in the country (Venkatesan & Swarnalata, 2013). It is seen that few court interventions are more to do with procedural wrangles on or about which rule or under which sections/subsections a given case involving such children with NDD must be taken up, presented or argued.

Despite the increasing incidence of children, adolescents, or adults with intellectual disabilities coming in contact with the justice system, there is still a lag in the manner in which the courts understand their problems or issues. To begin with, the nomenclature has changed (Carulla, Reed, Vaez-Azizi, Cooper, Leal, Bertelli, ... & Girimaji, 2011). It has been a long journey from early references to 'lunatics, idiots, imbeciles, and morons' in Indian Lunacy Act (1912). The Mental Healthcare Act (2017) refers to 'person' with mental illness, and 'The Rights of Persons with Disability Act' (2016) has also a changed terminology. The idea and intention are to eliminate the stigma and negative connotations that are conveyed through earlier terms like 'insane, dumb, deaf, blind, lame, crippled', or others. However, in actual practice, the use of non-stigmatizing, non-judgmental and neutral new terms is yet to gain acceptance in judicial practice. Personal experience of the first author (Box #3) has shown that the courts are still grappling at the basic level of attempting to understand the status role, scope of practice, the professional boundaries, their rules, duties, and responsibilities especially in the context of clinical populations with NDD. Probably, a meeting ground needs to be drawn between the judiciary and these helping professionals through a radical revision of curriculum during graduate and postgraduate training both in medical as well as law schools. There are provisions for the establishment of exclusive disability courts in the lines of 'courts' or 'police stations' exclusively for women' and/or 'children and juveniles' (Kumari, 2010). There is the office of Chief Commissioner for Persons with Disabilities who is vested with the power of a civil court under the Code of Civil Procedure under Sections 193 and 228 of the Indian Penal Code.

CHILDREN AND TEENAGERS IN CONFLICT WITH LAW

This refers to a population of anyone under eighteen who comes into contact with the justice system as a result of being suspected or accused of committing an offense. It may be petty crimes and minor offenses (also called status offenses) like vagrancy, truancy, begging, or alcohol use. Or it could also mean instances wherein they have engaged in serious criminal behavior at the behest or owing to coercion by adults. The juvenile justice system works on the principle of correction, repatriation, restoration, remediation or rehabilitation of such children and teenagers rather than meting out punishments as in the adults. It works on the lofty principle of presumption of innocence, dignity, and worth, right to be heard, the best interest of the juvenile, family responsibility, safety, use of positive measures, a fresh start, equality and non-discrimination, and non-waiver of rights. Therefore, such children are directed away from the adult judicial system towards community solutions, promoting restorative justice through reconciliation, restitution, and responsibility by giving alternatives to custodial sentencing like counseling, probation and community service by involving the child as well as their family members (Hansaria & Jose, 2010).

In India, the number of cases of juvenile delinquents has doubled since the 1990s to the post-millennium period. A part of this increase may be attributed to the changing definition of juveniles from 16 to 18 years. Nonetheless, more and more teenagers in the age group of 16-18 are coming into conflict with the law. The Juvenile Justice (Care and Protection of Children) Act of 2015 is the key legislation which provides a legal framework for juvenile justice in India. The Act provides a procedure for trial of children in conflict with the law and the orders that can be passed by Juvenile Justice Board when they are found guilty of commission of the offense. Such children are lodged in Observation Homes, Special

Homes or Place of Safety under the Act. The 2015 version of the law segregates children who have perpetrated heinous crimes and vests the discretion of the Board to decide whether the youth between 16-18 years is to be tried in the adult criminal justice system as opposed to the juvenile justice system. Offences against children with disabilities are made a special mention for being given priority under this Act (Mathur, 2017; Delhi Commission for Protection of Child Rights, 2015; Jacob, Golhar, Sheshadri, Mani, & Purushothaman, 2014; Konar, 2005).

Despite the absence of an agreed-upon definition or description of NDD, it is traditionally thought to be associated with brain changes at varying degrees of the organization since birth or early childhood. It is viewed as having enduring structural and functional consequences even until adolescent and adulthood. It is postulated as being genetic as well as environmental in origin. One view assumes that low dose exposure to neurotoxins like lead affect the developing brain in utero and during early childhood. This leads to later problems in cognition, communication, and behavior in NDD (Szpir, 2006). There is no complete or exhaustive agreed upon list of NDD. If one follows DSM-5, it can include intellectual disability, ASD, ADHD, tics, stereotypic movement disorder, developmental conduct disorder, communication disorders and specific learning difficulties. It would mean another list if one follows another classification.

It is shown that prevalence of NDD in prison populations of the United Kingdom is high (Underwood, Forrester, Chaplin, & McCarthy, 2013). For example, ADHD is present in 12-40% of prison population, which is 5-fold increase over the 4% of its prevalence in general population (Young, Moss, Sedgwick, Fridman, & Hodgkins, 2015; Ginsberg, Langstrom, Larsson, & Lichtenstein, 2014; Ginsberg & Lindefors, 2012; Ginsberg, Hirvikoski, & Lindefors, 2010; Rosler, Retz, Yaqoobi, & Retz-Junginger, 2009). It is shown that around 4.4% of persons with ASD in prisons and 1% of the general population with the condition have difficulties with establishing social relationships (Fazio, 2014). The distribution of ASD traits among prisoners appears to be normal and is not significantly higher than the rate found in population-based samples (Ashworth, 2016; Underwood, McCarthy, Chaplin, Forrester, Mills, & Murphy, 2016). Similarly, around 8-10% of the prison populations are reported as inmates with an intellectual disability having difficulties in comprehending rules and maintaining effective social relationships (Hayes, Shackell, Mottram, & Lancaster, 2007). There are grounds to suspect that about 5-10% of the offender, under-trial and/or inmate population in state prisons across countries might be persons with intellectual disabilities (Kebbell & Davies, 2003). There are instances of people with IQ as low as 25 (severe to profound intellectual disabilities) found within the penal system in the United States (Noble & Conley, 1992).

Venkatesan (2015) elicited data from 75 cases of persons with intellectual disabilities to compile 10 distinct areas, 37 themes and 7 levels of their contemplated and/or attempted engagements with the justice system covering areas of concern related to marriage, education, health, housing, employment, inheritance, citizenship, civil and political participation, legal capacity, decision-making, custody, reimbursement, and victimization. Although there was an apparent intent to seek judicial redress, their actual engagements with the formal justice system are minimal at 41% and the eventual 'verdict rate' is as low as 13%.

Children and adolescents with specific learning disabilities show greater proclivity towards offending risk or reoffending and may be associated with discipline and regime problems within the prison settings. Berman (1974) reported that half of the juvenile offenders showed signs of learning disabilities. Larson (1988) stated that youth with learning disabilities were adjudicated about twice as often as those without disabilities and delinquents with learning disabilities show a greater likelihood of recidivism and parole failure. Keilitz and Dunivant (1986) reported that youth with learning disabilities who had not been adjudicated were also more involved in delinquent acts than their peers who had no disabilities. Maughan et al (1985) found that 67% of their sample of adolescents with learning disabilities had records of juvenile delinquency. While observers agree that many children involved in juvenile delinquency cases have troubled schooling and academic problems (Unger, 1978; McKay & Brumback, 1980; Broder & Dunivant, 1981; Perlmutter, 1987; Waldie & Spreen, 1993), the issue of a link between learning disability and juvenile delinquency is far from being resolved (Broder & Dunivant, 1981; Larson, 1988; Crawford, 1996). The greater representation of children with learning disability in the population of juvenile delinquents does not necessarily make it a causal factor.

Juvenile delinquency in the background or context of NDD is an untouched area. Laypersons erroneously presume that children or teenagers who indulge in serious crimes like rape and murder are probably more mature for their age. Empirical evidence on adolescent brain and psychology contradict these assumptions. Neuroscience has shown that the pre-frontal cortex of the brain, which is responsible for performing higher mental functions like organizing, planning, strategizing, reasoning, judgment, decision making, and impulse control, is the slowest to mature. The process completes only by the age of twenty-five. Therefore, adolescents are more susceptible to negative influences and peer-pressure. They are less likely to focus on future outcomes, show poor impulse control, and are unable to evaluate risks and benefits of their actions. The adversarial adult criminal justice system is very inappropriate for juveniles in conflict with the law as they lack the capacity to participate in trials like adults (Scott & Steinberg, 2008; Cauffman & Steinberg, 2000).

The criminal doctrine distinguishes between adults and children or adolescents. This is even more true for those with intellectual or developmental disability. They are laggard in the light of their neural development. It would not be fair, in some sense, to expect them to do as an adult when they do not have the same cognitive capacity. They cannot be deemed as being inconsiderate of others on account of some moral deficiency. They are less considerate than mature adults because they are erroneously assumed to be wired differently. All this raises the issue whether they should be absolved of the crimes they indulge. For example, the courts generally prohibit the imposition of death penalty for even heinous crimes committed before age eighteen. Can neural under-development or immaturity become grounds for acquittal is a critical question? If the adolescent is less blameworthy because of diminished capacity; by the same token, adults with diminished capacity also should be less blameworthy. Admittedly, neuroscience is currently too imprecise to resolve this conundrum (Alces, 2018).

As mentioned earlier, children and adolescents can be roped in as perpetrators of crime as well as victims. Crimes reported on children as doers include assault resulting in grievous hurt, causing injury by rash driving, unlawful assembly, rioting, gambling, illegal betting, use of drugs, sexual harassment, attempting to outrage modesty of woman, voyeurism, stalking, theft, criminal trespass and burglary, robbery, dacoity and extortion, cheating, arson, forgery and counterfeiting. Crimes against children with NDD can include infanticide, feticide, abandonment, murder, rape, kidnap and abduction, abetment of suicide, attempt to commit murder, child/bonded labor, sexual harassment, use of a child for pornography, child marriage, sale and human trafficking. There are separate sections on crimes or atrocities against women, elderly, economic and cyber offenses, and those against the scheduled castes and tribes. However, there is no segment on crimes by or against children and adolescents with disabilities (NCRB, 2016). Their plight may be further aggravated by insensitive police dealing, long delays in the judicial process, the pendency of cases before Juvenile Justice Boards, inadequate rehabilitation mechanism and the paucity of aftercare facilities.

In sum, despite the doubts whether neurobiological underpinnings, those related to abnormal structure and function of amygdala and orbital-frontal cortex of early life, could have its effect on later life (Gao, Glenn, & Schug, 2009), there is consensus that prison populations of young adult offenders (age 18-25 years) met the official diagnostic criteria for ADHD and ASD in particular which are bracketed under NDD (Billstedt, Anckarsater, Wallinius, & Hofvander, 2017; McCarthy, Chaplin, Underwood, Forrester, Hayward, Sabet, Young, Asherson, Mills, & Murphy, 2016). There are indications that neurodevelopmental insults and psychopathy are not interrelated but are both directly and independently related to criminal violence and antisocial parenting (Harris, Rice, & Lalumiere, 2001). Some NDD, especially ASDs have elevated risk for subsequent violent criminality compared to matched unaffected controls (Lundstrom, 2014). A study reported that 28% of known multiple or serial killers had definite, highly probable or possible ASD, 22% had definite or suspected head injury, and 55% had experienced psychosocial stressors thereby concluding that there is lack of rigorous studies and that most of the literature is anecdotal and speculative (Allely, Minnis, Thompson, Wilson, & Gilberg, 2014).

Despite the advantages that it affords, there is a growing argument that the very public process or act of disability certification can be construed as invasion and infringement into the privacy of health information (Mishra, Parker, Nimgaonkar, & Deshpande, 2012). Anyone seeking a certificate from a specified government healthcare provider must submit personal details with a photograph which increase their risk of a breach in confidentiality in case the instrument is stolen, lost or even merely viewed by unauthorized persons. Further, the certificates usually give details of not only the diagnosis but also the degree, severity, or duration of their condition. While some visible disabilities are apparent, and cannot be concealed, there are others, such as, specific learning disability, paranoia, and/or obsessive-compulsive disorder which, one may not wish that others should come to know. While professionals are mandated not to disclose the private information of those who come to seek help, the issue of a disability certificate may become a distinctive and largely avoidable invasion of privacy.

Case Vignette #8

Reference is hereby made to Criminal Appeal Nos. 1217-1219 of 2017 between Ms. Eera through Dr. Manjula Krippendort (Appellant) versus State Government NCT of Delhi (Respondent) pertaining to the interpretation of Section 2(d) of the Protection of Children from Sexual Offences (POSCO) Act, 2012. The said section defines 'child' as any person below the age of 18 years. It was contended whether a 38-year old woman with an intellectual disability and cerebral palsy having a measured equivalent mental age of six to eight years, a victim of assault and rape, would be deemed as child or adult? The victim is intellectually in no position to depose on her own behalf and is, therefore, represented through and by her mother. The two main prayers were: (i) transfer the case to Special Court established under the POSCO Act as the functional age of the prosecutrix is six to eight years, and; (ii) that the case should be assigned to a trial court presided by a lady judge. It was submitted that a mentally retarded person may have the body mass, weight, and height which will match their physical or chronological age, but in reality behave like a child of their mental age. The submission was buttressed with similar cases. Clear distinctions between the terms 'mental retardation', 'developmental delay', and its measurements by means of 'mental age', 'intelligence quotient', 'development quotient' and 'social quotient' was enunciated. The verdict states that it is 'quite possible that a person with low IQ or mental age may possess the social and emotional capacities that will enable him or her to be a good parent'. It was stated that 'a developmental delay in mental intelligence should not be equated with mental incapacity and as far as possible the law should respect the decisions made by persons who are found to be in a state of mild to moderate "mental retardation" (Misra, 2017).

The Parliament has felt it appropriate to define the term 'age' by chronological or biological age as the safest yardstick than by referring to a person by his or her 'mental age'. This may be due to the fact that the standards of mental retardation are different and they require to be determined by an expert body. Their degree is also different. The Parliament, as it seems, has not included mental age…within the domain of legislative wisdom. By saying "age" would cover 'mental age' has the potential to create immense anomalous situations without there being any guidelines or statutory provisions. Needless to say, they are within the sphere of the legislature. The matter of providing compensation to the victim is viewed by the court as another matter that could seize for consideration by the respective District Legal Services Authority (DLSA).

PROBLEMS AND ISSUES

Despite the advantages that it affords, there is a growing argument that the very public process or act of disability certification can be construed as invasion and infringement into the privacy of health information (Mishra, Parker, Nimgaonkar, & Deshpande, 2012). Anyone seeking a certificate from a specified government healthcare provider must submit personal details with a photograph which increase their risk of a breach in confidentiality in case the instrument is stolen, lost or even merely viewed by unauthorized persons. Further, the certificates usually give details of not only the diagnosis but also the degree, severity, or duration of their condition. While some visible disabilities are apparent, and cannot be concealed, there are others, such as, specific learning disability, paranoia, and/or obsessive-compulsive disorder which, one may not wish that others should come to know. While professionals are mandated not to disclose the private information of those who come to seek help, the issue of a disability certificate may become a distinctive and largely avoidable invasion of privacy.

It must be noted that very little is being taught about disability and disability certification even at post-graduation levels across disciplines or specialties in India. There is need to create *national standards for training and certification* of rehabilitation specialists suitable for Indian conditions. Continuing education programs on this theme rarely happen. Periodic auditing of certificates issued by authorized persons or institutions by a competent authority must be in place to prevent errors as well as intended or unintended fraud. On many occasions, it occurs that a certificate issued by a competent authority is contested or even rejected by someone (such as school teacher or a ticket checker) owing to their own uninformed or prejudiced assumption that the person has no problem at all. At most, they were authorized only to verify the identity of the person by matching names or photograph of the person on the document. This amounts to trespassing limits of one's duties and responsibilities.

Another common problem encountered in clinical practice is related to *fraud by duplication*. There are instances wherein affected persons have availed certificates from two different doctors or institutions from the same discipline albeit with different estimations of their disability for securing benefits. Disability detection camps are being organized by various government and non-government organizations at various places to ensure the spread of certification to more beneficiaries. It is time-saving, economical and benefits persons or cases that cannot travel or reach out institution-based certification issue services. Although such one-shot or single-window schemes of issuing disability certificates appear temptingly advantageous, there are risks of over inclusion, false positive and undeserving persons receiving the benefits (Kashyap, Thunga, Rao, & Balamurali, 2012).

Another frequent challenge facing the practicing clinician authorized to issue disability certificate in Indian setting is *malingering*. Disability claims to receive pecuniary benefits, insurance gains, and to escape punishment is common. Malingering or illness deception refers to the intentional production of false or grossly exaggerated physical or psychological symptoms motivated by external incentives such as avoiding work, evading criminal prosecution, or for obtaining drugs. All this raises a doubt whether there some conscious plan to deceive. In the context of children, there is also the peril of what is called as malingering-by-proxy. It is the feigning of disability for compensation at the direction or pressure by others. At an extreme, it becomes a form of child abuse called Munchausen Syndrome-by-proxy, wherein a caregiver, usually the mother, induces illness or disability-like condition to gain attention for herself (Dumitrascu, Gallardo, & Caplan, 2015; Chafetz & Dufrene, 2014; Morrell & Tilley, 2012).

In Indian scene, malingering may be tutored by touts and peddlers who ensnare gullible customers and pre-indoctrinate on what questions would be asked by the certifying authorities or how they should maintain a façade of silence, unresponsiveness, and negativism to secure a financial benefit. It goes without saying that a good share of the pecuniary benefits goes into the pockets of these agents who throng the corridors of many government hospitals. They exploit people's wariness of the convoluted and time-consuming government processes to get the job done in no time for a price (Chandra, 2012; Nandi, 2010). In rare undetected cases, the beneficiary might have even reaped the advantage of a fake certificate before the long arm of the law can catch them (The Hindu, 2017b).

Ideally, disability estimation is not simply a matter of structural, bodily, or organic loss alone. It is not even enough to consider functional shortcomings in the affected person on what they can or cannot perform. Much more than that, a *person-in-the-environment perspective may need to be invoked* to take into account other soft parameters like extent of available accessibility, physical, social and attitudinal barriers, quality of life indices, availability of family, social and cultural supports, life satisfaction and happiness qualifiers, amount of discrimination, stigma and stereotyping in the milieu-which must be all factored into the final score (Goswami, Venkatesan, & Mathew, 2015; Subrahmanyam, 2007; Demeter & Andersson, 2003).

When the paradigm shift from medical models to right-based approach gathers momentum in the country, probably, the thrust should also move in the direction of empowering rehabilitation professionals along with medical specialists to certify individuals with a disability in their own merit. The rights-based certificate would cover protection for the affected individual across a variety of domains including education, work and employment, protection against violence, exploitation and abuse, health, home and family, culture, leisure and sport, legal capacity, life and living, protection and safety, liberty, privacy, freedom of speech and expression, live independently in community, right to exercise franchise, stand for election & hold public office, receive social security, etc.

Even though some rules are in place for identification and issue of officially recognized certificates of disability in deserving cases, there is scope and need for more empirical research on these lines. Fair and competent medico-legal reports must be issued by remaining within one's sphere of technical competence and avoiding professional trespassing. Navigating the disability certification process is a formidable task for the typical rural and non-ambulatory as well as the intellectually dependent affected persons who have to meander through the bureaucracy and red tape of several windows or desks to secure one certificate (Bilder & Mechanic, 2003). Cost-effective and time-saving practices or procedures are required in place for the issue of disability certificates for deserving cases. In a related study, it was shown that invisible and unaccounted costs incurred on the procurement of disability benefits from the government following official certification on intangibles like felt pain, stress, burden, social stigma and appeasement along with tangibles like time, effort and money were far exceeding (Venkatesan, 2010).

There is a concern related reliability and validity of the certification issued to persons with NDD. While there are grounds to believe that concurrent or simultaneous cross-sectional assessments between professionals and parents may have high congruence or correlation (Otenbacher, 2000; Venkatesan & Madhurao, 1990), what would be the consistency of diagnostic re-certification of the same persons over a period of time? What is the prospect that a child who was diagnosed as expressive speech delay during preschool years will be later diagnosed as academic delay during primary school and/or as learning disability during high school? Further, unlike in the west, there is no machinery or mechanism of any official body for periodic in-service training and certification of the specialists themselves who are authorized by law to issue such certificates for persons with NDD (Palmer, Percy, Tivnan, Jul, Tunnessen, & Scheiber, 2003).

Although textbooks make distinctions between various subtypes of NDD, in actual clinical practice one frequently encounters their co-existence or sharing of symptoms across disorders called as co-morbidity. The acronym ESSENCE (Early Symptomatic Syndromes Eliciting Neurodevelopmental Clinical Examinations) has been used to refer to the reality of children and their parents for especially young infants, toddlers, and preschoolers. Across domains of general development, language, and communication, social interrelationships, motor coordination, attention, activity, affect and sleep, there are several overlapping symptoms. When this is so, and a specialist sees the child, there is every possibility of their missing out the larger picture. It is deemed that there is no time to watch or wait. Something has to be done. Hence, the chances are that a hastened diagnosis may turn into an incorrect diagnosis (Gillberg, 2010).

SUMMARY

In sum, there is a need for perspective change in the certifying authorities to abandon the medical model of viewing impairment or disability as cause or consequence of the individual's condition. The disability certificate must take into account NOT only the percent of impairment but MORE SO the consequences impacting as a handicap. It is seen that mild or borderline multiple disability conditions can be even more impacting than moderate to severe singular conditions. Unfortunately, these are the conditions that do not even fall under the banner of those who are certified. There is a need for more research on: Evaluation of impact or outcomes of disability certification, environmental audits, and certification, cost-benefit analysis of certification, service delivery processes and benchmarking on certification, consumer behavior in service delivery systems, ecological and ethnographic studies covering ethnic, cultural or phenomenological perceptions in the certification processes.

REFERENCES

Aggrawal, A. (2015). Salient features regarding medico-legal certificate. *Medicolegal Corner*, *1*(1), 45–51. doi:10.4103/2394-7438.150068

Alces, P. A. (2018). *The moral conflict of law and neuroscience*. Chicago: The University of Chicago Press. doi:10.7208/chicago/9780226513676.001.0001

Allely, C. S., Minnis, H., Thompson, L., Wilson, P., & Gilberg, C. (2014). Neurodevelopmental and psychosocial risk factors in serial killers and mass murderers. *Aggression and Violent Behavior*, *19*(3), 288–301. doi:10.1016/j.avb.2014.04.004

Anand, R. (2001). *Manharan Singh Gill vs State of Punjab on 11 January, 2001*. Available at: https://indiankanoon.org/doc/145397/

Ashworth, S. (2016). Autism is underdiagnosed in prisoners. *British Medical Journal*, *353*, i3028. doi:10.1136/bmj.i3028 PMID:27255544

Balakrishnan, K. G., Sathasivam, P., & Chauhan, B. S. (2009). *Suchita Srivastava & Anr vs Chandigarh Administration on 28 August, 2009*. Available at: https://indiankanoon.org/doc/1500783/

Berman, A. (1974). Delinquents are disabled. In B. L. Kratoville (Ed.), *Youth in trouble* (pp. 34–43). San Rafael, CA: Academic Therapy.

Bilder, S., & Mechanic, D. (2003). Navigating the disability process: Persons with mental disorders applying for and receiving disability benefits. *The Milbank Quarterly*, *81*(1), 75–106. doi:10.1111/1468-0009.00039 PMID:12669652

Billstedt, E., Anckarsater, H., Wallinius, M., & Hofvander, B. (2017). Neurodevelopmental disorders in young violent offenders: Offenders and background characteristics. *Psychiatry Research*, *252*, 234–241. doi:10.1016/j.psychres.2017.03.004 PMID:28285251

Blau, T. H. (2001). *The psychologist as an expert witness*. Hoboken, NJ: Wiley.

Broder, P. K., & Dunivant, N. (1981). *Change in delinquent behavior as a function of learning disabilities: A two- year longitudinal study*. Williamsburg, VA: National Centre for State Courts.

Brodsky, S. L. (2013). *Testifying in court: Guidelines and maxims for the expert witness*. Washington, DC: American Psychological Association. doi:10.1037/14037-000

Carter, R. M. (2011). *The interaction between lawyers and physicians in litigation*. Edmonton, Alberta: The Law Society of Alberta.

Carulla, L. S., Reed, G. M., Vaez-Azizi, L. M., Cooper, S. A., Leal, R., Bertelli, M., ... Girimaji, S. C. (2011). Intellectual developmental disorders: Towards a new name, definition and framework for "mental retardation/intellectual disability" in ICD-11. *World Psychiatry; Official Journal of the World Psychiatric Association (WPA)*, *10*(3), 175–180. doi:10.1002/j.2051-5545.2011.tb00045.x PMID:21991267

Cauffman, E., & Steinberg, L. (2000). (Im)maturity of judgment in adolescence: Why adolescents may be less culpable than adults. *Behavioral Sciences & the Law*, *18*(6), 741–743. doi:10.1002/bsl.416 PMID:11180420

Chafetz, M., & Dufrene, M. (2014). Malingering-by-proxy: The need for child protection and guidance for reporting. *Child Abuse & Neglect*, *38*(11), 1755–1765. doi:10.1016/j.chiabu.2014.08.015 PMID:25236718

Chandra, N. (2012). 'Disability' on sale: Enjoy benefits for the handicapped as touts can get you fake certificates. *Mail Online India*. Retrieved from http://www.dailymail.co.uk/indiahome/indianews/article-2180685/Disability-sale-Enjoy-benefits-handicapped-touts-fake-certificates.html

Crawford, D. (1996). Review of research on learning disabilities and juvenile delinquency. In S. Cramer & W. Ellis (Eds.), *Learning Disabilities: Lifelong Issues*. Baltimore, MD: Paul H. Brookes Publishing Co.

Dahan-Oliel, N., Shikako-Thomas, K., & Majnemer, A. (2012). Quality of life and leisure participation in children with neurodevelopmental disabilities: A thematic analysis of the literature. *Quality of Life Research: An International Journal of Quality of Life Aspects of Treatment, Care and Rehabilitation*, *21*(3), 427–439. doi:10.100711136-011-0063-9 PMID:22101860

Delhi Commission for Protection of Child Rights. (2015). *Why children commit offences: Study on children in conflict with the law in Delhi*. New Delhi: Author.

Demeter, S. L., & Andersson, B. J. (2003). *Disability evaluation*. St. Louis, MO: Mosby.

Dumitrascu, C. I., Gallardo, K. E., & Caplan, J. P. (2015). Malingering imposed on another: A diagnosis that is missing in action? *Psychosomatics*, *56*(6), 609–614. doi:10.1016/j.psym.2015.07.006 PMID:26497617

Fazio, R. L., Pietz, C. A., & Denney, R. L. (2012). An estimate of the prevalence of autism spectrum disorders in an incarcerated population. *Open Access Journal of Forensic Psychology*, *4*, 69–80.

Folstein, M. F., Folstein, S. E., & McHugh, P. R. (1975). Mini-mental state, a practical method of grading the cognitive state of patients for the clinician. *Journal of Psychiatric Research*, *12*(3), 189–198. doi:10.1016/0022-3956(75)90026-6 PMID:1202204

Gao, Y., Glenn, A. L., Schug, R. A., Yang, Y., & Raine, A. (2009). The neurobiology of psychopathy: A neurodevelopmental perspective. *Canadian Journal of Psychiatry*, *54*(12), 813–823. doi:10.1177/070674370905401204 PMID:20047720

Gaur, S. (2012). *Jagjit Singh and Anr vs Delhi Development Authority on 26 November, 2012*. Available at: https://indiankanoon.org/doc/47289866/

Gillberg, C. (2010). The ESSENCE of child psychiatry: Early Symptomatic Syndromes Eliciting Neurodevelopmental Clinical Examinations (ESSENCE). *Research in Developmental Disabilities*, *31*(6), 1543–1551. doi:10.1016/j.ridd.2010.06.002 PMID:20634041

Ginsberg, Y., Hirvikoski, T., & Lindefors, N. (2010). Attention Deficit Hyperactivity Disorder (ADHD) among longer-term prison inmates is a prevalent, persistent and disabling disorder. *BMC Psychiatry*, *10*(1), 112. doi:10.1186/1471-244X-10-112 PMID:21176203

Ginsberg, Y., Langstrom, N., Larsson, H., & Lichtenstein, P. (2014). ADHD and criminality: Could treatment benefit prisoners with ADHD who are at higher risk of reoffending? *Expert Review of Neurotherapeutics*, *13*(4), 345–348. doi:10.1586/ern.13.22 PMID:23545049

Ginsberg, Y., & Lindefors, N. (2012). Methylphenidate treatment of adult male prison inmates with attention-deficit hyperactivity disorder: A randomised double-blind placebo-controlled trial with open-label extension. *The British Journal of Psychiatry*, *200*(1), 68–73. doi:10.1192/bjp.bp.111.092940 PMID:22075648

Goswami, S. P., Venkatesan, S., & Mathew, S. (2015). Disability certification: Issues and concerns. *Journal of All India Institute of Speech and Hearing*, *34*, 1–7.

Gutheil, T. G., & Drogin, E. Y. (2013). *The mental health professional in court: A survival guide*. Washington, DC: American Psychiatric Publishing.

Hansaria, V., & Jose, P. I. (2010). *Juvenile justice system: Working manual for stakeholders*. New Delhi: Universal Law Publishing.

Harris, G. T., Rice, M. E., & Lalumiere, M. (2001). The roles of psychopathy, neurodevelopmental insults, and antisocial parenting. *Criminal Justice and Behavior*, *28*(4), 402–426. doi:10.1177/009385480102800402

Hayes, S., Shackell, P., Mottram, P., & Lancaster, R. (2007). The prevalence of intellectual disability in a major UK prison. *British Journal of Learning Disabilities*, *35*(3), 162–167. doi:10.1111/j.1468-3156.2007.00461.x

IDEAS. (2002). *Indian Disability Evaluation Assessment Scale: A scale for measuring and quantifying disability in mental disorders*. Indian Psychiatric Society.

Jacob, P., Golhar, T., Sheshadri, S., Mani, R. N., & Purushothaman, K. (2014). Child and adolescent mental health in the juvenile justice system in India: Challenges and initiatives. *Adolescent Psychiatry*, *4*, 4. doi:10.2174/2210676604666141127205656

Jain, M., & Passi, G. R. (2005). Assessment of a modified mini-mental status scale for cognitive functions in children. *Indian Pediatrics*, *42*(9), 907–912. PMID:16208050

Kapardis, A. (2010). *Psychology and law: A critical introduction*. Cambridge, UK: Cambridge University Press.

Kashyap, K., Thunga, R., Rao, A. K., & Balamurali, N. P. (2012). Trends of utilization of government benefits among chronic mentally ill. *Indian Journal of Psychiatry*, *54*(1), 54–58. doi:10.4103/0019-5545.94648 PMID:22556439

Kasthuri, P., Sharan, R., Chandrashekar, H., & Kumar, S. (2016). Profile of psychiatric patients with certifiable disability in a general hospital psychiatry unit of Bangalore, South India. *Journal of Research in Psychiatry and Behavioural Sciences*, *2*(1), 7–10.

Kebbell, M. R., & Davies, D. G. (2003). People with intellectual disabilities in the investigation and prosecution crime. *Legal and Criminological Psychology*, *8*(2), 219–222. doi:10.1348/135532503322362988

Keilitz, I., & Dunivant, N. (1986). The relationship between learning disability and juvenile delinquency: Current state of knowledge. *Remedial and Special Education*, *7*(3), 18–26. doi:10.1177/074193258600700305

Khanna, S., & Misra, D. (2011). *Vibhor Anand vs Vice Chancellor, Guru Gobind ... on 3 March, 2011*. Available at: https://indiankanoon.org/doc/1838901/

Konar, D. (2005). Juvenile justice as a part of the child and adolescent care. *Journal of Indian Association of Child and Adolescent Mental Health*, *1*(3), 3.

Kumar, K. A. (2017). IDEAS and the IPS. *Indian Journal of Psychiatry*, *59*(1), 124–125. doi:10.4103/psychiatry.IndianJPsychiatry_68_17 PMID:28529373

Kumari, V. (2010). *The juvenile justice system in India: From welfare to rights*. New York: Oxford University Press.

Larson, K. A. (1988). A research review and alternative hypothesis explaining the link between learning disability and delinquency. *Journal of Learning Disabilities*, *21*(6), 357–363. doi:10.1177/002221948802100607 PMID:3047295

Lundstrom, S., Forsman, M., Larsson, H., Keekes, N., Serlachius, E., Langstrom, N., & Lichtenstein, P. (2014). Childhood neurodevelopmental disorders and violent criminality: A sibling control study. *Journal of Autism and Developmental Disorders*, *44*(11), 2707–2718. doi:10.100710803-013-1873-0 PMID:23807203

Mathur, A. (2017). *Living conditions in institutions for children in conflict with the law: Manual*. New Delhi: Delhi Commission for Protection of Child Rights, Ministry of Women and Child Development, Government of India.

Maughan, B., Gray, G., & Rutter, M. (1985). Reading retardation and antisocial behavior: A follow-up into employment. *Journal of Child Psychology and Psychiatry, and Allied Disciplines*, *26*(5), 741–758. doi:10.1111/j.1469-7610.1985.tb00588.x PMID:4044719

McCarthy, J., Chaplin, E., Underwood, L., Forrester, A., Hayward, H., Sabet, J., ... Murphy, D. (2016). Characteristics of prisoners with neurodevelopmental disorders and difficulties. *Journal of Intellectual Disability Research*, *60*(3), 201–206. doi:10.1111/jir.12237 PMID:26486964

McKay, S., & Brumback, R. A. (1980). Relationship between learning disabilities and juvenile delinquency. *Perceptual and Motor Skills*, *51*(3), 1223–1226. doi:10.2466/pms.1980.51.3f.1223 PMID:7220224

Meera, T. (2016). Medicolegal cases: What every doctor should know. *Journal of Medical Society*, *30*(3), 133–134. doi:10.4103/0972-4958.191174

Mishra, N. N., Parker, L. S., Nimgaonkar, V. L., & Deshpande, S. N. (2012). Disability certificates in India: A challenge to health privacy. *Indian Journal of Medical Ethics*, *9*(1), 43–45. PMID:22319852

Misra, D. (2017). *Ms. Eera Through Dr. Manjula ... vs State (Govt. Of NCT Of Delhi) on 21 July, 2017*. Available at: https://indiankanoon.org/doc/69624144/

Mohan, I., Tandon, R., Kalra, H., & Trivedi, J. K. (2005). Disability assessment of mental illnesses using Indian Disability Evaluation Assessment Scale (IDEAS). *The Indian Journal of Medical Research, 121*, 759–763. PMID:16037620

Morrell, B., & Tilley, D. S. (2012). The role of non-perpetrating fathers in Munchausen Syndrome by proxy: A review of the literature. *Journal of Pediatric Nursing, 27*(4), 328–335. doi:10.1016/j.pedn.2011.03.008 PMID:22703679

Morris, J. (2001). Impairment and disability: Constructing an ethics of care that promotes human rights. *Hypatia, 16*(4), 1–16. doi:10.1111/j.1527-2001.2001.tb00750.x

Mukherjee, S. K., & Sadhu, S. S. (2014). *An Application For Bail Under ... vs Sanjib Banerjee & Another on 2 May, 2014.* Available at: https://indiankanoon.org/doc/23091486/

Murali, T., Taly, A. B., & Srivastava, A. (2006). Neurological legal disability. *Annals of Indian Academy of Neurology, 9*(3), 184–186. doi:10.4103/0972-2327.27668

Nandi, J. (2010). Disability certificate for Rs. 3000 in Karnataka. *The Times of India*. Retrieved from https://timesofindia.indiatimes.com/india/Disability-certificate-for-Rs-3000-in-Karnataka/articleshow/6576215.cms

National Crime Records Bureau. (2016). *Crime in India: 2016. Ministry of Home Affairs, Government of India*. New Delhi: Author.

Nityanandam, G. (2013). *G. Nityanandam vs Tmt. D. Saritha on 16 April, 2013*. Available at: https://indiankanoon.org/doc/102909949/

Nizamie, S. H., Prakash, R., Praharaj, S. K., & Akhtar, S. (2009). Certification in psychiatry. *Indian Journal of Psychiatry, 51*(1), 35–81.

Noble, J. H., & Conley, R. W. (1992). Toward an epidemiology of relevant attributes. In R. W. Conley, R. Luckasson, & G. Bouthilet (Eds.), *The criminal justice system and mental retardation* (pp. 17–54). Baltimore, MD: Paul Brookes Publishing.

Otenbacher, K., Msall, M., Lyon, N., Duffy, L. C., Ziviani, J., Granger, C. V., & Braun, S. (2000). Functional assessment and care of children with neurodevelopmental disabilities. *American Journal of Physical Medicine & Rehabilitation, 79*(2), 114–123. doi:10.1097/00002060-200003000-00002 PMID:10744184

Palmer, F. B., Percy, A. K., Tivnan, P., Jul, D., Tunnessen, W. W., & Scheiber, S. C. (2003). Certification in neurodevelopmental disabilities: The development of a new subspecialty and results of the initial examinations. *Developmental Disabilities Research Reviews, 9*(2), 128–131. doi:10.1002/mrdd.10069 PMID:12784231

Perlmutter, B. F. (1987). Delinquency and learning disabilities: Evidence for compensatory behavior and adaptation. *Journal of Youth and Adolescence, 16*(2), 89–95. doi:10.1007/BF02138913 PMID:24277316

Perry, J., & Drogin, E. Y. (2007). *Mental disability law, evidence, and testimony: A comprehensive reference manual for lawyers, judges, and mental disability professionals*. Chicago: American Bar Association Publishing.

Radhakrishna, H. (2008). Neurological legal disability. *Annals of Indian Academy of Neurology*, *9*(2), 98–102. doi:10.4103/0972-2327.25981 PMID:19893646

Raveesh, B. N., Nayak, R. B., & Kumbar, S. F. (2016). Preventing Medicolegal issues in clinical practice. *Annals of Indian Academy of Neurology*, *19*(5S1), S15–S20. doi:10.4103/0972-2327.192886 PMID:27891020

Rosler, M., Retz, W., Yaqoobi, K., & Retz-Junginger, P. (2009). Attention deficit/hyperactivity disorder in female offenders: Prevalence, psychiatric comorbidity, and psychosocial implications. *European Archives of Psychiatry and Clinical Neuroscience*, *259*(2), 97–105. doi:10.100700406-008-0841-8 PMID:18806916

Scott, E. S., & Steinberg, L. (2008). Adolescent development and the regulation of youth crime. *The Future of Children*, *18*(2), 20–21. PMID:21337996

Sharma, R. K. (2008). *Medico-legal aspects of patient care*. New Delhi: Peepee Publishers.

Srivastava, P., & Kumar, P. (2015). Disability, its issues, and challenges and legal aspects in the Indian scenario. *Delhi Psychiatry Journal*, *18*(1), 195–205.

Stevens, B. A. (2008). *Crossfire: How to survive giving expert evidence as a psychologist. Bowen Hills*. Australian Academic Press.

Subrahmanyam, B. V. (2007). *Human disability evaluation: Personal injuries, principles, practices & law including disability consequent to medical negligence*. Allahabad: Law Publishers.

Swamy, L. N. (2014a). *Narayanaswamy vs State by Karnataka on 15 May, 2014*. Available at: https://indiankanoon.org/doc/36978708/

Swamy, L. N. (2014b). *Narayanaswamy vs State by Karnataka on 15 May, 2014*. Available at: https://indiankanoon.org/doc/1500783/

Szpir, M. (2006). New thinking on neurodevelopment. *Environmental Health Perspectives*, *114*(2), A100–A107. doi:10.1289/ehp.114-a100 PMID:16451834

Thara, R. (2005). Commentary: Measurement of psychiatric disability. *The Indian Journal of Medical Research*, *121*, 723–724. PMID:16037616

The Hindu. (2017a). *Cleaning up: On reviewing laws in India*. Retrieved from http://www.thehindu.com/opinion/editorial/cleaningup/article22084026.ece

The Hindu. (2017b). *Fake disability certificate: Action ordered against girl's father*. Retrieved from http://www.thehindu.com/news/cities/bangalore/fake-disability-certificate-action-ordered-against-girls-father/article17962726.ece

Underwood, L., Forrester, A., Chaplin, E., & McCarthy, J. (2013). Prisoners with neurodevelopmental disorders. *Journal of Intellectual Disabilities and Offending Behaviour*, *4*(1/2), 17–23. doi:10.1108/JIDOB-05-2013-0011

Underwood, L., McCarthy, J., Chaplin, E., Forrester, A., Mills, R., & Murphy, D. (2016). Autism spectrum disorder traits among prisoners. *Advances in Autism*, *2*(3), 106–117. doi:10.1108/AIA-11-2015-0023

Unger, K. V. (1978). Learning disabilities and juvenile delinquency. *Journal of Juvenile and Family Courts, 29*(1), 25–30. doi:10.1111/j.1755-6988.1978.tb01144.x

Upton, J. (2013). Mini-Mental State Examination. In M. D. Gellman & J. R. Turner (Eds.), *Encyclopaedia of Behavioural Medicine*. New York, NY: Springer.

Ustun, T. B., Kostanjsek, N., Chatterji, S., & Rehm, J. (2010). *Measuring health and disability: Manual for WHO Disability Assessment Scale (WHODAS 2.0)*. Geneva: World Health Organization.

Venkatesan, S. (2010). A case study on cost-benefit analysis for the government-sponsored scheme for persons with mental disabilities. *Asian Journal of Developmental Matters, 4*(1), 176–188.

Venkatesan, S. (2011). Blame game triangulation between parents, teachers, and children with academic problems. *Psychological Studies, 56*(2), 206–215. doi:10.100712646-011-0082-1

Venkatesan, S. (2014). Coercion tactics of parents on children with academic problems in India. *International Journal of Psychology and Psychiatry, 2*(1), 42–56. doi:10.5958/j.2320-6233.2.1.007

Venkatesan, S. (2015). Engagement between justice system vis-a-vis persons with intellectual and developmental disabilities. *International Journal of Psychology and Psychiatry, 3*(1), 30–56. doi:10.5958/2320-6233.2015.00003.6

Venkatesan, S., & Madhurao, P. (1990). The validity of parental estimates against actual test estimates in mentally handicapped individuals. *The Creative Psychologist, 2*(2), 71–75.

Venkatesan, S., & Swarnalata, G. V. (2013). Problem behaviors and academic grade level performance of adjudicated children with juvenile delinquency. *Disability, CBR and Inclusive Development, 24*(1), 99–114. doi:10.5463/dcid.v24i1.162

Waldie, K., & Spreen, O. (1993). The relationship between learning disabilities and persisting delinquency. *Journal of Learning Disabilities, 26*(6), 417–423. doi:10.1177/002221949302600608 PMID:8354946

Young, S., Moss, D., Sedgwick, O., Fridman, M., & Hodgkins, P. (2015). A meta-analysis of the prevalence of attention deficit hyperactivity disorder in incarcerated populations. *Psychological Medicine, 45*(2), 247–258. doi:10.1017/S0033291714000762 PMID:25066071

KEY TERMS AND DEFINITIONS

Affidavit: A written statement confirmed by oath or affirmation for use as evidence in court.

Amicus Curiae: An impartial adviser to a court of law in a particular case.

Assault: A physical attack.

Attorney: A lawyer appointed to act for another person on legal matters.

Battery: The infliction of unlawful personal violence on another person even when the contact does no harm.

Bullying: An unwanted, aggressive behavior that involves a real or perceived power imbalance.

Child Abuse: A physical maltreatment or sexual molestation of a child.

Civil Proceeding: A system of law based on regulation of private matters as distinct from criminal, political, or military matters.

Complainant (Syn. Plaintiff or Petitioner): The party who complains or sues in a civil action.

Confidentiality: A legally protected right that prohibits the health care provider from disclosing information communicated during the consultation to a third party about the patient.

Criminal Proceeding: A system of adjudication by law based on impeachment or using a charge or trial for misconduct which ends up in conviction or acquittal.

Defendant (Accused): A person accused of committing a crime or a person against whom some type of civil relief is being sought.

Delinquency: Person especially one below the age of eighteen when criminal prosecution is disallowed.

Disability: Usually a consequence of impairment, it is the functional inability of an individual to perform any activity in the manner or within the range considered "normal" for any human being.

Disorders: A group of disorders in which the developmental of the central nervous system is disturbed.

District Legal Services Authority: Based on the Legal Services Authority Act (1987), as amended in 1994, it constitutes a provision for free and competent legal services to the weaker sections (including the disabled) of the society. The tiers of these statutory bodies work at national, state, district and taluk levels, respectively.

Domestic Violence: A pattern of behavior which involves abuse or use of violence in marriage or cohabitation.

Expert Witness: A person whose level of specialized knowledge or skill in a particular field qualifies them to present their opinion about the facts of a case during legal proceedings.

Forensic Medicine: The application of medical knowledge to the investigation of crime.

Handicap: Is a disadvantage resulting or consequence of impairment or as well as disability.

Human Rights Model: Unlike the medical model which views the individual as a victim and the core of the problem, the social model views barriers as the source of problems for persons with disability.

Impairment: Any visible structural/anatomical loss of physical or sense organs in an individual.

Indian Penal Code: A comprehensive code in the country which is intended to cover all substantive aspects of criminal law.

Informed Consent: Permission granted in full knowledge of the possible consequences, typically that which is given by a patient to a doctor for treatment with knowledge of the possible risks and benefits.

Juvenile: The habitual committing of criminal acts or offences by a young.

Medical Jurisprudence: The branch of law relating to medicine.

Medical Model: Arising from the biomedical perception of disability, this model believes in identifying or listing symptoms, categorizing them, making a diagnosis, before seeking to cure them.

Medico-Legal Cases: Case of injury or ailment in which investigations by law enforcing agencies are essential to fix responsibility regarding the causation of the said injury or ailment.

Plaintiff: A person who brings a case against another in a court of law.

POCSO Act: The Protection of Children from Sexual Offences Act (2010) seeks to safeguard and protect children from pornography, assault, abuse, or harassment through child-friendly specially designated courts.

Public Prosecutor: A law officer who conducts criminal proceedings on behalf of the state or in public interest.

Rape: Sexual intercourse, or other forms of sexual penetration, committed by a perpetrator against a victim without their consent.

Sexual Harassment: Unwelcome sexual advances, requests for sexual favors, and other verbal or physical conduct.

Victimization: The action of singling out for cruel and unjust treatment.

Compilation of References

Abikoff, H. (1991). Cognitive training in ADHD children: Less to it than meets the eye. *Journal of Learning Disabilities*, *24*(4), 205–209. doi:10.1177/002221949102400404 PMID:1875155

Abrahams, B. S., & Geschwind, D. H. (2008). Advances in autism genetics: On the threshold of a new neurobiology. *Nature Reviews. Genetics*, *9*(5), 341–355. doi:10.1038/nrg2346 PMID:18414403

Acar, G. O., Yilmaz, M., Sekercioğlu, N., & Yüksel, A. (2010). Keutel syndrome in a patient presenting with hearing loss. *B-ENT*, *6*, 201–204. PMID:21090163

Acharya, P. S. R. S. (2008). *Yam, Niyam, Asana and Pranayam*. Mathura: Akhand Jyoti Sansthan.

Acosta, M. T., & Pearl, P. L. (2004, September). Imaging data in autism: From structure to malfunction. *Seminars in Pediatric Neurology*, *11*(3), 205–213. doi:10.1016/j.spen.2004.07.004 PMID:15575415

Aggrawal, A. (2015). Salient features regarding medico-legal certificate. *Medicolegal Corner*, *1*(1), 45–51. doi:10.4103/2394-7438.150068

Ahearn, W. H., Castine, T., Nault, K., & Green, G. (2001). An assessment of food acceptance in children with autism or pervasive developmental disorder-not otherwise specified. *Journal of Autism and Developmental Disorders*, *31*(5), 505–511. doi:10.1023/A:1012221026124 PMID:11794415

Akhtar, N. (2005). The robustness of learning through overhearing. *Developmental Science*, *8*(2), 199–209. doi:10.1111/j.1467-7687.2005.00406.x PMID:15720377

Alces, P. A. (2018). *The moral conflict of law and neuroscience*. Chicago: The University of Chicago Press. doi:10.7208/chicago/9780226513676.001.0001

Alexander, A. L., Lee, J. E., Lazar, M., Boudos, R., DuBray, M. B., Oakes, T. R., ... Bigler, E. D. (2007). Diffusion tensor imaging of the corpus callosum in Autism. *NeuroImage*, *34*(1), 61–73. doi:10.1016/j.neuroimage.2006.08.032 PMID:17023185

Alkhouri, N., Kaplan, B., Kay, M., Shealy, A., Crowe, C., Bauhuber, S., & Zenker, M. (2008). Johanson-Blizzard syndrome with mild phenotypic features confirmed by UBR1 gene testing. *World Journal of Gastroenterology*, *14*(44), 6863–6866. doi:10.3748/wjg.14.6863 PMID:19058315

Allely, C. S., Minnis, H., Thompson, L., Wilson, P., & Gilberg, C. (2014). Neurodevelopmental and psychosocial risk factors in serial killers and mass murderers. *Aggression and Violent Behavior*, *19*(3), 288–301. doi:10.1016/j.avb.2014.04.004

Allopenna, P. D., Magnuson, J. S., & Tanenhaus, M. K. (1998). Tracking the time course of spoken word recognition using eye movements: Evidence for continuous mapping models. *Journal of Memory and Language*, *38*(4), 419–439. doi:10.1006/jmla.1997.2558

Alloway, T. P., & Gathercole, S. E. (Eds.). (2006). *Working memory and neurodevelopmental disorders*. Hove, UK: Psychology Press.

Almashraki, N., Abdulnabee, M. Z., Sukalo, M., Alrajoudi, A., Sharafadeen, I., & Zenker, M. (2011). Johanson-Blizzard syndrome. *World Journal of Gastroenterology*, *17*(37), 4247–4250. doi:10.3748/wjg.v17.i37.4247 PMID:22072859

Alonso, P., Lopez-Sola, C., Real, E., Segalas, C., & Menchon, J. M. (2015). Animal models of obsessive-compulsive disorder: Utility and limitations. *Neuropsychiatric Disease and Treatment*, *11*, 1939–1955. doi:10.2147/NDT.S62785 PMID:26346234

Alworth, L. N., Plyler, P. N., Reber, M. B., & Johnstone, P. M. (2010). The effects of receiver placement on probe microphone, performance, and subjective measures with open canal hearing instruments. *Journal of the American Academy of Audiology*, *21*(4), 249–266. doi:10.3766/jaaa.21.4.4 PMID:20388451

Amaral, D. G., Schumann, C. M., & Nordahl, C. W. (2008). Neuroanatomy of autism. *Trends in Neurosciences*, *31*(3), 137–145. doi:10.1016/j.tins.2007.12.005 PMID:18258309

Amendah, D., Grosse, S. D., Peacock, G., & Mandell, D. S. (2011). The economic costs of autism: A review. In D. Amaral, D. Geschwind, & G. Dawson (Eds.), *Autism spectrum disorders* (pp. 1347–1360). New York, NY: Oxford University Press. doi:10.1093/med/9780195371826.003.0088

American Association on Intellectual and Developmental Disabilities. (2008). *Mental Retardation: Definition, Classification, and Systems of Supports* (10th ed.). Washington, DC: American Association on Intellectual and Developmental Disabilities.

American Psychiatric Association. (1980). *Diagnostic and Statistical Manual of Mental Disorders* (3rd ed.). Washington, DC: Author.

American Psychiatric Association. (2000). *Diagnostic and Statistical Manual of Mental Disorders-IV-TR*. Washington, DC: Author.

American Psychiatric Association. (2000). *DSM-IV-TR: Diagnostic and statistical manual of mental disorders, text revision*. Washington, DC: American Psychiatric Association.

American Psychiatric Association. (2013). *Diagnostic and statistical manual of mental disorders* (5th ed.). Arlington, VA: American Psychiatric Association.

American Psychiatric Association. (2013). Diagnostic and statistical manual of mental disorders (5th ed.). Arlington, VA: American Psychiatric Publishing.

American Psychiatric Association. (2013). *Diagnostic and statistical manual of mental disorders (DSM-5®)*. American Psychiatric Pub.

American Psychiatric Association. (2013). *Diagnostic and statistical manual of mental disorders: DSM-5* (5th ed.). Washington, DC: American Psychiatric Association.

American Psychiatric Association. (2013). Neuro-cognitive disorders. In The American Psychiatric Textbook of Psychiatry (5th ed.). Washington, DC: Author. doi:10.1176/appi.books.9781585625031.rh24

American Psychiatric Association. (2016). *Neuro-developmental disorders: DSM-5 selections*. Washington, DC: Author.

Amita, S., Prabhakar, S., Manoj, I., Harminder, S., & Pawan, T. (2009). Effect of yoga-nidra on blood glucose level in diabetic patients. *Indian Journal of Physiology and Pharmacology*, *53*(1), 97–101. PMID:19810584

Anand, R. (2001). *Manharan Singh Gill vs State of Punjab on 11 January, 2001*. Available at: https://indiankanoon.org/doc/145397/

Andrasik, F., & Lords, A. O. (2008). Biofeedback. In L. Freeman (Ed.), *Mosby's Complementary and Alternative Medicine: A research-based approach* (pp. 189–214). St. Louis, MO: Mosby Elsevier.

Andrews, G., Pine, D. S., Hobbs, M. J., Anderson, T. M., & Sunderland, M. (2009). Neurodevelopmental disorders: Cluster 2 of the proposed meta-structure for DSM-V and ICD-11. *Psychological Medicine*, *39*(2), 2013–2023. doi:10.1017/S0033291709990274 PMID:19796427

Andrienko, G., Andrienko, N., Burch, M., & Weiskopf, D. (2012). Visual analytics methodology for eye movement studies. *IEEE Transactions on Visualization and Computer Graphics*, *18*(12), 2889–2898. doi:10.1109/TVCG.2012.276 PMID:26357198

Angell, A. (2010). Selective eaters and tactile sensitivity: A review of classification and treatment methods that address anxiety and support a child's need for a sense of control. *ICAN: Infant, Child, &. Adolescent Nutrition*, *2*(5), 299–303.

Anjos, T., Altmäe, S., Emmett, P., Tiemeier, H., Closa-Monasterolo, R., Luque, V., & Egan, B. (2013). Nutrition and neurodevelopment in children: Focus on NUTRIMENTHE project. *European Journal of Nutrition*, *52*(8), 1825–1842. doi:10.100700394-013-0560-4 PMID:23884402

Archer, L. A., Rosenbaum, P. L., & Streiner, D. L. (1991). The children's eating behavior inventory: Reliability and validity results. *Journal of Pediatric Psychology*, *16*(5), 629–642. doi:10.1093/jpepsy/16.5.629 PMID:1744810

Archer, L. A., & Szatmari, P. (1990). Assessment and treatment of food aversion in a four year old boy: A multidimensional approach. *Canadian Journal of Psychiatry*, *35*(6), 501–505. doi:10.1177/070674379003500606 PMID:1698524

Aresti-Bartolome, N., & Garcia-Zapirain, B. (2014). Technologies as support tools for persons with autistic spectrum disorder: A systematic review. *International Journal of Environmental Research and Public Health*, *11*(8), 7767–7802. doi:10.3390/ijerph110807767 PMID:25093654

Arim, R. G., Kohen, D. E., Garner, R. E., Lach, L. M., Brehaut, J. C., MacKenzie, M. J., & Rosenbaum, P. L. (2015). Psychosocial functioning in children with neurodevelopmental disorders and externalizing behavior problems. *Disability and Rehabilitation*, *37*(4), 345–354. doi:10.3109/09638288.2014.919361 PMID:24840026

Armagan, O., Tascioglu, F., & Oner, C. (2003). Electromyographic biofeedback in the treatment of the hemiplegic hand: A placebo-controlled study. *American Journal of Physical Medicine & Rehabilitation*, *82*(11), 856–861. doi:10.1097/01.PHM.0000091984.72486.E0 PMID:14566153

Arndt, T. L., Stodgell, C. J., & Rodier, P. M. (2005). The teratology of autism. *The International Journal of Neuroscience*, *23*, 189–199. PMID:15749245

Arvedson, J., & Brodsky, L. (1993). Management of swallowing problems. *Pediatric Swallowing and Feeding: Assessment and Management*, 327–387.

Arvedson, J. C. (2013). Feeding children with cerebral palsy and swallowing difficulties. *European Journal of Clinical Nutrition*, *67*(S2), S9–S12. doi:10.1038/ejcn.2013.224 PMID:24301008

Ashwood, P., & Van de Water, J. (2004). Is autism an autoimmune disease? *Autoimmunity Reviews*, *3*(7–8), 557–562. doi:10.1016/j.autrev.2004.07.036 PMID:15546805

Ashworth, S. (2016). Autism is underdiagnosed in prisoners. *British Medical Journal*, *353*, i3028. doi:10.1136/bmj.i3028 PMID:27255544

Association for Play Therapy. (n.d.). Retrieved November 30, 2011, from http://www.a4pt.org/index.html

Ataalla, M. (2015). Behavioral, mental health issues and neurodevelopmental disorders. In O. Naga (Ed.), *Pediatric Board Study Guide* (pp. 29–43). Cham: Springer; doi:10.1007/978-3-319-10115-6_2

Auriemmo, J., Kuk, F., Lau, C., Dornan, B. K., Sweeton, S., Marshall, S., & Stenger, P. (2009). Efficacy of an adaptive directional microphone and a noise reduction system for school-aged children. *Journal of Educational Audiology*, *15*, 15–27.

Auriemmo, J., Kuk, F., & Stenger, P. (2008). Criteria for evaluating the performance of linear frequency transposition in children. *The Hearing Journal*, *61*(4), 50–52. doi:10.1097/01.HJ.0000315831.15143.9f

Aurobindo, S. (1917). *The synthesis of Yoga*. Pondicherry: Sri Aurobindo Ashram.

Autio, S., Louhimo, T., & Helenius, M. (1982). The clinical course of mannosidosis. *Annals of Clinical Research*, *14*, 93–97. PMID:7149616

Axline, V. M. (1947). *Play therapy: The inner dynamics of childhood*. Boston: Houghton Mifflin.

Axline, V. M. (1969). *Play therapy*. New York, NY: Ballenti.

Ayers, M. E. (1995). Long-term follow up of EEG neurofeedback with absence seizures. *Biofeedback and Self-Regulation*, *20*(3), 309–310.

Aylward, E. H., Minshew, N. J., Field, K., Sparks, B. F., & Singh, N. (2002). Effects of age on brain volume and head circumference in autism. *Neurology*, *59*(2), 175–183. doi:10.1212/WNL.59.2.175 PMID:12136053

Aylward, E. H., Minshew, N. J., Goldstein, G., Honeycutt, N. A., Augustine, A. M., Yates, K. O., ... Pearlson, G. D. (1999). MRI volumes of amygdala and hippocampus in non–mentally retarded autistic adolescents and adults. *Neurology*, *53*(9), 2145–2145. doi:10.1212/WNL.53.9.2145 PMID:10599796

Azeez, R., & Prakash, P. (2016). *Phonological and morphological processing in Urdu: An eye tracking investigation* (Unpublished Doctoral dissertation). University of Mysore, Mysore.

Babbitt, R. L., Hoch, T. A., Coe, D. A., Cataldo, M. F., Kelly, K. J., Stackhouse, C., & Perman, J. A. (1994). Behavioral assessment and treatment of pediatric feeding disorders. *Journal of Developmental and Behavioral Pediatrics*, *15*(4), 278–291. doi:10.1097/00004703-199408000-00011 PMID:7798374

Bachevalier, J. (1994). Medial temporal lobe structures and autism: A review of clinical and experimental findings. *Neuropsychologia*, *32*(6), 627–648. doi:10.1016/0028-3932(94)90025-6 PMID:8084420

Badalyan, V., & Schwartz, R. H. (2011). Feeding problems and GI dysfunction in children with Asperger syndrome or pervasive developmental disorder not otherwise specified; comparison with their siblings. *Open Journal of Pediatrics*, *1*(04), 51–63. doi:10.4236/ojped.2011.14014

Badano, J. L., Mitsuma, N., Beales, P. L., & Katsanis, N. (2006). The ciliopathies: An emerging class of human genetic disorders. *Annual Review of Genomics and Human Genetics*, *7*(1), 125–148. doi:10.1146/annurev.genom.7.080505.115610 PMID:16722803

Bahmad, F. Jr, Costa, C. S. A., Teixeira, M. S., de Barros Filho, J., Viana, L. M., & Marshall, J. (2014). Familial Alström syndrome: A rare cause of bilateral progressive hearing loss. *Revista Brasileira de Otorrinolaringologia (English Ed.)*, *80*(2), 99–104. doi:10.5935/1808-8694.20140023 PMID:24830966

Baio, J. (2012). Prevalence of autism spectrum disorders: Autism and developmental disabilities monitoring network, 14 sites, United States, 2008. *MMWR. Surveillance Summaries*, *61*(3), 1–19. PMID:22456193

Baird, G. (2013). Editorial: Classification of diseases and the neurodevelopmental disorders: The challenges for DSM-5 and ICD-11. *Developmental Medicine and Child Neurology*, *55*(3), 200–201. doi:10.1111/dmcn.12087 PMID:23398148

Bakhshayesh, A. R., Hansch, S., Wschkon, A., Rezai, M. J., & Esser, G. (2011). Neurofeedback in ADHD: A single-blind randomized controlled trial. *European Child & Adolescent Psychiatry*, *20*(9), 481–491. doi:10.100700787-011-0208-y PMID:21842168

Balakrishnan, K. G., Sathasivam, P., & Chauhan, B. S. (2009). *Suchita Srivastava & Anr vs Chandigarh Administration on 28 August, 2009*. Available at: https://indiankanoon.org/doc/1500783/

Balan, O., Moldoveanu, A., Moldoveanu, F., Morar, A., & Asavei, V. (2013). Assistive IT for Visually Impaired People. *Journal of Information Systems & Operations Management*, *7*(2), 391–403.

Baldovino, S., Moliner, A. M., Taruscio, D., Daina, E., & Roccatello, D. (2016). Rare diseases in Europe: From a wide to a local perspective. *The Israel Medical Association Journal*, *18*, 359–363. PMID:27468531

Bamford, J., & Saunders, E. (1992). Hearing impairment, auditory perception and language disability. *Child Language Teaching and Therapy*, *8*(2), 227–228. doi:10.1177/026565909200800218

Bamiou, D. E., Spraggs, P. R. D., Gibberd, F. B., Sidey, M. C., & Luxon, L. M. (2003). Hearing loss in adult Refsum's disease. *Clinical Otolaryngology and Allied Sciences*, *28*(3), 227–230. doi:10.1046/j.1365-2273.2003.00694.x PMID:12755761

Baranek, G. T., Boyd, B. A., Poe, M. D., David, F. J., & Watson, L. R. (2007). Hyper-responsive sensory patterns in young children with autism, developmental delay, and typical development. *American Journal of Mental Retardation*, *112*(4), 233–245. doi:10.1352/0895-8017(2007)112[233:HSPIYC]2.0.CO;2 PMID:17559291

Barker, D. J. P. (1998). *Mothers, babies and health in later life* (2nd ed.). Edinburgh, UK: Churchill Livingstone.

Barnea-Goraly, N., Kwon, H., Menon, V., Eliez, S., Lotspeich, L., & Reiss, A. L. (2004). White matter structure in autism: Preliminary evidence from diffusion tensor imaging. *Biological Psychiatry*, *55*(3), 323–326. doi:10.1016/j.biopsych.2003.10.022 PMID:14744477

Baron-Cohen, S., Leslie, A. M., & Frith, U. (1985). Does the autistic child have a "theory of mind"? *Cognition*, *21*(1), 37–46. doi:10.1016/0010-0277(85)90022-8 PMID:2934210

Bartlett, S. C., Armstrong, E., & Roberts, J. (2005). Linguistic resources of individuals with Asperger syndrome. *Clinical Linguistics & Phonetics*, *19*(3), 203–213. doi:10.1080/02699200410001698634 PMID:15823956

Barzegary, L., & Zamini, S. (2011). The effect of play therapy on children with ADHD. *Procedia: Social and Behavioral Sciences*, *30*, 2216–2218. doi:10.1016/j.sbspro.2011.10.432

Bashat, D. B., Kronfeld-Duenias, V., Zachor, D. A., Ekstein, P. M., Hendler, T., Tarrasch, R., & Sira, L. B. (2007). Accelerated maturation of white matter in young children with autism: A high b value DWI study. *NeuroImage*, *37*(1), 40–47. doi:10.1016/j.neuroimage.2007.04.060 PMID:17566764

Basmajian, J. V. (1989). *Biofeedback: Principles and practice for clinicians*. Philadelphia: Williams & Wilkins.

Bass, M. M., Duchowny, C. A., & Llabre, M. M. (2009). The effect of therapeutic horseback riding on social functioning in children with autism. *Journal of Autism and Developmental Disorders*, *39*(9), 1261–1267. doi:10.100710803-009-0734-3 PMID:19350376

Batool, A., & Arooj, M. (2016). Complex neurodevelopmental disorders and their genetic aetiologies. *International Journal of Scientific & Technology Research*, *5*(9), 57–67.

Bauman, M. L. (2010). Medical comorbidities in autism: Challenges to diagnosis and treatment. *Neurotherapeutics; the Journal of the American Society for Experimental NeuroTherapeutics*, *7*(3), 320–327. doi:10.1016/j.nurt.2010.06.001 PMID:20643385

Baxter, A., Brugha, T., Erskine, H., Scheurer, R., Vos, T., & Scott, J. (2015). The epidemiology and global burden of autism spectrum disorders. *Psychological Medicine*, *45*(3), 601–613. doi:10.1017/S003329171400172X PMID:25108395

Bazinet, R. P., & Layé, S. (2014). Polyunsaturated fatty acids and their metabolites in brain function and disease. *Nature Reviews. Neuroscience*, *15*(12), 771–785. doi:10.1038/nrn3820 PMID:25387473

Beatty, J., & Legewie, H. (1977). *Biofeedback and behavior*. London: Plenum Press. doi:10.1007/978-1-4684-2526-0

Becerra, J., Fernández, T., Harmony, T., Caballero, M. I., García, F., Fernández-Bouzas, A., ... Prado-Alcalá, R. A. (2006). Follow-up study of learning-disabled children treated with neurofeedback or placebo. *Clinical EEG and Neuroscience*, *37*(3), 198–203. doi:10.1177/155005940603700307 PMID:16929704

Becker, J. L., Rogers, E. C., & Burrows, B. (2017). Animal-assisted social skills training for children with autism spectrum disorders. *Anthrozoos*, *30*(2), 307–326. doi:10.1080/08927936.2017.1311055

Beck, M., Olsen, K. J., Wraith, J. E., Zeman, J., Michalski, J. C., Saftig, P., ... Malm, D. (2013). Natural history of alpha mannosidosis a longitudinal study. *Orphanet Journal of Rare Diseases*, *8*(1), 88. doi:10.1186/1750-1172-8-88 PMID:23786919

Behere, R. V., Arasappa, R., Jagannathan, A., Varambally, S., Venkatasubramanian, G., Thirthalli, J., ... Gangadhar, B. N. (2011). Effect of yoga therapy on facial emotion recognition deficits, symptoms and functioning in patients with schizophrenia. *Acta Psychiatrica Scandinavica*, *123*(2), 147–153. doi:10.1111/j.1600-0447.2010.01605.x PMID:20846271

Bekele, E., Wade, J., Bian, D., Fan, J., Swanson, A., Warren, Z., & Sarkar, N. (2016, March). Multimodal adaptive social interaction in a virtual environment (MASI-VR) for children with Autism spectrum disorders (ASD). In Virtual Reality (VR), 2016 IEEE (pp. 121-130). IEEE.

Belmonte, M. K., Allen, G., Beckel-Mitchener, A., Boulanger, L. M., Carper, R. A., & Webb, S. J. (2004). Autism and abnormal development of brain connectivity. *The Journal of Neuroscience*, *24*(42), 9228–9231. doi:10.1523/JNEUROSCI.3340-04.2004 PMID:15496656

Ben-Ari, Y. (2016). Progress in autism research and post-genomic studies. *Lancet Neurology*, *15*(2), 136. doi:10.1016/S1474-4422(15)00402-0 PMID:28463118

Benfatto, M. N., Seimyr, G. Ö., Ygge, J., Pansell, T., Rydberg, A., & Jacobson, C. (2016). Screening for dyslexia using eye tracking during reading. *PLoS One*, *11*(12), e0165508.

Benoit, D. (1993). Failure to thrive and feeding disorders. In C. H. Zeanah (Ed.), *Handbook of Infant Mental Health* (pp. 317–331). New York: Guilford Press.

Bentler, R. A. (2005). Effectiveness of directional microphones and noise reduction schemes in hearing aids: A systematic review of the evidence. *Journal of the American Academy of Audiology*, *16*(7), 473–484. doi:10.3766/jaaa.16.7.7 PMID:16295234

Bentler, R., & Chiou, L. K. (2006). Digital noise reduction: An overview. *Trends in Amplification*, *10*(2), 67–82. doi:10.1177/1084713806289514 PMID:16959731

Benton, D. (2010). The influence of dietary status on the cognitive performance of children. *Molecular Nutrition & Food Research*, *54*(4), 457–470. doi:10.1002/mnfr.200900158 PMID:20077417

Benton, D., & Donohoe, R. T. (1999). The effects of nutrients on mood. *Public Health Nutrition*, *2*(3a), 403–409. doi:10.1017/S1368980099000555 PMID:10610080

Berg, A. T., & Dobyns, W. B. (2015). Progress in autism and related disorders of brain development. *Lancet Neurology*, *14*(11), 1169–1170. doi:10.1016/S1474-4422(15)00048-4 PMID:25891008

Bergsmark, J., & Djupesland, G. (1968). Heredopathia Atactica Polyneuritiformis (Refsum's Disease) An Audiological Examination of two Patients. *European Neurology*, *1*(2), 122–130. doi:10.1159/000113655 PMID:4177049

Berlin, K. S., Davies, W. H., Silverman, A. H., Woods, D. W., Fischer, E. A., & Rudolph, C. D. (2010). Assessing children's mealtime problems with the Mealtime Behavior Questionnaire. *Children's Health Care*, *39*(2), 142–156. doi:10.1080/02739611003679956

Berman, A. (1974). Delinquents are disabled. In B. L. Kratoville (Ed.), *Youth in trouble* (pp. 34–43). San Rafael, CA: Academic Therapy.

Berninger, V. W., Abbot, R. D., & Nagy Carlisle, J. (2010). Growth in phonological, orthographic and morphological awareness in grades 1 to 6. *Journal of Psycholinguistic Research*, *39*(2), 141–163. doi:10.100710936-009-9130-6 PMID:19826956

Berry, R. C., Novak, P., Withrow, N., Schmidt, B., Rarback, S., Feucht, S., & Sharp, W. G. (2015). Nutrition management of gastrointestinal symptoms in children with autism spectrum disorder: Guideline from an expert panel. *Journal of the Academy of Nutrition and Dietetics*, *115*(12), 1919–1927. doi:10.1016/j.jand.2015.05.016 PMID:26164551

Bertelli, M. O., Merli, M. P., Bradley, E., Keller, R., Varrucciu, N., Furia, C. D., & Panocchia, N. (2015). The diagnostic boundary between autism spectrum disorder, intellectual developmental disorder, and schizophrenia spectrum disorders. *Advances in Mental Health and Intellectual Disabilities*, *9*(5), 243–264. doi:10.1108/AMHID-05-2015-0024

Berthier, M. L., Starkstein, S. E., & Leiguarda, R. (1990). Developmental cortical anomalies in Asperger's syndrome: Neuroradiological findings in two patients. *The Journal of Neuropsychiatry and Clinical Neurosciences*, *2*(2), 197–201. doi:10.1176/jnp.2.2.197 PMID:2136076

Bettelheim, B. (1967). *The empty fortress: Infantile autism and the birth of the self.* New York: Free Press.

Bettison, S. (1996). The long-term effects of auditory training on children with autism. *Journal of Autism and Developmental Disorders*, *26*(3), 361–374. doi:10.1007/BF02172480 PMID:8792266

Bhasin, M. K., Dusek, J. A., Chang, B. H., Joseph, M. G., Denninger, J. W., Fricchione, G. L., ... Libermann, T. A. (2013). Relaxation response induces temporal transcriptome changes in energy metabolism, insulin secretion and inflammatory pathways. *PLoS One*, *8*(5), e62817. doi:10.1371/journal.pone.0062817 PMID:23650531

Bhatnagar, S., & Taneja, S. (2001). Zinc and cognitive development. *British Journal of Nutrition*, *85*(S2), S139–S145. doi:10.1079/BJN2000306 PMID:11509102

Bhide, P., Gund, P., & Kar, A. (2016). Prevalence of congenital anomalies in an Indian maternal cohort: Healthcare, prevention, and surveillance implications. *PLoS One*, 11. PMID:27832123

Bhuyan, A. (2017, May 26). *Government submits rare disease policy to Delhi HC, recommends Rs 100 Crore for genetic diseases*. Retrieved from https://thewire.in/140229/rare-disease-policy/

Bilbo, S. D., & Schwartz, J. M. (2012). The immune system and developmental programming of brain and behavior. *Frontiers in Neuroendocrinology*, *33*(3), 267–286. doi:10.1016/j.yfrne.2012.08.006 PMID:22982535

Bilder, S., & Mechanic, D. (2003). Navigating the disability process: Persons with mental disorders applying for and receiving disability benefits. *The Milbank Quarterly*, *81*(1), 75–106. doi:10.1111/1468-0009.00039 PMID:12669652

Billstedt, E., Anckarsater, H., Wallinius, M., & Hofvander, B. (2017). Neurodevelopmental disorders in young violent offenders: Offenders and background characteristics. *Psychiatry Research*, *252*, 234–241. doi:10.1016/j.psychres.2017.03.004 PMID:28285251

Birbaumer, N., & Kimmel, H. D. (Eds.). (1979). *Biofeedback and self regulation*. Hillsdale, NJ: Erlbaum.

Bishop, D., & Rutter, M. (2008). Neurodevelopmental disorders: conceptual issues. Rutter's child and adolescent psychiatry, 32-41.

Bishop, D. V. M. (2010). Which neurodevelopmental disorders get researched and why? *PLoS One*, *5*(11), e15112. doi:10.1371/journal.pone.0015112 PMID:21152085

Biswas, P., & Langdon, P. (2014). Eye-gaze Tracking Based Interaction in India. *Procedia Computer Science*, *39*, 59–66. doi:10.1016/j.procs.2014.11.010

Blanco, P., & Ray, D. (2011). Play therapy in the schools: A best practice for improving academic achievement. *Journal of Counseling and Development*, *89*(2), 235–242. doi:10.1002/j.1556-6678.2011.tb00083.x

Blankenship, K., & Lawver, T. (2008). Play therapy: A case-based example of a nondirective approach. *Psychiatry (Edgmont)*, *5*(10), 24–28. PMID:19724720

Blau, T. H. (2001). *The psychologist as an expert witness*. Hoboken, NJ: Wiley.

Blaxter, M. (1990). *Health and lifestyles*. London: Routledge. doi:10.4324/9780203393000

Blumberg, S. J., Bramlett, M. D., Kogan, M. D., Schieve, L. A., Jones, J. R., & Lu, M. C. (2013). *Changes in prevalence of parent-reported autism spectrum disorder in school-aged U.S. children: 2007 to 2011-2012*. Hyattsville, MD: National Center for Health Statistics.

Boddaert, N., Belin, P., Chabane, N., Poline, J. B., Barthélémy, C., Mouren-Simeoni, M. C., & Zilbovicius, M. (2003). Perception of complex sounds: Abnormal pattern of cortical activation in autism. *The American Journal of Psychiatry*, *160*(11), 2057–2060. doi:10.1176/appi.ajp.160.11.2057 PMID:14594758

Boddaert, N., Chabane, N., Belin, P., Bourgeois, M., Royer, V., Barthelemy, C., & Zilbovicius, M. (2004). Perception of complex sounds in autism: Abnormal auditory cortical processing in children. *The American Journal of Psychiatry*, *161*(11), 2117–2120. doi:10.1176/appi.ajp.161.11.2117 PMID:15514415

Bogdanowiez, K. (2006). *A short introduction to dyslexia*. Available: http://www.jezykangielski.org/teacher6

Bölte, S., & Hallmayer, J. (Eds.). (2011). *Autism spectrum conditions: FAQs on autism, Asperger syndrome, and atypical autism answered by international experts*. Hogrefe Publishing.

Bölte, S., Schipper, E., Robison, J. E., Wong, V. C., Selb, M., Singhal, N., ... Zwaigenbaum, L. (2014). Classification of functioning and impairment: The development of ICF core sets for autism spectrum disorder. *Autism Research*, *7*(1), 167–172. doi:10.1002/aur.1335 PMID:24124074

Bondemark, L., & Ruf, S. (2015). Randomized controlled trial: The gold standard or unobtainable fallacy. *European Journal of Orthodontics*, *37*(5), 457–461. doi:10.1093/ejo/cjv046 PMID:26136438

Bonis, S. (2016). Stress and parents of children with autism: A review of the literature. *Issues in Mental Health Nursing*, *37*(3), 153–163. doi:10.3109/01612840.2015.1116030 PMID:27028741

Boothroyd, A. (1984). Auditory perception of speech contrasts by subjects with sensorineural hearing loss. *Journal of Speech, Language, and Hearing Research: JSLHR*, *27*(1), 134–144. doi:10.1044/jshr.2701.134 PMID:6716999

Boraston, Z., & Blakemore, S. J. (2007). The application of eye-tracking technology in the study of autism. *The Journal of Physiology*, *581*(3), 893–898. doi:10.1113/jphysiol.2007.133587 PMID:17430985

Bortolini, U., Caselli, M. C., Deevy, P., & Leonard, L. B. (2002). Specific language impairment in Italian: The first steps in the search for a clinical marker. *International Journal of Language & Communication Disorders*, *37*(2), 77–93. doi:10.1080/13682820110116758 PMID:12012618

Boyle, C. A., Boulet, S., Schieve, L. A., Cohen, R. A., Blumberg, S. J., Yeargin-Allsopp, M., ... Kogan, M. D. (2011). Trends in the prevalence of developmental disabilities in US children, 1997–2008. *Pediatrics*, *127*(6), 1034–1042. doi:10.1542/peds.2010-2989 PMID:21606152

Bradley, L., & Bryant, P. E. (1983). Categorizing sounds and learning to read-A causal connection. *Nature*, *301*(3), 419–421. doi:10.1038/301419a0

Branton, M. H., Schiffmann, R., Sabnis, S. G., Murray, G. J., Quirk, J. M., Altarescu, G., ... Kopp, J. B. (2002). Natural history of Fabry renal disease: Influence of alpha-galactosidase: A activity and genetic mutations on clinical course. *Medicine*, *81*(2), 122–138. doi:10.1097/00005792-200203000-00003 PMID:11889412

Bratton, S. C., & Ferebee, K. W. (1999). The use of structured expressive art activities in group activity therapy with preadolescents. In D. S. Sweeny & L. E. Homeyer (Eds.), *The handbook of group play therapy: How to do it, how it works, whom it's best for* (pp. 192–214). San Francisco, CA: Jossey-Bass.

Braud, L. W., Lupin, M. N., & Braud, W. G. (1975). The use of electromyographic biofeedback in the control of hyperactivity. *Journal of Learning Disabilities*, *8*(7), 420–452. doi:10.1177/002221947500800704

Braun, J., Lerner, A., & Gershoni-Baruch, R. (1991). The temporal bone in the Johanson-Blizzard syndrome. *Pediatric Radiology*, *21*(8), 580–583. doi:10.1007/BF02012603 PMID:1815181

Broder, P. K., & Dunivant, N. (1981). *Change in delinquent behavior as a function of learning disabilities: A two- year longitudinal study*. Williamsburg, VA: National Centre for State Courts.

Brodsky, S. L. (2013). *Testifying in court: Guidelines and maxims for the expert witness*. Washington, DC: American Psychological Association. doi:10.1037/14037-000

Brody, D. M., Nelon, B. A., & Brody, J. F. (1975). The use of visual feedback in establishing normal vocal intensity in two mildly retarded adults. *The Journal of Speech and Hearing Disorders*, *40*(4), 602–507. doi:10.1044/jshd.4004.502 PMID:1234966

Brook, S. L., & Bowler, D. M. (1992). Autism by another name? Semantic and pragmatic impairments in children. *Journal of Autism and Developmental Disorders*, *22*(1), 61–81. doi:10.1007/BF01046403 PMID:1592765

Brown, B. B. (1977). *Stress and the art of biofeedback*. New York: Harper & Row.

Brown, R. (1973). *A first language: The early stages*. Oxford, UK: Harvard University Press. doi:10.4159/harvard.9780674732469

Bruce, S. K. (2011). Academic underachievement: A neurodevelopmental perspective. *Revista Médica Clínica Las Condes*, *22*(2), 211–217. doi:10.1016/S0716-8640(11)70415-1

Brugha, T. S., McManus, S., Bankart, J., Scott, F., Purdon, S., Smith, J., & Meltzer, H. (2011). Epidemiology of autism spectrum disorders in adults in the community in England. *Archives of General Psychiatry*, *68*(5), 459–465. doi:10.1001/archgenpsychiatry.2011.38 PMID:21536975

Bruneau, D., Sasse, M. A., & McCarthy, J. D. (2002, April).The eyes never lie: The use of eye tracking data in HCI research. *Proceedings of the CHI*, 2, 25.

Bryson, S. E., Wainwright-Sharp, J. A., & Smith, I. M. (1990). Autism: A developmental spatial neglect syndrome? *Advances in Psychology*, *69*, 405–427. doi:10.1016/S0166-4115(08)60468-9

Budzynski, T., Stoyva, J., & Adler, C. (1970). Feedback induced relaxation: Application to tension headache. *Journal of Behavior Therapy and Experimental Psychiatry*, *1*(3), 205–211. doi:10.1016/0005-7916(70)90004-2

Buhrman, D., Thakkar, K., Poe, M., & Escolar, M. L. (2014). Natural history of Sanfilippo syndrome type A. *Journal of Inherited Metabolic Disease*, *37*(3), 431–437. doi:10.100710545-013-9661-8 PMID:24271936

Bulling, A., & Roggen, D., & Tröster, G. (2009). Wearable EOG goggles: Seamless sensing and context-awareness in everyday environments. *Journal of Ambient Intelligence and Smart Environments*, *1*, 157–171.

Bury, M. (2004). Researching patient/professional interactions. *Journal of Health Services Research & Policy*, *9*(1), 48–54. doi:10.1258/135581904322724130 PMID:15006228

Busch, C., Tucha, L., Talarovicova, A., Fuermaier, A. B. M., Lewis-Evans, B., & Tucha, O. (2016). Animal-assisted interventions for children with attention-deficit/hyperactivity disorder: A theoretical review and consideration of future research directions. *Psychological Reports*, *118*(1), 292–331. doi:10.1177/0033294115626633 PMID:29693527

Buschkens, J., Graham, D., & Cottrell, D. (2010). Well-being Under chronic stress: Is morningness an advantage? *Stress and Health*, *26*(4), 330–340. doi:10.1002mi.1300

Bush, G., Valera, E. M., & Seidman, L. J. (2005). Functional neuroimaging of attention-deficit/hyperactivity disorder: A review and suggested future directions. *Biological Psychiatry*, *57*(11), 1273–1284. doi:10.1016/j.biopsych.2005.01.034 PMID:15949999

Butler, F. (1978). *Biofeedback: A survey of literature*. New York: Plenum Publishing Corporation.

Butler, F., & Stoyva, J. (1973). *Biofeedback and self-regulation: A bibliography*. Colorado: Biofeedback Research Society.

Bylund, C. L., Weiss, E. S., Michaels, M., Patel, S., D'Agostino, T. A., Peterson, E. B., ... McKee, M. D. (2017). Primary care physicians' attitudes and beliefs about cancer clinical trials. *Clinical Trials*, *14*(5), 518–525. doi:10.1177/1740774517717722 PMID:28693389

Byrne, D., Sinclair, S., & Noble, W. (1998). Open earmold fittings for improving aided auditory localization for sensorineural hearing losses with good high-frequency hearing. *Ear and Hearing*, *19*(1), 62–71. doi:10.1097/00003446-199802000-00004 PMID:9504273

Byrne, M. D., Anderson, J. R., Douglass, S., & Matessa, M. (1999). Eye tracking the visual search of click-down menus. In *Proceedings of the SIGCHI conference on Human Factors in Computing Systems* (pp. 402-409). ACM. 10.1145/302979.303118

Calder, P. C. (2013). Omega-3 polyunsaturated fatty acids and inflammatory processes: Nutrition or pharmacology? *British Journal of Clinical Pharmacology*, *75*(3), 645–662. doi:10.1111/j.1365-2125.2012.04374.x PMID:22765297

Campbell, J. M., Morgan, S. B., & Jackson, J. N. (2004). Autism spectrum disorders and mental retardation. In R. T. Brown (Ed.), *Handbook of pediatric psychology in school settings*. Lawrence Erlbaum Associates.

Cannell, J. J. (2008). Autism and vitamin D. *Medical Hypotheses*, *70*(4), 750–759. doi:10.1016/j.mehy.2007.08.016 PMID:17920208

Card, R., & Dodd, B. (2006). The phonological awareness abilities of children with cerebral palsy who do not speak. *Augmentative and Alternative Communication*, *22*(3), 149–159. doi:10.1080/07434610500431694 PMID:17114160

Carper, R. A., & Courchesne, E. (2000). Inverse correlation between frontal lobe and cerebellum sizes in children with autism. *Brain*, *123*(4), 836–844. doi:10.1093/brain/123.4.836 PMID:10734014

Carper, R. A., Moses, P., Tigue, Z. D., & Courchesne, E. (2002). Cerebral lobes in autism: Early hyperplasia and abnormal age effects. *NeuroImage*, *16*(4), 1038–1051. doi:10.1006/nimg.2002.1099 PMID:12202091

Carroll, L. S., & Owen, M. J. (2009). Genetic overlap between autism, schizophrenia and bipolar disorder. *Genome Medicine*, *1*(102), 1–7. PMID:19886976

Carter, R. M. (2011). *The interaction between lawyers and physicians in litigation*. Edmonton, Alberta: The Law Society of Alberta.

Caruana, N., Stieglitz Ham, H., Brock, J., Woolgar, A., Kloth, N., Palermo, R., & McArthur, G. (2017). Joint attention difficulties in autistic adults: An interactive eye-tracking study. *Autism*, 1362361316676204. PMID:28423919

Carulla, L. S., Reed, G. M., Vaez-Azizi, L. M., Cooper, S. A., Leal, R., Bertelli, M., ... Girimaji, S. C. (2011). Intellectual developmental disorders: Towards a new name, definition and framework for "mental retardation/intellectual disability" in ICD-11. *World Psychiatry; Official Journal of the World Psychiatric Association (WPA)*, *10*(3), 175–180. doi:10.1002/j.2051-5545.2011.tb00045.x PMID:21991267

Carver, R. H., & Nash, J. G. (2009). *Doing data analysis with SPSS: Version 20*. Belmont, CA: Brooks/Cole Cengage Learning.

Castelli, F., Frith, C., Happé, F., & Frith, U. (2002). Autism, Asperger syndrome and brain mechanisms for the attribution of mental states to animated shapes. *Brain*, *125*(8), 1839–1849. doi:10.1093/brain/awf189 PMID:12135974

Castren, E., Elgersma, Y., Maffel, L., & Hagerman, R. (2012). Treatment of neurodevelopmental disorders in adulthood. *The Journal of Neuroscience*, *32*(41), 14074–14079. doi:10.1523/JNEUROSCI.3287-12.2012 PMID:23055475

Cataltepe, S., & Tuncbilek, E. (1992). A family with one child with acrocallosal syndrome, one child with anencephaly-polydactyly, and parental consanguinity. *European Journal of Pediatrics*, *151*(4), 288–290. doi:10.1007/BF02072231 PMID:1499582

Cauffman, E., & Steinberg, L. (2000). (Im)maturity of judgment in adolescence: Why adolescents may be less culpable than adults. *Behavioral Sciences & the Law*, *18*(6), 741–743. doi:10.1002/bsl.416 PMID:11180420

Centers for Disease Control and Prevention. (2016, March 31). *CDC estimates 1 in 68 school-aged children have autism: No change from previous estimate*. Retrieved from https://www.cdc.gov/media/releases/2016/p0331-children-autism.html

Centers for Disease Control and Prevention. (2017, March 10). Autism spectrum disorder (ASD). Retrieved from https://www.cdc.gov/ncbddd/autism/data.html

Cermak, S. A., Curtin, C., & Bandini, L. G. (2010). Food selectivity and sensory sensitivity in children with autism spectrum disorders. *Journal of the Academy of Nutrition and Dietetics*, *110*(2), 238–246. PMID:20102851

Chafetz, M., & Dufrene, M. (2014). Malingering-by-proxy: The need for child protection and guidance for reporting. *Child Abuse & Neglect*, *38*(11), 1755–1765. doi:10.1016/j.chiabu.2014.08.015 PMID:25236718

Chailangkarn, T., Trujillo, C. A., Freitas, B. C., Hrvoj-Mihic, B., Herai, R. H., Diana, X. Y., ... Stefanacci, L. (2016). A human neurodevelopmental model for Williams syndrome. *Nature*, *536*(7616), 338–343. doi:10.1038/nature19067 PMID:27509850

Chandler, C. K. (2012). *Animal-assisted therapy in counseling*. New York, NY: Taylor & Francis.

Chandler, S., Howlin, P., Simonoff, E., Kennedy, J., & Baird, G. (2016). Comparison of the parental estimate of developmental age with measured IQ in children with neurodevelopmental disorders. *Child: Care, Health and Development*, *42*(4), 486–493. doi:10.1111/cch.12346 PMID:27126521

Chandra, N. (2012). 'Disability' on sale: Enjoy benefits for the handicapped as touts can get you fake certificates. *Mail Online India*. Retrieved from http://www.dailymail.co.uk/indiahome/indianews/article-2180685/Disability-sale-Enjoy-benefits-handicapped-touts-fake-certificates.html

Chapman, R. S., Schwartz, S. E., & Bird, E. K. R. (1991). Language skills of children and adolescents with Down syndrome: I. Comprehension. *Journal of Speech and Hearing Research*, *34*(5), 1106–1120. doi:10.1044/jshr.3405.1106 PMID:1836243

Chapman, R. S., Seung, H. K., Schwartz, S. E., & Bird, E. K. R. (1998). Language skills of children and adolescents with Down syndrome: II. Production deficits. *Journal of Speech, Language, and Hearing Research: JSLHR*, *41*(4), 861–873. doi:10.1044/jslhr.4104.861 PMID:9712133

Chatfield, K. C., Schrier, S. A., Li, J., Clark, D., Kaur, M., Kline, A. D., ... Krantz, I. D. (2012). Congenital heart disease in Cornelia de Lange syndrome: Phenotype and genotype analysis. *American Journal of Medical Genetics. Part A*, *158A*(10), 2499–2505. doi:10.1002/ajmg.a.35582 PMID:22965847

Chawarska, K., Macari, S., & Shic, F. (2012). Context modulates attention to social scenes in toddlers with autism. *Journal of Child Psychology and Psychiatry, and Allied Disciplines*, *53*(8), 903–913. doi:10.1111/j.1469-7610.2012.02538.x PMID:22428993

Chazan, S., & Cohen, E. (2010). Adaptive and defensive strategies in post-traumatic play of young children exposed to violent attacks. *Journal of Child Psychotherapy*, *36*(2), 133–151. doi:10.1080/0075417X.2010.495024

Chen, C., Chen, H., Hong, W., Yang, F. G., Yang, L., & Wu, C. (2010). Oromotor variability in children with mild spastic cerebral palsy: A kinematic study of speech motor control. *Journal of Neuroengineering and Rehabilitation*, *7*(1), 54. doi:10.1186/1743-0003-7-54 PMID:20979638

Cheng, M. F. (1992). For whom does the female dove coo? A case for the role of vocal self-stimulation. *Animal Behaviour*, *43*(6), 1035–1044. doi:10.1016/S0003-3472(06)80016-3

Cheng, M. F. (2003). Vocal self-stimulation: From the ring dove story to emotion-based vocal communication. *Advances in the Study of Behavior*, *33*, 309–353. doi:10.1016/S0065-3454(03)33007-4

Chennamma, H. R., & Yuan, X. (2013). *A survey on eye-gaze tracking techniques*. arXiv preprint arXiv:1312.6410

Chew, E., Ghosh, M., & McCulloch, C. (1982). Amiodarone-induced cornea verticillata. *Canadian Journal of Ophthalmology. Journal Canadien D'ophtalmologie*, *17*, 96–99. PMID:7116220

Chinnery, P. F., Elliott, C., Green, G. R., Rees, A., Coulthard, A., Turnbull, D. M., & Griffiths, T. D. (2000). The spectrum of hearing loss due to mitochondrial DNA defects. *Brain*, *123*(1), 82–92. doi:10.1093/brain/123.1.82 PMID:10611123

Chiri, G., & Warfield, M. (2012). Unmet need and problems accessing core health care services for children with autism spectrum disorder. *Maternal and Child Health Journal*, *16*(5), 1081–1091. doi:10.100710995-011-0833-6 PMID:21667201

Chiu, P. H., Kayali, M. A., Kishida, K. T., Tomlin, D., Klinger, L. G., Klinger, M. R., & Montague, P. R. (2008). Self responses along cingulate cortex reveal quantitative neural phenotype for high-functioning autism. *Neuron*, *57*(3), 463–473. doi:10.1016/j.neuron.2007.12.020 PMID:18255038

Chuang, L. H., Soares, M. O., Tilbrook, H., Cox, H., Hewitt, C. E., Aplin, J., ... Torgerson, D. J. (2012). A pragmatic multicentered randomized controlled trial of yoga for chronic low back pain: Economic evaluation. *Spine*, *37*(18), 1593–1601. doi:10.1097/BRS.0b013e3182545937 PMID:22433499

Chugani, D. C., Muzik, O., Rothermel, R., Behen, M., Chakraborty, P., Mangner, T., & Chugani, H. T. (1997). Altered serotonin synthesis in the dentatothalamocortical pathway in autistic boys. *Annals of Neurology*, *42*(4), 666–669. doi:10.1002/ana.410420420 PMID:9382481

Ciechanover, A. (1994). The ubiquitin-mediated proteolytic pathway: Mechanisms of action and cellular physiology. *Biological Chemistry Hoppe-Seyler*, *375*, 565–581. PMID:7840898

Ciechanover, A., & Iwai, K. (2004). The ubiquitin system: From basic mechanisms to the patient bed. *IUBMB Life*, *56*(4), 193–201. doi:10.1080/15216540420000223616 PMID:15230346

Cioni, G., Inguaggiato, E., & Sgandurra, G. (2016). Early intervention in neurodevelopmental disorders: Underlying neural mechanisms. *Developmental Medicine and Child Neurology*, *58*(S4), 61–66. doi:10.1111/dmcn.13050 PMID:27027609

Clausen, J. M., Ruff, S. C., Wiederhold, W. V., & Heineman, T. V. (2012). For as long as it takes: Relationship-based play therapy for children in foster care. *Psychoanalytic Social Work*, *19*(1-2), 43–53. doi:10.1080/15228878.2012.666481

Clegg, J., Gillott, A., & Jones, J. (2013). Conceptual issues in neurodevelopmental disorders: Lives out of synch. *Current Opinion in Psychiatry*, *28*, 1–3. doi:10.1097/ YCO.ObO13e32835f6771 PMID:23519204

Cloud, H., Ekvall, S. W., & Hicks, L. (2005). Feeding problems of the child with special health-care needs. In S. W. Ekvall & V. K. Ekvall (Eds.), *Pediatric Nutrition in Chronic Diseases and Developmental Disorders: Prevention, assessment and treatment* (2nd ed., pp. 172–182). New York: Oxford University Press.

Coben, R., & Myers, T. E. (2010). The relative efficacy of connectivity guided and symptom-based EEG biofeedback for autistic disorders. *Applied Psycho-physiological Biofeedback*, *35*(1), 13–23. doi:10.100710484 009-9102-5 PMID:19649702

Cogan, D. G., Chu, F. C., & Reingold, D. B. (1982). Ocular signs of cerebellar disease. *Archives of Ophthalmology*, *100*(5), 755–760. doi:10.1001/archopht.1982.01030030759007 PMID:7082205

Coi, A., Santoro, M., Pierini, A., Marrucci, S., Pieroni, F., & Bianchi, F. (2017). Prevalence estimates of rare congenital anomalies by integrating two population-based registries in Tuscany, Italy. *Public Health Genomics*, *20*(4), 229–234. doi:10.1159/000481358 PMID:29045944

Coleman, P. D., Romano, J., Lapham, L., & Simon, W. (1985). Cell counts in cerebral cortex of an autistic patient. *Journal of Autism and Developmental Disorders*, *15*(3), 245–255. doi:10.1007/BF01531496 PMID:4030660

Collins, B. C., & Collins, T. M. (2005). *Crisis and trauma: Developmental-ecological intervention.* Boston: Houghton Mifflin.

Collins, T. (2005). Health policy analysis: A simple tool for policy makers. *Public Health*, *119*(3), 192–196. doi:10.1016/j.puhe.2004.03.006 PMID:15661129

Congenital Anomalies: Prevalence and Risk Factors. (n.d.). Retrieved March 31, 2018, from https://www.researchgate.net/publication/259526843_Congenital_Anomalies_Prevalence_and_Risk_Factors

Connan, F., Campbell, I. C., Katzman, M., Lightman, S. L., & Treasure, J. (2003). A neurodevelopmental model for anorexia nervosa. *Physiology & Behavior*, *79*(1), 13–24. doi:10.1016/S0031-9384(03)00101-X PMID:12818706

Connor, K., & Miller, J. (2000). Animal-assisted therapy: An in-depth look. *Dimensions of Critical Care Nursing*, *19*(3), 20–26. doi:10.1097/00003465-200019030-00006 PMID:11998003

Conrad, S., & Rout, A. (2013). Perceived Occlusion and Comfort in Receiver-in-the-Ear Hearing Aids. *American Journal of Audiology*, *22*(2), 283–290. doi:10.1044/1059-0889(2013/11-0025) PMID:23824427

Coonrod, E. E., & Stone, W. L. (2005). Screening for autism in young children. In F. R. Volkmar, R. Paul, A. Klin, & D. Cohen (Eds.), Handbook of Autism and Pervasive Developmental Disorders (pp. 707–729). New York: Wiley; doi:10.1002/9780470939352.ch1

Cooper, S. A. (1997). Deficient health and social services for elderly people with learning disabilities. *Journal of Intellectual Disability Research*, *41*(4), 331–338. doi:10.1111/j.1365-2788.1997.tb00717.x PMID:9297611

Cornelissen, R. M. M. (2004). The evolution of consciousness in Sri Aurobindo's cosmo-psychology. In H. Wautischer (Ed.), *Ontology of consciousness: Percipient action* (pp. 1–29). Boston: The MIT Press.

Cornish, K., Scerif, G., & Karmiloff-Smith, A. (2007). Tracing syndrome-specific trajectories of attention across the lifespan. *Cortex*, *43*(6), 672–685. doi:10.1016/S0010-9452(08)70497-0 PMID:17710820

Coulson-Thomas, V. J., Gesteira, T. F., Esko, J., & Kao, W. (2014). Heparan sulfate regulates hair follicle and sebaceous gland morphogenesis and homeostasis. *The Journal of Biological Chemistry*, *289*(36), 25211–25226. doi:10.1074/jbc.M114.572511 PMID:25053416

Courchesne, E., Hesselink, J. R., Jernigan, T. L., & Yeung-Courchesne, R. (1987). Abnormal neuroanatomy in a nonretarded person with autism: Unusual findings with magnetic resonance imaging. *Archives of Neurology*, *44*(3), 335–341. doi:10.1001/archneur.1987.00520150073028 PMID:3827686

Courchesne, E., Karns, C. M., Davis, H. R., Ziccardi, R., Carper, R. A., Tigue, Z. D., & Lincoln, A. J. (2001). Unusual brain growth patterns in early life in patients with autistic disorder an MRI study. *Neurology*, *57*(2), 245–254. doi:10.1212/WNL.57.2.245 PMID:11468308

Courchesne, E., & Pierce, K. (2005). Brain overgrowth in autism during a critical time in development: Implications for frontal pyramidal neuron and interneuron development and connectivity. *International Journal of Developmental Neuroscience*, *23*(2-3), 153–170. doi:10.1016/j.ijdevneu.2005.01.003 PMID:15749242

Courchesne, E., Saitoh, O., Yeung-Courchesne, R., Press, G. A., Lincoln, A. J., Haas, R. H., & Schreibman, L. (1994). Abnormality of cerebellar vermian lobules VI and VII in patients with infantile autism: Identification of hypoplastic and hyperplastic subgroups with MR imaging. *AJR. American Journal of Roentgenology*, *162*(1), 123–130. doi:10.2214/ajr.162.1.8273650 PMID:8273650

Couriel, J. M., Bisse, R., Miller, R., Thomas, A., & Clarke, M. (1993). Assessment of feeding problems in neurodevelopmental handicap: A team approach. *Archives of Disease in Childhood*, *69*(5), 609–613. doi:10.1136/adc.69.5.609 PMID:7504911

Courtens, W., Vamos, E., Christophe, C., & Schinzel, A. (1998). Acrocallosal syndrome in Algerian boy born to consanguineous parents: Review of the literature and further delineation of the syndrome. *American Journal of Medical Genetics*, *69*(1), 17–22. doi:10.1002/(SICI)1096-8628(19970303)69:1<17::AID-AJMG4>3.0.CO;2-Q PMID:9066878

Craig, A. R., & Cleary, P. J. (1982). Reduction of stuttering by young male stutterers using EMG feedback. *Biofeedback and Self-Regulation*, *7*(3), 241–255. doi:10.1007/BF00998918 PMID:7171633

Craig, F., Operto, F. F., De Giacomo, A., Margari, L., Frolli, A., Conson, M., ... Margari, F. (2016). Parenting stress among parents of children with neurodevelopmental disorders. *Psychiatry Research*, *242*, 121–129. doi:10.1016/j.psychres.2016.05.016 PMID:27280521

Crawford, H., Moss, J., Oliver, C., Elliot, N., Anderson, G. M., & McCleery, J. P. (2016). Visual preference for social stimuli in individuals with autism or neurodevelopmental disorders: An eye-tracking study. *Molecular Autism,* 7- 24. doi:10.118613229-016-0084-x

Crawford, D. (1996). Review of research on learning disabilities and juvenile delinquency. In S. Cramer & W. Ellis (Eds.), *Learning Disabilities: Lifelong Issues*. Baltimore, MD: Paul H. Brookes Publishing Co.

Crawley, J. N. (2012). Translational animal models of autism and neurodevelopmental disorders. *Dialogues in Clinical Neuroscience*, *14*(3), 293–305. PMID:23226954

Crie, M. (2005). *Teaching today: Helping dyslexic students succeed.* Available: http://www.glencoe.com/sec/teachingtoday/educationupclose.phtml/46

Cristino, A. S., Williams, S. M., Hawi, Z., An, J.-Y., Bellgrove, M. A., Schwartz, C. E., ... Claudianos, C. (2014). Neurodevelopmental and neuropsychiatric disorders represent an interconnected molecular system. *Molecular Psychiatry*, *19*(3), 297–301. doi:10.1038/mp.2013.16 PMID:23439483

Crist, W., McDonnell, P., Beck, M., Gillespie, C. T., Barrett, P., & Mathews, J. (1994). Behavior at mealtimes and the young child with cystic fibrosis. *Journal of Developmental and Behavioral Pediatrics*, *15*(3), 157–161. doi:10.1097/00004703-199406000-00001

Crist, W., & Napier-Phillips, A. (2001). Mealtime behaviors of young children: A comparison of normative and clinical data. *Journal of Developmental and Behavioral Pediatrics*, *22*(5), 279–286. doi:10.1097/00004703-200110000-00001 PMID:11718230

Critchley, H. D., Daly, E. M., Bullmore, E. T., Williams, S. C., Van Amelsvoort, T., Robertson, D. M., & Murphy, D. G. (2000). The functional neuroanatomy of social behaviour: Changes in cerebral blood flow when people with autistic disorder process facial expressions. *Brain*, *123*(11), 2203–2212. doi:10.1093/brain/123.11.2203 PMID:11050021

Croughan, M. (2001). Factors influencing physician participation in practice-based research network studies: A call for further research. [Commentary]. *The Journal of Family Practice*, *50*(11), 978. PMID:11711017

Cruz, I., Vicaria, I., Wang, N.-Y., Niparko, J., & Quittner, A. L. (2012). Language and behavioral outcomes in children with developmental disabilities using cochlear implants. *Otology & Neurotology*, *33*(5), 751–760. doi:10.1097/MAO.0b013e3182595309 PMID:22699986

Cryan, J. F., & Dinan, T. G. (2015). More than a gut feeling: The microbiota regulates neurodevelopment and behavior. *Neuropsychopharmacology*, *40*(1), 241–242. doi:10.1038/npp.2014.224 PMID:25482171

Crystal, D. (1986). Pasado, presente y futuro de la linguïsticaclinica [The past, present and future of clinical linguistics]. In M. Montfort (Ed), Investigaccion y logopedia (pp. 34-42). Madrid: Ciencias de la EducacionPreescolar y Especial, III LogopedicsCongess, Madrid.

Crystal, D. (1984). *Linguistic Encounters with language handicapped.* Oxford, UK: Blackwell.

Cullen, L., Titler, M., & Drahozal, R. (1999). Family and pet visitation in the critical care unit. *Critical Care Nurse*, *19*(3), 84. PMID:10661096

Cumine, V., Leach, J., & Stevenson, G. (2000). *Autism in the early years: A practical guide.* London: David Fulton.

Cumine, V., Leach, J., & Stevenson, G. (2000). *The pre-school child with autism.* London: David Fulton.

Cunningham, M., & Murphy, P. (1981). The effects of bilateral EEG biofeedback on verbal, visuospatial and creative skills in LD male adolescents. *Journal of Learning Disabilities*, *14*(4), 204–208. doi:10.1177/002221948101400406 PMID:7229554

Cuschieri, T., Khaled, R., Farrugia, V. E., Martinez, H. P., & Yannakakis, G. N. (2014 September). The iLearnRW Game: Support for Students with Dyslexia in Class and at Home. In *Games and Virtual Worlds for Serious Applications (VS-GAMES), 2014 6th International Conference on* (pp. 1-2). IEEE.

Dahan-Oliel, N., Shikako-Thomas, K., & Majnemer, A. (2012). Quality of life and leisure participation in children with neurodevelopmental disabilities: A thematic analysis of the literature. *Quality of Life Research: An International Journal of Quality of Life Aspects of Treatment, Care and Rehabilitation*, *21*(3), 427–439. doi:10.100711136-011-0063-9 PMID:22101860

Daly, D. A., & Cantrell, R. P. (2006). *Cluttering: Characteristics labelled as diagnostically significant by 60 fluency experts.* Paper presented at the 6th IFA world congress on disorders of fluency, Dublin, Ireland.

Damasio, A. R., & Maurer, R. G. (1978). A neurological model for childhood autism. *Archives of Neurology*, *35*(12), 777–786. doi:10.1001/archneur.1978.00500360001001 PMID:718482

Davidson, P. W., Myers, G. J., & Weiss, B. (2004). Mercury exposure and child development outcomes. *Pediatrics*, *113*(Supplement 3), 1023–1029. PMID:15060195

Davies, W. H., Ackerman, L. K., Davies, C. M., Vannatta, K., & Noll, R. B. (2007). About your child's eating: Factor structure and psychometric properties of a feeding relationship measure. *Eating Behaviors*, *8*(4), 457–463. doi:10.1016/j.eatbeh.2007.01.001 PMID:17950934

Dawson, G. (2008). Early behavioral intervention, brain plasticity, and the prevention of autism spectrum disorder. *Development and Psychopathology*, *20*(3), 775–803. doi:10.1017/S0954579408000370 PMID:18606031

Dawson, G., Munson, J., Webb, S. J., Nalty, T., Abbott, R., & Toth, K. (2007). Rate of head growth decelerates and symptoms worsen in the second year of life in autism. *Biological Psychiatry*, *61*(4), 458–464. doi:10.1016/j.biopsych.2006.07.016 PMID:17137564

Dawson, G., Osterling, J., Meltzoff, A. N., & Kuhl, P. (2000). Case study of the development of an infant with autism from birth to two years of age. *Journal of Applied Developmental Psychology*, *21*(3), 299–313. doi:10.1016/S0193-3973(99)00042-8 PMID:23667283

De Felice, A., Ricceri, L., Venerosi, A., Chiarotti, F., & Calamandrei, G. (2015). Multifactorial origin of neurodevelopmental disorders: Approaches to understanding complex aetiologies. *Toxics*, *3*(1), 89–129. doi:10.3390/toxics3010089 PMID:29056653

De Luca, M., Di Pace, E., Judica, A., Spinelli, D., & Zoccolotti, P. (1999). Eye movement patterns in linguistic and non-linguistic tasks in developmental surface dyslexia. *Neuropsychologia*, *37*(12), 1407–1420. doi:10.1016/S0028-3932(99)00038-X PMID:10606014

De Souza, A. S., Fernandes, F. S., & Tavares do Carmo, M. D. G. (2011). Effects of maternal malnutrition and postnatal nutritional rehabilitation on brain fatty acids, learning, and memory. *Nutrition Reviews*, *69*(3), 132–144. doi:10.1111/j.1753-4887.2011.00374.x PMID:21348877

Delhi Commission for Protection of Child Rights. (2015). *Why children commit offences: Study on children in conflict with the law in Delhi.* New Delhi: Author.

Delpech, J. C., Thomazeau, A., Madore, C., Bosch-Bouju, C., Larrieu, T., Lacabanne, C., & Layé, S. (2015). Dietary n-3 PUFAs deficiency increases vulnerability to inflammation-induced spatial memory impairment. *Neuropsychopharmacology, 40*(12), 2774–2787. doi:10.1038/npp.2015.127 PMID:25948102

Demeter, S. L., & Andersson, B. J. (2003). *Disability evaluation*. St. Louis, MO: Mosby.

Desikachar, T. K. V. (1999). *The heart of Yoga: Developing a personal practice*. Rochester, VT: Inner Traditions International.

DeSilva, M. D. K., Kooknoor, V., Shetty, H. N., & Thontadarya, S. (2016). Effect of multichannel and channels free hearing aid signal processing on phoneme recognition in quiet and noise. *International Journal of Health Sciences and Research, 6*(3), 248–257.

Desroches, A. S., Joanisse, M. F., & Robertson, E. K. (2006). Specific phonological impairments in dyslexia revealed by eye tracking. *Cognition, 100*(3), B32–B42. doi:10.1016/j.cognition.2005.09.001 PMID:16288732

Di Stasi, L. L., Catena, A., Canas, J. J., Macknik, S. L., & Martinez-Conde, S. (2013). Saccadic velocity as an arousal index in naturalistic tasks. *Neuroscience and Biobehavioral Reviews, 37*(5), 968–975. doi:10.1016/j.neubiorev.2013.03.011 PMID:23541685

Dicara, L. V., & Miller, N. E. (1968). Instrumental learning of vasomotor responses by rats: Learning to respond differentially in the two ears. *Science, 159*(3822), 1485–1486. doi:10.1126cience.159.3822.1485 PMID:5732491

Dickinson, A., Gregor, P., & Newell, A. F. (2002, July). Ongoing investigation of the ways in which some of the problems encountered by some dyslexics can be alleviated using computer techniques. In *Proceedings of the fifth international ACM conference on Assistive technologies* (pp. 97-103). ACM. 10.1145/638249.638268

Diehl, J. J., Schmitt, L. M., Villano, M., & Crowell, C. R. (2012). The clinical use of robots for individuals with Autism Spectrum Disorders: A critical review. *Research in Autism Spectrum Disorders, 6*(1), 249–262. doi:10.1016/j.rasd.2011.05.006 PMID:22125579

Dillon, A., Kelly, M., Robertson, I. H., & Robertson, D. A. (2016). Smartphone applications utilizing biofeedback can aid stress reduction. *Frontiers in Psychology, 7*, 832. doi:10.3389/fpsyg.2016.00832 PMID:27378963

Dillon, H., Keidser, G., O'Brien, A., & Silberstein, H. (2003). Sound quality comparisons of advanced hearing aids. *The Hearing Journal, 56*(4), 30–40. doi:10.1097/01.HJ.0000293908.50552.34

Ding, Y., Leng, J., Fan, F., Xia, B., & Xu, P. (2013). The role of mitochondrial DNA mutations in hearing loss. *Biochemical Genetics, 51*(7-8), 588–602. doi:10.100710528-013-9589-6 PMID:23605717

Diwan, S., & Diwan, J. (2013). A study of feeding problems in children with cerebral palsy. *National Journal of Integrated Research in Medicine, 4*, 78–86.

Dodd, B. (1975). Recognition and reproduction of words by Down's syndrome and non-Down's syndrome retarded children. *American Journal of Mental Deficiency, 80*(3), 306–311. PMID:127529

Dodrill, P. (2014). Feeding problems and oropharyngeal dysphagia in children. *Journal of Gastroenterology and Hepatology Research, 3*(5).

Doemberg, E., & Hollander, E. (2016). Neurodevelopmental disorders (ASD and ADHD): DSM-5, ICD-10, and ICD-11. *CNS Spectrums, 21*(4), 295–299. doi:10.1017/S1092852916000262 PMID:27364515

Dollaghan, C. A. (2007). *The handbook for evidence-based practice in communication disorders*. Paul H. Brookes Pub.

Donaldson, G. W., Moinpour, C. M., Bush, N. E., Chapko, M., Jocom, J., Siadak, M., & Sullivan, K. M. (1999). Physician participation in research surveys: A randomized study of inducements to return mailed research questionnaires. *Evaluation & the Health Professions*, *22*(4), 427–441. doi:10.1177/01632789922034392 PMID:10623399

Dossetor, D. R. (2007). 'All that glitters is not gold': Misdiagnosis of psychosis in pervasive developmental disorders-A case series. *Clinical Child Psychology and Psychiatry*, *12*(4), 537–548. doi:10.1177/1359104507078476 PMID:18095536

Drusch, G., Bastien, J. C., & Paris, S. (2014). Analysing eye-tracking data: From scanpaths and heatmaps to the dynamic visualization of areas of interest. *Advances in Science, Technology. Higher Education and Society in the Conceptual Age: STHESCA*, *20*, 205.

Duchowski, A. T. (2007). Eye tracking methodology. *Theory into Practice*, 328.

Duchowski, A. T. (2007). *Eye Tracking Methodology: Theory and Practice*. New York: Springer-Verlag Inc.

Duchowski, A. T., Driver, J., Jolaoso, S., Tan, W., Ramey, B. N., & Robbins, A. (2010). Scanpath comparison revisited. In *Proceedings of the 2010 symposium on eye-tracking research & applications* (pp. 219-226). ACM. 10.1145/1743666.1743719

Dumitrascu, C. I., Gallardo, K. E., & Caplan, J. P. (2015). Malingering imposed on another: A diagnosis that is missing in action? *Psychosomatics*, *56*(6), 609–614. doi:10.1016/j.psym.2015.07.006 PMID:26497617

Durand, V. M., & Barlow, D. (2009). *Abnormal psychology: An integrative approach*. Belmont, CA: Wadsworth Cengage Learning.

Dusek, J. A., Otu, H. H., Wohlhueter, A. L., Bhasin, M., Zerbini, L. F., Joseph, M. G., ... Libermann, T. A. (2008). Genomic counter-stress changes induced by the relaxation response. *PLoS One*, *3*(7), e2576. doi:10.1371/journal.pone.0002576 PMID:18596974

Dykens, E. M. (2015). Family adjustment and interventions in neurodevelopmental disorders. *Current Opinion in Psychiatry*, *28*(2), 121–126. doi:10.1097/YCO.0000000000000129 PMID:25594421

Eapen, V., Nicholls, L., Spagnol, V., & Mathew, N. E. (2017). Current status of biological treatment options in autism spectrum disorder. *Asian Journal of Psychiatry*, *30*, 1–10. doi:10.1016/j.ajp.2017.07.025 PMID:28704714

Ecker, C., Bookheimer, S. Y., & Murphy, D. G. M. (2015). Neuroimaging in autism spectrum disorder: Brain structure and function across life span. *Lancet Neurology*, *14*(11), 1121–1134. doi:10.1016/S1474-4422(15)00050-2 PMID:25891007

Edwards, L. (2010). Learning Disabilities in Deaf and Hard-of-Hearing Children. In M. Marschark & P. E. Spencer (Eds.), *The Oxford handbook of deaf studies, language and education* (Vol. 2). Oxford University Press. doi:10.1093/oxfordhb/9780195390032.013.0028

Egaas, B., Courchesne, E., & Saitoh, O. (1995). Reduced size of corpus callosum in autism. *Archives of Neurology*, *52*(8), 794–801. doi:10.1001/archneur.1995.00540320070014 PMID:7639631

Egelund, E. P. (1987). Congenital hearing loss in patients with Cornelia de Lange syndrome (a report of two cases). *The Journal of Laryngology and Otology*, *101*(12), 1276–1279. doi:10.1017/S0022215100103652 PMID:3323381

Eigsti, I. M., & Bennetto, L. (2009). Grammaticality judgments in autism: Deviance or delay. *Journal of Child Language*, *36*(5), 999–1021. doi:10.1017/S0305000909009362 PMID:19224652

Ekinci, O., Arman, A. R., Işık, U., Bez, Y., & Berkem, M. (2010). EEG abnormalities and epilepsy in autistic spectrum disorders: Clinical and familial correlates. *Epilepsy & Behavior*, *17*(2), 178–182. doi:10.1016/j.yebeh.2009.11.014 PMID:20042370

Elder, L. M., Dawson, G., Toth, K., Fein, D., & Munson, J. (2008). Head circumference as an early predictor of autism symptoms in younger siblings of children with autism spectrum disorder. *Journal of Autism and Developmental Disorders, 38*(6), 1104–1111. doi:10.100710803-007-0495-9 PMID:18058011

Elfenbein, J. L., Hardin-Jones, M. A., & Davis, J. M. (1994). Oral communication skills of children who are hard of hearing. *Journal of Speech, Language, and Hearing Research: JSLHR, 37*(1), 216–226. doi:10.1044/jshr.3701.216 PMID:8170125

Elia, J., Ambrosini, P. J., & Rapoport, J. L. (1999). Treatment of attention-deficit-hyperactivity disorder. *The New England Journal of Medicine, 340*(10), 780–788. doi:10.1056/NEJM199903113401007 PMID:10072414

Ellery, K. M., & Erdman, S. H. (2014). Johanson-Blizzard Syndrome: Expanding the Phenotype of Exocrine Pancreatic Insufficiency. *Journal of the Pancreas, 15*(4), 388–390. PMID:25076350

Elnakib, A., Casanova, M. F., Gimelrfarb, G., Switala, A. E., & El-Baz, A. (2012). Dyslexia diagnostics by 3-D shape analysis of the corpus callosum. *IEEE Transactions on Information Technology in Biomedicine, 16*(4), 700–708. doi:10.1109/TITB.2012.2187302 PMID:22334032

Elsabbagh, M., Divan, G., Koh, Y. J., Kim, Y. S., Kauchali, S., Marcín, C., ... Yasamy, M. T. (2012). Global prevalence of autism and other pervasive developmental disorders. *Autism Research, 5*(3), 160–179. doi:10.1002/aur.239 PMID:22495912

Enck, P., Van Der Voort, I. R., & Klosterhalfen, S. (2009). Biofeedback therapy for fecal incontinence and constipation. *Neurogastroenterology and Motility, 21*(11), 1133–1141. doi:10.1111/j.1365-2982.2009.01345.x PMID:19566591

Erick, P. (1993). Biofeedback training in disordered defecation: A critical review. *Digestive Diseases and Sciences, 38*(11), 1953–1960. doi:10.1007/BF01297069 PMID:8223066

Erny, D., de Angelis, A. L. H., Jaitin, D., Wieghofer, P., Staszewski, O., David, E., & Schwierzeck, V. (2015). Host microbiota constantly control maturation and function of microglia in the CNS. *Nature Neuroscience, 18*(7), 965–977. doi:10.1038/nn.4030 PMID:26030851

Esmaili, S. K., Shafaroodi, N., & Zardkhaneh, S. A. (2017). Effect of play based therapy on meta-cognitive and behavioral aspects of executive functions: A randomised, controlled, clinical trial on the students with learning disabilities. *Basic and Clinical Neuroscience, 8*(3), 2003–2012.

Estes, A., Zwaigenbaum, L., Gu, H., John, T. S., Paterson, S., Elison, J. T., & Kostopoulos, P. (2015). Behavioral, cognitive, and adaptive development in infants with autism spectrum disorder in the first 2 years of life. *Journal of Neurodevelopmental Disorders, 7*(1), 24. doi:10.118611689-015-9117-6 PMID:26203305

Falck-Ytter, T., Bölte, S., & Gredebäck, G. (2013). Eye tracking in early autism research. *Journal of Neurodevelopmental Disorders, 5*(1), 28. doi:10.1186/1866-1955-5-28 PMID:24069955

Farmer, M. E., & Klein, R. M. (1995). The evidence for a temporal processing deficit linked to dyslexia: A review. *Psychonomic Bulletin & Review, 2*(4), 460–493. doi:10.3758/BF03210983 PMID:24203785

Farran, E. K., & Karmiloff-Smith, A. (2012). *Neurodevelopmental disorders across the lifespan: A neuro-constructive approach.* Oxford, UK: Oxford University Press.

Fatemi, S. H., & Folsom, T. D. (2009). The neurodevelopmental hypothesis of schizophrenia revisited. *Schizophrenia Bulletin, 35*(1), 528–548. doi:10.1093chbulbn187 PMID:19223657

Fayter, D., McDaid, C., Ritchie, G., Stirk, L., & Eastwood, A. (2006). *Systematic review of barriers, modifiers and benefits involved in participation in cancer clinical trials. Research Report. CRD Report (31).* University of York NHS Centre for Reviews & Dissemination.

Fazio, R. L., Pietz, C. A., & Denney, R. L. (2012). An estimate of the prevalence of autism spectrum disorders in an incarcerated population. *Open Access Journal of Forensic Psychology*, *4*, 69–80.

Fernándezm, T., Harmony, T., Fernández-Bouzas, A., Díaz-Comas, L., Prado-Alcalá, R. A., Valdés-Sosa, P., ... García-Martínez, F. (2007). Changes in EEG current sources induced by neurofeedback in learning disabled children: An exploratory study. *Applied Psychophysiology and Biofeedback*, *32*(3-4), 169–183. doi:10.100710484-007-9044-8 PMID:17978869

Fine, A. H. (2015). *Handbook on Animal-Assisted Therapy: Foundations and Guidelines for Animal-Assisted Interventions*. New York, NY: Academic Press.

Fishbein, D. H., Rose, E. J., Darcey, V. L., Belcher, A. M., & VanMeter, J. W. (2016). Neurodevelopmental precursors and consequences of substance use during adolescence: Promises and pitfalls of longitudinal neuroimaging strategies. *Frontiers in Human Neuroscience*, *10*, 296. doi:10.3389/fnhum.2016.00296 PMID:27445743

Flahive, M., & Ray, D. (2007). Effect of group sand tray therapy with preadolescents in a school setting. *Journal for Specialists in Group Work*, *32*(4), 362–382. doi:10.1080/01933920701476706

Fleischman, M. J., & Othmer, S. (2005). Case study: Improvements in IQ score and maintenance of gains following EEG biofeedback with mildly developmentally delayed twins. *Journal of Neurotherapy*, *9*(4), 35–46. doi:10.1300/J184v09n04_03

Fleiss, J. L. (1981). *Statistical methods for rates and proportions*. New York: John Wiley.

Fleiss, J. L., & Cohen, J. (1973). The equivalence of weighted kappa and the intra-class correlation coefficient as measures of reliability. *Educational and Psychological Measurement*, *33*(1), 613–619. doi:10.1177/001316447303300309

Folen, R. A., James, L. C., Earles, J. E., & Andrasik, F. (2001). Biofeedback via telehealth: A new frontier for applied psychophysiology. *Applied Psychophysiology and Biofeedback*, *26*(3), 195–204. doi:10.1023/A:1011346103638 PMID:11680283

Foley, J. F., & Moertel, C. G. (1991). Improving accrual into cancer clinical trials. *Journal of Cancer Education*, *6*(3), 165–173. doi:10.1080/08858199109528114 PMID:1931596

Folstein, M. F., Folstein, S. E., & McHugh, P. R. (1975). Mini-mental state, a practical method of grading the cognitive state of patients for the clinician. *Journal of Psychiatric Research*, *12*(3), 189–198. doi:10.1016/0022-3956(75)90026-6 PMID:1202204

Foucault, M. (1973). *The birth of clinic*. London: Tavistock.

Fraker, C., Fishbein, M., Cox, S., & Walbert, L. (2009). *Food chaining: The proven 6-step plan to stop picky eating, solve feeding problems, and expand your child's diet*. Da Capo Lifelong Books.

Franca, M. C., & Bass-Ringdahi, S. (2015). A clinical demonstration of the application of audiovisual biofeedback in the treatment of puberphonia. *International Journal of Pediatric Otorhinolaryngology*, *79*(6), 912–920. doi:10.1016/j.ijporl.2015.04.013 PMID:25912681

Franck, B. A., van Kreveld-Bos, C. S., Dreschler, W. A., & Verschuure, H. (1999). Evaluation of spectral enhancement in hearing aids, combined with phonemic compression. *The Journal of the Acoustical Society of America*, *106*(3 Pt 1), 1452–1464. doi:10.1121/1.428055 PMID:10489703

Frank, D. L., Khorshid, L., Kiffer, J. F., Moravec, C. S., & McKee, M. G. (2010). Biofeedback in medicine: Who, when, why and how? *Mental Health in Family Medicine*, *7*(2), 85–91. PMID:22477926

Frank, M. C., Vul, E., & Saxe, R. (2012). Measuring the Development of Social Attention Using Free-Viewing. *Infancy*, *17*(4), 355–375. doi:10.1111/j.1532-7078.2011.00086.x

Frazier, T. W., Klingemier, E. W., Beukemann, M., Speer, L., Markowitz, L., Parikh, S., & Ahuja, V. (2016). Development of an objective autism risk index using remote eye tracking. *Journal of the American Academy of Child and Adolescent Psychiatry, 55*(4), 301–309. doi:10.1016/j.jaac.2016.01.011 PMID:27015721

Freedman, E. G., & Foxe, J. J. (2017). Eye movements, sensorimotor adaptation and cerebellar-dependent learning in autism: Toward potential biomarkers and subphenotypes. *The European Journal of Neuroscience*, *47*(6), 549–555. doi:10.1111/ejn.13625 PMID:28612953

Freitag, C. M. (2007). The genetics of autistic disorders and its clinical relevance: A review of the literature. *Molecular Psychiatry, 12*(1), 2–22. doi:10.1038j.mp.4001896 PMID:17033636

Freud, A. (1928). *Introduction to the technique of Child Analysis* (L. P. Clark, Trans.). New York: Nervous and Mental Disease Publishing.

Freud, A. (1946). *The psycho-analytical treatment of children*. New York: International Universities.

Freud, S. (1909). Analysis of a Phobia in a Five-Year-Old Boy. *The Standard Edition of the Complete Psychological Works of Sigmund Freud*, *X*, 3–149.

Friedmann, E., Son, H., & Saleem, M. (2015). The animal–human bond: Health and wellness. In A. H. Fine (Ed.), *Handbook on Animal-Assisted Therapy: Foundations and Guidelines for Animal-Assisted Interventions* (4th ed., pp. 73–88). Burlington, MA: Academic Press. doi:10.1016/B978-0-12-801292-5.00007-9

Friedmann, I., Spellacy, E., Crow, J., & Watts, R. W. (1985). Histopathological studies of the temporal bones in Hurler's disease. *The Journal of Laryngology and Otology*, *99*(01), 29–41. doi:10.1017/S0022215100096250 PMID:3918131

Frölander, H. E., Möller, C., Rudner, M., Mishra, S., Marshall, J. D., Piacentini, H., & Lyxell, B. (2015). Theory-of-mind in individuals with Alström syndrome is related to executive functions, and verbal ability. *Frontiers in Psychology*, *6*, 1426. doi:10.3389/fpsyg.2015.01426 PMID:26441796

Fuglestad, A. J., Rao, R., & Georgieff, M. K. (2008). The role of nutrition in cognitive development. In C. A. Nelson & M. Luciana (Eds.), *Handbook in Developmental Cognitive Neuroscience* (2nd ed.; pp. 623–641). Cambridge, MA: MIT Press.

Fung, S. C. (2017). An observational study on canine-assisted play therapy for children with autism: Move towards the phrase of manualization and protocol development. *Global Journal of Health Science*, *9*(7), 67. doi:10.5539/gjhs.v9n7p67

Gabriele, M., Tobon, L., D'Agostino, G., & Testa, G. (2018). The chromatin basis of neurodevelopmental disorders: Rethinking dysfunction along the molecular and temporal axes. *Progress in Neuro-psychopharmacology and Biological Psychiatry, S0278-5846*(17), 30538-30539. doi:10.1016/j.pnpbp.2017.12.013

Gabriels, R. L., Agnew, J. A., Holt, K. D., Shoffner, A., Zhaoxing, P., Ruzzano, S., ... Mesibov, G. (2012). Pilot study measuring the effects of therapeutic horseback riding on school-age children and adolescents with autism spectrum disorders. *Research in Autism Spectrum Disorders*, *6*(2), 578–588. doi:10.1016/j.rasd.2011.09.007

Gagnon, J., Bouchard, F., Landry, M., Belles-Isles, M., Fortier, M., & Fillion, L. (2004). Implementing a hospital-based animal therapy program for children with cancer: A descriptive study. *Canadian Oncology Nursing Journal/Revue canadienne de soins infirmiers en oncologie, 14*(4), 217-222.

Gale, C. R., Martyn, C. N., Marriott, L. D., Limond, J., Crozier, S., Inskip, H. M., ... Robinson, S. M. (2009). Dietary patterns in infancy and cognitive and neuropsychological function in childhood. *Journal of Child Psychology and Psychiatry, and Allied Disciplines*, *50*(7), 816–823. doi:10.1111/j.1469-7610.2008.02029.x PMID:19236526

Gall, M. D., Borg, W. R., & Gall, J. P. (1996). *Educational Research*. White Plains.

Gallo-Lopez, L., & Rubin, L. C. (2012). *Play-Based Interventions for Children and Adolescents with Autism Spectrum Disorders*. New York: Routledge.

Gammonley, J., & Yates, J. (1991). Pet projects: Animal assisted therapy in nursing homes. *Journal of Gerontological Nursing*, *17*(1), 12–15. doi:10.3928/0098-9134-19910101-05 PMID:1899683

Gangil, A., Patwari, A. K., Aneja, S., Ahuja, B., & Anand, V. K. (2001). Feeding problems in children with cerebral palsy. *Indian Pediatrics*, *38*(8), 839–846. PMID:11520994

Ganz, M. L. (2007). The lifetime distribution of the incremental societal costs of autism. *Archives of Pediatrics & Adolescent Medicine*, *161*(4), 343–349. doi:10.1001/archpedi.161.4.343 PMID:17404130

Gao, Y., Glenn, A. L., Schug, R. A., Yang, Y., & Raine, A. (2009). The neurobiology of psychopathy: A neurodevelopmental perspective. *Canadian Journal of Psychiatry*, *54*(12), 813–823. doi:10.1177/070674370905401204 PMID:20047720

Garber, H. J., & Ritvo, E. R. (1992). Magnetic resonance imaging of the posterior fossa in autistic adults. *The American Journal of Psychiatry*, *149*(2), 245–247. doi:10.1176/ajp.149.2.245 PMID:1734747

Garber, H. J., Ritvo, E. R., Chiu, L. C., Griswold, V. J., & Kashanian, A. (1989). A magnetic resonance imaging study of autism: Normal fourth ventricle size and absence of pathology. *The American Journal of Psychiatry*, *146*(4), 532–534. doi:10.1176/ajp.146.4.532 PMID:2929757

García, F. M. S., & Teruya-Feldstein, J. (2014). The diagnosis and treatment of dyskeratosis congenita: A review. *Journal of Blood Medicine*, *5*, 157–167. PMID:25170286

Gardener, H., Spiegelman, D., & Buka, S. L. (2011). Perinatal and neonatal risk factors for autism: A comprehensive meta-analysis. *Pediatrics*, *128*(2), 344–355. doi:10.1542/peds.2010-1036 PMID:21746727

Gathercole, S. E., & Alloway, T. P. (2006). Practitioner review: Short-term and working memory impairments in neurodevelopmental disorders: Diagnosis and remedial support. *Journal of Child Psychology and Psychiatry, and Allied Disciplines*, *47*(1), 4–15. doi:10.1111/j.1469-7610.2005.01446.x PMID:16405635

Gaur, S. (2012). *Jagjit Singh and Anr vs Delhi Development Authority on 26 November, 2012*. Available at: https://indiankanoon.org/doc/47289866/

Geary, D. C., Hoard, M. K., Nugent, L., & Bailey, D. H. (2012). Mathematical cognitive deficits in children with learning disabilities and persistent low achievement: A five-year prospective study. *Journal of Educational Psychology*, *104*(1), 206–233. doi:10.1037/a0025398 PMID:27158154

Geladé, K., Bink, M., Janssen, T. W., Van Mourik, R., Maras, A., & Oosterlaan, J. (2017). An RCT into the effects of neurofeedback on neurocognitive functioning compared to stimulant medication and physical activity in children with ADHD. *European Child & Adolescent Psychiatry*, *26*(4), 457–468. doi:10.100700787-016-0902-x PMID:27665293

George, A., & Routray, A. (2015). *Design and Implementation of Real-time Algorithms for Eye Tracking and PERCLOS Measurement for on board Estimation of Alertness of Drivers*. arXiv preprint arXiv:1505.06162

George, M. S., Costa, D. C., Kouris, K., Ring, H. A., & Ell, P. J. (1992). Cerebral blood flow abnormalities in adults with infantile autism. *The Journal of Nervous and Mental Disease*, *180*(7), 413–417. doi:10.1097/00005053-199207000-00002 PMID:1624921

Germain, D. P., Avan, P., Chassaing, A., & Bonfils, P. (2002). Patients affected with Fabry disease have an increased incidence of progressive hearing loss and sudden deafness: An investigation of twenty-two hemizygous male patients. *BMC Medical Genetics*, *3*(1), 10. doi:10.1186/1471-2350-3-10 PMID:12377100

Geschwind, D. H. (2009). Advances in autism. *Annual Review of Medicine*, *60*(1), 367–380. doi:10.1146/annurev.med.60.053107.121225 PMID:19630577

Geschwind, D. H., & State, M. W. (2015). Gene hunting in autism spectrum disorder: On the path to precision medicine. *Lancet Neurology*, *14*(11), 1109–1120. doi:10.1016/S1474-4422(15)00044-7 PMID:25891009

Ghayas, N., Naz, S., Fazil, H., & Sulman, N. (2014). Identification of oromotor impairments perceived by parents related to feeding difficulties in children with cerebral palsy. *International Journal of Physical and Social Sciences*, *4*(7), 229.

Gil, A., & Gil, F. (2015). Fish, a Mediterranean source of n-3 PUFA: Benefits do not justify limiting consumption. *British Journal of Nutrition*, *113*(S2), S58–S67. doi:10.1017/S0007114514003742 PMID:26148923

Gillam, R. B., Logan, K. J., & Pearson, N. A. (2009). *Test of Childhood Stuttering (TOCS)*. Pearson Inc.

Gillberg, C. (2010). The ESSENCE of child psychiatry: Early Symptomatic Syndromes Eliciting Neurodevelopmental Clinical Examinations (ESSENCE). *Research in Developmental Disabilities*, *31*(6), 1543–1551. doi:10.1016/j.ridd.2010.06.002 PMID:20634041

Gillberg, I. C., Bjure, J., Uvebrant, P., Vestergren, E., & Gillberg, C. (1993). SPECT (single photon emission computed tomography) in 31 children and adolescents with autism and autistic-like conditions. *European Child & Adolescent Psychiatry*, *2*(1), 50–59. doi:10.1007/BF02098830 PMID:21590529

Ginott, H. (1960). A rationale for selecting toys in play therapy. *Journal of Consulting Psychology*, *24*(3), 243–246. doi:10.1037/h0043980 PMID:13850211

Ginsberg, Y., Hirvikoski, T., & Lindefors, N. (2010). Attention Deficit Hyperactivity Disorder (ADHD) among longer-term prison inmates is a prevalent, persistent and disabling disorder. *BMC Psychiatry*, *10*(1), 112. doi:10.1186/1471-244X-10-112 PMID:21176203

Ginsberg, Y., Langstrom, N., Larsson, H., & Lichtenstein, P. (2014). ADHD and criminality: Could treatment benefit prisoners with ADHD who are at higher risk of reoffending? *Expert Review of Neurotherapeutics*, *13*(4), 345–348. doi:10.1586/ern.13.22 PMID:23545049

Ginsberg, Y., & Lindefors, N. (2012). Methylphenidate treatment of adult male prison inmates with attention-deficit hyperactivity disorder: A randomised double blind placebo-controlled trial with open-label extension. *The British Journal of Psychiatry*, *200*(1), 68–73. doi:10.1192/bjp.bp.111.092940 PMID:22075648

Glascoe, F. P., & Sandler, H. (1995). Value of parents' estimate of children's developmental ages. *The Journal of Pediatrics*, *127*(5), 831–835. doi:10.1016/S0022-3476(95)70184-2 PMID:7472847

Glass, R. P., & Wolf, L. S. (1992). *Feeding and swallowing disorders in infancy: Assessment and management*. San Antonio, TX: Therapy Skill Builders.

Glenk, L. M. (2017). Current perspectives on therapy dog welfare in animal-assisted interventions. *Animals (Basel)*, *7*(2), 7. doi:10.3390/ani7020007 PMID:28157145

Gnanavel, S. (2017). Biomarkers in autism spectrum disorders: An illusion or promising reality. *Indian Journal of Psychological Medicine*, *39*(5), 714–715. doi:10.4103/IJPSYM.IJPSYM_122_17 PMID:29200579

Gnewikow, D., & Moss, M. (2006). Hearing aid outcomes with open and closed canal fittings. *The Hearing Journal*, *59*(11), 66–72. doi:10.1097/01.HJ.0000286220.14835.13

Goepfert, E., Mule, C., von Hahn, E., Visco, Z., & Siegel, M. (2015). Family systems interventions for families of children with autism spectrum disorder. *Child and Adolescent Psychiatric Clinics of North America*, *24*(3), 571–583. doi:10.1016/j.chc.2015.02.009 PMID:26092740

Gökdoğan, Ç., Altinyay, Ş., Gökdoğan, O., Tutar, H., Gündüz, B., Okur, İ., ... Kemaloğlu, Y. K. (2016). Audiologic evaluations of children with mucopolysaccharidosis. *Revista Brasileira de Otorrinolaringologia (English Ed.)*, *82*(3), 281–284. doi:10.1016/j.bjorl.2015.05.007 PMID:26601996

Goldberg, H. J., & Kotval, X. P. (1999). Computer interface evaluation using eye movements: Methods and constructs. *International Journal of Industrial Ergonomics*, *24*(6), 631–645. doi:10.1016/S0169-8141(98)00068-7

Goldberg, H. J., & Wichansky, A. M. (2003). Eye tracking in usability evaluation: A practitioner's guide. In J. Hyönä, R. Radach, & H. Deubel (Eds.), *The mind's eye: Cognitive and applied aspects of eye movement research* (pp. 493–516). Amsterdam: Elsevier. doi:10.1016/B978-044451020-4/50027-X

Goldstein, P., Ziegler, W., Vogel, M., & Hoole, P. (1994). Combined palatal-lift and EPG-feedback therapy in dysarthria: A case study. *Clinical Linguistics & Phonetics*, *8*(3), 201–218. doi:10.3109/02699209408985307

Gorlin, R. J., Toriello, H. V., & Cohen, M. M. (1995). *Hereditary hearing loss and its syndromes*. New York: Oxford University Press.

Goswami, S. P., Venkatesan, S., & Mathew, S. (2015). Disability certification: Issues and concerns. *Journal of All India Institute of Speech and Hearing*, *34*, 1–7.

Goswami, U. (1999). Causal connections in beginning reading: The importance of rhyme. *Journal of Research in Reading*, *22*(3), 217–240. doi:10.1111/1467-9817.00087

Graef, J. W., Wolfsdorf, J. I., & Greenes, D. S. (Eds.). (2008). *Manual of pediatric therapeutics* (7th ed.). Philadelphia: Lippincott Williams & Wilkins.

Graham, J. T., & Graham, L. W. (1971). Language behaviour of the mentally retarded: Syntactic characteristics. *American Journal of Mental Deficiency*, *75*(5), 623–629. PMID:5551507

Granet, D. B., Castro, E. F., & Gomi, C. F. (2006). Reading: Do the eyes have it? *The American Orthoptic Journal*, *56*(1), 44–49. doi:10.3368/aoj.56.1.44

Grantham-McGregor, S. M., Lira, P. I., Ashworth, A., Morris, S. S., & Assunçao, A. M. (1998). The development of low birth weight term infants and the effects of the environment in northeast Brazil. *The Journal of Pediatrics*, *132*(4), 661–666. doi:10.1016/S0022-3476(98)70357-9 PMID:9580767

Gravel, J. S., Fausel, N., Liskow, C., & Chobot, J. (1999). Children's speech recognition in noise using omni-directional and dual-microphone hearing aid technology. *Ear and Hearing*, *20*(1), 1–11. doi:10.1097/00003446-199902000-00001 PMID:10037061

Green, L. (2009). Morphology and literacy: Getting our heads in the game. *Language, Speech, and Hearing Services in Schools, 40*(3), 283–285. doi:10.1044/0161-1461(2009/08-0091)

Green, E., & Green, A. (1977). *Beyond biofeedback*. New York: Delacorte Press/Seymour.

Greider, C. W. (1996). Telomere length regulation. *Annual Review of Biochemistry*, *65*(1), 337–365. doi:10.1146/annurev.bi.65.070196.002005 PMID:8811183

Greydanus, D. E. (2005). Pharmacologic treatment of attention-deficit hyperactivity disorder. *Indian Journal of Pediatrics*, *72*(11), 953–960. doi:10.1007/BF02731672 PMID:16391451

Grohol, J. M. (2013). *DSM-5 Changes: Neurodevelopmental Disorders*. Retrieved November 14, 2017, from pro.psychcentral.com/dsm-5-changes-neurodevelopmental-disorders/004366.html

Grund, M., Naumann, C. L., & Haug, G. (2004). Diagnostischer Rechtschreibtest f¨ur 5. Klassen: DRT 5; *Manual. Deutsche Schultests*. Beltz Test, G¨ottingen, 2., aktual. aufl. in neuerrechtschreibung edition.

Grunwell, P. (1985). *Phonological Assessment of Child Speech (PACS)*. Windsor: NFER-Nelson.

Grunwell, P. (1993). *Analysing cleft palate speech*. London: Whurr Publishers Ltd.

Grupp-Phelan, J., Harman, J. S., & Kelleher, K. J. (2007). Trends in mental health and chronic condition visits by children presenting for care at U.S. emergency departments. *Public Health Reports*, *122*(1), 55–61. doi:10.1177/003335490712200108 PMID:17236609

Guerney, B. Jr. (1964). Filial therapy: Description and rationale. *Journal of Consulting Psychology*, *28*(4), 304–310. doi:10.1037/h0041340 PMID:14198792

Guillon, Q., Hadjikhani, N., Baduel, S., & Rogé, B. (2014). Visual social attention in autism spectrum disorder: Insights from eye tracking studies. *Neuroscience and Biobehavioral Reviews*, *42*, 279–297. doi:10.1016/j.neubiorev.2014.03.013 PMID:24694721

Guitar, B. (1975). Reduction of stuttering frequency using analog electromyographic feedback. *Journal of Speech and Hearing Research*, *18*(4), 672–685. doi:10.1044/jshr.1804.672 PMID:1207099

Gulati, S., Menon, S., Kabra, M., & Kalra, V. (2003). Schinzel Acrocallosal syndrome. *Indian Journal of Pediatrics*, *70*(2), 173–176. doi:10.1007/BF02723749 PMID:12661815

Guldberg-Kjar, T., Sehlin, S., & Johansson, B. (2013). ADHD symptoms across life span in population-based Swedish sample aged 65-80. *International Psychogeriatrics*, *29*(4), 667–675. doi:10.1017/S1041610212002050 PMID:23237190

Gupta, A., Gupta, R., Sood, S., & Arkham, M. (2014). Pranayam for treatment of chronic obstructive pulmonary disease: Results from a randomized controlled trial. *Integrative Medicine: A Clinician's Journal, 13*(1), 26-31.

Gupta, S. K., & Venkatesan, S. (2014b). Efficacy of training program on executive functions in children with learning disability. *Guru Journal of Behavioral and Social Sciences, 2*(2), 283-291. Retrieved from http://gjbss.org/wp-content/uploads/2014/03/gjbss_Vol2_Issue2_Paper1.pdf

Gupta, S., & Kulhara, P. (2010). What is schizophrenia: A neurodevelopmental or neurodegenerative disorder or a combination of both? A critical analysis. *Indian Journal of Psychiatry, 52*(1), 21-27. doi: 14.4103/0019-6645.68891

Gupta, S. K., & Venkatesan, S. (2014a). Reappraisal of research on executive function training in children with learning disabilities. *International Journal of Psychology and Psychiatry*, *2*(1), 7–18. doi:10.5958/j.2320-6233.2.1.002

Gutheil, T. G., & Drogin, E. Y. (2013). *The mental health professional in court: A survival guide*. Washington, DC: American Psychiatric Publishing.

Hagerman, R. J., & Hendren, R. L. (2014). *Treatment of neurodevelopmental disorders: Targeting neurobiological mechanisms*. Oxford, UK: Oxford University Press. doi:10.1093/med/9780199937806.001.0001

Hagerman, R. J., Ligsay, A., & Goldberg, J. (2016). Aging with neurodevelopmental disorders: On-call assessment and future directions. In *On-Call Geriatric Psychiatry: Handbook of Principles and Practice* (pp. 341–351). New York: Springer International Publishing; doi:10.1007/978-3-319-30346-8_26

Hailesellasie, M., & Hasan, S. R. (2017, May). A fast FPGA-based deep convolutional neural network using pseudo-parallel memories. In *Circuits and Systems (ISCAS), 2017 IEEE International Symposium on* (pp. 1-4). IEEE. 10.1109/ISCAS.2017.8050317

Hall, J. W., Prentice, C. H., Smiley, G., & Werkhaven, J. (1995). Auditory dysfunction in selected syndromes and patterns of malformations : Review and case findings. *Journal of the American Academy of Audiology*, *6*, 80–92. PMID:7696681

Hallmayer, J., Cleveland, S., Torres, A., Phillips, J., Cohen, B., Torigoe, T., & Lotspeich, L. (2011). Genetic heritability and shared environmental factors among twin pairs with autism. *Archives of General Psychiatry*, *68*(11), 1095–1102. doi:10.1001/archgenpsychiatry.2011.76 PMID:21727249

Hall, T. M., Kaduson, H. G., & Schaefer, C. E. (2002). Fifteen effective play therapy techniques. *Professional Psychology, Research and Practice*, *33*(6), 515–522. doi:10.1037/0735-7028.33.6.515

Halpin, C., Owen, G., Gutiérrez-Espeleta, G. A., Sims, K., & Rehm, H. L. (2005). Audiologic features of Norrie disease. *The Annals of Otology, Rhinology, and Laryngology*, *114*(7), 533–538. doi:10.1177/000348940511400707 PMID:16134349

Hames, E. C., Murphy, B., Rajmohan, R., Anderson, R. C., Baker, M., Zupancic, S., ... Richman, D. (2016). Visual, Auditory, and Cross Modal Sensory Processing in Adults with Autism: An EEG Power and BOLD fMRI Investigation. *Frontiers in Human Neuroscience*, *10*, 167. doi:10.3389/fnhum.2016.00167 PMID:27148020

Hamilton, D. R. (2015). Treatment of neurodevelopmental disorders: Targeting neurobiological mechanisms. *Journal of Developmental and Behavioral Pediatrics*, *36*(6), 425. doi:10.1097/DBP.0000000000000183

Hammond, D. C. (2008). Comprehensive Neuro-feedback Bibliography: 2007 Update. *Journal of Neurotherapy*, *11*(3), 45–60. doi:10.1080/10874200802126241

Hanna, R., Wilfling, F., & McNeill, B. (1975). A biofeedback treatment for stuttering. *The Journal of Speech and Hearing Disorders*, *40*(2), 270–273. doi:10.1044/jshd.4002.270 PMID:1234938

Hansaria, V., & Jose, P. I. (2010). *Juvenile justice system: Working manual for stakeholders*. New Delhi: Universal Law Publishing.

Happe, F., & Charlton, R. A. (2012). Aging in autism spectrum disorders: A mini review. *Gerontology*, *58*(1), 70–78. doi:10.1159/000329720 PMID:21865667

Harding, J. E. (2001). The nutritional basis of the fetal origins of adult disease. *International Journal of Epidemiology*, *30*(1), 15–23. doi:10.1093/ije/30.1.15 PMID:11171842

Hariprasad, V. R., Arasappa, R., Varambally, S., Srinath, S., & Gangadhar, B. N. (2013). Feasibility and efficacy of yoga as an add-on intervention in attention deficit-hyperactivity disorder: An exploratory study. *Indian Journal of Psychiatry*, *55*(7S3), S379–S384. doi:10.4103/0019-5545.116317 PMID:24049203

Harris, A., & Williams, J. M. (2017). The impact of a horse riding intervention on the social functioning of children with autism spectrum disorder. *International Journal of Environmental Research and Public Health*, *14*(4), E776. doi:10.3390/ijerph14070776 PMID:28708075

Harris, G. T., Rice, M. E., & Lalumiere, M. (2001). The roles of psychopathy, neurodevelopmental insults, and antisocial parenting. *Criminal Justice and Behavior*, *28*(4), 402–426. doi:10.1177/009385480102800402

Harris, J. C. (2014). A new classification of neurodevelopmental disorders in DSM-5. *Current Opinion in Psychiatry*, *27*(2), 95–97. doi:10.1097/YCO.0000000000000042 PMID:24441422

Harrison, L. J., Manocha, R., & Rubia, K. (2004). Sahaja yoga meditation as a family treatment programme for children with attention deficit-hyperactivity disorder. *Clinical Child Psychology and Psychiatry*, *9*(4), 479–497. doi:10.1177/1359104504046155

Hartfiel, N., Clarke, G., Havenhand, J., Phillips, C., & Edwards, R. (2017). Cost-effectiveness of yoga for managing musculoskeletal conditions in the workplace. *Occupational Medicine*, *67*(9), 1–9. doi:10.1093/occmed/kqx161 PMID:29202204

Harvey, J. N., & Barnett, D. (1992). Endocrine dysfunction in Kearns-Sayre syndrome. *Horumon To Rinsho*, *37*, 97–103. PMID:1424198

Harvey, S. (2006). Dynamic play therapy. In C. E. Schaefer & H. G. Kaduson (Eds.), *Contemporary play therapy: Theory* (pp. 55–81). Research, and Practice.

Hashimoto, T., Tayama, M., Murakawa, K., Yoshimoto, T., Miyazaki, M., Harada, M., & Kuroda, Y. (1995). Development of the brainstem and cerebellum in autistic patients. *Journal of Autism and Developmental Disorders*, *25*(1), 1–18. doi:10.1007/BF02178163 PMID:7608030

Hatch, A. (2007). The view from all fours: A look at an animal-assisted activity program from the animals' perspective. *Anthrozoos*, *20*(1), 37–50. doi:10.2752/089279307780216632

Haubenhofer, D. K., & Kirchengast, S. (2006). Austrian and American approaches to animal-based health care services. *Anthrozoos*, *19*(4), 365–373. doi:10.2752/089279306785415484

Hawelka, S., & Wimmer, H. (2005). Impaired visual processing of multielement arrays is associated with increased number of eye movements in dyslexic reading. *Vision Research*, *45*(7), 855–863. doi:10.1016/j.visres.2004.10.007 PMID:15644226

Hayes, S., Shackell, P., Mottram, P., & Lancaster, R. (2007). The prevalence of intellectual disability in a major UK prison. *British Journal of Learning Disabilities*, *35*(3), 162–167. doi:10.1111/j.1468-3156.2007.00461.x

Hazlett, E. A., Buchsbaum, M. S., Hsieh, P., Haznedar, M. M., Platholi, J., LiCalzi, E. M., ... Hollander, E. (2004). Regional glucose metabolism within cortical Brodmann areas in healthy individuals and autistic patients. *Neuropsychobiology*, *49*(3), 115–125. doi:10.1159/000076719 PMID:15034226

Hazlett, H. C., Poe, M. D., Gerig, G., Smith, R. G., & Piven, J. (2006). Cortical gray and white brain tissue volume in adolescents and adults with autism. *Biological Psychiatry*, *59*(1), 1–6. doi:10.1016/j.biopsych.2005.06.015 PMID:16139816

Hazlett, H. C., Poe, M., Gerig, G., Smith, R. G., Provenzale, J., Ross, A., & Piven, J. (2005). Magnetic resonance imaging and head circumference study of brain size in autism: Birth through age 2 years. *Archives of General Psychiatry*, *62*(12), 1366–1376. doi:10.1001/archpsyc.62.12.1366 PMID:16330725

Haznedar, M. M., Buchsbaum, M. S., Wei, T. C., Hof, P. R., Cartwright, C., Bienstock, C. A., & Hollander, E. (2000). Limbic circuitry in patients with autism spectrum disorders studied with positron emission tomography and magnetic resonance imaging. *The American Journal of Psychiatry*, *157*(12), 1994–2001. doi:10.1176/appi.ajp.157.12.1994 PMID:11097966

Healey, E. C., Reid, R., & Donaher, J. (2005). Treatment of the child who stutters with co-existing learning, behavioral, and cognitive challenges. In R. Lees & C. Stark (Eds.), *The treatment of stuttering in the young school-aged child* (pp. 178–196). London: Whurr Publishers.

Heimlich, K. (2001). Animal-assisted therapy and the severely disabled child: A quantitative study. *Journal of Rehabilitation*, *67*(4), 48.

Heindel, J. J., & Vandenberg, L. N. (2015). Developmental origins of health and disease: A paradigm for understanding disease etiology and prevention. *Current Opinion in Pediatrics*, *27*(2), 248–253. doi:10.1097/MOP.0000000000000191 PMID:25635586

Heldermon, C. D., Hennig, A. K., Ohlemiller, K. K., Ogilvie, J. M., Herzog, E. D., Breidenbach, A., ... Sands, M. S. (2007). Development of sensory, motor and behavioral deficits in the murine model of sanfilippo syndrome type B. *PLoS One*, *2*(8), e772. doi:10.1371/journal.pone.0000772 PMID:17712420

Helps, S. (2016). Systemic psychotherapy with families where someone has an autism spectrum condition. *NeuroRehabilitation*, *38*(3), 223–230. doi:10.3233/NRE-161314 PMID:27030899

Hendren, R. L., Goldani, A., & Hagerman, R. J. (2014). Overview of neurodevelopmental processes and the assessment of patients with neurodevelopmental disorders. In R. J. Hagerman & R. L. Hendren (Eds.), *Treatment of neurodevelopmental disorders: Targeting neurobiological mechanisms*. Oxford, UK: Oxford University Press. doi:10.1093/med/9780199937806.003.0001

Henschen, T. L., & Burton, N. G. (1978). Treatment of spastic dysphonia by EMG biofeedback. *Biofeedback and Self-Regulation*, *3*(1), 91–96. doi:10.1007/BF00998566 PMID:667194

Herbert, A., & Esparham, A. (2017). Mind–Body Therapy for children with attention deficit hyperactivity disorder. *Children*, *4*(5), 31. doi:10.3390/children4050031 PMID:28441363

Herbert, M. R., Harris, G. J., Adrien, K. T., Ziegler, D. A., Makris, N., Kennedy, D. N., & Takeoka, M. (2002). Abnormal asymmetry in language association cortex in autism. *Annals of Neurology*, *52*(5), 588–596. doi:10.1002/ana.10349 PMID:12402256

Herbert, M. R., Ziegler, D. A., Deutsch, C. K., O'brien, L. M., Lange, N., Bakardjiev, A., & Kennedy, D. (2003). Dissociations of cerebral cortex, subcortical and cerebral white matter volumes in autistic boys. *Brain*, *126*(5), 1182–1192. doi:10.1093/brain/awg110 PMID:12690057

Herold, S., Frackowiak, R. S. J., Le Couteur, A., Rutter, M., & Howlin, P. (1988). Cerebral blood flow and metabolism of oxygen and glucose in young autistic adults. *Psychological Medicine*, *18*(4), 823–831. doi:10.1017/S0033291700009752 PMID:3270827

Hersher, L. (1980). Hearing loss and learning disability. *American Journal of Diseases of Children*, *134*, 94. PMID:7350794

Herwegen, J. V., Riby, D., & Farran, E. K. (2015). Neurodevelopmental disorders: Definitions and issues. In J. V. Herwegen & D. Riby (Eds.), *Neurodevelopmental disorders: Research challenges and solutions* (pp. 3–19). New York: Psychology Press.

Herzer, K. R., & Pronovost, P. J. (2015). Physician motivation: Listening to what pay for performance programs and quality improvement collaboratives are telling us. *Joint Commission Journal on Quality and Patient Safety*, *41*(11), 522–528. doi:10.1016/S1553-7250(15)41069-4 PMID:26484685

Hessels, R. S., Niehorster, D. C., Kemner, C., & Hooge, I. T. (2017). Noise-robust fixation detection in eye movement data: Identification by two-means clustering (I2MC). *Behavior Research Methods*, *49*(5), 1802–1823. doi:10.375813428-016-0822-1 PMID:27800582

Hibbeln, J. R., Davis, J. M., Steer, C., Emmett, P., Rogers, I., Williams, C., & Golding, J. (2007). Maternal seafood consumption in pregnancy and neurodevelopmental outcomes in childhood (ALSPAC study): An observational cohort study. *Lancet*, *369*(9561), 578–585. doi:10.1016/S0140-6736(07)60277-3 PMID:17307104

Hill, A. (2006). Play therapy with sexually abused children: Including parents in therapeutic play. *Child & Family Social Work, 11*(4), 316–324. doi:10.1111/j.1365-2206.2006.00411.x

Hirvikoski, T., Mittendorfer-Rutz, E., Boman, M., Larsson, H., Lichtenstein, P., & Bolte, S. (2016). Premature mortality in autism spectrum disorder. *The British Journal of Psychiatry, 208*(3), 232–238. doi:10.1192/bjp.bp.114.160192 PMID:26541693

Hoffman, D. J., Benda, N. C., Fairbanks, R. J., & Auguste, T. C. (2017). Simulated motivations: Understanding influences on medical professionals' decision making to participate in human factors research studies. *Proceedings of the International Symposium on Human Factors and Ergonomics in Health Care, 6*(1), 9-12. 10.1177/2327857917061003

Hoffmann, B., Beck, M., Sunder-Plassmann, G., Borsini, W., Ricci, R., & Mehta, A. (2007). Nature and prevalence of pain in Fabry disease and its response to enzyme replacement therapy: A retrospective analysis from the Fabry Outcome Survey. *The Clinical Journal of Pain, 23*(6), 535–542. doi:10.1097/AJP.0b013e318074c986 PMID:17575495

Hollander, E., Anagnostou, E., Chaplin, W., Esposito, K., Haznedar, M. M., Licalzi, E., & Buchsbaum, M. (2005). Striatal volume on magnetic resonance imaging and repetitive behaviors in autism. *Biological Psychiatry, 58*(3), 226–232. doi:10.1016/j.biopsych.2005.03.040 PMID:15939406

Holmqvist, K., Nyström, M., Andersson, R., Dewhurst, R., Jarodzka, H., & Van de Weijer, J. (2011). *Eye tracking: A comprehensive guide to methods and measures.* Oxford, UK: Oxford University.

Homberg, J. R., Kyzar, E. J., Stewart, A. M., Nguyen, M., Poudel, M. K., Echevarria, D. J., ... Pittman, J. (2016). Improving treatment of neurodevelopmental disorders: Recommendations based on preclinical studies. *Expert Opinion on Drug Discovery, 11*(1), 11–25. doi:10.1517/17460441.2016.1115834 PMID:26558752

Hong, W. H., Chen, C. L., Yang, L. Y., & Chen, H. C. (2007). Kinematic analysis of speech motor control in children with cerebral palsy. In F. Ibrahim, N. A. A. Osman, J. Usman, & N. A. Kadri (Eds.), *Third Kuala Lumpur International Conference on Biomedical Engineering 2006. IFMBE Proceedings,* Vol 15. Berlin: Springer. 10.1007/978-3-540-68017-8_52

Hoppe, S., & Bulling, A. (2016). *End-to-end eye movement detection using convolutional neural networks.* arXiv preprint arXiv:1609.02452

Hossain, M. D., Ahmed, H. U., Uddin, M. J., Chowdhury, W. A., Iqbal, M. S., Kabir, R. I., ... Hossain, S. W. (2017). Autism Spectrum disorders (ASD) in South Asia: A systematic review. *BMC Psychiatry, 17*(1), 281. doi:10.118612888-017-1440-x PMID:28826398

Houge, G., & Skarbøvik, A. J. (2005). [Fabry disease--a diagnostic and therapeutic challenge]. *Tidsskrift for Den Norske Laegeforening: Tidsskrift for Praktisk Medicin. Ny Raekke, 125,* 1004–1006.

Hristova, E., Gerganov, A., Todorova, E., & Georgieva, S. (2010, January). Eye-Movements of Dyslexic Children Reading in Regular Orthography: Exploring word frequency and length effects. *Proceedings of the Annual Meeting of the Cognitive Science Society,* 32.

Hsiao, E. Y., McBride, S. W., Hsien, S., Sharon, G., Hyde, E. R., McCue, T., & Patterson, P. H. (2013). Microbiota modulate behavioral and physiological abnormalities associated with neurodevelopmental disorders. *Cell, 155*(7), 1451–1463. doi:10.1016/j.cell.2013.11.024 PMID:24315484

Hua, H., Krishnaswamy, P., & Rolland, J. P. (2006). Video-based eyetracking methods and algorithms in head-mounted displays. *Optics Express, 14*(10), 4328–4350. doi:10.1364/OE.14.004328 PMID:19516585

Huang, H., Wolf, S. L., & He, J. (2006). Recent developments in biofeedback of neuro-motor rehabilitation. *Journal of Neuroengineering and Rehabilitation, 3*(1), 11. doi:10.1186/1743-0003-3-11 PMID:16790060

Hudspeth, W. J., & Pribram, K. H. (1992). Psychophysiological indices of cerebral maturation. *International Journal of Psychophysiology, 12*(1), 19–29. doi:10.1016/0167-8760(92)90039-E PMID:1740399

Hug-Hellmuth, H. V. (1921). On the technique of Child-Analysis. *The International Journal of Psycho-Analysis, 2*, 287–305.

Hur, D. J., Raymond, G. V., Kahler, S. G., Riegert-Johnson, D. L., Cohen, B. A., & Boyadjiev, S. A. (2005). A novel MGP mutation in a consanguineous family: Review of the clinical and molecular characteristics of Keutel syndrome. *American Journal of Medical Genetics. Part A, 135A*(1), 36–40. doi:10.1002/ajmg.a.30680 PMID:15810001

Hutchinson, H. (1999). Feeding problems in young children: Report of three cases and review of the literature. *Journal of Human Nutrition and Dietetics, 12*(4), 337–343. doi:10.1046/j.1365-277x.1999.00171.x

Hutzler, F., Kronbichler, M., Jacobs, A. M., & Wimmer, H. (2006). Perhaps correlational but not causal: No effect of dyslexic readers' magnocellular system on their eye movements during reading. *Neuropsychologia, 44*(4), 637–648. doi:10.1016/j.neuropsychologia.2005.06.006 PMID:16115655

Hutzler, F., & Wimmer, H. (2004). Eye movements of dyslexic children when reading in a regular orthography. *Brain and Language, 89*(1), 235–242. doi:10.1016/S0093-934X(03)00401-2 PMID:15010255

Hu, W. F., Chahrour, M. H., & Walsh, C. A. (2014). The diverse genetic landscape of neurodevelopmental disorders. *Annual Review of Genomics and Human Genetics, 15*(1), 195–213. doi:10.1146/annurev-genom-090413-025600 PMID:25184530

Hyönä, J., & Olson, R. K. (1995). Eye fixation patterns among dyslexic and normal readers: Effects of word length and word frequency. *Journal of Experimental Psychology. Learning, Memory, and Cognition, 21*(6), 1430–1440. doi:10.1037/0278-7393.21.6.1430 PMID:7490575

Iannuzzi, D., & Rowan, A. N. (1991). Ethical issues in animal-assisted therapy programs. *Anthrozoos, 4*(3), 154–163. doi:10.2752/089279391787057116

IDEAS. (2002). *Indian Disability Evaluation Assessment Scale: A scale for measuring and quantifying disability in mental disorders*. Indian Psychiatric Society.

Illingworth, R. S., & Lister, J. (1964). The critical or sensitive period, with special reference to certain feeding problems in infants and children. *The Journal of Pediatrics, 65*(6), 839–848. doi:10.1016/S0022-3476(64)80006-8 PMID:14244090

Ismail, R., & Jaafar, A. (2011, November). Interactive Screen-Based design for dyslexic Children. In *User Science and Engineering (i-USEr), 2011 International Conference on* (pp. 168-171). IEEE. 10.1109/iUSEr.2011.6150559

Ito, H., Mori, K., Hashimoto, T., Miyazaki, M., Hori, A., Kagami, S., & Kuroda, Y. (2005). Findings of brain 99mTc-ECD SPECT in high-functioning autism-3-dimensional stereotactic ROI template analysis of brain SPECT. *The Journal of Medical Investigation, 52*(1-2), 49-56.

Ivarsson, T., Weidle, B., Skarphedinsson, G., & Valderhaug, R. (2017). Neurobiological and neurodevelopmental perspectives on OCD and their clinical implications. In J. S. Abramowitz, D. McKay, & E. A. Storch (Eds.), *The Wiley Handbook of Obsessive Compulsive Disorders*. Chichester, UK: John Wiley & Sons; doi:10.1002/9781118890233.ch15

Iyengar, B. K. S. (1993). *Light on the Yogasutras of Patanjali*. New Delhi: Harper Collins.

Jackson, G. M., & Eberly, D. A. (1982). Facilitation of performance on an arithmetic task as a result of the application of a biofeedback procedure to suppress alpha wave activity. *Biofeedback and Self-Regulation, 7*(2), 211–221. doi:10.1007/BF00998784 PMID:7138953

Jackson, L., Kline, A. D., Barr, M. A., & Koch, S. (1993). de Lange syndrome: A clinical review of 310 individuals. *American Journal of Medical Genetics, 47*(7), 940–946. doi:10.1002/ajmg.1320470703 PMID:8291537

Jacob, P., Golhar, T., Sheshadri, S., Mani, R. N., & Purushothaman, K. (2014). Child and adolescent mental health in the juvenile justice system in India: Challenges and initiatives. *Adolescent Psychiatry*, *4*, 4. doi:10.2174/2210676604666141127205656

Jacob, S., & Brinda, V. (2017). The effect of non-directive play therapy on development among mentally challenged children in selected institutions of Coimbatore. *Asian Journal of Nursing Education and Research*, *7*(4), 482–490. doi:10.5958/2349-2996.2017.00094.5

Jain, S., Dwarakanath, V. M., & Suresh, S. (2014). Audiological profile of a patient with MPS type IVA. *Rare Diseases and Orphan Drugs, 1*. Retrieved from http://rarejournal.org/rarejournal/article/view/30

Jain, A., Spencer, D., Yang, W., Kelly, J. P., Newschaffer, C. J., Johnson, J., ... Dennen, T. (2014). Injuries among children with autism spectrum disorder. *Academic Pediatrics*, *14*(4), 390–397. doi:10.1016/j.acap.2014.03.012 PMID:24976351

Jain, M., & Passi, G. R. (2005). Assessment of a modified mini-mental status scale for cognitive functions in children. *Indian Pediatrics*, *42*(9), 907–912. PMID:16208050

Jain, S., & Dinesh, N. (2016). A rare manifestation of specific learning disability in a child with Aicardi syndrome. *Acta Oto-Laryngologica Case Reports*, *1*(1), 17–23. doi:10.1080/23772484.2016.1192949

Jakobson, R. (1971). Linguistics in relation to other sciences. In *Selected writings, Word and language* (pp. 655–696). Mouton.

James, I. A., Mukaetova-Ladinska, E., Reichelt, F. K., Briel, R., & Scully, A. (2006). Diagnosing Asperger's syndrome in the elderly: A series of case presentations. *International Journal of Geriatric Psychiatry*, *21*(10), 951–960. doi:10.1002/gps.1588 PMID:16927399

James, W. D., Berger, T. G., Elston, D. M., & Odom, R. B. (2006). *Andrews' diseases of the skin: Clinical dermatology* (10th ed.). Philadelphia: Saunders Elsevier.

Janek, K. C., Smith, D. F., Kline, A. D., Benke, J. R., Chen, M. L., Kimball, A., & Ishman, S. L. (2016). Improvement in hearing loss over time in Cornelia de Lange syndrome. *International Journal of Pediatric Otorhinolaryngology*, *87*, 203–207. doi:10.1016/j.ijporl.2016.06.032 PMID:27368472

Janicki, M. P., Dalton, A. J., Henderson, C. M., & Davidson, P. W. (1999). Mortality and morbidity among older adults with intellectual disability: Health services considerations. *Disability and Rehabilitation*, *21*(5-6), 284–294. doi:10.1080/096382899297710 PMID:10381241

Jarmulowicz, L., & Hay, S. E. (2009). Derivational morphophonology: Exploring errors in third graders' productions. *Language, Speech, and Hearing Services in Schools, 40*(3), 299–311. doi:10.1044/0161-1461(2008/08-0006)

Jelm, J. M. (1990). Oral-motor/feeding rating scale. Tucson, AZ: Therapy skill builders.

Jensen, M., & Girirajan, S. (2017). Mapping a shared genetic basis for neurodevelopmental disorders. *Genome Medicine*, *9*(1), 109. doi:10.118613073-017-0503-4 PMID:29241461

Jenstad, L. M., Seewald, R. C., Cornelisse, L. E., & Shantz, J. (1999). Comparison of linear gain and wide dynamic range compression hearing aid circuits: Aided speech perception measures. *Ear and Hearing*, *20*(2), 117–126. doi:10.1097/00003446-199904000-00003 PMID:10229513

Jernberg, A. M. (1979). *Theraplay: A new treatment using structured play for problem children and their families.* Academic Press.

Jeste, S. S., Frohlich, J., & Loo, S. K. (2015). Electrophysiological biomarkers of diagnosis and outcome in neurodevelopmental disorders. *Current Opinion in Neurology*, *28*(2), 110–116. doi:10.1097/WCO.0000000000000181 PMID:25710286

Jeter, P., Slutsky, J., Singh, N., & Khalsa, S. B. (2015). Yoga as a therapeutic intervention: A bibliometric analysis of published research studies from 1967 to 2013. *Journal of Alternative and Complementary Medicine (New York, N.Y.)*, *21*(10), 586–592. doi:10.1089/acm.2015.0057 PMID:26196166

Johanson, A., & Blizzard, R. (1971). A syndrome of congenital aplasia of the alae nasi, deafness, hypothyroidism, dwarfism, absent permanent teeth, and malabsorption. *The Journal of Pediatrics*, *79*(6), 982–987. doi:10.1016/S0022-3476(71)80194-4 PMID:5171616

Johnson, J. (2017). Social learning theory as a framework for recreational therapy intervention in children with neurodevelopmental disorders. *Illuminare: A Student Journal in Recreation, Parks, and Tourism Studies, 15*(1).

Johnson, E. E. (2006). Segmenting dispensers: Factors in selecting open-canal fittings. *The Hearing Journal*, *59*(11), 58–64. doi:10.1097/01.HJ.0000286219.07211.99

Jones, P. B., & Kerwin, R. W. (1990). Left temporal lobe damage in Asperger's syndrome. *The British Journal of Psychiatry*, *156*(4), 570–572. doi:10.1192/bjp.156.4.570 PMID:2386870

Jones, S., Howard, L., & Thornicroft, G. (2008). Diagnostic overshadowing: Worse physical health care for people with mental illness. *Acta Psychiatrica Scandinavica*, *118*(3), 169–171. doi:10.1111/j.1600-0447.2008.01211.x PMID:18699951

Josefi, O., & Ryan, V. (2009). Non-directive play therapy for young children with autism: A case study. *Clinical Child Psychology and Psychiatry*, *9*(4), 533–551. doi:10.1177/1359104504046158

Juranek, J., Filipek, P. A., Berenji, G. R., Modahl, C., Osann, K., & Spence, M. A. (2006). Association between amygdala volume and anxiety level: Magnetic resonance imaging (MRI) study in autistic children. *Journal of Child Neurology*, *21*(12), 1051–1058. doi:10.1177/7010.2006.00237 PMID:17156697

Just, M. A., & Carpenter, P. A. (1980). A theory of reading: From eye fixations to comprehension. *Psychological Review*, *87*(4), 329–354. doi:10.1037/0033-295X.87.4.329 PMID:7413885

Just, M. A., Cherkassky, V. L., Keller, T. A., Kana, R. K., & Minshew, N. J. (2006). Functional and anatomical cortical underconnectivity in autism: Evidence from an fMRI study of an executive function task and corpus callosum morphometry. *Cerebral Cortex*, *17*(4), 951–961. doi:10.1093/cercor/bhl006 PMID:16772313

Kachalaki, S. M., & Faghirpour, M. (2015). The effect of play therapy in the development of cognitive skills, social and motor educable mentally retarded students. *Journal UMP Social Sciences and Technology Management*, *3*, 3.

Kaduson, H., & Schaefer, C. (Eds.). (1997). *101 favorite play therapy techniques*. Northvale, NJ: Jason Aronson.

Kahlert, S., Schönfeld, P., & Reiser, G. (2005). The Refsum disease marker phytanic acid, a branched chain fatty acid, affects Ca2+ homeostasis and mitochondria, and reduces cell viability in rat hippocampal astrocytes. *Neurobiology of Disease*, *18*(1), 110–118. doi:10.1016/j.nbd.2004.08.010 PMID:15649701

Kail, R. A. (1994). A method for studying the generalized slowing hypothesis in children with specific language impairment. *Journal of Speech Language and Hearing Research*, *37*(2), 418–421. doi:10.1044/jshr.3702.418 PMID:8028323

Kalejaiye, A., Giri, N., Brewer, C. C., Zalewski, C. K., King, K. A., Adams, C. D., ... Alter, B. P. (2016). Otologic manifestations of Fanconi anemia and other inherited bone marrow failure syndromes. *Pediatric Blood & Cancer*, *63*(12), 2139–2145. doi:10.1002/pbc.26155 PMID:27428025

Kalyani, B. G., Venkatasubramanian, G., Arasappa, R., Rao, N. P., Kalmady, S. V., Behere, R. V., ... Gangadhar, B. N. (2011). Neurohemodynamic correlates of 'OM'chanting: A pilot functional magnetic resonance imaging study. *International Journal of Yoga*, *4*(1), 3–6. doi:10.4103/0973-6131.78171 PMID:21654968

Kamioka, H., Okada, S., Tsutani, K., Park, H., Okuizumi, H., Handa, S., ... Abe, T. (2014). Effectiveness of animal-assisted therapy: A systematic review of randomized controlled trials. *Complementary Therapies in Medicine*, *22*(2), 371–390. doi:10.1016/j.ctim.2013.12.016 PMID:24731910

Kamiya, J. (1968). Conscious control of brain waves. *Psychology Today*, *1*, 56–60.

Kana, R. K., Keller, T. A., Cherkassky, V. L., Minshew, N. J., & Just, M. A. (2006). Sentence comprehension in autism: Thinking in pictures with decreased functional connectivity. *Brain*, *129*(9), 2484–2493. doi:10.1093/brain/awl164 PMID:16835247

Kancherla, V., Van Naarden Braun, K., & Yeargin-Allsopp, M. (2013). Childhood vision impairment, hearing loss and co-occurring autism spectrum disorder. *Disability and Health Journal*, *6*(4), 333–342. doi:10.1016/j.dhjo.2013.05.003 PMID:24060256

Kanner, L. (1949). Problems of nosology and psychodynamics of early infantile autism. *The American Journal of Orthopsychiatry*, *19*(3), 416–426. doi:10.1111/j.1939-0025.1949.tb05441.x PMID:18146742

Kapardis, A. (2010). *Psychology and law: A critical introduction*. Cambridge, UK: Cambridge University Press.

Kapur, M., John, A., Rozario, J., & Oommen, A. (2002). NIMHANS index of specific learning disabilities. In U. Hirisave, A. Oommen, & M. Kapur (Eds.), *Psychological Assessment of Children in the Clinical Setting* (pp. 88–126). Bangalore: Department of Clinical Psychology, National Institute of Mental Health and Neurosciences.

Karande, S. (2011). Book Review: Toy kit for kids with developmental disabilities: User manual. Indian Paediatrics, 48(10), 830.

Karande, S., & Kulkarni, M. (2005). Poor school performance. *Indian Journal of Pediatrics*, *72*(11), 961–967. doi:10.1007/BF02731673 PMID:16391452

Karen, J. K., Hale, E. K., & Ma, L. (2005). Angiokeratoma corporis diffusum (Fabry disease). *Dermatology Online Journal*, *11*, 8. PMID:16403380

Karstad, S. B., Kvello, O., Wichstrom, L., & Berg-Nielsen, T. S. (2014). What do parents know about their children's comprehension of emotions? The accuracy of parental estimates in a community sample of pre-schoolers. *Child: Care, Health and Development*, *40*(3), 346–353. doi:10.1111/cch.12071 PMID:23601022

Kashyap, K., Thunga, R., Rao, A. K., & Balamurali, N. P. (2012). Trends of utilization of government benefits among chronic mentally ill. *Indian Journal of Psychiatry*, *54*(1), 54–58. doi:10.4103/0019-5545.94648 PMID:22556439

Kasthuri, P., Sharan, R., Chandrashekar, H., & Kumar, S. (2016). Profile of psychiatric patients with certifiable disability in a general hospital psychiatry unit of Bangalore, South India. *Journal of Research in Psychiatry and Behavioural Sciences*, *2*(1), 7–10.

Katbamna, B., & Crumpton, T. (2011). Impact of Neurodevelopmental Disorders on Hearing in Children and Adolescents. In D. R. Patel, D. E. Greydanus, H. A. Omar, & J. Merrick (Eds.), *Neurodevelopmental Disabilities* (pp. 297–320). Dordrecht: Springer Netherlands. doi:10.1007/978-94-007-0627-9_19

Kaufmann, W. E., Cooper, K. L., Mostofsky, S. H., Capone, G. T., Kates, W. R., Newschaffer, C. J., & Lanham, D. C. (2003). Specificity of cerebellar vermian abnormalities in autism: A quantitative magnetic resonance imaging study. *Journal of Child Neurology*, *18*(7), 463–470. doi:10.1177/08830738030180070501 PMID:12940651

Kebbell, M. R., & Davies, D. G. (2003). People with intellectual disabilities in the investigation and prosecution crime. *Legal and Criminological Psychology, 8*(2), 219–222. doi:10.1348/135532503322362988

Keen, D. V. (2008). Childhood autism, feeding problems and failure to thrive in early infancy. *European Child & Adolescent Psychiatry, 17*(4), 209–216. doi:10.100700787-007-0655-7 PMID:17876499

Keilitz, I., & Dunivant, N. (1986). The relationship between learning disability and juvenile delinquency: Current state of knowledge. *Remedial and Special Education, 7*(3), 18–26. doi:10.1177/074193258600700305

Keilmann, A., Hegemann, S., Conti, G., & Hajioff, D. (2006). Fabry disease and the ear. In A. Mehta, M. Beck, & G. Sunder-Plassmann (Eds.), *Fabry Disease: Perspectives from 5 Years of FOS*. Oxford, UK: Oxford PharmaGenesis. Retrieved from http://www.ncbi.nlm.nih.gov/books/NBK11606/

Kelleher, E., & Corvin, A. (2015). Overlapping aetiology of neurodevelopmental disorders. In K. J. Mitchell (Ed.), *The genetics of neurodevelopmental disorders*. Hoboken, NJ: John Wiley & Sons. Mitchell. doi:10.1002/9781118524947.ch2

Keller, T. A., Kana, R. K., & Just, M. A. (2007). A developmental study of the structural integrity of white matter in autism. *Neuroreport, 18*(1), 23–27. doi:10.1097/01.wnr.0000239965.21685.99 PMID:17259855

Keller, W. D., Tillery, K. L., & McFadden, S. L. (2006). Auditory processing disorder in children diagnosed with nonverbal learning disability. *American Journal of Audiology, 15*(2), 108–113. doi:10.1044/1059-0889(2006/014) PMID:17182875

Kelly, D. P., Kelly, B. J., Jones, M. L., Moulton, N. J., Verhulst, S. J., & Bell, S. A. (1993). Attention deficits in children and adolescents with hearing loss: A survey. *American Journal of Diseases of Children, 147*(7), 737–741. doi:10.1001/archpedi.1993.02160310039014 PMID:8322743

Kelly, J. R., Minuto, C., Cryan, J. F., Clarke, G., & Dinan, T. G. (2017). Cross talk: The microbiota and neurodevelopmental disorders. *Frontiers in Neuroscience, 15*(11), 490. doi:10.3389/fnins.2017.00490 PMID:28966571

Kemper, T. L., & Bauman, M. L. (1993). The contribution of neuropathologic studies to the understanding of autism. *Neurologic Clinics, 11*(1), 175–187. doi:10.1016/S0733-8619(18)30176-2 PMID:8441369

Kennedy, D. P., Redcay, E., & Courchesne, E. (2006). Failing to deactivate: Resting functional abnormalities in autism. *Proceedings of the National Academy of Sciences of the United States of America, 103*(21), 8275–8280. doi:10.1073/pnas.0600674103 PMID:16702548

Kenner, C., & McGrath, J. M. (Eds.). (2010). *Developmental care of newborns and infants: A guide for health professionals* (2nd ed.). St. Louis, MO: Mosby.

Kenny, D. J., Koheil, R. M., Greenberg, J., Reid, D., Milner, M., Moran, R., & Judd, P. L. (1989). Development of a multidisciplinary feeding profile for children who are dependent feeders. *Dysphagia, 4*(1), 16–28. doi:10.1007/BF02407398 PMID:2534818

Kenny, M. C., & Winick, C. B. (2000). An integrative approach to play therapy with an autistic girl. *International Journal of Play Therapy, 9*(1), 11–33. doi:10.1037/h0089438

Kern, J. K., & Jones, A. M. (2006). Evidence of toxicity, oxidative stress, and neuronal insult in autism. *Journal of Toxicology and Environmental Health. Part B, 9*(6), 485–499.

Keshavan, M. S. (1999). Development, disease, and degeneration in schizophrenia: A unitary pathophysiological model. *Journal of Psychiatric Research, 33*(6), 513–521. doi:10.1016/S0022-3956(99)00033-3 PMID:10628528

Keutel, J., Jörgensen, G., & Gabriel, P. (1971). Ein neues autosomal-rezessiv vererbbares Syndrom. *Deutsche Medizinische Wochenschrift, 96*(43), 1676–1681, passim. doi:10.1055-0028-1110200 PMID:5099199

Khachatryan, H., & Rihn, A. L. (2014). *Eye-tracking methodology and applications in consumer research.* Retrived from https://edis.ifas.ufl.edu/pdffiles/FE/FE94700.pdf

Khaledi, S., Pak, A. V., Mirkhan, I., & Atai, M. (2014). The positive impact of play therapy on writing performance of students with dysgraphia. *International Journal of School Health, 1*(2), e22655. doi:10.17795/intjsh-22655

Khanna, S., & Misra, D. (2011). *Vibhor Anand vs Vice Chancellor, Guru Gobind ... on 3 March, 2011.* Available at: https://indiankanoon.org/doc/1838901/

Khansari, P. S., & Sperlagh, B. (2012). Inflammation in neurological and psychiatric diseases. *Inflammopharmacology, 20*(3), 103–107. doi:10.100710787-012-0124-x PMID:22361843

Khazan, I. Z. (2013). *The clinical handbook of biofeedback: A step-by-step guide for training and practice with mindfulness.* Sussex, UK: Wiley-Blackwell. doi:10.1002/9781118485309

Khoshali, A. K., & Venkatesan, S. (2007). Play behaviors of children with mental retardation. *Psychological Studies, 52*(1), 90–94.

Khosroshahi, H. e., Sahin, S., Akyuz, Y., & Ede, H. (2014). Long term follow-up of four patients with Keutel syndrome. *American Journal of Medical Genetics. Part A, 164*(11), 2849–2856. doi:10.1002/ajmg.a.36699 PMID:25123378

Kiely, B. T., Kohler, J. L., Coletti, H. Y., Poe, M. D., & Escolar, M. L. (2017). Early disease progression of Hurler syndrome. *Orphanet Journal of Rare Diseases, 12*(1), 32. doi:10.118613023-017-0583-7 PMID:28193245

Kim, B. N., Lee, J. S., Shin, M. S., Cho, S. C., & Lee, D. S. (2002). Regional cerebral perfusion abnormalities in attention deficit/hyperactivity disorder. *European Archives of Psychiatry and Clinical Neuroscience, 252*(5), 219–225. doi:10.100700406-002-0384-3 PMID:12451463

Kim, J., Kim, E. Y., Lee, J. S., Lee, W. S., & Kim, H. N. (2008). Temporal bone CT findings in Cornelia de Lange syndrome. *AJNR. American Journal of Neuroradiology, 29*(3), 569–573. doi:10.3174/ajnr.A0888 PMID:18065514

Kim, J., Yu, A., Choi, B. Y., Nam, J. H., Kim, M. K., Oh, D. H., & Yang, Y. J. (2015). Dietary patterns derived by cluster analysis are associated with cognitive function among Korean older adults. *Nutrients, 7*(6), 4154–4169. doi:10.3390/nu7064154 PMID:26035243

Kimmel, H. D. (1974). Instrumental conditioning of autonomically mediated responses in human beings. *The American Psychologist, 29*(5), 325–335. doi:10.1037/h0037621 PMID:4847492

Kimmel, H. D. (1981). The relevance of experimental studies to clinical applications of biofeedback. *Biofeedback and Self-Regulation, 6*(2), 263–271. doi:10.1007/BF00998874 PMID:7260190

Kim, S. D. (2017). Psychological effects of yoga nidra in women with menstrual disorders: A systematic review of randomized controlled trials. *Complementary Therapies in Clinical Practice, 28*, 4–8. doi:10.1016/j.ctcp.2017.04.001 PMID:28779936

Kim, Y. S., & State, M. W. (2014). Recent challenges to the psychiatric diagnostic nosology: A focus on the genetics and genomics of neurodevelopmental disorders. *International Journal of Epidemiology, 43*(2), 465–475. doi:10.1093/ije/dyu037 PMID:24618187

King, B. H. (2016). Psychiatric comorbidities in neurodevelopmental disorders. *Current Opinion in Neurology, 29*(2), 113–117. doi:10.1097/WCO.0000000000000299 PMID:26840045

Kleinhans, N. M., Johnson, L. C., Richards, T., Mahurin, R., Greenson, J., Dawson, G., & Aylward, E. (2009). Reduced neural habituation in the amygdala and social impairments in autism spectrum disorders. *The American Journal of Psychiatry*, *166*(4), 467–475. doi:10.1176/appi.ajp.2008.07101681 PMID:19223437

Klein, M. (1955). The psychoanalytic play technique. *The American Journal of Orthopsychiatry*, *25*(2), 223–227. doi:10.1111/j.1939-0025.1955.tb00131.x PMID:14376493

Kliegman, R., & Stanton, R. (2011). *Nelson textbook of pediatrics*. Philadelphia, PA: Elsevier Saunders.

Klin, A., Chawarska, K., Paul, R., Rubin, E., Morgan, T., Wiesner, L., & Volkmar, F. (2004). Autism in a 15-month-old child. *The American Journal of Psychiatry*, *161*(11), 1981–1988. doi:10.1176/appi.ajp.161.11.1981 PMID:15514396

Klin, A., & Jones, W. (2008). Altered face scanning and impaired recognition of biological motion in a 15-month-old infant with autism. *Developmental Science*, *11*(1), 40–46. doi:10.1111/j.1467-7687.2007.00608.x PMID:18171365

Kline, A. D., Krantz, I. D., Sommer, A., Kliewer, M., Jackson, L. G., FitzPatrick, D. R., ... Selicorni, A. (2007). Cornelia de Lange syndrome: Clinical review, diagnostic and scoring systems, and anticipatory guidance. *American Journal of Medical Genetics. Part A*, *143A*(12), 1287–1296. doi:10.1002/ajmg.a.31757 PMID:17508425

Klingberg, T., Fernell, E., Olesen, P. J., Johnson, M., Gustafsson, P., Dahlström, K., ... Westerberg, H. (2005). Computerized training of working memory in children with ADHD-A randomized, controlled trial. *Journal of the American Academy of Child and Adolescent Psychiatry*, *44*(2), 177–186. doi:10.1097/00004583-200502000-00010 PMID:15689731

Klingberg, T., Forssberg, H., & Westerberg, H. (2002). Training of working memory in children with ADHD. *Journal of Clinical and Experimental Neuropsychology*, *24*(6), 781–791. doi:10.1076/jcen.24.6.781.8395 PMID:12424652

Knell, S. (1993). *Cognitive-behavioral play therapy*. Northvale, NJ: Aronson.

Kochunov, P., & Hong, L. E. (2014). Neurodevelopmental and neurodegenerative models of schizophrenia: White matter at the center stage. *Schizophrenia Bulletin*, *40*(4), 721–728. doi:10.1093chbulbu070 PMID:24870447

Kodak, T., & Piazza, C. C. (2008). Assessment and behavioral treatment of feeding and sleeping disorders in children with autism spectrum disorders. *Child and Adolescent Psychiatric Clinics*, *17*(4), 887–905. doi:10.1016/j.chc.2008.06.005 PMID:18775376

Kodiyath, G. K., Mohan, K. M., & Bellur, R. (2017). Influence of channel and ChannelFree™ processing technology on the vocal parameters in hearing-impaired individuals. *Indian Journal of Otology*, *23*(1), 21–26. doi:10.4103/0971-7749.199506

Koegel, R. L., Bharoocha, A. A., Ribnick, C. B., Ribnick, R. C., Bucio, M. O., Fredeen, R. M., & Koegel, L. K. (2012). Using individualized reinforcers and hierarchical exposure to increase food flexibility in children with autism spectrum disorders. *Journal of Autism and Developmental Disorders*, *42*(8), 1574–1581. doi:10.100710803-011-1392-9 PMID:22042309

Kogan, M. D., Blumberg, S. J., Schieve, L. A., Boyle, C. A., Perrin, J. M., Ghandour, R. M., & van Dyck, P. C. (2009). Prevalence of parent-reported diagnosis of autism spectrum disorder among children in the US, 2007. *Pediatrics*, *124*(5), 1395–1403. doi:10.1542/peds.2009-1522 PMID:19805460

Kogan, M. D., Strickland, B. B., Blumberg, S. J., Singh, G. K., Perrin, J. M., & Van Dyck, P. C. (2008). A national profile of the health care experiences and family impact of autism spectrum disorder among children in the United States, 2005-2006. *Pediatrics*, *122*(6), e1149–e1158. doi:10.1542/peds.2008-1057 PMID:19047216

Kolevzon, A., Gross, R., & Reichenberg, A. (2007). Prenatal and perinatal risk factors for autism: A review and integration of findings. *Archives of Pediatrics & Adolescent Medicine, 161*(4), 326–333. doi:10.1001/archpedi.161.4.326 PMID:17404128

Konar, D. (2005). Juvenile justice as a part of the child and adolescent care. *Journal of Indian Association of Child and Adolescent Mental Health, 1*(3), 3.

Koning, C., & Magill-Evans, J. (2001). Social and Language Skills in Adolescent Boys with Asperger Syndrome. *Autism, 5*(1), 23–36. doi:10.1177/1362361301005001003 PMID:11708387

Korkmaz, B. (2011). Theory of mind and neurodevelopmental disorders of childhood. *Pediatric Research, 69*(5 Part 2), 101R–108R. doi:10.1203/PDR.0b013e318212c177 PMID:21289541

Kornblum, C., Broicher, R., Walther, E., Herberhold, S., Klockgether, T., Herberhold, C., & Schröder, R. (2005). Sensorineural hearing loss in patients with chronic progressive external ophthalmoplegia or Kearns-Sayre syndrome. *Journal of Neurology, 252*(9), 1101–1107. doi:10.100700415-005-0827-7 PMID:15827867

Koshino, H., Carpenter, P. A., Minshew, N. J., Cherkassky, V. L., Keller, T. A., & Just, M. A. (2005). Functional connectivity in an fMRI working memory task in high-functioning autism. *NeuroImage, 24*(3), 810–821. doi:10.1016/j.neuroimage.2004.09.028 PMID:15652316

Koshino, H., Kana, R. K., Keller, T. A., Cherkassky, V. L., Minshew, N. J., & Just, M. A. (2007). fMRI investigation of working memory for faces in autism: Visual coding and underconnectivity with frontal areas. *Cerebral Cortex, 18*(2), 289–300. doi:10.1093/cercor/bhm054 PMID:17517680

Kouijzer, M. E., van Schie, H. T., Gerrits, B. J., Buitelaar, J. K., & de Moor, J. M. (2013). Is EEG-biofeedback an effective treatment in autism spectrum disorders? A randomized controlled trial. *Applied Psychophysiology and Biofeedback, 38*(1), 17–28. doi:10.100710484-012-9204-3 PMID:22903518

Kozlowski, A. M., Matson, J. L., Fodstad, J. C., & Moree, B. N. (2011). Feeding therapy in a child with autistic disorder: Sequential food presentation. *Clinical Case Studies, 10*(3), 236–246. doi:10.1177/1534650111405189

Kranitz, L., & Lehrer, P. (2004). *Biofeedback applications in the treatment of cardiovascular diseases*. Academic Press. doi:10.1097/01.crd.0000107893.17799.95

Kricoss, B. P., & Seyfried, D. N. (1996). Speech and language characteristics, assessment and management issues. In R. L. Schow & M. A. Nerbonne (Eds.), *Introduction to aural rehabilitation* (pp. 168–229). Boston: Allyn & Bacon.

Kruger, K. A., & Serpell, J. A. (2010). Animal-assisted interventions in mental health: Definitions and theoretical foundations. In A. H. Fine (Ed.), *Handbook on Animal-Assisted Therapy: Foundations And Guidelines For Animal-Assisted Interventions* (3rd ed.; pp. 33–48). Burlington, MA: Academic Press; doi:10.1016/B978-0-12-381453-1.10003-0

Kubota, M., Ohta, S., Ando, A., Koyama, A., Terashima, H., Kashii, H., ... Hayashi, M. (2015). Nationwide survey of Cockayne syndrome in Japan: Incidence, clinical course and prognosis. *Pediatrics International, 57*(3), 339–347. doi:10.1111/ped.12635 PMID:25851792

Kuk, F., Keenan, D., & Ludvigsen, C. (2005). Efficacy of an open fitting hearing aid. *Hearing Review, 12*(4), 26–32.

Kumar, D., Dutta, A., Das, A., & Lahiri, U. (2016). SmartEye: Developing a novel eye tracking system for quantitative assessment of oculomotor abnormalities. *IEEE Transactions on Neural Systems and Rehabilitation Engineering, 24*(10), 1051–1059. doi:10.1109/TNSRE.2016.2518222 PMID:26780816

Kumari, V. (2010). *The juvenile justice system in India: From welfare to rights*. New York: Oxford University Press.

Kumar, K. A. (2017). IDEAS and the IPS. *Indian Journal of Psychiatry*, *59*(1), 124–125. doi:10.4103/psychiatry.IndianJPsychiatry_68_17 PMID:28529373

Kummer, A. (2008). *Cleft palate & craniofacial anomalies: Effects on speech and resonance* (2nd ed.). New York, NY: Cengage Learning.

Kuruvilla, K. (2010). India contribution to behavior therapy. *Indian Journal of Psychiatry*, *52*(7S1), S371–S377. doi:10.4103/0019-5545.69271 PMID:21836708

Kuskowski, M. A. (1988). Eye movements in progressive cerebral neurological disease. In C. W. Johnston & F. J. Pirozzolo (Eds.), *Neuropsychology of Eye Movements* (pp. 146–176). Hillsdale, NJ: Psychology Press.

Lacey, G., Taylor, G. W., & Areibi, S. (2016). *Deep learning on FPGAS: Past, present, and future.* arXiv preprint arXiv:1602.04283

Lach, L. M., Kohen, D. E., Garner, R. E., Brehaut, J. C., Miller, A. R., Klassen, A. F., & Rosenbaum, P. L. (2009). The health and psychosocial functioning of caregivers of children with neurodevelopmental disorders. *Disability and Rehabilitation*, *31*(8), 607–618. doi:10.1080/09638280802242163 PMID:19360498

Lachowska, M., Pastuszka, A., Łukaszewicz-Moszyńska, Z., Mikołajewska, L., & Niemczyk, K. (2016). Cochlear implantation in autistic children with profound sensorineural hearing loss. *Revista Brasileira de Otorrinolaringologia (English Ed.)*, *84*(1), 15–19. doi:10.1016/j.bjorl.2016.10.012 PMID:27939998

Lai, M. C., Lombardo, M. V., Suckling, J., Ruigrok, A. N. V., Chakrabarti, B., Ecker, C., ... Baron-Cohen, S. (2013). Biological sex affects the neurobiology of autism. *Brain*, *136*(9), 2799–2815. doi:10.1093/brain/awt216 PMID:23935125

Lai, M. L., Tsai, M. J., Yang, F. Y., Hsu, C. Y., Liu, T. C., Lee, S. W. Y., & Tsai, C. C. (2013). A review of using eye-tracking technology in exploring learning from 2000 to 2012. *Educational Research Review*, *10*, 90–115. doi:10.1016/j.edurev.2013.10.001

Lainhart, J. E., Piven, J., Wzorek, M., Landa, R., Santangelo, S. L., Coon, H., & Folstein, S. E. (1997). Macrocephaly in children and adults with autism. *Journal of the American Academy of Child and Adolescent Psychiatry*, *36*(2), 282–290. doi:10.1097/00004583-199702000-00019 PMID:9031582

Landa, R. (2000). Social language use in Asperger syndrome and high-functioning autism. In A. Klin, F. R. Volkmar, & S. S. Sparrow (Eds.), *Asperger syndrome* (pp. 125–155). New York: Guilford Press.

Landis, J. R., & Koch, G. G. (1977). The measurement of observer agreement for categorical data. *Biometrics, 33*(1), 159-174.

Landreth, G. L. (1991). Play therapy: The art of the relationship. Accelerated Development.

Landreth, G. L. (1996). *Play therapy interventions with children's problems.* Northvale, NJ: Aronson.

Landreth, G. L. (2002). *Play therapy: The art of the relationship.* New York: Routledge.

Landrigan, P. J. (2010). What causes autism? Exploring the environmental contribution. *Current Opinion in Pediatrics*, *22*(2), 219–225. doi:10.1097/MOP.0b013e328336eb9a PMID:20087185

Landrigan, P. J., Lambertini, L., & Birnbaum, L. S. (2012). A research strategy to discover the environmental causes of autism and neurodevelopmental disorders. *Environmental Health Perspectives*, *120*(7), a258–a260. doi:10.1289/ehp.1104285 PMID:22543002

Lane, A. E., Young, R. L., Baker, A. E., & Angley, M. T. (2010). Sensory processing subtypes in autism: Association with adaptive behavior. *Journal of Autism and Developmental Disorders*, *40*(1), 112–122. doi:10.100710803-009-0840-2 PMID:19644746

Larson, K. A. (1988). A research review and alternative hypothesis explaining the link between learning disability and delinquency. *Journal of Learning Disabilities*, *21*(6), 357–363. doi:10.1177/002221948802100607 PMID:3047295

Larsson, L., Nyström, M., Andersson, R., & Stridh, M. (2015). Detection of fixations and smooth pursuit movements in high-speed eye-tracking data. *Biomedical Signal Processing and Control*, *18*, 145–152. doi:10.1016/j.bspc.2014.12.008

Lask, B., Gordon, I., Christie, D., Frampton, I., Chowdhury, U., & Watkins, B. (2005). Functional neuroimaging in early-onset anorexia nervosa. *International Journal of Eating Disorders*, *37*(1), 49–51. doi:10.1002/eat.20117 PMID:15852320

Laud, R. B., Girolami, P. A., Boscoe, J. H., & Gulotta, C. S. (2009). Treatment outcomes for severe feeding problems in children with autism spectrum disorder. *Behavior Modification*, *33*(5), 520–536. doi:10.1177/0145445509346729 PMID:19748900

Laugel, V. (2013). Cockayne syndrome: The expanding clinical and mutational spectrum. *Mechanisms of Ageing and Development*, *134*(5-6), 161–170. doi:10.1016/j.mad.2013.02.006 PMID:23428416

LaVaque, T. J., Hammond, D. C., Trudeau, D., Monastra, V. J., Perry, J., Lehrer, P., ... Sherman, R. (2002). Template for developing guidelines for the evaluation of the clinical efficacy of psycho-physiological interventions. *Applied Psychophysiology and Biofeedback*, *27*(4), 273–281. doi:10.1023/A:1021061318355 PMID:12557455

Lavelle, T. A., Weinstein, M. C., Newhouse, J. P., Munir, K., Kuhlthau, K. A., & Prosser, L. A. (2014). Economic burden of autism spectrum disorders. *Pediatrics*, *133*(3), e520–e529. doi:10.1542/peds.2013-0763 PMID:24515505

Lee, J. E., Bigler, E. D., Alexander, A. L., Lazar, M., DuBray, M. B., Chung, M. K., & Lu, J. (2007). Diffusion tensor imaging of white matter in the superior temporal gyrus and temporal stem in autism. *Neuroscience Letters*, *424*(2), 127–132. doi:10.1016/j.neulet.2007.07.042 PMID:17714869

Lefebvre, S. L., Golab, G. C., Christensen, E., Castrodale, L., Aureden, K., Bialachowski, A., ... Weese, J. S. (2008). Writing panel of working group. Guidelines for animal-assisted interventions in health care facilities. *American Journal of Infection Control*, *36*(2), 78–85. doi:10.1016/j.ajic.2007.09.005 PMID:18313508

Lehrer, P., & Vaschilio, E. (2006). Heart rate variability biofeedback: Effects on age of heart rate variability, baroreflex gain, and asthma. *Chest Journal*, *129*(2), 278–384. doi:10.1378/chest.129.2.278 PMID:16478842

Leins, U., Goth, G., Hinterberger, T., Klinger, C., Rumpf, N., & Strehl, U. (2007). EEG biofeedback for children with ADHD: A comparison of SCP and theta/beta protocols. *Applied Psychophysiology and Biofeedback*, *32*(2), 73–88. doi:10.100710484-007-9031-0 PMID:17356905

Leonard, L. B. (2014). *Children with specific language impairment*. Cambridge, MA: MIT Press.

Leslie, P., & Crawford, H. (2017). *The Concise Guide to Decision Making and Ethics in Dysphagia*. Guildford, UK: J&R Press Ltd.

Leventakou, V., Roumeliotaki, T., Sarri, K., Koutra, K., Kampouri, M., Kyriklaki, A., & Chatzi, L. (2016). Dietary patterns in early childhood and child cognitive and psychomotor development: The Rhea mother–child cohort study in Crete. *British Journal of Nutrition*, *115*(8), 1431–1437. doi:10.1017/S0007114516000246 PMID:26887648

Levine, A., Bachar, L., Tsangen, Z., Mizrachi, A., Levy, A., Dalal, I., ... Boaz, M. (2011). Screening criteria for diagnosis of infantile feeding disorders as a cause of poor feeding or food refusal. *Journal of Pediatric Gastroenterology and Nutrition*, *52*(5), 563–568. doi:10.1097/MPG.0b013e3181ff72d2 PMID:21464761

Levitt, H. (1987). Interrelationships among the speech and language measures. *ASHA Monographs, 26*, 123–139. PMID:3509665

Levy, D. M. (1938). Release therapy in young children. *Psychiatry, 1*(3), 387–389. doi:10.1080/00332747.1938.11022205

Levy, S. E., Frasso, R., Colantonio, S., Reed, H., Stein, G., Barg, F. K., ... Fiks, A. G. (2016). Shared decision making and treatment decisions for young children with autism spectrum disorder. *Academic Pediatrics, 16*(6), 571–578. doi:10.1016/j.acap.2016.04.007 PMID:27132050

Lewis, J. D., & Elman, J. L. (2008). Growth-related neural reorganization and the autism phenotype: A test of the hypothesis that altered brain growth leads to altered connectivity. *Developmental Science, 11*(1), 135–155. doi:10.1111/j.1467-7687.2007.00634.x PMID:18171375

Lewis, M. H., Tanimura, Y., Lee, L. W., & Bodfish, J. W. (2007). Animal models of restricted repetitive behavior autism. *Behavioural Brain Research, 176*(1), 66–74. doi:10.1016/j.bbr.2006.08.023 PMID:16997392

Lewis, S. W., & Murray, R. M. (1987). Is schizophrenia a neurodevelopmental disorder? *British Medical Journal (Clinical Research Ed.), 296*, 681–682. PMID:3117295

Li, G., & Qiu, S. (2014). Neurodevelopmental underpinnings of Angelman Syndrome. *Journal of Bioanalysis & Biomedicine, 6*(6), 52–56. doi:10.4172/1948-593X.1000111 PMID:26491538

Lima, S. D., & Inhoff, A. W. (1985). Lexical access during eye fixations in reading: Effects of word-initial letter sequence. *Journal of Experimental Psychology. Human Perception and Performance, 11*(3), 272–285. doi:10.1037/0096-1523.11.3.272

Lindberg, L., Bohlin, G., & Hagekull, B. (1991). Early feeding problems in a normal population. *International Journal of Eating Disorders, 10*(4), 395–405. doi:10.1002/1098-108X(199107)10:4<395::AID-EAT2260100404>3.0.CO;2-A

Linder, D. E., Siebens, H. C., Mueller, M. K., Gibbs, D. M., & Freeman, L. M. (2017). Animal-assisted interventions: A national survey of health and safety policies in hospitals, eldercare facilities, and therapy animal organizations. *American Journal of Infection Control, 45*(8), 883–887. doi:10.1016/j.ajic.2017.04.287 PMID:28673680

Linscheid, T. R. (1983). Eating problems in children. In C. E. Walker & M. C. Roberts (Eds.), *Handbook of clinical child psychology*. New York: Wiley.

Liu, C., Conn, K., Sarkar, N., & Stone, W. (2008). Online affect detection and robot behavior adaptation for intervention in children with autism. *IEEE Transactions on Robotics, 24*(4), 883–896. doi:10.1109/TRO.2008.2001362

Liu, X., Liu, J., Xiong, X., Yang, T., Hou, N., Liang, X., ... Li, T. (2016). Correlation between nutrition and symptoms: Nutritional survey of children with autism spectrum disorder in Chongqing, China. *Nutrients, 8*(5), 294. doi:10.3390/nu8050294 PMID:27187463

Livingston, L. A., & Happe, F. (2017). Conceptualizing compensation in neurodevelopmental disorders: Reflections from autism spectrum disorders. *Neuroscience and Biobehavioral Reviews, 80*, 729–742. doi:10.1016/j.neubiorev.2017.06.005 PMID:28642070

Logemann, J. (1998). Mechanisms of normal and abnormal swallowing. In *Otolaryngology Head and Neck Surgery* (pp. 1844–1849). St. Louis, MO: Mosby.

Logemann, J. A. (1995). Dysphagia: Evaluation and treatment. *Folia Phoniatrica et Logopaedica, 47*(3), 140–164. doi:10.1159/000266348 PMID:7640720

Lombardo, M. V., Chakrabarti, B., Bullmore, E. T., Sadek, S. A., Pasco, G., Wheelwright, S. J., & Baron-Cohen, S. (2009). Atypical neural self-representation in autism. *Brain, 133*(2), 611–624. doi:10.1093/brain/awp306 PMID:20008375

López-Gallardo, E., López-Pérez, M. J., Montoya, J., & Ruiz-Pesini, E. (2009). CPEO and KSS differ in the percentage and location of the mtDNA deletion. *Mitochondrion, 9*(5), 314–317. doi:10.1016/j.mito.2009.04.005 PMID:19410662

Lotspeich, L. J., Kwon, H., Schumann, C. M., Fryer, S. L., Goodlin-Jones, B. L., Buonocore, M. H., ... Reiss, A. L. (2004). Investigation of neuroanatomical differences between autism and Asperger syndrome. *Archives of General Psychiatry, 61*(3), 291–298. doi:10.1001/archpsyc.61.3.291 PMID:14993117

Lozoff, B., & Georgieff, M. K. (2006). Iron deficiency and brain development. *Seminars in Pediatric Neurology, 13*(3), 158–165. doi:10.1016/j.spen.2006.08.004 PMID:17101454

Lubar, J. F. (1991). Discourse on the development of EEG diagnostics and biofeedback for attention-deficit/hyperactivity disorders. *Biofeedback and Self-Regulation, 16*(3), 201–225. doi:10.1007/BF01000016 PMID:1932259

Lukens, C. T., & Linscheid, T. R. (2008). Development and validation of an inventory to assess mealtime behavior problems in children with autism. *Journal of Autism and Developmental Disorders, 38*(2), 342–352. doi:10.100710803-007-0401-5 PMID:17578658

Luna, B., Minshew, N. J., Garver, K. E., Lazar, N. A., Thulborn, K. R., Eddy, W. F., & Sweeney, J. A. (2002). Neocortical system abnormalities in autism An fMRI study of spatial working memory. *Neurology, 59*(6), 834–840. doi:10.1212/WNL.59.6.834 PMID:12297562

Lundstrom, S., Forsman, M., Larsson, H., Kerekes, N., Serlachius, E., Langstrom, N., & Lichtenstein, P. (2014). Childhood neurodevelopmental disorders and violent criminality: A sibling control study. *Journal of Autism and Developmental Disorders, 44*(11), 2707–2718. doi:10.100710803-013-1873-0 PMID:23807203

Lupu, R. G., & Ungureanu, F. (2013). A survey of eye tracking methods and applications. *Buletinul Institutului Politehnic din Iaşi,* 71-86.

Luthe, W., & Schultz, J. H. (1969). *Autogenic therapy: Applications in psychotherapy*. New York: Grune & Stratton.

Lynch, M. P., Oller, D. K., Steffens, M. L., & Levine, S. L. (1995). Onset of speech-like vocalizations in infants with Down syndrome. *American Journal of Mental Retardation, 100*(1), 68–86. PMID:7546639

Madeira, J., Silva, C., Marcelino, L., & Ferreira, P. (2015). Assistive Mobile Applications for Dyslexia. *Procedia Computer Science, 64*, 417–424. doi:10.1016/j.procs.2015.08.535

Madipakkam, A. R., Rothkirch, M., Dziobek, I., & Sterzer, P. (2017). Unconscious avoidance of eye contact with autism spectrum disorder. *Scientific Reports, 7*(1), 13378. doi:10.103841598-017-13945-5 PMID:29042641

Madore, C., Nadjar, A., Delpech, J. C., Sere, A., Aubert, A., Portal, C., ... Layé, S. (2014). Nutritional n-3 PUFAs deficiency during perinatal periods alters brain innate immune system and neuronal plasticity-associated genes. *Brain, Behavior, and Immunity, 41*, 22–31. doi:10.1016/j.bbi.2014.03.021 PMID:24735929

Maenner, M. J., & Durkin, M. S. (2010). Trends in the prevalence of autism on the basis of special education data. *Pediatrics, 126*(5), 1018–1025. doi:10.1542/peds.2010-1023 PMID:20974790

Magnusson, L., Claesson, A., Persson, M., & Tengstrand, T. (2013). Speech recognition in noise using bilateral open-fit hearing aids: The limited benefit of directional microphones and noise reduction. *International Journal of Audiology, 52*(1), 29–36. doi:10.3109/14992027.2012.707335 PMID:22928919

Magrelli, S., Jermann, P., Basilio, N., Ansermet, F., Hentsch, F., Nadel, J., & Billard, A. (2013). Social orienting of children with autism to facial expressions and speech: A study with a wearable eye-tracker in naturalistic settings. *Frontiers in Psychology, 4*, 840. doi:10.3389/fpsyg.2013.00840 PMID:24312064

Mahdi, S., Viljoen, M., Yee, T., Selb, M., Singhal, N., Almodayfer, O., ... Bölte, S. (2017). An international qualitative study of functioning in autism spectrum disorder using the World Health Organization international classification of functioning, disability and health framework. *Autism Research, 11*(3), 463–475. doi:10.1002/aur.1905 PMID:29226604

Makkonen, I., Riikonen, R., Kokki, H., Airaksinen, M. M., & Kuikka, J. T. (2008). Serotonin and dopamine transporter binding in children with autism determined by SPECT. *Developmental Medicine and Child Neurology, 50*(8), 593–597. doi:10.1111/j.1469-8749.2008.03027.x PMID:18754896

Malavika, A. (2015). *An Investigation of the Feeding Problems in Children with Down Syndrome* (Unpublished Master's dissertation). University of Mysore, Mysore.

Malchiodi, C. A. (Ed.). (2005). *Expressive Therapies*. Guilford Publications.

Malm, D., & Nilssen, Ø. (2008). Alpha-mannosidosis. *Orphanet Journal of Rare Diseases, 3*(1), 21. doi:10.1186/1750-1172-3-21 PMID:18651971

Maltese, A., Gallai, B., Marotta, R., Lavano, F., Lavano, S. M., Tript, G., & Romano, P., D'Oro, & Salerno, M. (2017). The syntactive theory of development: The keyword for neurodevelopmental disorders. *Acta Medica Mediterranea, 33*, 1257. doi:10.19193/0393-6384_2017_2S_194

Manschreck, T. C., Kalotkin, M., & Jacobson, A. M. (1980). Utility of electro-myographic biological feedback in chronic stuttering: A clinical study with follow-up. *Perceptual and Motor Skills, 51*(2), 535–540. doi:10.2466/pms.1980.51.2.535 PMID:7443374

Marazziti, D., Baroni, S., Picchetti, M., Landi, P., Silvestri, S., Vatteroni, E., & Catena Dell'Osso, M. (2012). Psychiatric disorders and mitochondrial dysfunctions. *European Review for Medical and Pharmacological Sciences, 16*(2), 270–275. PMID:22428481

Marchisio, P., Selicorni, A., Pignataro, L., Milani, D., Baggi, E., Lambertini, L., ... Principi, N. (2008). Otitis media with effusion and hearing loss in children with Cornelia de Lange syndrome. *American Journal of Medical Genetics. Part A, 146A*(4), 426–432. doi:10.1002/ajmg.a.32183 PMID:18203151

Marinacci, A. A. (1955). *Clinical electromyography: A brief review of the electrophysiology of the motor unit and its application to the diagnosis of lower motor neuron diseases, peripheral neuropathy and the myopathies*. Los Angeles, CA: San Lucas Press.

Marino, L., & Lilienfeld, S. O. (2007). Dolphin-assisted therapy: More flawed data and more flawed conclusions. *Anthrozoos, 20*(3), 239–249. doi:10.2752/089279307X224782

Marler, J. A., Elfenbein, J. L., Ryals, B. M., Urban, Z., & Netzloff, M. L. (2005). Sensorineural hearing loss in children and adults with Williams syndrome. *American Journal of Medical Genetics. Part A, 138*(4), 318–327. doi:10.1002/ajmg.a.30970 PMID:16222677

Marriage, J. E., & Moore, B. C. (2003). New speech tests reveal benefit of widedynamic-range, fast-acting compression for consonant discrimination in children with moderate-to-profound hearing loss. *International Journal of Audiology, 42*(7), 418–425. doi:10.3109/14992020309080051 PMID:14582638

Marshall, S. P. (2000, July). *Method and apparatus for eye tracking and monitoring pupil dilation to evaluate cognitive activity*. U.S. Patent 6,090,051.

Marshall, J., Hill, R. J., Ziviani, J., & Dodrill, P. (2014). Features of feeding difficulty in children with Autism Spectrum Disorder. *International Journal of Speech-Language Pathology*, *16*(2), 151–158. doi:10.3109/17549507.2013.808700 PMID:24001171

Martell, L., Lau, K., Mei, M., Burnett, V., Decker, C., & Foehr, E. D. (2011). Biomarker analysis of Morquio syndrome: Identification of disease state and drug responsive markers. *Orphanet Journal of Rare Diseases*, *6*(1), 84. doi:10.1186/1750-1172-6-84 PMID:22176730

Martens, G. J. M., & van Loo, K. M. J. (2007). Genetic and environmental factors in complex neurodevelopmental disorders. *Current Genomics*, *8*(7), 429–444. doi:10.2174/138920207783591717 PMID:19412416

Martin, F., & Farnum, J. (2002). Animal-assisted therapy for children with pervasive developmental disorders. *Western Journal of Nursing Research*, *24*(6), 657–670. doi:10.1177/019394502320555403 PMID:12365766

Maryn, Y., De Bodt, M., & Van Cauwenberge, P. (2006). Effects of biofeedback in phonatory disorders and phonatory performance: A systematic literature. *Applied Psychophysiology and Biofeedback*, *31*(1), 65–83. doi:10.100710484-006-9005-7 PMID:16514557

Mason, S., Tovey, P., & Long, A. F. (2002). Evaluating complementary medicine: Methodological challenges of randomised controlled trials. *British Medical Journal*, *325*(7368), 832–834. doi:10.1136/bmj.325.7368.832 PMID:12376448

Mathur, A. (2017). *Living conditions in institutions for children in conflict with the law: Manual*. New Delhi: Delhi Commission for Protection of Child Rights, Ministry of Women and Child Development, Government of India.

Matin, E. (1974). Saccadic suppression: A review and an analysis. *Psychological Bulletin*, *81*(12), 899 917. doi:10.1037/h0037368

Matos, R. (2010). *Designing eye-tracking experiments to measure human behavior*. Retrived from http://www.measuringbehavior.org/files/tutorials/Tobii_MB2010_tutorial_handouts.pdf

Matson, J. L., & Fodstad, J. C. (2009). Issues in identifying the etiology of food refusal in young children. *Journal of Pediatric Gastroenterology and Nutrition*, *48*(3), 274–275. doi:10.1097/MPG.0b013e31818af6b6 PMID:19242285

Matson, J. L., Gardner, W. I., Coe, D. A., & Sovner, R. (1991). A scale for evaluating emotional disorders in severely and profoundly mentally retarded persons development of the diagnostic assessment for the severely handicapped (DASH) scale. *The British Journal of Psychiatry*, *159*(3), 404–409. doi:10.1192/bjp.159.3.404 PMID:1958951

Matson, J. L., Nebel-Schwalm, M., & Matson, M. L. (2007). A review of methodological issues in the differential diagnosis of autism spectrum disorders in children. *Research in Autism Spectrum Disorders*, *1*(1), 38–54. doi:10.1016/j.rasd.2006.07.004

Mattson, M. P. (2015). What doesn't kill you? *Scientific American*, *313*(1), 40–45. doi:10.1038cientificamerican0715-40 PMID:26204714

Mattson, M. P., Allison, D. B., Fontana, L., Harvie, M., Longo, V. D., Malaisse, W. J., ... Seyfried, T. N. (2014). Meal frequency and timing in health and disease. *Proceedings of the National Academy of Sciences of the United States of America*, *111*(47), 16647–16653. doi:10.1073/pnas.1413965111 PMID:25404320

Matuszek, S. (2010). Animal-facilitated therapy in various patient populations: Systematic literature review. *Holistic Nursing Practice*, *24*(4), 187–203. doi:10.1097/HNP.0b013e3181e90197 PMID:20588128

Maughan, B., Gray, G., & Rutter, M. (1985). Reading retardation and antisocial behavior: A follow-up into employment. *Journal of Child Psychology and Psychiatry, and Allied Disciplines*, *26*(5), 741–758. doi:10.1111/j.1469-7610.1985.tb00588.x PMID:4044719

Mazefsky, C. A., Pelphrey, K. A., & Dahl, R. E. (2012). The need for a broader approach to emotion regulation research in autism. *Child Development Perspectives*, *6*(1), 92–97. doi:10.1111/j.1750-8606.2011.00229.x PMID:22639681

McCarthy, J., Chaplin, E., Underwood, L., Forrester, A., Hayward, H., Sabet, J., ... Murphy, D. (2016). Characteristics of prisoners with neurodevelopmental disorders and difficulties. *Journal of Intellectual Disability Research*, *60*(3), 201–206. doi:10.1111/jir.12237 PMID:26486964

McKay, S., & Brumback, R. A. (1980). Relationship between learning disabilities and juvenile delinquency. *Perceptual and Motor Skills*, *51*(3), 1223–1226. doi:10.2466/pms.1980.51.3f.1223 PMID:7220224

McLaren, J., & Bryson, S. E. (1987). Review of recent epidemiological studies of mental retardation: Prevalence, associated disorders, and etiology. *American Journal of Mental Retardation*, *92*(3), 243–254. PMID:3322329

McLeavey, B. C., Toomey, J. F., & Dempsey, P. J. (1982). Nonretarded and mentally retarded children's control over syntactic structures. *American Journal of Mental Deficiency*, *86*(5), 485–494. PMID:7124802

McNamara, R. K., & Strawn, J. R. (2013). Role of long chain omega-3 fatty acids in psychiatric practice. *PharmaNutrition*, *1*(2), 41–49. doi:10.1016/j.phanu.2012.10.004 PMID:23607087

McNeil, S. E. (2017). Editorial: Disorders in children and adolescents: Challenges in diagnosis and treatment with an emphasis on neurodevelopmental disorders. The *American Journal of Psychiatry*. *Resident's Journal*, *12*(9), 2–2. doi:10.1176/appi.ajp-rj.2017.120901

McPartland, J. C. (2016). Considerations in biolmarker development for neurodevelopmental disorders. *Current Opinion in Neurology*, *29*(2), 118–122. doi:10.1097/WCO.0000000000000300 PMID:26844621

Meera, T. (2016). Medicolegal cases: What every doctor should know. *Journal of Medical Society*, *30*(3), 133–134. doi:10.4103/0972-4958.191174

Meier, M., Weng, L. P., Alexandrakis, E., Rüschoff, J., & Goeckenjan, G. (2001). Tracheobronchial stenosis in Keutel syndrome. *The European Respiratory Journal*, *17*(3), 566–569. doi:10.1183/09031936.01.17305660 PMID:11405537

Meikle, P. J., Hopwood, J. J., Clague, A. E., & Carey, W. F. (1999). Prevalence of lysosomal storage disorders. *Journal of the American Medical Association*, *281*(3), 249–254. doi:10.1001/jama.281.3.249 PMID:9918480

Meng-Chieh, Y., Huan, W., & Ming-Sui, L. (2012). Multimedia assisted breath-walk aware system. *IEEE Transactions on Biomedical Engineering*, *59*(12), 3276–3282. doi:10.1109/TBME.2012.2208747 PMID:23203771

Merenstein, G. B., & Gardner, S. L. (2002). *Handbook of Neonatal Intensive Care*. St. Louis, MO: Mosby.

Mesolella, M., Cimmino, M., Cantone, E., Marino, A., Cozzolino, M., Casa, R., ... Iengo, M. (2013). Management of otolaryngological manifestations in mucopolysaccharidoses: Our experience. *Acta Otorhinolaryngologica Italica*, *33*, 267–272. PMID:24043915

Meyerson, B. J., Wilkins, S. E., & Sawyer, C. H. (1969). Effects of estrogen on self-stimulation behavior in ovariectomized rats. *Physiology & Behavior*, *4*(3), 291–296. doi:10.1016/0031-9384(69)90177-2

Michalski, J.-C., & Klein, A. (1999). Glycoprotein lysosomal storage disorders: A- and β-mannosidosis, fucosidosis and α-N-acetylgalactosaminidase deficiency. *Biochimica et Biophysica Acta (BBA) -. Molecular Basis of Disease*, *1455*(2-3), 69–84. doi:10.1016/S0925-4439(99)00077-0 PMID:10571005

Micheletti, S., Palestra, F., Martelli, P., Accorsi, P., Alli, J., Glordano, L., ... Fazzi, E. (2016). Neurodevelopmental profile in Angelman syndrome: More than low intelligence quotient. *Italian Journal of Pediatrics*, *42*(1), 91. doi:10.118613052-016-0301-4 PMID:27769316

Miles, S., & Chapman, R. S. (2002). Narrative content as described by individuals with Down syndrome and typically developing children. *Journal of Speech, Language, and Hearing Research, 45*(1), 175–189. doi:10.1044/1092-4388(2002/013)

Miller, A. J. (1982). Deglutition. *Physiological Reviews, 62*(1), 129–184. doi:10.1152/physrev.1982.62.1.129 PMID:7034008

Miller, H., & Kiani, R. (2008). Inter-relationships between hearing impairment, learning disability services and mental health: Are learning disability services 'deaf' to hearing impairments? *Advances in Mental Health and Learning Disabilities, 2*(2), 25–30. doi:10.1108/17530180200800014

Miller, N. E., & Dworkin, B. (1974). Visceral learning: Recent difficulties with curarized rats and significant problems for human research. In P. A. Obrist, A. H. Black, J. Brener, & L. V. DiCara (Eds.), *Cardiovascular psychophysiology* (pp. 312–331). New York: Aldine.

Ministry of Home Affairs, Government of India. (2011). *Census of India, 2011*. Retrieved from: http://censusindia.gov.in/ 2011-common/censusdataonline.html

Minshew, N. J., Sweeney, J. A., Bauman, M. L., & Webb, S. J. (2005). Neurologic aspects of autism. In F. R., Volkmar, R. Paul, A. Klin, & D. J. Cohen (Eds.), Handbook of autism and pervasive developmental disorders, diagnosis, development, neurobiology, and behavior (3rd ed.; vol. 1, pp. 473-514). John Wiley & Sons, Inc. doi:10.1002/9780470939345.ch18

Minshew, N. J., & Williams, D. L. (2007). The new neurobiology of autism: Cortex, connectivity, and neuronal organization. *Archives of Neurology, 64*(7), 945–950. doi:10.1001/archneur.64.7.945 PMID:17620483

Mishra, N. N., Parker, L. S., Nimgaonkar, V. L., & Deshpande, S. N. (2012). Disability certificates in India: A challenge to health privacy. *Indian Journal of Medical Ethics, 9*(1), 43–45. PMID:22319852

Misra, D. (2017). *Ms. Eera Through Dr. Manjula ... vs State (Govt. Of NCT Of Delhi) on 21 July, 2017*. Available at: https://indiankanoon.org/doc/69624144/

Misra, S. (2012). Randomized double-blind placebo control studies, the 'Gold Standard' in intervention-based studies. *Indian Journal of Sexually Transmitted Diseases, 33*(2), 131–134. doi:10.4103/0253-7184.102130 PMID:23188942

Mogford, K. (1993). Oral Language acquisition in the prelinguistically deaf. In D. Bishop & K. Mogford (Eds.), *Language Development in Exceptional Circumstances* (pp. 110–131). Hove, UK: Erlbaum.

Moghanloo, M., Vafaie, M. E. A., Rostami, R., & Farahani, H. (2014). Determination of the effects of neurofeedback training in the neuropsychological rehabilitation in inattentive and combined subtypes of attention-deficit/hyperactivity disorder. *NeuroRegulaton, 1*(2), 131–150. doi:10.15540/nr.1.2.131

Mohan, I., Tandon, R., Kalra, H., & Trivedi, J. K. (2005). Disability assessment of mental illnesses using Indian Disability Evaluation Assessment Scale (IDEAS). *The Indian Journal of Medical Research, 121*, 759–763. PMID:16037620

Molfese, M. L. (2000). Predicting dyslexia at 8 years of age using neonatal brain responses. *Brain and Language, 72*(3), 238–245. doi:10.1006/brln.2000.2287 PMID:10764519

Monastra, V. J. (2008). Quantitative electroencephalography and attention-deficit/hyperactivity disorder: Implications for clinical practice. *Current Psychiatry Reports, 10*(5), 432–438. doi:10.100711920-008-0069-3 PMID:18803918

Monastra, V. J., Lynn, S., Linden, M., Lubar, J. F., Gruzelier, J., & LaVaque, T. J. (2006). Electroencephalographic biofeedback in the treatment of attention-deficit/ hyperactivity disorder. *Journal of Neurotherapy, 9*(4), 5–34. doi:10.1300/J184v09n04_02

Monika, S. U., Ghildiyal, A., Kala, S., & Srivastava, N. (2012). Effect of Yoga Nidra on physiological variables in patients of menstrual disturbances of reproductive age group. *Indian Journal of Physiology and Pharmacology*, *56*(2), 161–167. PMID:23387245

Montes, G., & Halterman, J. S. (2008). Association of autism spectrum disorders and loss of family income. *Pediatrics*, *121*(4), 1594. doi:10.1542/peds.2007-1594 PMID:18381511

Montgomery, J. (2003). Working memory and comprehension in children with SLI: What do we know so far? *Journal of Communication Disorders*, *36*, 221–231. doi:10.1016/S0021-9924(03)00021-2 PMID:12742669

Moore, B. C., & Glasberg, B. R. (1986). A comparison of two-channel and single-channel compression hearing aids. *Audiology*, *25*(5), 210–226. doi:10.3109/00206098609078387 PMID:3566630

Moqasale, V., Paul, D. V., Patil, M. N., & Mogasale, V. (2012). Prevalence of specific learning disabilities among primary school children in South Indian city. *Indian Journal of Pediatrics*, *79*(3), 432–347. PMID:21887581

Morais, J. (2003). Levels of phonological representation in skilled reading and learning to read. *Reading and Writing*, *16*(1/2), 123–151. doi:10.1023/A:1021702307703

Moretto, M. J., Pereira, T. de S., & de Aguiar, S. M. H. C. Á. (2012). Case Report: Cornelia de Lange Syndrome (CDLS). *Archives of Health Investigation*, *1*, 78.

Morrell, B., & Tilley, D. S. (2012). The role of non-perpetrating fathers in Munchausen Syndrome by proxy: A review of the literature. *Journal of Pediatric Nursing*, *27*(4), 328–335. doi:10.1016/j.pedn.2011.03.008 PMID:22703679

Morris, S. E., & Klein, M. D. (1987). Pre-feeding skills: A comprehensive resource for feeding development. Tucson, AZ: Therapy Skill Builders.

Morris, J. (2001). Impairment and disability: Constructing an ethics of care that promotes human rights. *Hypatia*, *16*(4), 1–16. doi:10.1111/j.1527-2001.2001.tb00750.x

Morrison, G. M., & Cosden, M. A. (1997). Risk, resilience, and adjustment of individuals with learning disabilities. *Learning Disability Quarterly*, *20*(1), 43–60. doi:10.2307/1511092

Morrison, M. L. (2007). Health benefits of animal-assisted interventions. *Complementary Health Practice Review*, *12*(1), 51–62. doi:10.1177/1533210107302397

Morrison, T. L., & Newcomer, B. L. (1975). Effects of directive vs. nondirective play therapy with institutionalized mentally retarded children. *American Journal of Mental Deficiency*, *79*, 666–669. PMID:1146857

Morris, S. E. (1989). Development of oral-motor skills in the neurologically impaired child receiving non-oral feedings. *Dysphagia*, *3*(3), 135–154. doi:10.1007/BF02407132 PMID:2517923

Morris, S. E., & Klein, M. D. (2000). *Pre-feeding skills: A comprehensive resource for mealtime development*. San Antonio, TX: Therapy Skill Builders.

Motamedi, M., Gysel, P., Akella, V., & Ghiasi, S. (2016). Design space exploration of -based deep convolutional neural networks. In *Design Automation Conference (ASP-DAC), 2016 21st Asia and South Pacific*(pp. 575-580). IEEE. 10.1109/ASPDAC.2016.7428073

Mould, M. S., Foster, D. H., Amano, K., & Oakley, J. P. (2012). A simple nonparametric method for classifying eye fixations. *Vision Research*, *57*, 18–25. doi:10.1016/j.visres.2011.12.006 PMID:22227608

Mountz, J. M., Tolbert, L. C., Lill, D. W., Katholi, C. R., & Liu, H. G. (1995). Functional deficits in autistic disorder: Characterization by technetium-99m-HMPAO and SPECT. *Journal of Nuclear Medicine*, *36*(7), 1156–1162. PMID:7790938

Moustakas, C. E. (1959). *Psychotherapy with children: The living relationship*. New York: Harper & Brothers.

Mueller, G. H., & Bentler, R. A. (2005). Fitting hearing aids using clinical measures of loudness discomfort levels: An evidence-based review of effectiveness. *Journal of the American Academy of Audiology, 16*(7), 461–472. doi:10.3766/jaaa.16.7.6 PMID:16295233

Mueller, K. L., & Tomblin, J. B. (2012). Examining the comorbidity of language disorders and ADHD. *Topics in Language Disorders, 32*, 228–246. doi:10.1097/TLD.0b013e318262010d PMID:25505812

Mukaetova-Ladinska, E. B., Perry, E., Baron, M., & Povey, C. (2012). Ageing in people with autism spectrum disorder. *International Journal of Geriatric Psychiatry, 27*(2), 109–118. doi:10.1002/gps.2711 PMID:21538534

Mukherjee, S. K., & Sadhu, S. S. (2014). *An Application For Bail Under ... vs Sanjib Banerjee & Another on 2 May, 2014*. Available at: https://indiankanoon.org/doc/23091486/

Munir, K. M. (2016). The co-occurrence of mental disorders in children and adolescents with intellectual disability/intellectual developmental disorder. *Current Opinion in Psychiatry, 29*(2), 95–102. doi:10.1097/YCO.0000000000000236 PMID:26779862

Munson, J., Dawson, G., Abbott, R., Faja, S., Webb, S. J., Friedman, S. D., & Dager, S. R. (2006). Amygdalar volume and behavioral development in autism. *Archives of General Psychiatry, 63*(6), 686–693. doi:10.1001/archpsyc.63.6.686 PMID:16754842

Murali, T., Taly, A. B., & Srivastava, A. (2006). Neurological legal disability. *Annals of Indian Academy of Neurology, 9*(3), 184–186. doi:10.4103/0972-2327.27668

Murphy, M., & Donovan, S. (1999). *The physical and psychological effects of meditation: A review of contemporary research with a comprehensive bibliography 1931-1996 (2nd ed.)*. Sausalito, CA: Institute of Noetic Sciences.

Nacewicz, B. M., Dalton, K. M., Johnstone, T., Long, M. T., McAuliff, E. M., Oakes, T. R., & Davidson, R. J. (2006). Amygdala volume and nonverbal social impairment in adolescent and adult males with autism. *Archives of General Psychiatry, 63*(12), 1417–1428. doi:10.1001/archpsyc.63.12.1417 PMID:17146016

Naderi, F., Heidarie, L. B., & Asgari, P. (2010). The efficacy of play therapy on ADHD, anxiety and social maturity in 8 to 12 years aged clientele children of Ahwaz metropolitan counseling clinics. *Journal of Applied Sciences (Faisalabad), 10*(3), 189–195. doi:10.3923/jas.2010.189.195

Nadon, G., Feldman, D., & Gisel, E. (2013). Feeding issues associated with the autism spectrum disorders. In *Recent Advances in Autism Spectrum Disorders* (Vol. 1, pp. 614–616). IntechOpen Publications; doi:10.5772/53644

Nagai, Y., & Matsuura, M. (2011). Biofeedback treatment for epilepsy. *Brain and Nerve, 63*(4), 385–392. PMID:21441642

Nakamura, K., Sekine, Y., Ouchi, Y., Tsujii, M., Yoshikawa, E., Futatsubashi, M., & Matsuzaki, H. (2010). Brain serotonin and dopamine transporter bindings in adults with high-functioning autism. *Archives of General Psychiatry, 67*(1), 59–68. doi:10.1001/archgenpsychiatry.2009.137 PMID:20048223

Nakano, T., Kato, N., & Kitazawa, S. (2011). Lack of eyeblink entrainments in autism spectrum -disorders. *Neuropsychologia, 49*(9), 2784–2790. doi:10.1016/j.neuropsychologia.2011.06.007 PMID:21699907

Nandi, J. (2010). Disability certificate for Rs. 3000 in Karnataka. *The Times of India*. Retrieved from https://timesofindia.indiatimes.com/india/Disability-certificate-for-Rs-3000-in-Karnataka/articleshow/6576215.cms

National Crime Records Bureau. (2016). *Crime in India: 2016. Ministry of Home Affairs, Government of India*. New Delhi: Author.

National Institutes of Health. (2017, September 24). Complementary, alternative, or integrative health: What's in a name? Retrieved from https://nccih.nih.gov/health/integrative-health

National Organization for Rare Disorders (Ed.). (2003). *NORD guide to rare disorders*. Philadelphia: Lippincott Williams & Wilkins.

Nazir, T. A., Heller, D., & Sussmann, C. (1992). Letter visibility and word recognition: The optimal viewing position in printed words. *Perception & Psychophysics*, *52*(3), 315–328. doi:10.3758/BF03209148 PMID:1408642

Nazir, T. A., O'regan, J. K., & Jacobs, A. M. (1991). On words and their letters. *Bulletin of the Psychonomic Society*, *29*(2), 171–174. doi:10.3758/BF03335227

Neill, C. A., & Dingwall, M. M. (1950). A Syndrome Resembling Progeria: A Review of Two Cases. *Archives of Disease in Childhood*, *25*(123), 213–223. doi:10.1136/adc.25.123.213 PMID:14783428

Nelson, L. A. (2007). The role of biofeedback in stroke rehabilitation: Past and future directions. *Topics in Stroke Rehabilitation*, *14*(4), 59–66. doi:10.1310/tsr1404-59 PMID:17698458

Nestoriuc, Y., Martin, A., Rief, W., & Andrasik, F. (2008). Biofeedback treatment for headache disorders: A comprehensive efficacy review. *Applied Psychophysiology and Biofeedback*, *33*(3), 125–140. doi:10.100710484-008-9060-3 PMID:18726688

Newfield, M. U., & Schlanger, B. B. (1968). The acquisition of English morphology by normal and educable mentally retarded children. *Journal of Speech, Language, and Hearing Research: JSLHR*, *11*(4), 693–706. doi:10.1044/jshr.1104.693 PMID:5719224

Newschaffer, C. J., Croen, L. A., Daniels, J., Giarelli, E., Grether, J. K., Levy, S. E., ... Windham, G. C. (2007). The epidemiology of autism spectrum disorders. *Annual Review of Public Health*, *28*(1), 235–258. doi:10.1146/annurev.publhealth.28.021406.144007 PMID:17367287

Nimer, J., & Lundahl, B. (2007). Animal-assisted therapy: A meta-analysis. *Anthrozoos*, *20*(3), 225–238. doi:10.2752/089279307X224773

Nityanandam, G. (2013). *G. Nityanandam vs Tmt. D. Saritha on 16 April, 2013*. Available at: https://indiankanoon.org/doc/102909949/

Nizamie, S. H., Prakash, R., Praharaj, S. K., & Akhtar, S. (2009). Certification in psychiatry. *Indian Journal of Psychiatry*, *51*(1), 35–81.

Noble, J. H., & Conley, R. W. (1992). Toward an epidemiology of relevant attributes. In R. W. Conley, R. Luckasson, & G. Bouthilet (Eds.), *The criminal justice system and mental retardation* (pp. 17–54). Baltimore, MD: Paul Brookes Publishing.

Nogueira, C., Meehan, T., & O'Donoghue, G. (2014). Refsum's Disease and Cochlear Implantation. *The Annals of Otology, Rhinology, and Laryngology*, *123*(6), 425–427. doi:10.1177/0003489414526846 PMID:24690989

Norbury, C. F., & Sparks, A. (2013). Difference or disorder? Cultural issues in understanding neurodevelopmental disorders. *Developmental Psychology*, *49*(1), 45–58. doi:10.1037/a0027446 PMID:22390668

Northstone, K., Joinson, C., Emmett, P., Ness, A., & Paus, T. (2012). Are dietary patterns in childhood associated with IQ at 8 years of age? A population-based cohort study. *Journal of Epidemiology and Community Health*, *66*(7), 624–628. doi:10.1136/jech.2010.111955 PMID:21300993

Nowell, M. A., Hackney, D. B., Muraki, A. S., & Coleman, M. (1990). Varied MR appearance of autism: Fifty-three pediatric patients having the full autistic syndrome. *Magnetic Resonance Imaging*, *8*(6), 811–816. doi:10.1016/0730-725X(90)90018-W PMID:2266809

Ntourou, K., Conture, E. G., & Lipsey, M. W. (2011). Language abilities of children who stutter: A meta-analytical review. *American Journal of Speech-Language Pathology*, *20*(3), 163–179. doi:10.1044/1058-0360(2011/09-0102) PMID:21478281

Nyaradi, A., Foster, J. K., Hickling, S., Li, J., Ambrosini, G. L., Jacques, A., & Oddy, W. H. (2014). Prospective associations between dietary patterns and cognitive performance during adolescence. *Journal of Child Psychology and Psychiatry, and Allied Disciplines*, *55*(9), 1017–1024. doi:10.1111/jcpp.12209 PMID:24673485

Nyaradi, A., Li, J., Hickling, S., Foster, J., & Oddy, W. H. (2013). The role of nutrition in children's neurocognitive development, from pregnancy through childhood. *Frontiers in Human Neuroscience*, *7*, 97. doi:10.3389/fnhum.2013.00097 PMID:23532379

O' Shea, S., & McInnis, M. G. (2016). Neurodevelopmental origins of bipolar disorder: IPSC models. *Molecular and Cellular Neurosciences*, *73*, 63–73. doi:10.1016/j.mcn.2015.11.006 PMID:26608002

O'Brien, S., Repp, A. C., Williams, G. E., & Christophersen, E. R. (1991). Pediatric feeding disorders. *Behavior Modification*, *15*(3), 394–418. doi:10.1177/01454455910153007 PMID:1953626

O'Haire, M. E. (2013). Animal-assisted intervention for autism spectrum disorder: A systematic literature review. *Journal of Autism and Developmental Disorders*, *43*(7), 1606–1622. doi:10.100710803-012-1707-5 PMID:23124442

O'Haire, M. E., McKenzie, S. J., Beck, A. M., & Slaughter, V. (2013). Social behaviors increase in children with autism in the presence of animals compared to toys. *PLoS One*, *68*(2), e57010. doi:10.1371/journal.pone.0057010 PMID:23468902

O'Haire, M. E., McKenzie, S. J., McCune, S., & Slaughter, V. (2014). Effects of classroom animal-assisted activities on social functioning in children with autism spectrum disorder. *Journal of Alternative and Complementary Medicine (New York, N.Y.)*, *20*(3), 162–168. doi:10.1089/acm.2013.0165 PMID:24156772

O'Hearn, K., Asato, M., Ordaz, S., & Luna, B. (2008). Neurodevelopment and executive function in autism. *Development and Psychopathology*, *20*(4), 1103–1132. doi:10.1017/S0954579408000527 PMID:18838033

O'Regan, J. K., & Jacobs, A. M. (1992). Optimal viewing position effect in word recognition: A challenge to current theory. *Journal of Experimental Psychology. Human Perception and Performance*, *18*(1), 185–197. doi:10.1037/0096-1523.18.1.185

O'Regan, J. K., & Lévy-Schoen, A. (1987). Eye-movement strategy and tactics in word recognition and reading. In M. Coltheart (Ed.), *Attention and performance 12: The psychology of reading* (pp. 363–383). Hillsdale, NJ: Lawrence Erlbaum Associates, Inc.

Oddi, D., Crusio, W. E., D'amato, F. R., & Pietropaolo, S. (2013). Monogenic mouse models of social dysfunction: Implications for autism. *Behavioural Brain Research*, *251*, 75–84. doi:10.1016/j.bbr.2013.01.002 PMID:23327738

Odell, D., Maciulis, A., Cutler, A., Warren, L., McMahon, W. M., Coon, H., ... Torres, A. (2005). Confirmation of the association of the C4B null allelle in autism. *Human Immunology*, *66*(2), 140–145. doi:10.1016/j.humimm.2004.11.002 PMID:15694999

Oghan, F., Harputluoglu, U., Guclu, E., Guvey, A., Turan, N., & Ozturk, O. (2007). Permanent t-tube insertion in two patients with Hurler's syndrome. *International Journal of Audiology*, *46*(2), 94–96. doi:10.1080/14992020600975287 PMID:17365060

Ohnishi, T., Matsuda, H., Hashimoto, T., Kunihiro, T., Nishikawa, M., Uema, T., & Sasaki, M. (2000). Abnormal regional cerebral blood flow in childhood autism. *Brain, 123*(9), 1838–1844. doi:10.1093/brain/123.9.1838 PMID:10960047

Okugawa, G., Sedvall, G. C., & Agartz, I. (2003). Smaller cerebellar vermis but not hemisphere volumes in patients with chronic schizophrenia. *The American Journal of Psychiatry, 160*(9), 1614–1617. doi:10.1176/appi.ajp.160.9.1614 PMID:12944335

Oliveira, L. S., de, Brosco, K. C., Oliveira, E. B., Alvarenga, K. de F., Oliveira, L. S., de, & Brosco, K. C., … Alvarenga, K. de F. (2017). Cochlear implant in Kearns-Sayre syndrome: Case study of twin sisters. *Audiology - Communication Research*, 22.

Olson, R. K., Kliegl, R., & Davidson, B. J. (1983). Dyslexic and normal readers' eye movements. *Journal of Experimental Psychology. Human Perception and Performance*, *9*(5), 816–825. doi:10.1037/0096-1523.9.5.816 PMID:6227691

Orphanet: Cockayne syndrome. (2011). Retrieved April 12, 2018, from http://www.orpha.net/consor/cgi-bin

Orphanet: Dyskeratosis congenita. (2011). Retrieved April 12, 2018, from http://www.orpha.net/consor/cgi-bin

Otake, M., Schull, W. J., & Yoshimaru, H. (1991). Brain damage among the prenatally exposed. *Journal of Radiation Research, 32*(1SUPPLEMENT), 249–264. doi:10.1269/jrr.32.SUPPLEMENT_249 PMID:1762113

Otenbacher, K., Msall, M., Lyon, N., Duffy, L. C., Ziviani, J., Granger, C. V., & Braun, S. (2000). Functional assessment and care of children with neurodevelopmental disabilities. *American Journal of Physical Medicine & Rehabilitation, 79*(2), 114–123. doi:10.1097/00002060-200003000-00002 PMID:10744184

Ottenbacher, K., Bundy, A., & Short, M. A. (1983). The development and treatment of oral-motor dysfunction: A review of clinical research. *Physical & Occupational Therapy in Pediatrics*, *3*(2), 1–13. PMID:27541087

Ovtcharov, K., Ruwase, O., Kim, J. Y., Fowers, J., Strauss, K., & Chung, E. S. (2015). Accelerating deep convolutional neural networks using specialized hardware. *Microsoft Research Whitepaper, 2*(11).

Oysu, C., Aslan, I., Basaran, B., & Baserer, N. (2001). The site of the hearing loss in Refsum's disease. *International Journal of Pediatric Otorhinolaryngology, 61*(2), 129–134. doi:10.1016/S0165-5876(01)00559-6 PMID:11589979

Ozonoff, S., Iosif, A. M., Young, G. S., Hepburn, S., Thompson, M., Colombi, C., & Rogers, S. J. (2011). Onset patterns in autism: Correspondence between home video and parent report. *Journal of the American Academy of Child and Adolescent Psychiatry, 50*(8), 796–806. doi:10.1016/j.jaac.2011.03.012 PMID:21784299

Packman, J., & Bratton, S. C. (2003). A school-based group play/activity therapy intervention with learning disabled preadolescents exhibiting behavior problems. *International Journal of Play Therapy, 12*(2), 7–29. doi:10.1037/h0088876

Palley, L. S., O'Rourke, P. P., & Niemi, S. M. (2010). Mainstreaming animal-assisted therapy. *ILAR Journal, 51*(3), 199–207. doi:10.1093/ilar.51.3.199 PMID:21131720

Palmen, S. J., Pol, H. E. H., Kemner, C., Schnack, H. G., Durston, S., Lahuis, B. E., & Van Engeland, H. (2005). Increased gray-matter volume in medication-naive high-functioning children with autism spectrum disorder. *Psychological Medicine, 35*(4), 561–570. doi:10.1017/S0033291704003496 PMID:15856726

Palmer, C. V., & Grimes, A. M. (2005). Effectiveness of signal processing strategies for the pediatric population: A systematic review of the evidence. *Journal of the American Academy of Audiology, 16*(7), 505–514. doi:10.3766/jaaa.16.7.10 PMID:16295237

Palmer, F. B., Percy, A. K., Tivnan, P., Jul, D., Tunnessen, W. W., & Scheiber, S. C. (2003). Certification in neurodevelopmental disabilities: The development of a new subspecialty and results of the initial examinations. *Developmental Disabilities Research Reviews*, *9*(2), 128–131. doi:10.1002/mrdd.10069 PMID:12784231

Palmer, M. M., Crawley, K., & Blanco, I. A. (1993). Neonatal Oral-Motor Assessment scale: A reliability study. *Journal of Perinatology*, *13*(1), 28–35. PMID:8445444

Palombo, J., Bendicsen, H. K., & Koch, B. J. (2009). *Guide to psychoanalytic developmental theories*. New York: Springer.

Papagiannopoulou, E. A., Chitty, K. M., Hermens, D. F., Hickie, I. B., & Lagopoulos, J. (2014). A systematic review and meta-analysis of eye-tracking studies in children with autism spectrum disorders. *Social Neuroscience*, *9*(6), 610–632. PMID:24988218

Pardini, M., Elia, M., Garaci, F. G., Guida, S., Coniglione, F., Krueger, F., & Gialloreti, L. E. (2012). Long-term cognitive and behavioral therapies, combined with augmentative communication, are related to uncinate fasciculus integrity in autism. *Journal of Autism and Developmental Disorders*, *42*(4), 585–592. doi:10.100710803-011-1281-2 PMID:21573693

Parker, N., & O' Brien, P. (2011). A play therapy reaching the child with autism. *International Journal of Special Education*, *26*(1), 80–87.

Parker, R. I., Vannest, K. J., & Brown, L. (2009). The improvement rate difference for single-case research. *Exceptional Children*, *75*(2), 135–150. doi:10.1177/001440290907500201

Parmar, H., Blaser, S., Unger, S., Yoo, S.-J., Papsin, B., Parmar, H., ... Yoo, S.-J. (2006). Petrified ears in a patient with Keutel syndrome: Temporal bone CT findings. *Pediatric Radiology*, *36*(3), 241–243. doi:10.100700247-005-0036-7 PMID:16328322

Pastor, P. N., & Reuben, C. A. (2008). Diagnosed attention deficit hyperactivity disorder and learning disability: United States, 2004-2006. *Vital and Health Statistics. Series 10, Data from the National Health Survey*, (237): 1–14. PMID:18998276

Patel, P., Goldberg, D., & Moss, S. (1993). Psychiatric morbidity in older people with moderate and severe learning disability. II: The prevalence study. *The British Journal of Psychiatry*, *163*(4), 481–491. doi:10.1192/bjp.163.4.481 PMID:8252287

Patel, V. B., Preedy, V. R., & Martin, C. R. (2014). *Comprehensive guide to autism*. New York, NY: Springer. doi:10.1007/978-1-4614-4788-7

Patja, K., Livanainen, M., Vesala, H., Oksanen, H., & Ruoppila, I. (2000). Life expectancy of people with intellectual disability: A 35-year old follow-up study. *Journal of Intellectual Disability Research*, *44*(5), 591–599. doi:10.1046/j.1365-2788.2000.00280.x PMID:11079356

Patterson, P. H. (2011). Maternal infection and immune involvement in autism. *Trends in Molecular Medicine*, *17*(7), 389–394. doi:10.1016/j.molmed.2011.03.001 PMID:21482187

Pavan, M. H. (1996). Disorders of feeding and swallowing in infants and children: Pathophysiology, diagnosis, and treatment. *Archives of Pediatrics & Adolescent Medicine*, *150*(8), 886–886. doi:10.1001/archpedi.1996.02170330112028

Pavlidis, G. T. (1983). The "dyslexia syndrome" and its objective diagnosis by erratic eye movements. In Eye movements in reading: Perceptual and language Processes (pp.441–466). Academic Press.

Pavlidis, G. T. (1981). Do eye movements hold the key to dyslexia? *Neuropsychologia*, *19*(1), 57–64. doi:10.1016/0028-3932(81)90044-0 PMID:7231665

Pearson, N. (1962). Self-stimulation in the goat. *Acta Physiologica (Oxford, England), 55*(2-3), 276–285. doi:10.1111/J.1748-1716.1962.tb02441.x PMID:14485613

Peeters, M., Verhoeven, L., de Moor, J., & van Balkom, H. (2009). Importance of speech production for phonological awareness and word decoding: The case of children with cerebral palsy. *Research in Developmental Disabilities, 30*(4), 712–726. doi:10.1016/j.ridd.2008.10.002 PMID:19026521

Pelphrey, K. A., Sasson, N. J., Reznick, J. S., Paul, G., Goldman, B. D., & Piven, J. (2002). Visual scanning of faces in autism. *Journal of Autism and Developmental Disorders, 32*(4), 249–261. doi:10.1023/A:1016374617369 PMID:12199131

Penagarikano, O., Abrahams, B. S., Herman, E. I., Winden, K. D., Gdalyahu, A., Dong, H., & Golshani, P. (2011). Absence of CNTNAP2 leads to epilepsy, neuronal migration abnormalities, and core autism-related deficits. *Cell, 147*(1), 235–246. doi:10.1016/j.cell.2011.08.040 PMID:21962519

Pence, P. G., Katz, L. S., Huffman, C., & Cojucar, G. (2014). Delivering Integrative Restoration-Yoga Nidra Meditation (iRest®) to women with sexual trauma at a Veteran's Medical Center: A pilot study. *International Journal of Yoga Therapy, 24*, 53–62. PMID:25858651

Peper, E., & Shaffer, F. (2010). Biofeedback history: An alternative view. *Biofeedback, 38*(4), 142–147. doi:10.5298/1081-5937-38.4.03

Perlmutter, B. F. (1987). Delinquency and learning disabilities: Evidence for compensatory behavior and adaptation. *Journal of Youth and Adolescence, 16*(2), 89–95. doi:10.1007/BF02138913 PMID:24277316

Perreau-Linck, E., Lessard, N., Levesque, J., & Beauregard, M. (2010). Effects of neurofeedback training on inhibitory capacities in ADHD children: A single-blind, randomized, placebo-controlled study. *Journal of Neurotherapy, 14*(3), 229–242. doi:10.1080/10874208.2010.501514

Perry, J., & Drogin, E. Y. (2007). *Mental disability law, evidence, and testimony: A comprehensive reference manual for lawyers, judges, and mental disability professionals*. Chicago: American Bar Association Publishing.

Peshawaria, R., & Venkatesan, S. (1992a). *Behavioral approaches to teaching mentally handicapped children: A manual for teachers*. National Institute for the Mentally Handicapped.

Peshawaria, R., & Venkatesan, S. (1992b). *Behavioral assessment scales for Indian children with mental retardation (BASIC-MR)*. National Institute for the Mentally Handicapped.

Peshawaria, R., Venkatesan, S., & Menon, D. K. (1988). Consumer demand for services by parents of mentally handicapped individuals. *Indian Journal of Disability & Rehabilitation, 2*(2), 43–57.

Peshawaria, R., Venkatesan, S., & Menon, D. K. (1990). Behavior problems in mentally handicapped persons: An analysis of parent needs. *Indian Journal of Clinical Psychology, 17*(2), 63–70.

Peshawaria, R., Venkatesan, S., Mohapatra, B., & Menon, D. K. (1990). Teachers' perception of problem behaviors among mentally handicapped persons in special school settings. *Indian Journal of Disability & Rehabilitation, 4*(1), 23–30.

Piaget, J. (1962). *Play, dreams, and imitation in childhood*. New York: Norton.

Picciano, M. F. (2003). Pregnancy and lactation: Physiological adjustments, nutritional requirements and the role of dietary supplements. *The Journal of Nutrition, 133*(6), 1997S–2002S. doi:10.1093/jn/133.6.1997S PMID:12771353

Pierce, K., Marinero, S., Hazin, R., McKenna, B., Barnes, C. C., & Malige, A. (2016). Eye tracking reveals an abnormal visual preference for geometric images as an early biomarker of an autism spectrum disorder subtype associated with increased symptom severity. *Biological Psychiatry, 79*(8), 657–666. doi:10.1016/j.biopsych.2015.03.032 PMID:25981170

Pierce, K., Müller, R. A., Ambrose, J., Allen, G., & Courchesne, E. (2001). Face processing occurs outside the fusiformface area in autism: Evidence from functional MRI. *Brain*, *124*(10), 2059–2073. doi:10.1093/brain/124.10.2059 PMID:11571222

Pietropaolo, S., Goubran, M., Joffre, C., Aubert, A., Lemaire-Mayo, V., Crusio, W. E., & Laye, S. (2014). Dietary supplementation of omega-3 fatty acids rescues fragile X phenotypes in Fmr1-Ko mice. *Psychoneuroendocrinology*, *49*, 119–129. doi:10.1016/j.psyneuen.2014.07.002 PMID:25080404

Pijl, S., & Westerberg, B. D. (2008). Cochlear implantation results in patients with Kearns-sayre syndrome. *Ear and Hearing*, *29*(3), 472–475. doi:10.1097/01.aud.0000310791.83193.62 PMID:18382375

Pillion, J. P., Rawool, V. W., Bibat, G., & Naidu, S. (2003). Prevalence of hearing loss in Rett syndrome. *Developmental Medicine and Child Neurology*, *45*(5), 338–343. doi:10.1111/j.1469-8749.2003.tb00405.x PMID:12729148

Pink, D. H. (2011). *Drive: The surprising truth about what motivates us*. New York, NY: Penguin Group.

Pirozzolo, F. J., & Rayner, K. (1979). The neural control of eye movements in acquired and developmental reading disorders. In Studies in Neurolinguistics (vol. 4, pp. 97-123). Academic Press. doi:10.1016/B978-0-12-746304-9.50009-4

Piven, J., Bailey, J., Ranson, B. J., & Arndt, S. (1998). No difference in hippocampus volume detected on magnetic resonance imaging in autistic individuals. *Journal of Autism and Developmental Disorders*, *28*(2), 105–110. doi:10.1023/A:1026084430649 PMID:9586772

Piven, J., & Rabins, P. (2011). Autism spectrum disorders in older adults: Toward defining a research agenda. *Journal of the American Geriatrics Society*, *59*(11), 2151–2155. doi:10.1111/j.1532 5415.2011.03632.x PMID:22091837

Platt, L. J., Andrews, G., & Howie, P. M. (1980). Dysarthria of adult cerebral palsy: II. Phonemic analysis of articulation errors. *Journal of Speech and Hearing Research*, *23*(1), 41–55. doi:10.1044/jshr.2301.41 PMID:7442183

Ploeger, A., & Galis, F. (2011). Evolutionary approaches to autism: An overview and integration. *McGill Journal of Medicine*, *13*(2), 38. PMID:22363193

Pomplun, M., & Sunkara, S. (2003, June). Pupil dilation as an indicator of cognitive workload in human-computer interaction. *Proceedings of the International Conference on HCI.*

Poole, A., & Ball, L. J. (2006). Eye tracking in HCI and usability research. Encyclopedia of Human-Computer Interaction, 1, 211-219.

Port, R. G., Anwar, A. R., Ku, M., Carlson, G. C., Siegel, S. J., & Roberts, T. P. (2015). Prospective MEG biomarkers in ASD: Pre-clinical evidence and clinical promise of electrophysiological signatures. *The Yale Journal of Biology and Medicine*, *88*(1), 25. PMID:25745372

Powers, N. R., Eicher, J. D., Butter, F., Kong, Y., Miller, L. L., Ring, S. M., ... Gruen, J. R. (2013). Alleles of a polymorphic ETV6 binding site in DCDC2 confer risk of reading and language impairment. *American Journal of Human Genetics*, *93*(1), 19–28. doi:10.1016/j.ajhg.2013.05.008 PMID:23746548

Prado, C., Dubois, M., & Valdois, S. (2007). The eye movement of dyslexic children during reading and visual search: Impact of the visual attention span. *Vision Research*, *47*(19), 2521–2530. doi:10.1016/j.visres.2007.06.001 PMID:17719073

Prado, E. L., & Dewey, K. G. (2014). Nutrition and brain development in early life. *Nutrition Reviews*, *72*(4), 267–284. doi:10.1111/nure.12102 PMID:24684384

Prat, C., Lemaire, O., Bret, J., Zabraniecki, L., & Fournié, B. (2008). Morquio syndrome: Diagnosis in an adult. *Joint, Bone, Spine. Revue du Rhumatisme*, *75*, 495–498. PMID:18456538

Prehn-Kristensen, A., Cooke, R., Baving, L., & Schumann, C. (2012). Neurodevelopmental disorders. In T. Bartsch (Ed.), The clinical neurobiology of the hippocampus: An integrated view. Oxford, UK: Oxford Scholarship Online/Oxford University Press. doi:10.1093/acprof:oso/9780199592388.003.0010

Prevalence and incidence of rare diseases: Bibilographic data. (2016). Retrieved on April 17, 2018, from http://www.orphadata.org/cgi-bin/index.php/

Prinsloo, G. E., Raunch, H. G. L., & Derman, W. E. (2014). A brief review and clinical applications of heart rate variability biofeedback in sports, exercise and rehabilitation medicine. *The Physician and Sportsmedicine*, *42*(2), 88–99. doi:10.3810/psm.2014.05.2061 PMID:24875976

Prosek, R. A., Montgomery, A. A., Walden, B. E., & Schwartz, D. M. (1978). EMG biofeedback in the treatment of hyperfunctional voice disorders. *The Journal of Speech and Hearing Disorders*, *43*(3), 282–294. doi:10.1044/jshd.4303.282 PMID:692095

Prothmann, A., & Fine, A. H. (2011). Animal-assisted interventions in child psychiatry. In P. McCardle, S. McCune, J. A. Griffin, L. Esposito, & L. S. Freund (Eds.), *Animals in our lives: Human animal interaction in family, community and therapeutic settings* (pp. 143–162). Baltimore, MD: Paul H. Brooks Publishing.

Psillas, G., & Daniilidis, J. (2003). Low-frequency hearing assessment by middle latency responses in children with pervasive developmental disorder. *International Journal of Pediatric Otorhinolaryngology*, *67*(6), 613–619. doi:10.1016/S0165-5876(03)00071-5 PMID:12745154

Pugh, K. R., Mencl, W. E., Jenner, A. R., Katz, L., Frost, S. J., Lee, J. R., ... Shaywitz, B. A. (2001). Neurobiological studies of reading and reading disability. *Journal of Communication Disorders*, *34*(6), 479–492. doi:10.1016/S0021-9924(01)00060-0 PMID:11725860

Quiegley, S. P., & King, C. M. (1980). Syntactic performance of Hearing Impaired and normal hearing individuals. *Applied Psycholinguistics*, *1*(4), 329–356. doi:10.1017/S0142716400000990

Racine, E., Caron, R., & Stanton-Jean, M. (2018). Justice and neurodevelopmental disorders: Moral-political philosophies, policies, and their outcomes. *Seminars in Pediatric Neurology*, *25*, 1. doi:10.1016/j.spen.2018.03.006 PMID:29735107

Rack, J. P., Snowling, M., & Olson, R. (1992). The non-word reading deficit in developmental dyslexia: A review. *Reading Research Quarterly*, *27*(1), 29–53. doi:10.2307/747832

Radant, A. D., & Hommer, D. W. (1992). A quantitative analysis of saccades and smooth pursuit during visual pursuit tracking. A comparison of schizophrenics with normals and substance abusing controls. *Schizophrenia Research*, *6*(3), 225–235. doi:10.1016/0920-9964(92)90005-P PMID:1349241

Rahman, S., Majumder, M. A. A., Shaban, S. F., Rahman, N., Ahmed, M., Abdulrahman, K. B., & D'Souza, U. J. (2011). Physician participation in clinical research and trials: Issues and approaches. *Advances in Medical Education and Practice*, *2*, 85–93. doi:10.2147/AMEP.S14103 PMID:23745079

Rakesh, A., & Srinath, S. (2010). Play therapy: Voice of a silent scream. *Journal of Indian Association for Child and Adolescent Mental Health*, *6*(1), 13–18.

Ramaa, S. (2000). Two decades of research on learning disabilities in India. *Dyslexia (Chichester, England)*, *6*(4), 268–283. doi:10.1002/1099-0909(200010/12)6:4<268::AID-DYS177>3.0.CO;2-A PMID:11129452

Ramos, S., Ramos, H. F., Ramos, R. F., Peixoto, C. A. M., & Ramos, B. F. (2010). Johanson-Blizzard syndrome. *Revista Brasileira de Otorrinolaringologia (English Ed.)*, *76*, 794–794. PMID:21180950

Ramsay, M., Martel, C., Porporino, M., & Zygmuntowicz, C. (2011). The Montreal Children's Hospital Feeding Scale: A brief bilingual screening tool for identifying feeding problems. *Paediatrics & Child Health*, *16*(3), 147–e17. doi:10.1093/pch/16.3.147 PMID:22379377

Ramteke, V. V., Darole, P. A., Shaikh, Z. F., Padwal, N. J., Agrawal, B., Shrivastava, M. S., & Kamath, S. (2011). Acrocallosal syndrome in a young hypertensive male. *BMJ Case Reports*, *2011*(apr27 1), bcr1220103648. doi:10.1136/bcr.12.2010.3648 PMID:22696705

Rao, K. (2002). Stress and its management. In P. Jose (Ed.), *Indian health –A reference document* (pp. 433–435). Kerala: Deepika Publishers.

Rapin, I., Weidenheim, K., Lindenbaum, Y., Rosenbaum, P., Merchant, S. N., Krishna, S., & Dickson, D. W. (2006). Cockayne syndrome in adults: Review with clinical and pathologic study of a new case. *Journal of Child Neurology*, *21*(11), 991–1006. doi:10.1177/08830738060210110101 PMID:17092472

Rappley, M. D. (2005). Clinical practice: Attention deficit-hyperactivity disorder. *The New England Journal of Medicine*, *352*(2), 165–173. doi:10.1056/NEJMcp032387 PMID:15647579

Rare Diseases Act of 2002 (2002 - H.R. 4013). (n.d.). Retrieved November 14, 2017, from https://www.govtrack.us/congress/bills/107/hr4013

Rare Diseases India. (n.d.). Retrieved November 14, 2017, from http://www.rarediseasesindia.org/

Raveesh, B. N., Nayak, R. B., & Kumbar, S. F. (2016). Preventing Medicolegal issues in clinical practice. *Annals of Indian Academy of Neurology*, *19*(5S1), S15–S20. doi:10.4103/0972-2327.192886 PMID:27891020

Ray, D. C., Armstrong, S., Balkin, R., & Jayne, K. (2015). Child centered play therapy in the schools: Review and meta-analysis. *Psychology in the Schools*, *52*(2), 107–123. doi:10.1002/pits.21798

Ray, D. C., Schottelkorb, A., & Tsai, M. H. (2007). Play therapy with children exhibiting symptoms of ADHD. *Inter national Journal of Play Therapy*, *16*(2), 95–111. doi:10.1037/1555-6824.16.2.95

Rayner, K. (1998). Eye Movements in Reading and Information Processing: *20* Years of Research. *Psychological Bulletin*, *124*(3), 372–422. doi:10.1037/0033-2909.124.3.372 PMID:9849112

Rayner, K., & Duffy, S. A. (1986). Lexical complexity and fixation times in reading: Effects of word frequency, verb complexity, and lexical ambiguity. *Memory & Cognition*, *14*(3), 191–201.

Rayner, K., Inhoff, A. W., Morrison, R. E., Slowiaczek, M. L., & Bertera, J. H. (1981). Masking of foveal and parafoveal vision during eye fixations in reading. *Journal of Experimental Psychology. Human Perception and Performance*, *7*(1), 167–179. doi:10.1037/0096-1523.7.1.167

Rayner, K., Well, A. D., Pollatsek, A., & Bertera, J. H. (1982). The availability of useful information to the right of fixation in reading. *Perception & Psychophysics*, *31*(6), 537–550.

Read, J., Fosse, R., Moskowitz, A., & Perry, B. (2014). The traumagenic neurodevelopmental model of psychosis revisited. *Neuropsychiatry*, *4*(1), 65–79. doi:10.2217/npy.13.89

Reau, N. R., Senturia, Y. D., Lebailly, S. A., & Christoffel, K. K. (1996). Infant and toddler feeding patterns and problems: Normative data and a new direction. *Journal of Developmental and Behavioral Pediatrics*, *17*(3), 149–153. doi:10.1097/00004703-199606000-00002 PMID:8783060

Redcay, E., & Courchesne, E. (2005). When is the brain enlarged in autism? A meta-analysis of all brain size reports. *Biological Psychiatry*, *58*(1), 1–9. doi:10.1016/j.biopsych.2005.03.026 PMID:15935993

Redefer, L. A., & Goodman, J. F. (1989). Brief report: Pet-facilitated therapy with autistic children. *Journal of Autism and Developmental Disorders, 19*(3), 461–467. doi:10.1007/BF02212943 PMID:2793790

Redmond, S. M., Ash, A. C., & Hogan, T. P. (2015). Consequences of co-occurring attention-deficit/hyperactivity disorder on children's language impairments. *Language, Speech, and Hearing Services in Schools, 46*(2), 68–80. doi:10.1044/2014_LSHSS-14-0045 PMID:25381450

Rees, S., & Inder, T. (2005). Fetal and neonatal origins of altered brain development. *Early Human Development, 81*(9), 753–761. doi:10.1016/j.earlhumdev.2005.07.004 PMID:16107304

Rehm, H. L., Zhang, D. S., Brown, M. C., Burgess, B., Halpin, C., Berger, W., ... Chen, Z. Y. (2002). Vascular defects and sensorineural deafness in a mouse model of Norrie disease. *The Journal of Neuroscience, 22*(11), 4286–4292. doi:10.1523/JNEUROSCI.22-11-04286.2002 PMID:12040033

Reilly, S. M., Skuse, D. H., Wolke, D., & Stevenson, J. (1999). Oral-motor dysfunction in children who fail to thrive: Organic or non-organic? *Developmental Medicine and Child Neurology, 41*(2), 115–122. doi:10.1017/S0012162299000225 PMID:10075097

Reiss, S., Levitan, G., & Szyszko, G. W. (1982). Emotional disturbance and mental retardation: Diagnostic overshadowing. *American Journal of Mental Deficiency, 86*(6), 567–574. PMID:7102729

Reiss, S., & Szyszko, J. (1983). Diagnostic overshadowing and professional experience with mentally retarded persons. *American Journal of Mental Deficiency, 87*(4), 396–402. PMID:6829617

Rello, L., Baeza-Yates, R., Dempere, L., & Saggion, H. (2013). Frequent words improve readability and short words improve understandability for people with dyslexia. Proc. INTERACT '13. doi:10.1007/978-3-642-40498-6_15

Rello, L. (2014). Design of Word Exercises for children with dyslexia. *Procedia Computer Science, 27*, 74–83. doi:10.1016/j.procs.2014.02.010

Rello, L., Bayarri, C., & Gorriz, A. (2012, October). What is wrong with this word? Dyseggxia: A game for children with dyslexia. In *Proceedings of the 14th international ACM SIGACCESS conference on Computers and accessibility* (pp. 219-220). ACM. 10.1145/2384916.2384962

Riccig, C. A., & Hynd, G. W. (1996). Relationship between ADHD and central auditory processing disorder: A review of the literature. *School Psychology International, 17*(3), 235–252. doi:10.1177/0143034396173001

Rice, K., Moriuchi, J. M., Jones, W., & Klin, A. (2012). Parsing heterogeneity in autism spectrum disorders: Visual scanning of dynamic social scenes in school aged children. *Journal of the American Academy of Child and Adolescent Psychiatry, 51*(3), 238–248. doi:10.1016/j.jaac.2011.12.017 PMID:22365460

Rice, M. L., Wexler, K., & Cleave, P. L. (1995). Specific language impairment as a period of extended optional infinitive. *Journal of Speech and Hearing Research, 38*(4), 850–863. doi:10.1044/jshr.3804.850 PMID:7474978

Ricketts, T., Galster, J., & Tharpe, A. M. (2007). Directional benefit in simulated classroom environments. *American Journal of Audiology, 16*(2), 130-144. doi:(2007/017 doi:10.1044/1059-0889

Rickles, W. H., Sandweiss, J. H., Jacobs, D. W., Grove, R. N., & Criswell, E. (Eds.). (1983). *Biofeedback and family practice medicine*. London: Plenum Press. doi:10.1007/978-1-4684-1173-7

Riedner, E. D., & Levin, L. S. (1977). Hearing patterns in Morquio's syndrome (mucopolysaccharidosis IV). *Archives of Otolaryngology, 103*(9), 518–520. doi:10.1001/archotol.1977.00780260048003 PMID:409383

Rigby, S. N., Stoesz, B. M., & Jakobson, L. S. (2016). Gaze patterns during scene processing in typical adults and adults with autism spectrum disorders. *Research in Autism Spectrum Disorders*, *25*, 24–36. doi:10.1016/j.rasd.2016.01.012

Riley, G. (1981). *SPI: Stuttering Prediction Instrument*. Austin, TX: Pro-Ed.

Riley, G. (1994). *SSI-3: Stuttering Severity Instrument* (3rd ed.). Austin, TX: Pro-Ed.

Riordan, M. M., Iwata, B. A., Finney, J. W., Wohl, M. K., & Stanley, A. E. (1984). Behavioral assessment and treatment of chronic food refusal in handicapped children. *Journal of Applied Behavior Analysis*, *17*(3), 327–341. doi:10.1901/jaba.1984.17-327 PMID:6239853

Riva, D., Bellugi, U., & Denckla, M. B. (2005). *Neurodevelopmental disorders: cognitive/behavioral phenotypes*. Montrouge, France: John Libbey Eurotext.

Robinson, A., Simpson, C., & Hott, B. L. (2017). The effects of child centered play therapy on the behavioral performance of three first grade students with ADHD. *International Journal of Play Therapy*, *26*(2), 73–83. doi:10.1037/pla0000047

Robinson, E. B., Koenen, K. C., McCormick, M. C., Munir, K., Hallett, V., Happé, F., & Ronald, A. (2012). A multivariate twin study of autistic traits in 12-year-olds: Testing the fractionable autism triad hypothesis. *Behavior Genetics*, *42*(2), 245–255. doi:10.100710519-011-9500-3 PMID:21927971

Roces, D. P., Lüllmann-Rauch, R., Peng, J., Balducci, C., Andersson, C., Tollersrud, O., ... von Figura, K. (2004). Efficacy of enzyme replacement therapy in alpha-mannosidosis mice: A preclinical animal study. *Human Molecular Genetics*, *13*(18), 1979–1988. doi:10.1093/hmg/ddh220 PMID:15269179

Roche, D. J. O., & King, A. C. (2010). Alcohol impairment of saccadic and smooth pursuit eye movements: Impact of risk factors for alcohol dependence. *Psychopharmacology*, *212*(1), 33–44. doi:10.100700213-010-1906-8 PMID:20635179

Roeser, K., Obergfell, F., Meule, A., Vögele, C., Schlarb, A. A., & Kübler, A. (2012). Of larks and hearts—morningness/eveningness, heart rate variability and cardiovascular stress response at different times of day. *Physiology & Behavior*, *106*(2), 151–157. doi:10.1016/j.physbeh.2012.01.023 PMID:22330324

Rogers, B., Arvedson, J., Buck, G., Smart, P., & Msall, M. (1994). Characteristics of dysphagia in children with cerebral palsy. *Dysphagia*, *9*(1), 69–73. doi:10.1007/BF00262762 PMID:8131428

Rogers, C. (1951). *Client-centered therapy*. Boston: Houghton Mifflin Co.

Rogers, L. G., Magill-Evans, J., & Rempel, G. R. (2012). Mothers' challenges in feeding their children with autism spectrum disorder-Managing more than just picky eating. *Journal of Developmental and Physical Disabilities*, *24*(1), 19–33. doi:10.100710882-011-9252-2

Romano, E., Cosentino, L., Laviola, G., & De Filippis, B. (2016). Genes and sex hormones interaction in neurodevelopmental disorders. *Neuroscience and Biobehavioral Reviews*, *67*, 9–24. doi:10.1016/j.neubiorev.2016.02.019 PMID:26952805

Ronald, A., & Hoekstra, R. A. (2011). Autism spectrum disorders and autistic traits: A decade of new twin studies. *American Journal of Medical Genetics. Part B, Neuropsychiatric Genetics*, *156*(3), 255–274. doi:10.1002/ajmg.b.31159 PMID:21438136

Rondal, J. A. (2009). Spoken language in persons with Down syndrome: A life span perspective. *International Journal of Early Childhood Special Education*, *1*(2), 138–155.

Rondal, J. A. (2013). Explaining grammatical difficulties in intellectual disabilities. *Revista de Logopedia, Foniatría y Audiología*, *33*(2), 64–68. doi:10.1016/j.rlfa.2013.04.002

Rosanowski, F., Hoppe, U., Hies, T., & Eysholdt, U. (1998). Das Johanson-Blizzard- Syndrom. *HNO*, *46*(10), 876–878. doi:10.1007001060050328 PMID:9846268

Roseboom, T. J., Painter, R. C., van Abeelen, A. F., Veenendaal, M. V., & de Rooij, S. R. (2011). Hungry in the womb: What are the consequences? Lessons from the Dutch famine. *Maturitas*, *70*(2), 141–145. doi:10.1016/j.maturitas.2011.06.017 PMID:21802226

Rosenbaum, P., Paneth, N., Leviton, A., Goldstein, M., Bax, M., Damiano, D., ... Jacobsson, B. (2007). A report: The definition and classification of cerebral palsy April 2006. *Developmental Medicine and Child Neurology*, *109*(suppl 109), 8–14. PMID:17370477

Rosenberg, D. R., & Keshavan, M. S. (1998). Toward a neurodevelopmental model of obsessive-compulsive disorder. *Biological Psychiatry*, *43*(9), 623–640. doi:10.1016/S0006-3223(97)00443-5 PMID:9582996

Rosenhall, U., Nordin, V., Sandström, M., Ahlsén, G., & Gillberg, C. (1999). Autism and hearing loss. *Journal of Autism and Developmental Disorders*, *29*(5), 349–357. doi:10.1023/A:1023022709710 PMID:10587881

Rosler, M., Retz, W., Yaqoobi, K., & Retz-Junginger, P. (2009). Attention deficit/hyperactivity disorder in female offenders: Prevalence, psychiatric comorbidity, and psychosocial implications. *European Archives of Psychiatry and Clinical Neuroscience*, *259*(2), 97–105. doi:10.100700406-008-0841-8 PMID:18806916

Rossetti, J., & King, C. (2010). Use of animal-assisted therapy with psychiatric patients: A literature review. *Journal of Psychosocial Nursing and Mental Health Services*, *48*(11), 44–48. doi:10.3928/02793695-20100831-05 PMID:20873700

Rossiter, T. (2004). The effectiveness of EEG biofeedback and stimulant drugs in treating AD/HD: Part II. Replication. *Applied Psychophysiology and Biofeedback*, *29*(4), 233–243. doi:10.100710484-004-0383-4 PMID:15707253

Rotzer, S., Loenneker, T., Kucian, K., Martin, E., Klaver, P., & Von Aster, M. (2009). Dysfunctional neural network of spatial working memory contributes to developmental dyscalculia. *Neuropsychologia*, *47*(13), 2859-2865. doi:psychologia.2009.06.009 doi:10.1016/j.neuro

Rubenstein, J. L., & Merzenich, M. M. (2003). Model of autism: Increased ratio of excitation/inhibition in key neural systems. *Genes Brain & Behavior*, *2*(5), 255–267. doi:10.1034/j.1601-183X.2003.00037.x PMID:14606691

Ruckenstein, M. J., Macdonald, R. E., Clarke, J. T., & Forte, V. (1991). The management of otolaryngological problems in the mucopolysaccharidoses: A retrospective review. *The Journal of Otolaryngology*, *20*, 177–183. PMID:1908026

Rudra, A., Belmonte, M. K., Soni, P. K., Banerjee, S., Mukerji, S., & Chakrabarti, B. (2017). Prevalence of autism spectrum disorder and autistic symptoms in a school-based cohort of children in Kolkata, India. *Autism Research*, *10*(10), 1597–1605. doi:10.1002/aur.1812 PMID:28544637

Rugari, S. M., Hunter, C. L., & Carswell, B. M. (2017). Animal-assisted therapy and activities in the critical care setting. *Nursing 2017. Critical Care (London, England)*, *12*(6), 32–40. Retrieved from http://journals.lww.com/nursingcriticalcare/Fulltext/2017/11000/Animal_assisted_therapy_and_activities_in_the.5.aspx

Rumsey, J. M., Duara, R., Grady, C., Rapoport, J. L., Margolin, R. A., Rapoport, S. I., & Cutler, N. R. (1985). Brain metabolism in autism: Resting cerebral glucose utilization rates as measured with positron emission tomography. *Archives of General Psychiatry*, *42*(5), 448–455. doi:10.1001/archpsyc.1985.01790280026003 PMID:3872650

Russell, W., Power, D., & Quigley, S. P. (1976). Linguistics and deaf children. Washington, DC: A. G. Bell Association for the deaf.

Russell, V. A. (2007). Neurobiology of animal models of attention-deficit hyperactivity disorder. *Journal of Neuroscience Methods*, *161*(2), 185–198. doi:10.1016/j.jneumeth.2006.12.005 PMID:17275916

Russell, V. A., Sagvolden, T., & Johansen, E. B. (2005). Animal models of attention-deficit hyperactivity disorder. *Behavioral and Brain Functions*, *1*(1), 9. doi:10.1186/1744-9081-1-9 PMID:16022733

Rutter, M. (1983). Cognitive deficits in the pathogenesis of autism. *Journal of Child Psychology and Psychiatry, and Allied Disciplines*, *24*(4), 513–531. doi:10.1111/j.1469-7610.1983.tb00129.x PMID:6630326

Ryu, Y. H., Lee, J. D., Yoon, P. H., Kim, D. I., Lee, H. B., & Shin, Y. J. (1999). Perfusion impairments in infantile autism on technetium-99m ethyl cysteinate dimer brain single-photon emission tomography: Comparison with findings on magnetic resonance imaging. *European Journal of Nuclear Medicine*, *26*(3), 253–259. doi:10.1007002590050385 PMID:10079316

Sachs, D. A., Martin, J. E., & Fitch, J. L. (1972). The effect of visual feedback on a digital exercise in a functionally deaf cerebral palsied child. *Journal of Behavior Therapy and Experimental Psychiatry*, *3*(3), 217–222. doi:10.1016/0005-7916(72)90078-X

Sadowski, B., & Dembiriska, M. (1973). Some characteristics of self-stimulation behavior of dogs. *Acta Neurobiologiae Experimentalis*, *33*(4), 757–769. PMID:4205636

Saitoh, O., Courchesne, E., Egaas, B., Lincoln, A. J., & Schreibman, L. (1995). Cross-sectional area of the posterior hippocampus in autistic patients with cerebellar and corpus callosum abnormalities. *Neurology*, *45*(2), 317–324. doi:10.1212/WNL.45.2.317 PMID:7854533

Salmon, P., Lush, E., Jablonski, M., & Sephton, S. E. (2009). Yoga and mindfulness: Clinical aspects of an ancient mind/body practice. *Cognitive and Behavioral Practice*, *16*(1), 59–72. doi:10.1016/j.cbpra.2008.07.002

Salvador-Carulla, L., Bertelli, M., & Martinez-Leal, R. (2018). The road to the 11th edition of the International Classification of Diseases: Trajectories of scientific consensus and contested science in the classification of intellectual disability/intellectual developmental disorders. Current Opinions in Psychiatry, 31(2), 79-87. doi: .0000000000000396 doi:10.1097/YCO

Salvucci, D. D., & Goldberg, J. H. (2000). Identifying fixations and saccades in eye-tracking protocols. In *Proceedings of the 2000 Symposium on Eye Tracking Research & Applications* (pp. 71-78). ACM. 10.1145/355017.355028

Samfira, M., & Petroman, I. (2011). Therapeutic value of the human being-animal relationship. *Lucrari Stiintifice. Zootehnie si Biotehnologii*, *44*(2), 512–515.

Sampson, P. D., Streissguth, A. P., Bookstein, F. L., Little, R. E., Clarren, S. K., Dehaene, P., ... Graham, J. M. (1997). Incidence of fetal alcohol syndrome and prevalence of alcohol-related neurodevelopmental disorder. *Teratology*, *56*(5), 317–326. doi:10.1002/(SICI)1096-9926(199711)56:5<317::AID-TERA5>3.0.CO;2-U PMID:9451756

Sams, M. J., Fortney, E. V., & Willenbring, S. (2006). Occupational therapy incorporating animals for children with autism: A pilot investigation. *The American Journal of Occupational Therapy*, *60*(3), 268–274. doi:10.5014/ajot.60.3.268 PMID:16776394

Sanfilippo, S. J., Podosin, R., Langer, L., & Good, R. A. (1963). Mental retardation associated with acid mucopolysaccharíduria (heparitin sulfate type). *The Journal of Pediatrics*, *63*(4), 837–838. doi:10.1016/S0022-3476(63)80279-6

Santos, S., López, L., González, L., & Domínguez, M. J. (2011). Hearing loss and airway problems in children with Mucopolysaccharidoses. *Acta Otorrinolaringologica Espanola*, 411–417. doi:10.1016/j.otorri.2011.05.003 PMID:21757178

Saraiva, J. M. (2000). Dysgenesis of corpus callosum in Lenz-Majewski hyperostotic dwarfism. *American Journal of Medical Genetics*, *91*(3), 198–200. doi:10.1002/(SICI)1096-8628(20000320)91:3<198::AID-AJMG8>3.0.CO;2-4 PMID:10756342

Saraswati, S. S. (1996). *Asana, Panayama, Mudra Bandh*. Munger: Yog Publications Trust.

Sarkar, S., Patra, C., Dasgupta, M. K., Nayek, K., & Karmakar, P. R. (2013). Prevalence of congenital anomalies in neonates and associated risk factors in a tertiary care hospital in eastern India. *Journal of Clinical Neonatology*, *2*(3), 131–134. doi:10.4103/2249-4847.119998 PMID:24251257

Sarpoulaki, B., & Kolahi, P. (2016). Role of play therapy on aggression and learning disabilities in students: A Quasi-experimental design. *International Journal of Indian Psychology*, *3*(4), 57.

Sasson, N. J., & Elison, J. T. (2012). Eye tracking young children with autism. *Journal of Visualized Experiments*, *61*, 3675. PMID:22491039

Sasson, N. J., & Touchstone, E. W. (2014). Visual attention to competing social and object images by preschool children with autism spectrum disorder. *Journal of Autism and Developmental Disorders*, *44*(3), 584–592. doi:10.100710803-013-1910-z PMID:23918441

Sasson, N. J., Turner-Brown, L. M., Holtzclaw, T. N., Lam, K. S., & Bodfish, J. W. (2008). Children with autism demonstrate circumscribed attention during passive viewing of complex social and nonsocial picture arrays. *Autism Research*, *1*(1), 31–42. doi:10.1002/aur.4 PMID:19360648

Savage, S. A. (2013). Dyskeratosis Congenita. In *Gene Review* (1st ed.). Seattle, WA: University of Washington, Seattle.

Schaefer, C. E. (2003). *Foundations of play therapy*. Hoboken, NJ: John Wiley & Sons.

Schaefer, C. E. (2010). *Play therapy for preschool children*. Washington, DC: American Psychological Association. doi:10.1037/12060-000

Schaefer, C. E., & O'Connor, J. K. (1982). *Handbook of Play Therapy* (Vol. 1). Somerset, NJ: John Wiley & Sons, Inc.

Schanen, N. C. (2006). Epigenetics of autism spectrum disorders. *Human Molecular Genetics*, *15*(2), R138–R150. doi:10.1093/hmg/ddl213 PMID:16987877

Schiffman, H. R. (2001). Fundamental visual functions and phenomena. *Sensation and Perception*, 89-115.

Schinzel, A. (1979). Postaxial polydactyly, hallux duplication, absence of the corpus callosum, macrencephaly and severe mental retardation: A new syndrome? *Helvetica Paediatrica Acta*, *34*, 141–146. PMID:457430

Schmidt, R. J., Hansen, R. L., Hartiala, J., Allayee, H., Schmidt, L. C., Tancredi, D. J., & Hertz-Picciotto, I. (2011). Prenatal vitamins, one-carbon metabolism gene variants, and risk for autism. *Epidemiology (Cambridge, Mass.)*, *22*(4), 476–485. doi:10.1097/EDE.0b013e31821d0e30 PMID:21610500

Schmithorst, V. J., Plante, E., & Holland, S. (2014). Unilateral deafness in children affects development of multi-modal modulation and default mode networks. *Frontiers in Human Neuroscience*, *8*, 164. doi:10.3389/fnhum.2014.00164 PMID:24723873

Schmitt, L. M., Cook, E. H., Sweeney, J. A., & Mosconi, M. W. (2014). Saccadic eye movement abnormalities in autism spectrum disorder indicate dysfunctions in cerebellum and brainstem. *Molecular Autism*, *5*(1), 47. doi:10.1186/2040-2392-5-47 PMID:25400899

Schreck, K. A., & Williams, K. (2006). Food preferences and factors influencing food selectivity for children with autism spectrum disorders. *Research in Developmental Disabilities*, *27*(4), 353–363. doi:10.1016/j.ridd.2005.03.005 PMID:16043324

Schreck, K. A., Williams, K., & Smith, A. F. (2004). A comparison of eating behaviors between children with and without autism. *Journal of Autism and Developmental Disorders*, *34*(4), 433–438. doi:10.1023/B:JADD.0000037419.78531.86 PMID:15449518

Schultz, R. T. (2005). Developmental deficits in social perception in autism: The role of the amygdala and fusiform face area. *International Journal of Developmental Neuroscience*, *23*(2–3), 125–141. doi:10.1016/j.ijdevneu.2004.12.012 PMID:15749240

Schultz, R. T., Gauthier, I., Klin, A., Fulbright, R. K., Anderson, A. W., Volkmar, F., & Gore, J. C. (2000). Abnormal ventral temporal cortical activity during face discrimination among individuals with autism and Asperger syndrome. *Archives of General Psychiatry*, *57*(4), 331–340. doi:10.1001/archpsyc.57.4.331 PMID:10768694

Schumann, C. M., Hamstra, J., Goodlin-Jones, B. L., Lotspeich, L. J., Kwon, H., Buonocore, M. H., & Amaral, D. G. (2004). The amygdala is enlarged in children but not adolescents with autism; the hippocampus is enlarged at all ages. *The Journal of Neuroscience*, *24*(28), 6392–6401. doi:10.1523/JNEUROSCI.1297-04.2004 PMID:15254095

Schwartz, M., & Andrasik, F. (2016). *Biofeedback: A practitioner's guide* (4th ed.). New York: Guilford Publications.

Schwarz, S. M. (2003). Feeding disorders in children with developmental disabilities. *Infants and Young Children*, *16*(4), 317–330. doi:10.1097/00001163-200310000-00005

Scott, C. M., & Windsor, J. (2000). General language performance measures in spoken and written narrative and expository discourse of school-age children with language learning disabilities. *Journal of Speech, Language, and Hearing Research: JSLHR*, *43*(2), 324–339. doi:10.1044/jslhr.4302.324 PMID:10757687

Scott, E. S., & Steinberg, L. (2008). Adolescent development and the regulation of youth crime. *The Future of Children*, *18*(2), 20–21. PMID:21337996

Sears, L. L., Vest, C., Mohamed, S., Bailey, J., Ranson, B. J., & Piven, J. (1999). An MRI study of the basal ganglia in autism. *Progress in Neuro-Psychopharmacology & Biological Psychiatry*, *23*(4), 613–624. doi:10.1016/S0278-5846(99)00020-2 PMID:10390720

Seddon, P. C., & Khan, Y. (2003). Respiratory problems in children with neurological impairment. *Archives of Disease in Childhood*, *88*(1), 75–78. doi:10.1136/adc.88.1.75 PMID:12495971

Seidenberg, M. S., Tanenhaus, M. K., Leiman, J. M., & Bienkowski, M. (1982). Automatic access of the meanings of ambiguous words in context: Some limitations of knowledge-based processing. *Cognitive Psychology*, *14*(4), 489–537.

Seiverling, L., Hendy, H. M., & Williams, K. (2011). The screening tool of feeding problems applied to children (STEP-CHILD): Psychometric characteristics and associations with child and parent variables. *Research in Developmental Disabilities*, *32*(3), 1122–1129. doi:10.1016/j.ridd.2011.01.012 PMID:21316919

Seung, H. K. (2007). Linguistic characteristics of individuals with high functioning autism and Asperger syndrome. *Clinical Linguistics & Phonetics*, *21*(4), 247–259. doi:10.1080/02699200701195081 PMID:17453867

Shah, N., Parwar, A., & Shah, L. P. (1998). Specific learning disability. *Converse*, *2*(2), 5–12.

Shapiro, S., Schwartz, G., & Santerre, C. (2002). Meditation and positive psychology. In C. R. Snyder & S. J. Lopez (Eds.), *Handbook of positive psychology* (pp. 632–645). New York: Oxford University Press.

Sharma, R. K. (2008). *Medico-legal aspects of patient care*. New Delhi: Peepee Publishers.

Sharma, S., Woolfson, L. M., & Hunter, S. C. (2012). Confusion and inconsistency in diagnosis of Asperger syndrome: A review of studies from 1981 to 2010. *Autism*, *16*(5), 465–486. doi:10.1177/1362361311411935 PMID:21810909

Sharp, W. G., Berry, R. C., McCracken, C., Nuhu, N. N., Marvel, E., Saulnier, C. A., & Jaquess, D. L. (2013). Feeding problems and nutrient intake in children with autism spectrum disorders: A meta-analysis and comprehensive review of the literature. *Journal of Autism and Developmental Disorders*, *43*(9), 2159–2173. doi:10.100710803-013-1771-5 PMID:23371510

Sharp, W. G., Jaquess, D. L., Morton, J. F., & Herzinger, C. V. (2010). Pediatric feeding disorders: A quantitative synthesis of treatment outcomes. *Clinical Child and Family Psychology Review*, *13*(4), 348–365. doi:10.100710567-010-0079-7 PMID:20844951

Shaw, R. J., Garcia, M., Thorn, M., Farley, C. A., & Flanagan, G. (2003). Treatment of feeding disorders in children with Down syndrome. *Clinical Child Psychology and Psychiatry*, *8*(1), 105–117. doi:10.1177/1359104503008001010

Shaywitz, B. A., Shaywitz, S. E., Pugh, K. R., Mencl, W. E., Fulbright, R. K., Skudlarski, P., ... Gore, J. C. (2002). Disruption of posterior brain systems for reading in children with developmental dyslexia. *Biological Psychiatry*, *52*(2), 101–110. doi:10.1016/S0006-3223(02)01365-3 PMID:12114001

Shaywitz, S. E. (1998). Dyslexia. *The New England Journal of Medicine*, *338*(5), 307–312. doi:10.1056/NEJM199801293380507 PMID:9445412

Shaywitz, S. E., & Shaywitz, B. A. (2005). Dyslexia (Specific Reading Disability*). Biological Psychiatry*, *57*(11), 1301–1309. doi:10.1016/j.biopsych.2005.01.043 PMID:15950002

Shcheglovitov, A., Shcheglovitova, O., Yazawa, M., Portmann, T., Shu, R., Sebastiano, V., & Dolmetsch, R. E. (2013). SHANK3 and IGF1 restore synaptic deficits in neurons from 22q13 deletion syndrome patients. *Nature*, *503*(7475), 267–271. doi:10.1038/nature12618 PMID:24132240

Shemen, L. J., Mitchell, D. P., & Farkashidy, J. (1984). Cockayne syndrome: An audiologic and temporal bone analysis. *The American Journal of Otology*, *5*, 300–307. PMID:6720882

Shen, M. D., Nordahi, C. W., Young, G. S., Wotton-Gorges, S. L., Lee, A., Liston, S. E., ... Amarai, D. G. (2013). Early brain enlargement and elevated extra-axial fluid in infants who develop autism spectrum disorder. *Brain*, *136*(Pt9), 2825–2835. doi:10.1093/brain/awt166 PMID:23838695

Sheppard, J. J., Hochman, R., & Baer, C. (2014). The dysphagia disorder survey: Validation of an assessment for swallowing and feeding function in developmental disability. *Research in Developmental Disabilities*, *35*(5), 929–942. doi:10.1016/j.ridd.2014.02.017 PMID:24637033

Sherlin, L., Arns, M., Lubar, J., & Sokhadze, E. (2010). A position paper on neurofeedback for the treatment of ADHD. *Journal of Neurotherapy*, *14*(2), 66–78. doi:10.1080/10874201003773880

Shic, F., Bradshaw, J., Klin, A., Scassellati, B., & Chawarska, K. (2011). Limited activity monitoring in toddlers with autism spectrum disorder. *Brain Research*, *1380*, 246–254. doi:10.1016/j.brainres.2010.11.074 PMID:21129365

Shic, F., Macari, S., & Chawarska, K. (2014). Speech disturbs face scanning in 6-month-old infants who develop autism spectrum disorder. *Biological Psychiatry*, *75*(3), 231–237. doi:10.1016/j.biopsych.2013.07.009 PMID:23954107

Shic, F., Scassellati, B., & Chawarska, K. (2008, March). The incomplete fixation measure. In *Proceedings of the 2008 Symposium on Eye Tracking Research & Applications* (pp. 111-114). ACM. 10.1145/1344471.1344500

Shimabukuro, T. T., Grosse, S. D., & Rice, C. (2008). Medical expenditures for children with an autism spectrum disorder in a privately insured population. *Journal of Autism and Developmental Disorders*, *38*(3), 546–552. doi:10.100710803-007-0424-y PMID:17690969

Shimmin, L. C., Ramirez, C., Matheson, A. T., & Dennis, P. P. (1989). Sequence alignment and evolutionary comparison of the L10 equivalent and L12 equivalent ribosomal proteins from archaebacteria, eubacteria, and eucaryotes. *Journal of Molecular Evolution*, *29*(5), 448–462. doi:10.1007/BF02602915 PMID:2515294

Shin, J. J., & Hartnick, C. J. (2004). Otologic manifestations of ectodermal dysplasia. *Archives of Otolaryngology--Head & Neck Surgery*, *130*(9), 1104–1107. doi:10.1001/archotol.130.9.1104 PMID:15381599

Shi, X., Gillespie, P. G., & Nuttall, A. L. (2007). Apical phosphatidylserine externalization in auditory hair cells. *Molecular Membrane Biology*, *24*(1), 16–27. doi:10.1080/09687860600926883 PMID:17453410

Shouse, M. N., & Lubar, J. F. (1979). Operant conditioning of EEG rhythms and Ritalin in the treatment of hyper-kinesis. *Biofeedback and Self-Regulation*, *4*(4), 299–312. doi:10.1007/BF00998960 PMID:526475

Shriberg, L. D., & Widder, C. J. (1990). Speech and prosody characteristics of adults with mental retardation. *Journal of Speech and Hearing Research*, *33*(4), 627–653. doi:10.1044/jshr.3304.627 PMID:2273880

Siegel, L. J. (1982). Classical and operant procedures in the treatment of a case of food aversion in a young child. *Journal of Clinical Child and Adolescent Psychology*, *11*(2), 167–172. doi:10.120715374424jccp1102_12

Silberberg, D., Arora, N., Bhutani, V., Durkin, M., Gulati, S., Nair, M., & Pinto-Martin, J. (2014). Neuro-Developmental Disorders in India - From Epidemiology to Public Policy (I10-1.006). *Neurology*, *82*(S10), I10–I11.

Silberberg, D., Arora, N., Bhutani, V., Durkin, M., Gulati, S., Nair, M., & Pinto-Martin, J. (2014). Neuro-developmental disorders in India-From epidemiology to public policy (I10-1.006). *Neurology*, *82*(10Supplement), I10–I11.

Sillery, J., Hargreaves, J., Marin, P., Lerma, E., Kuznia, C., & Abbe, C. (2004). Pasteurella multocida peritonitis another risk of animal-assisted therapy. *Infection Control and Hospital Epidemiology*, *25*(1), 5–6. doi:10.1086/503486 PMID:14756211

Silva, K., Correia, R., Lima, M., Magalhães, A., & de Sousa, L. (2011). Can dogs prime autistic children for therapy? Evidence from a single case study. *Journal of Alternative and Complementary Medicine (New York, N.Y.)*, *17*(7), 655–659. doi:10.1089/acm.2010.0436 PMID:21689015

Simmons, M. A., Bruce, I. A., Penney, S., Wraith, E., & Rothera, M. P. (2005). Otorhinolaryngological manifestations of the mucopolysaccharidoses. *International Journal of Pediatric Otorhinolaryngology*, *69*(5), 589–595. doi:10.1016/j.ijporl.2005.01.017 PMID:15850680

Singal, R., Pandit, S., Saini, A., Singh, P., & Dhawan, N. (2014). The Acrocallosal syndrome in a neonate with further widening of phenotypic expression. *Iranian Journal of Child Neurology*, *8*, 60–64. PMID:24949054

Singh, A. P. (2017). Effectiveness of yogic lifestyle for promoting mental health and well-being: Implications for therapeutic value and school health-care policy. In A. Dubey & A. Shukla (Eds.), Mental health: Psychosocial perspectives (vol. 4). New Delhi: Concept.

Singh, A. P., & Misra, G. (2012). Adolescent lifestyle in India: Prevalence of risk and health-promotive factors. *Psychology and Developing Societies*, *24*(2), 145–160. doi:10.1177/097133361202400203

Singh, A. P., & Misra, G. (2015). Pattern of leisure-lifestyles in Indian school adolescents: Contextual influences and implications for health concerns. *Cognitive Psychology*, *2*(1), 1–11. doi:10.1080/23311908.2015.1050779

Singh, A. P., & Misra, G. (2016). Gender difference in life Style: Results of a survey among Indian school adolescents. *Social Change*, *46*(3), 1–16. doi:10.1177/0049085716654816

Singleton, C., & Simmons, F. (2001). An evaluation of Wordshark in the classroom. *British Journal of Educational Technology*, *32*(3), 317–330. doi:10.1111/1467-8535.00201

Sismanis, A., Polisar, I. A., Ruffy, M. L., & Lambert, J. C. (1979). Rare congenital syndrome associated with profound hearing loss. *Archives of Otolaryngology*, *105*(4), 222–224. doi:10.1001/archotol.1979.00790160056015 PMID:426713

Skiada, R., Soroniati, E., Gardeli, A., & Zissis, D. (2014). EasyLexia: A mobile application for children with learning difficulties. *Procedia Computer Science*, *27*, 218–228. doi:10.1016/j.procs.2014.02.025

Sklar, B., Hanley, J., & Simmons, W. W. (1973). A Computer Analysis of EEG Spectral Signatures from Normal and Dyslexic Children. *IEEE Transactions on Biomedical Engineering*, *1*(1), 20–26. doi:10.1109/TBME.1973.324247 PMID:4681806

Skuse, D., Stevenson, J., Reilly, S., & Mathisen, B. (1995). Schedule for oral-motor assessment (SOMA): Methods of validation. *Dysphagia*, *10*(3), 192–202. doi:10.1007/BF00260976 PMID:7614861

Smith, B. L., & Stoel-gammon, C. (1996). A quantitative analysis of reduplicated and variegated babbling in vocalizations by Down syndrome infants. *Clinical Linguistics & Phonetics*, *10*(2), 119–129. doi:10.3109/02699209608985166

Smithers, L. G., Golley, R. K., Mittinty, M. N., Brazionis, L., Northstone, K., Emmett, P., & Lynch, J. W. (2012). Dietary patterns at 6, 15 and 24 months of age are associated with IQ at 8 years of age. *European Journal of Epidemiology*, *27*(7), 525–535. doi:10.100710654-012-9715-5 PMID:22810299

Smithers, L. G., Golley, R. K., Mittinty, M. N., Brazionis, L., Northstone, K., Emmett, P., & Lynch, J. W. (2013). Do dietary trajectories between infancy and toddlerhood influence IQ in childhood and adolescence? Results from a prospective birth cohort study. *PLoS One*, *8*(3), e58904. doi:10.1371/journal.pone.0058904 PMID:23516574

Smith, J., Dann, M., & Brown, P. M. (2009). An evaluation of frequency transposition for hearing-impaired school-age children. *Deafness & Education International*, *11*(2), 62–82. doi:10.1179/146431509790559633

Smith, K. (2013). Evidence-informed policy in public health. In K. Smith (Ed.), *Beyond evidence-based policy in public health: The interplay of ideas* (pp. 42–69). London: Palgrave Macmillan UK; doi:10.1057/9781137026583_2

Smith, S. E., Li, J., Garbett, K., Mirnics, K., & Patterson, P. H. (2007). Maternal immune activation alters fetal brain development through interleukin-6. *The Journal of Neuroscience*, *27*(40), 10695–10702. doi:10.1523/JNEUROSCI.2178-07.2007 PMID:17913903

Smyth, J. F., Mossman, J., Hall, R., Hepburn, S., Pinkerton, R., Richards, M., ... Box, J. (1994). Conducting clinical research in the new NHS: The model of cancer. *British Medical Journal*, *309*(6952), 457–461. doi:10.1136/bmj.309.6952.457 PMID:7920132

Snider, L., Korner-Bitensky, N., Kammann, C., Warner, S., & Saleh, M. (2007). Horseback riding as therapy for children with cerebral palsy: Is there evidence of its effectiveness? *Physical & Occupational Therapy in Pediatrics*, *27*(2), 5–23. PMID:17442652

Snowling, M. J. (1995). Phonological processing and developmental dyslexia. *Journal of Research in Reading*, *18*(2), 132–138. doi:10.1111/j.1467-9817.1995.tb00079.x

Sokhadze, T. M., Cannon, R. L., & Trudeau, D. L. (2008). EEG biofeedback as a treatment for substance use disorders: Review, a rating of efficiency, and recommendations for further research. *Applied Psychophysiology and Biofeedback*, *33*(1), 1–28. doi:10.100710484-007-9047-5 PMID:18214670

Solomon, J. C. (1938). Active play therapy. *The American Journal of Orthopsychiatry*, *8*(3), 479–498. doi:10.1111/j.1939-0025.1938.tb06398.x

Solomon, M., Hessl, D., Chiu, S., Olsen, E., & Hendren, R. L. (2009). Towards a neurodevelopmental model of clinical case formulation. *Psychiatria Clinica*, *32*(1), 199–211. PMID:19248925

Solomon, O. (2010). What a dog can do: Children with autism and therapy dogs in social interaction. *ETHOS Journal of the Society of Psychological Anthropology*, *38*(1), 143–166.

Sontheimer, H. (2015). *Diseases of the nervous system*. Amsterdam: Elsevier Academic Press.

Sousa, S. B., Jenkins, D., Chanudet, E., Tasseva, G., Ishida, M., Anderson, G., ... Moore, G. E. (2014). Gain-of-function mutations in the phosphatidylserine synthase 1 (PTDSS1) gene cause Lenz-Majewski syndrome. *Nature Genetics*, *46*(1), 70–76. doi:10.1038/ng.2829 PMID:24241535

Souter, M. A., & Miller, M. D. (2007). Do animal-assisted activities effectively treat depression? A meta-analysis. *Anthrozoos*, *20*(2), 167–180. doi:10.2752/175303707X207954

Sparks, B. F., Friedman, S. D., Shaw, D. W., Aylward, E. H., Echelard, D., Artru, A. A., & Dager, S. R. (2002). Brain structural abnormalities in young children with autism spectrum disorder. *Neurology*, *59*(2), 184–192. doi:10.1212/WNL.59.2.184 PMID:12136055

Speer, L. L., Cook, A. E., McMahon, W. M., & Clark, E. (2007). Face processing in children with autism: Effects of stimulus contents and type. *Autism*, *11*(3), 265–277. doi:10.1177/1362361307076925 PMID:17478579

Sperdin, H. F., & Schaer, M. (2016). Aberrant development of speech processing in young children with autism: New insights from neuroimaging biomarkers. *Frontiers in Neuroscience*, *10*, 393. doi:10.3389/fnins.2016.00393 PMID:27610073

Srivastava, A. K. (2011). Book Review: Toy kit for kids with developmental disabilities: User manual. *Journal of Disability Management and Special Education*, *1*(1), 87–88.

Srivastava, K., Raman, M., & Bhattacharya, A. (2016). A study on comparison of anthropometrics of autism spectrum disorder children with normal children. *International Journal of Innovative Research and Development*, *5*(6), 484–487.

Srivastava, P., & Kumar, P. (2015). Disability, its issues, and challenges and legal aspects in the Indian scenario. *Delhi Psychiatry Journal*, *18*(1), 195–205.

Srushti, S., & Swapna, N. (2014). *Development and validation of feeding handicap index in children* (Unpublished Master's dissertation). University of Mysore, Mysore.

Stanfield, A. C., McIntosh, A. M., Spencer, M. D., Philip, R., Gaur, S., & Lawrie, S. M. (2008). Towards a neuroanatomy of autism: A systematic review and meta-analysis of structural magnetic resonance imaging studies. *European Psychiatry*, *23*(4), 289–299. doi:10.1016/j.eurpsy.2007.05.006 PMID:17765485

Stankovic, L. (2011). Transforming trauma: A qualitative feasibility study of integrative restoration (iRest) yoga Nidra on combat-related post-traumatic stress disorder. *International Journal of Yoga Therapy*, *21*, 23–37. PMID:22398342

Starling, P., Charlton, K., McMahon, A. T., & Lucas, C. (2015). Fish intake during pregnancy and fetal neurodevelopment: A systematic review of the evidence. *Nutrients*, *7*(3), 2001–2014. doi:10.3390/nu7032001 PMID:25793632

State, M. W., & Levitt, P. (2011). The conundrums of understanding genetic risks for autism spectrum disorders. *Nature Neuroscience*, *14*(12), 1499–1506. doi:10.1038/nn.2924 PMID:22037497

Stein, J. (2001). The Magnocellular theory of developmental dyslexia. *Dyslexia (Chichester, England)*, *7*(1), 12–36. doi:10.1002/dys.186 PMID:11305228

Stelmachowicz, P. G., Hoover, B. M., Lewis, D. E., Kortekaas, R. W., & Pittman, A. L. (2000). The relation between stimulus context, speech audibility, and perception for normal-hearing and hearing-impaired children. *Journal of Speech, Language, and Hearing Research: JSLHR*, *43*(4), 902–914. doi:10.1044/jslhr.4304.902 PMID:11386477

Stelmachowicz, P. G., Pittman, A. L., Hoover, B. M., Lewis, D. E., & Moeller, M. P. (2004). The importance of high-frequency audibility in the speech and language development of children with hearing loss. *Archives of Otolaryngology--Head & Neck Surgery*, *130*(5), 556–562. doi:10.1001/archotol.130.5.556 PMID:15148176

Sterne, A., & Goswami, U. (2000). Phonological awareness of syllables, rhymes, and phonemes in deaf children. *Journal of Child Psychology and Psychiatry, and Allied Disciplines*, *41*(5), 609–625. doi:10.1111/1469-7610.00648 PMID:10946753

Stevens, B. A. (2008). *Crossfire: How to survive giving expert evidence as a psychologist. Bowen Hills.* Australian Academic Press.

Stevenson, R. D., & Allaire, J. H. (1991). The development of normal feeding and swallowing. *Pediatric Clinics of North America*, *38*(6), 1439–1453. doi:10.1016/S0031-3955(16)38229-3 PMID:1945550

Stewart, P. A., Hyman, S. L., Schmidt, B. L., Macklin, E. A., Reynolds, A., Johnson, C. R., & Manning-Courtney, P. (2015). Dietary supplementation in children with autism spectrum disorders: Common, insufficient, and excessive. *Journal of the Academy of Nutrition and Dietetics*, *115*(8), 1237–1248. doi:10.1016/j.jand.2015.03.026 PMID:26052041

Stiles, J., & Jernigan, T. L. (2010). The basics of brain development. *Neuropsychology Review*, *20*(4), 327–348. doi:10.100711065-010-9148-4 PMID:21042938

Stoel-Gammon, C. (1980). Phonological analysis of four Down's syndrome children. *Applied Psycholinguistics*, *1*(01), 31–48. doi:10.1017/S0142716400000710

Stoel-Gammon, C. (2001). Down syndrome phonology: Developmental patterns and intervention strategies. *Down's syndrome, Research, and Practice. The Journal of the Sarah Duffen Centre*, *7*(3), 93–100. PMID:11721538

Strydom, A., Hassiotis, A., King, M., & Livingston, G. (2009). The relationship of dementia prevalence in older adults with intellectual disability (ID) to age and severity of ID. *Psychological Medicine*, *39*(1), 13–21. doi:10.1017/S0033291708003334 PMID:18410700

Strydom, A., Livingston, G., King, M., & Hassiotis, A. (2007). Prevalence of dementia in intellectual disability using different diagnostic criteria. *The British Journal of Psychiatry*, *191*(2), 150–157. doi:10.1192/bjp.bp.106.028845 PMID:17666500

Subrahmanyam, B. V. (2007). *Human disability evaluation: Personal injuries, principles, practices & law including disability consequent to medical negligence.* Allahabad: Law Publishers.

Sullivan, G. M. (2011). Getting off the 'Gold Standard': Randomized controlled trials and education research. *Journal of Graduate Medical Education*, *3*(3), 285–289. doi:10.4300/JGME-D-11-00147.1 PMID:22942950

Summers, J. (2012). Neurodevelopmental outcomes in children with Angelman syndrome after 1 year of behavioral intervention. *Developmental Neurorehabilitation*, *15*(4), 239–252. doi:10.3109/17518423.2012.676101 PMID:22646082

Suntjens, E., Dreschler, W. A., Hess-Erga, J., Skrunes, R., Wijburg, F. A., Linthorst, G. E., ... Biegstraaten, M. (2017). Hearing loss in children with Fabry disease. *Journal of Inherited Metabolic Disease*, *40*(5), 725–731. doi:10.100710545-017-0051-5 PMID:28567540

Swamy, L. N. (2014a). *Narayanaswamy vs State by Karnataka on 15 May, 2014*. Available at: https://indiankanoon.org/doc/36978708/

Swamy, L. N. (2014b). *Narayanaswamy vs State by Karnataka on 15 May, 2014*. Available at: https://indiankanoon.org/doc/1500783/

Swan, K., & Ray, D. (2014). Effects of child-centered play therapy on irritability and hyperactivity behaviors of children with intellectual disabilities. *Journal of Humanistic Counseling*, *53*(2), 120–133. doi:10.1002/j.2161-1939.2014.00053.x

Swapna, N., & Srushti, S. (2015). Validation of Feeding handicap index in children with Intellectual Disability and Autism Spectrum Disorder. Unpublished ARF Project funded by the All India Institute of Speech and Hearing, Mysore.

Swapna, N., & Srushti, S. (2017). *Manual of Feeding Handicap Index for Children (FHI-C)*. Mysore: All India Institute of Speech and Hearing.

Szpir, M. (2006). New thinking on neurodevelopment. *Environmental Health Perspectives*, *114*(2), A100–A107. doi:10.1289/ehp.114-a100 PMID:16451834

Takarae, Y., Minshew, N. J., Luna, B., & Sweeney, J. A. (2004). Oculomotor abnormalities parallel cerebellar histopathology in autism. *Journal of Neurology, Neurosurgery, and Psychiatry*, *75*(9), 1359–1361. doi:10.1136/jnnp.2003.022491 PMID:15314136

Taksande, A., & Vilhekar, K. (2008). Hurler syndrome or Morquio syndrome: Intelligence required for diagnosing the case. *The Indian Journal of Radiology & Imaging*, *18*(2), 175. doi:10.4103/0971-3026.40306

Taksande, A., Vilhekar, K., Chaturvedi, P., & Jain, M. (2010). Congenital malformations at birth in Central India: A rural medical college hospital based data. *Indian Journal of Human Genetics*, *16*(3), 159–163. doi:10.4103/0971-6866.73412 PMID:21206705

Talge, N. M., Neal, C., & Glover, V. (2007). Early Stress, translational research and prevention science network: Fetal and neonatal experience on child and adolescent mental health. Antenatal maternal stress and long-term effects on child neurodevelopment: How and why? *Journal of Child Psychology and Psychiatry, and Allied Disciplines*, *48*(3-4), 245–261. doi:10.1111/j.1469-7610.2006.01714.x PMID:17355398

Tanaka, M., Adachi, N., Asanuma, S., & Sakata, H. (2011). Characteristics of cases with comorbid profound deafness and pervasive developmental disorders. *Pediatric Otorhinolaryngology Japan*, *32*, 91–95.

Tan, G., Thornby, J., Hammond, C., Strehl, U., Canady, B., Arnemann, K., & Kaiser, D. A. (2009). Meta-analysis of EEG biofeedback in treating epilepsy. *Clinical EEG and Neuroscience*, *40*(3), 180–189. doi:10.1177/155005940904000310 PMID:19715180

Tanner, K., Dixon, R., & Verenikina, I. (2010, June). The digital technology in the learning of students with autism spectrum disorders (ASD) in applied classroom settings. In *EdMedia: World Conference on Educational Media and Technology* (pp. 2586-2591). Association for the Advancement of Computing in Education (AACE).

Tannock, R., Purvis, K. L., & Schachar, R. J. (1993). Narrative abilities in children with attention deficit hyperactivity disorder and normal peers. *Journal of Abnormal Child Psychology*, *21*(1), 103–117. doi:10.1007/BF00910492 PMID:8463500

Tansey, M. (1985). Brain wave signatures: An index reflexive of the brain's functional neuroanatomy: Further findings on the effect of EEG sensorimotor rhythm biofeedback training on the neurological precursors of learning disabilities. *International Journal of Psychophysiology*, *3*(2), 85–99. doi:10.1016/0167-8760(85)90030-3 PMID:4077617

Tanu, W., & Kakkar, D. (2018). A Study on Machine Learning Based Generalized Automated Seizure Detection System. In *Proceedings of 8th International Conference on Cloud Computing, Data Science and Engineering. CONFLUENCE 2018*. (pp. 20), IEEE.

Taylor, B. (2006). Real-world satisfaction and benefit with opencanal fittings. *The Hearing Journal*, *59*(11), 74–82. doi:10.1097/01.HJ.0000286222.91963.39

Taylor, D. D., & Bratton, S. C. (2014). Developmentally appropriate practice: Adlerian play therapy with preschool children. *Journal of Individual Psychology*, *70*(3), 205–219. doi:10.1353/jip.2014.0019

Taylor, W. D., Hsu, E., Krishnan, K. R. R., & MacFall, J. R. (2004). Diffusion tensor imaging: Background, potential, and utility in psychiatric research. *Biological Psychiatry*, *55*(3), 201–207. doi:10.1016/j.biopsych.2003.07.001 PMID:14744459

Temple, G., & Johnson, C. (2005). *Animals in translation. Using the mysteries of autism to decode animal behavior*. New York: Scribner Book Company.

Thapar, A., Cooper, M., Eyre, O., & Langley, K. (2013). Practitioner review: What have we learned about the causes of ADHD? *Journal of Child Psychology and Psychiatry, and Allied Disciplines*, *54*(1), 3–16. doi:10.1111/j.1469-7610.2012.02611.x PMID:22963644

Thapar, A., Cooper, M., Jefferies, R., & Stergiakouli, E. (2012). What causes attention deficit hyperactivity disorder? *Archives of Disease in Childhood*, *97*(3), 260–265. doi:10.1136/archdischild-2011-300482 PMID:21903599

Thara, R. (2005). Commentary: Measurement of psychiatric disability. *The Indian Journal of Medical Research*, *121*, 723–724. PMID:16037616

The Hindu. (2017a). *Cleaning up: On reviewing laws in India*. Retrieved from http://www.thehindu.com/opinion/editorial/cleaningup/article22084026.ece

The Hindu. (2017b). *Fake disability certificate: Action ordered against girl's father*. Retrieved from http://www.thehindu.com/news/cities/bangalore/fake-disability-certificate-action-ordered-against-girls-father/article17962726.ece

Thompson, R. A., & Nelson, C. A. (2001). Developmental science and the media: Early brain development. *The American Psychologist*, *56*(1), 5–15. doi:10.1037/0003-066X.56.1.5 PMID:11242988

Thoyre, S. M., Pados, B. F., Park, J., Estrem, H., Hodges, E. A., McComish, C., ... Murdoch, K. (2014). Development and content validation of the pediatric eating assessment tool (Pedi-EAT). *American Journal of Speech-Language Pathology*, *23*(1), 46–59. doi:10.1044/1058-0360(2013/12-0069) PMID:24097795

Thoyre, S. M., Shaker, C. S., & Pridham, K. F. (2005). The early feeding skills assessment for preterm infants. *Neonatal Network: The Journal of Neonatal Nursing*, *24*(3), 7–16. doi:10.1891/0730-0832.24.3.7 PMID:15960007

Tiadi, A., Seassau, M., Gerard, C. L., & Bucci, M. P. (2016). Differences between dyslexic and non-dyslexic children in the performance of phonological visual-auditory recognition task: An eye tracking study. *PLoS One*, *11*(7), e0159190. doi:10.1371/journal.pone.0159190 PMID:27438352

Tielsch-Goddard, A., & Gilmer, M. J. (2015). The role and impact of animals with patients. *Nursing*, *41*(2), 65–71. PMID:26292453

Tognini, P. (2017). Gut microbiota: A potential regulator of neurodevelopment. *Frontiers in Cellular Neuroscience*, *11*, 25. doi:10.3389/fncel.2017.00025 PMID:28223922

Tomchek, S. D., & Dunn, W. (2007). Sensory processing in children with and without autism: A comparative study using the short sensory profile. *The American Journal of Occupational Therapy*, *61*(2), 190–200. doi:10.5014/ajot.61.2.190 PMID:17436841

Tranel, D., & de Haan, E. (2007). Selective developmental neuropsychological disorders. *Cortex*, *43*(6), 667–671. doi:10.1016/S0010-9452(08)70496-9 PMID:17710819

Trottier, G., Srivastava, L., & Walker, C.-D. (1999). Etiology of infantile autism: A review of recent advances in genetic and neurobiological research. *Journal of Psychiatry & Neuroscience*, *24*(2), 103–115. PMID:10212552

Tsai, L. Y. (1989). Recent neurobiological findings in autism. In *Diagnosis and treatment of autism* (pp. 83–104). Boston, MA: Springer. doi:10.1007/978-1-4899-0882-7_7

Tsang, V. (2018). Eye-tracking study on facial emotion recognition tasks in individuals with high-functioning autism spectrum disorders. *Autism*, *22*(2), 161–170. doi:10.1177/1362361316667830 PMID:29490486

Tseng, P. H., Cameron, I. G., Pari, G., Reynolds, J. N., Munoz, D. P., & Itti, L. (2013). High-throughput classification of clinical populations from natural viewing eye movements. *Journal of Neurology*, *260*(1), 275–284. doi:10.100700415-012-6631-2 PMID:22926163

Turk, D., Meichenbaum, D. H., & Berman, W. H. (1979). Application of biofeedback for the regulation of pain: A critical review. *Psychological Bulletin*, *86*(6), 1322–1338. doi:10.1037/0033-2909.86.6.1322 PMID:515286

Twachtman-Reilly, J., Amaral, S. C., & Zebrowski, P. P. (2008). Addressing feeding disorders in children on the autism spectrum in school-based settings: Physiological and behavioral issues. *Language, Speech, and Hearing Services in Schools*, *39*(2), 261–272. doi:10.1044/0161-1461(2008/025) PMID:18420528

Tye, C., McLoughlin, G., Kuntsi, J., & Asherson, P. (2011). Electrophysiological markers of genetic risk for attention deficit hyperactivity disorder. *Expert Reviews in Molecular Medicine*, *13*, e9. doi:10.1017/S1462399411001797 PMID:21426626

Tye, C., Rijsdijk, F., Greven, C. U., Kuntsi, J., Asherson, P., & McLoughlin, G. (2012). Shared genetic influences on ADHD symptoms and very low-frequency EEG activity: A twin study. *Journal of Child Psychology and Psychiatry, and Allied Disciplines*, *53*(6), 706–715. doi:10.1111/j.1469-7610.2011.02501.x PMID:22118296

Underwood, L., Forrester, A., Chaplin, E., & McCarthy, J. (2013). Prisoners with neurodevelopmental disorders. *Journal of Intellectual Disabilities and Offending Behaviour*, *4*(1/2), 17–23. doi:10.1108/JIDOB-05-2013-0011

Underwood, L., McCarthy, J., Chaplin, E., Forrester, A., Mills, R., & Murphy, D. (2016). Autism spectrum disorder traits among prisoners. *Advances in Autism*, *2*(3), 106–117. doi:10.1108/AIA-11-2015-0023

Unger, K. V. (1978). Learning disabilities and juvenile delinquency. *Journal of Juvenile and Family Courts*, *29*(1), 25–30. doi:10.1111/j.1755-6988.1978.tb01144.x

United States Environmental Protective Agency. (2015). America's children and the environment: Neurodevelopmental Disorders (excerpt from the. In C. Croft (Ed.), *Environmental hazards and neurodevelopment: Where ecology and well being connect* (3rd ed.; pp. 3–40). Oakville, ON: Apple Academic Press.

Upton, J. (2013). Mini-Mental State Examination. In M. D. Gellman & J. R. Turner (Eds.), *Encyclopaedia of Behavioural Medicine*. New York, NY: Springer.

Ustun, T. B., Kostanjsek, N., Chatterji, S., & Rehm, J. (2010). *Measuring health and disability: Manual for WHO Disability Assessment Scale (WHODAS 2.0)*. Geneva: World Health Organization.

Utari, A., Adams, E., Berry-Kravis, E., Chavez, A., Scaggs, F., Ngotran, L., ... Tartaglia, N. (2010). Aging in fragile X syndrome. *Journal of Neurodevelopmental Disorders*, *2*(2), 70–76. doi:10.100711689-010-9047-2 PMID:20585378

Vallortigara, G., Snyder, A., Kaplan, G., Bateson, P., Clayton, N. S., & Rogers, L. J. (2008). Are animals autistic savants. *PLoS Biology*, *6*(2), e42. doi:10.1371/journal.pbio.0060042 PMID:18288892

van der Lely, H. K. J. (2003). Do heterogeneous deficits require hetero-geneous theories? SLI subgroups and the RDDR hypothesis. In Y. Levy & J. Schaeffer (Eds.), *Language competence across populations: Toward a definition of specific language impairment* (pp. 97–133). Mahwah, NJ: Lawrence Erlbaum Associate.

Van Dyke, D. C., Peterson, L. L., & Hoffman, M. N. (1990). Problems in feeding. In *Clinical Perspectives in the Management of Down Syndrome* (pp. 102–106). New York, NY: Springer. doi:10.1007/978-1-4613-9644-4_8

Van Heijst, B. F., & Geurts, H. M. (2015). Quality of life in autism across the lifespan: A meta-analysis. *Autism*, *19*(2), 158–160. doi:10.1177/1362361313517053 PMID:24443331

van Niekerk, M. E. H., Groen, W., Vissers, C. T. W. M., van-Driel-de Jong, D., Kan, C. C., & Oude Voshaar, R. C. (2011). Diagnosing autism spectrum disorders in elderly people. *International Psychogeriatrics*, *23*(5), 700–710. doi:10.1017/S1041610210002152 PMID:21110908

van Viersen, S., Slot, E. M., Kroesbergen, E. H., van't Noordende, J. E., & Leseman, P. P. (2013). The added value of eye-tracking in diagnosing dyscalculia: A case study. *Frontiers in Psychology*, *4*, 679. doi:10.3389/fpsyg.2013.00679 PMID:24098294

Vargas-Cuentas, N. I., Roman-Gonzalez, A., Gilman, R. H., Barrientos, F., Ting, J., Hidalgo, D., ... Zimic, M. (2017). Developing an eye-tracking algorithm as a potential tool for early diagnosis of autism spectrum disorder in children. *PLoS One*, *12*(11), e0188826. doi:10.1371/journal.pone.0188826 PMID:29190703

Varghese, R. T., & Venkatesan, S. (2013). A comparative study of maternal burnout in autism and hearing impairment. *International Journal of Psychology & Psychiatry*, *1*(2), 101–108. doi:10.5958/j.2320-6233.1.2.016

Vargo, F. E. (2012). *Neurodevelopmental disorders: A definitive guide for educators*. New York, NY: W. W. Norton & Company.

Vashistha, I., Aseri, Y., Singh, B. K., & Verma, P. C. (2016). Prevalence of hearing impairment in high risk infants. *Indian Journal of Otolaryngology and Head and Neck Surgery*, *68*(2), 214–217. doi:10.100712070-015-0869-9 PMID:27340640

Vellutino, F. R., Fletcher, J. M., Snowling, M. J., & Scanlon, D. M. (2004). Specific reading disability (dyslexia): What have we learned in the past four decades? *Journal of Child Psychology and Psychiatry, and Allied Disciplines*, *45*(1), 2–40. doi:10.1046/j.0021-9630.2003.00305.x PMID:14959801

Vellutino, F. R., & Scanlon, D. M. (1987). Phonological coding, phonological awareness, and reading ability: Evidence from a longitudinal and experimental study. *Merrill-Palmer Quarterly*, 321–363.

Vempati, R. P., & Telles, S. (2002). Yoga-based guided relaxation reduces sympathetic activity judged from baseline levels. *Psychological Reports*, *90*(2), 487–494. doi:10.2466/pr0.2002.90.2.487 PMID:12061588

Venkatesan, S. (2017b). Analysis of attributes in the official definitions for learning disability. *The International Journal of Indian Psychology, 4*(2), 46-57. doi: 18.01.027/20170402

Venkatesan, S. (2000). Play activities in children with mental retardation. *Indian Journal of Clinical Psychology, 27*(1), 124–128.

Venkatesan, S. (2004a). Activity log of preschool children with developmental disabilities and autism spectrum disorders. *Disability, CBR and Inclusive Development, 15*(2), 58–66.

Venkatesan, S. (2004b). Efficacy of home training program in skill enhancement of children with developmental disabilities. *Indian Journal of Clinical Psychology, 31*(1), 121–127.

Venkatesan, S. (2004c). *Children with developmental disabilities: A training guide for parents, teachers, and caregivers. New Delhi: Sage* Publications.

Venkatesan, S. (2004d). *Toy Kit for Kids with Developmental Disabilities: User Manual.* Mysore: All India Institute of Speech and Hearing.

Venkatesan, S. (2007). Professional help-seeking behaviors in parents of children with developmental disabilities. *Journal of All India Institute of Speech and Hearing, 26*(1), 72–75.

Venkatesan, S. (2009). Barriers to optimizing home training programs for children with developmental disabilities. *Journal of All India Institute of Speech and Hearing, 28*(1), 128–134.

Venkatesan, S. (2009b). *Ethical guidelines for biobehavioral research.* Mysore: All India Institute of Speech and Hearing.

Venkatesan, S. (2010). A case study on cost-benefit analysis for the government-sponsored scheme for persons with mental disabilities. *Asian Journal of Developmental Matters, 4*(1), 176–188.

Venkatesan, S. (2011). Blame game triangulation between parents, teachers, and children with academic problems. *Psychological Studies, 56*(2), 206–215. doi:10.100712646-011-0082-1

Venkatesan, S. (2012). Utility analysis of assembled toy kits for kids with developmental disabilities. *Journal of Disability Management and Special Education, 2*(2), 27–37.

Venkatesan, S. (2014). Availability of toys for children with developmental disabilities. *Journal of Disability Management and Special Education, 4*(1), 58–70.

Venkatesan, S. (2014). Coercion tactics of parents on children with academic problems in India. *International Journal of Psychology and Psychiatry, 2*(1), 42–56. doi:10.5958/j.2320-6233.2.1.007

Venkatesan, S. (2015). Engagement between justice system vis-a-vis persons with intellectual and developmental disabilities. *International Journal of Psychology and Psychiatry, 3*(1), 30–56. doi:10.5958/2320-6233.2015.00003.6

Venkatesan, S. (2015a). A growing trend in pseudo-diagnosis: A field study on children frequently mistaken for autism in India. *Psychological Studies, 60*(1), 91–100. doi:10.100712646-015-0302-1

Venkatesan, S. (2015b). *Problem behavior survey schedule.* Bangalore: Psychotronics.

Venkatesan, S. (2015c). Revisiting goal setting for children with developmental disabilities. *Journal of Disability Management and Special Education, 5*(2), 19–27.

Venkatesan, S. (2015d). Evaluation of teaching objectives earmarked for children with developmental disabilities. *Disabilities & Impairments, 29*(2), 85–95.

Venkatesan, S. (2016). A concept analysis of learning disability based on research articles published in India. *Indian Journal of Clinical Psychology, 43*(2), 97–107.

Venkatesan, S. (2017a). Analysis of bibliography on specific learning disability in India. *Disability, CBR and Inclusive Development, 28*(2), 59–73. doi:10.5463/dcid.v28i2.540

Venkatesan, S. (2017c). Diagnostic decision tree for a specific learning disability. *International Journal of Education and Psychological Research, 6*(2), 121–127.

Venkatesan, S. (2017d). Consequence mapping of problem behaviors in children with developmental delays. *Disabilities and Impairments, 31*(1), 47–64.

Venkatesan, S. (2017e). Barriers and facilitators in home-based problem behavior interventions for children. *Indian Journal of Health and Wellbeing, 8*(5), 345–351.

Venkatesan, S., & Das, A. K. (1994). The reported burden on family members in receiving/implementing home-based training programs for children with mental handicaps. *Journal of Psychological Researches, 38*(1 & 2), 39–45.

Venkatesan, S., & Madhurao, P. (1990). The validity of parental estimates against actual test estimates in mentally handicapped individuals. *The Creative Psychologist, 2*(2), 71–75.

Venkatesan, S., & Purusotham, P. (2008). A profile of etiological and therapeutic searches by netizen parents/caregivers of children on the autism spectrum. *Journal of All India Institute of Speech and Hearing, 27*(1), 89–94.

Venkatesan, S., & Rao, P. H. (1996). The significance of some birth factors in mental retardation. *Disabilities & Impairments, 10*(2), 53–64.

Venkatesan, S., & Ravindran, N. (2012). Play behaviors and activities in siblings of children with developmental disabilities. *Journal of the Indian Academy of Applied Psychology, 38*(1), 69–78.

Venkatesan, S., & Swarnalata, G. V. (2013). Problem behaviors and academic grade level performance of adjudicated children with juvenile delinquency. *Disability, CBR and Inclusive Development, 24*(1), 99–114. doi:10.5463/dcid.v24i1.162

Venkatesan, S., & Yashodhara Kumar, G. Y. (2016). Leisure and community exposure in persons with disabilities. *Journal of Disability Management and Special Education, 6*(1), 1–14.

Venkatesan, S., & Yashodhara Kumar, G. Y. (2017a). Toy index of children with or without developmental disabilities. *Indian Journal of Clinical Psychology, 44*(1), 60–67.

Venkatesan, S., & Yashodhara Kumar, G. Y. (2017b). Parent opinions and attitudes on toys for children with or without developmental disabilities. *The International Journal of Indian Psychology, 4*(4), 6–20. doi:10.25215/0404.061

Venkatesan, S., Yashodharakumar, G. Y., Gupta, S. K., & Vasudha, H. H. (2015). Gap analysis for evaluation of individualized education programs for children with developmental disabilities. *International Journal of Psychology and Psychiatry, 13*(2), 64–76. doi:10.5958/2320-6233.2015.00017.6

Verma, P. K., Ranganath, P., Dalal, A. B., & Phadke, S. R. (2012). Spectrum of Lysosomal storage disorders at a medical genetics center in northern India. *Indian Pediatrics, 49*(10), 799–804. doi:10.100713312-012-0192-4 PMID:22791670

Vernon, D., Frick, A., & Gruzelier, J. (2004). Neurofeedback as a treatment for ADHD: A methodological review with implications for future research. *Journal of Neurotherapy, 8*(2), 53–82. doi:10.1300/J184v08n02_04

Vidal, M., Turner, J., Bulling, A., & Gellersen, H. (2012). Wearable Eye Tracking for Mental Health Monitoring. *Computer Communications, 35*(11), 1306–1311. doi:10.1016/j.comcom.2011.11.002

Villar, J., Merialdi, M., Gulmezoglu, A. M., Abalos, E., Carroli, G., Kulier, R., & de Onis, M. (2003). Nutritional interventions during pregnancy for the prevention or treatment of maternal morbidity and preterm delivery: An overview of randomized controlled trials. *The Journal of Nutrition*, *133*(5), 1606S–1625S. doi:10.1093/jn/133.5.1606S PMID:12730475

Vivanti, G., Trembath, D., & Dissanayake, C. (2014). Atypical monitoring and responsiveness to goal-directed gaze in autism spectrum disorder. *Experimental Brain Research*, *232*(2), 695–701. doi:10.100700221-013-3777-9 PMID:24292493

Voineagu, I., Wang, X., Johnston, P., Lowe, J. K., Tian, Y., Horvath, S., & Geschwind, D. H. (2011). Transcriptomic analysis of autistic brain reveals convergent molecular pathology. *Nature*, *474*(7351), 380–384. doi:10.1038/nature10110 PMID:21614001

Volkmar, F., Siegel, M., Woodbury-Smith, M., King, B., McCracken, J., & State, M. (2014). Practice parameter for the assessment and treatment of children and adolescents with autism spectrum disorder. *Journal of the American Academy of Child and Adolescent Psychiatry*, *53*(2), 237–257. doi:10.1016/j.jaac.2013.10.013 PMID:24472258

Vollebregt, M. A., van Dongen-Boomama, M., Bultelaar, J. K., & Slaats-Willemse, D. (2014a). Does EEG-neurofeedback improve neurocognitive functioning in children with attention-deficit/hyperactivity disorder? A systematic review and a double-blind placebo-controlled study. *Journal of Clinical Psychology and Psychiatry*, *55*(5), 460–472. doi:10.1111/jcpp.12143 PMID:24168522

Vollebregt, M. A., van Dongen-Boomama, M., Slaats-Willemse, D., & Bultelaar, J. K. (2014b). What future research should bring to help resolving the debate about the efficacy of EEG-neurofeedback in children with ADHD. *Frontiers in Human Neuroscience*, *8*, 321. doi:10.3389/fnhum.2014.00321 PMID:24860487

Vulliamy, T., Marrone, A., Goldman, F., Dearlove, A., Bessler, M., Mason, P. J., & Dokal, I. (2001). The RNA component of telomerase is mutated in autosomal dominant dyskeratosis congenita. *Nature*, *413*(6854), 432–435. doi:10.1038/35096585 PMID:11574891

Wakefield, A. J., Murch, S. H., Anthony, A., Linnell, J., Casson, D. M., Malik, M., ... Harvey, P. (1998). RETRACTED: Ileal-lymphoid-nodular hyperplasia, non-specific colitis, and pervasive developmental disorder in children. *Lancet*, *351*(9103), 637–641. doi:10.1016/S0140-6736(97)11096-0 PMID:9500320

Waldie, K., & Spreen, O. (1993). The relationship between learning disabilities and persisting delinquency. *Journal of Learning Disabilities*, *26*(6), 417–423. doi:10.1177/002221949302600608 PMID:8354946

Wang, A. T., Dapretto, M., Hariri, A. R., Sigman, M., & Bookheimer, S. Y. (2004). Neural correlates of facial affect processing in children and adolescents with autism spectrum disorder. *Journal of the American Academy of Child and Adolescent Psychiatry*, *43*(4), 481–490. doi:10.1097/00004583-200404000-00015 PMID:15187809

Wang, K., Wang, S., & Ji, Q. (2016, March). Deep eye fixation map learning for calibration-free eye gaze tracking. In *Proceedings of the Ninth Biennial ACM Symposium on Eye Tracking Research & Applications* (pp. 47-55). ACM. 10.1145/2857491.2857515

Wang, S., Jiang, M., Duchesne, X. M., Laugeson, E. A., Kennedy, D. P., Adolphs, R., & Zhao, Q. (2015). Atypical visual saliency in autism spectrum disorder quantified through model-based eye tracking. *Neuron*, *88*(3), 604–616. doi:10.1016/j.neuron.2015.09.042 PMID:26593094

Ward, J. (1994). General practitioners' experience of research. *Family Practice*, *11*(4), 418–423. doi:10.1093/fampra/11.4.418 PMID:7895971

Wardle, J., Guthrie, C. A., Sanderson, S., & Rapoport, L. (2001). Development of the children's eating behaviour questionnaire. *Journal of Child Psychology and Psychiatry, and Allied Disciplines*, *42*(7), 963–970. doi:10.1111/1469-7610.00792 PMID:11693591

Ware, J. N. (2014). *Play Therapy for Children with Autism Spectrum Disorder: A Single-Case Design (Doctor of Philosophy)*. Counseling.

Warren, R. P., Singh, V. K., Cole, P., Odell, J. D., Pingree, C. B., Warren, W. L., & White, E. (1991). Increased frequency of the null allele at the complement C4b locus in autism. *Clinical and Experimental Immunology*, *83*(3), 438–440. doi:10.1111/j.1365-2249.1991.tb05657.x PMID:2004485

Wass, S. V., & Porayska-Pomsta, K. (2014). The uses of cognitive training technologies in the treatment of autism spectrum disorders. *Autism*, *18*(8), 851–871. doi:10.1177/1362361313499827 PMID:24129912

Wästlund, E., Shams, P., Löfgren, M., Witell, L., & Gustafsson, A. (2010). Consumer perception at point of purchase: Evaluating proposed package designs in an eye-tracking lab. *Journal of Business and Retail Management Research*, *5*(1), 41–50.

Webb, N. (2011). Play therapy for bereaved children: Adapting strategies to community, school, and home settings. *School Psychology International*, *32*(2), 132–143. doi:10.1177/0143034311400832

Webb, S. J., Nalty, T., Munson, J., Brock, C., Abbott, R., & Dawson, G. (2007). Rate of head circumference growth as a function of autism diagnosis and history of autistic regression. *Journal of Child Neurology*, *22*(10), 1182–1190. doi:10.1177/0883073807306263 PMID:17940244

Weber-Spickschen, T. S., Colcuc, C., Hanke, A., Clausen, J. D., James, P. A., & Horstmann, H. (2017). Fun during knee rehabilitation: Feasibility and acceptability testing of a new Android-based training device. *The Open Medical Informatics Journal*, *11*(1), 29–36. doi:10.2174/1874431101711010029 PMID:29081870

Weinberger, D. R. (1987). The implication of normal brain development for the pathogenesis of schizophrenia. *Archives of General Psychiatry*, *44*(7), 660–669. doi:10.1001/archpsyc.1987.01800190080012 PMID:3606332

Weismer, E. S. (2000). Intervention for children with developmental language delay. In D. V. M. Bishop & L. B. Leonard (Eds.), *Specific language impairments in children: Causes, characteristics, intervention and outcome* (pp. 157–176). Hove, UK: Psychology Press.

Wexler, K. (1994). Optional infinitives, head movement and the economy of derivations. In N. Hornstein & D. Lightfoot (Eds.), *Verb movement* (pp. 305–350). New York: Cambridge University Press. doi:10.1017/CBO9780511627705.016

Whitehouse, A. J., Coon, H., Miller, J., Salisbury, B., & Bishop, D. V. (2010). Narrowing the broader autism phenotype: A study using the Communication Checklist-Adult Version (CC-A). *Autism*, *14*(6), 559–574. doi:10.1177/1362361310382107 PMID:20923891

White, J., & Allers, C. T. (1994). Play therapy with abused children: A review of the literature. *Journal of Counseling and Development*, *72*(4), 390–394. doi:10.1002/j.1556-6676.1994.tb00955.x

WHO. (n.d.). Retrieved November 14, 2017, from http://www.who.int/en/

Wilkinson, G. S. (1993). *WRAT-3: Wide range achievement test administration manual*. Wide Range, Incorporated.

Williams, K. E., & Foxx, R. M. (2007). *Treating eating problems of children with autism spectrum disorders and developmental disabilities: Interventions for professionals and parents*. Pro-ed.

Williams, K. E., & Seiverling, L. (2010). Eating problems in children with autism spectrum disorders. *Topics in Clinical Nutrition*, *25*(1), 27–37. doi:10.1097/TIN.0b013e3181d10958

Williams, P. G., Dalrymple, N., & Neal, J. (2000). Eating habits of children with autism. *Pediatric Nursing*, *26*(3), 259–264. PMID:12026389

Wilska, M. L., & Kaski, M. K. (2001). Why and how to assess the aetiological diagnosis of children with intellectual disability/mental retardation and other neurodevelopmental disorders: Description of the Finnish approach. *European Journal of Paediatric Neurology*, *5*(1), 7–13. doi:10.1053/ejpn.2001.0398 PMID:11277365

Wilson, B. T., Stark, Z., Sutton, R. E., Danda, S., Ekbote, A. V., Elsayed, S. M., ... Wilson, I. J. (2016). The Cockayne Syndrome Natural History (CoSyNH) study: Clinical findings in 102 individuals and recommendations for care. *Genetics in Medicine*, *18*(5), 483–493. doi:10.1038/gim.2015.110 PMID:26204423

Wimmer, H. (1996). The nonword reading deficit in developmental dyslexia: Evidence from children learning to read German. *Journal of Experimental Psychology*, *61*, 80–90. PMID:8812031

Wing, L., Gould, J., & Gillberg, C. (2011). Autism spectrum disorders in the DSM-V: Better or worse than the DSM-IV? *Research in Developmental Disabilities*, *32*(2), 768–773. doi:10.1016/j.ridd.2010.11.003 PMID:21208775

Wolk, L., Edwards, M. L., & Conture, E. G. (1993). Coexistence of stuttering and disordered phonology in young children. *Journal of Speech, Language, and Hearing Research: JSLHR*, *36*(5), 906–917. doi:10.1044/jshr.3605.906 PMID:8246479

Wong, J. M. Y., & Collins, K. (2006). Telomerase RNA level limits telomere maintenance in X-linked dyskeratosis congenita. *Genes & Development*, *20*(20), 2848–2858. doi:10.1101/gad.1476206 PMID:17015423

Won, H., Mah, W., & Kim, E. (2013). Autism spectrum disorder causes, mechanisms, and treatments: Focus on neuronal synapses. *Frontiers in Molecular Neuroscience*, *6*, 19. doi:10.3389/fnmol.2013.00019 PMID:23935565

Woolfendon, S., Sarkozy, V., Ridley, G., & Williams, K. (2012). A systematic review of the diagnostic stability of autism spectrum disorder. *Research in Autism Spectrum Disorders*, *6*(1), 345–354. doi:10.1016/j.rasd.2011.06.008

World Health Organization. (1993). *The ICD-10 Classification of Mental and Behavioural Disorders: Clinical descriptions and diagnostic guidelines*. Geneva: Author.

World Health Organization. (2001). *International Classification of Functioning, Disability and Health: ICF*. World Health Organization.

World Health Organization. (2002). *ICF: The international classification of functioning, disability, and health. Towards a common language for functioning, disability, and health*. Retrieved May 9, 2018. from: http://www.who.int/classifications/icf/training/icfbeginnersguide.pdf

World Health Organization. (2007). *International Classification of Functioning, Disability, and Health-Children and Youth Version (ICF-CY)*. Geneva: Author.

World Health Organization. (2008). *The ICD-10 classification of mental and behavioral disorders descriptions and diagnostic guidelines*. Geneva: Author.

World Health Organization. (2011). *World Report on Disability 2011*. Retrieved from: http://www.unicef.org/protection/World_report_on_disability_eng.pdf

World Medical Association. (2015). *WMA Declaration of Helsinki-Ethical principles for medical research involving human subjects*. Author.

Worley, J. A., Matson, J. L., & Kozlowski, A. M. (2011). The effects of hearing impairment on symptoms of autism in toddlers. *Developmental Neurorehabilitation*, *14*(3), 171–176. doi:10.3109/17518423.2011.564600 PMID:21548858

Wright, K. B., Sparks, L., & O'Hair, H. D. (2013). *Health communication in the 21st century*. New York, NY: John Wiley & Sons.

Wu, A. S., Niedra, R., Pendergast, L., & McCrindle, B. W. (2002). Acceptability and impact of pet visitation on a cardiology inpatient unit. *Journal of Nursing, 17*(5), 354–362. PMID:12395303

Yairi, E., & Ambrose, N. (2005). *Early childhood stuttering for clinicians by clinicians*. Austin, TX: PRO-ED.

Yamasoba, T., Someya, S., Yamada, C., Weindruch, R., Prolla, T. A., & Tanokura, M. (2007). Role of mitochondrial dysfunction and mitochondrial DNA mutations in age-related hearing loss. *Hearing Research, 226*(1-2), 185–193. doi:10.1016/j.heares.2006.06.004 PMID:16870370

Yanagawa, H., Kishuku, M., Akaike, M., Azuma, H., & Irahara, M. (2010). View of physicians on and barriers to patient enrollment in a multicenter clinical trial: Experience in a Japanese rural area. *International Archives of Medicine, 3*(7). doi:10.1186/1755-7682-3-7 PMID:20525325

Yan-bin, W. (2009). Impact of Lev Vygotsky on special education. *Canadian Social Science, 5*(5), 100–103.

Yeates, S. (1998). Hearing Loss in People with Learning Disabilities. *Tizard Learning Disability Review, 3*(2), 20–28. doi:10.1108/13595474199800014

Ye, X., Smallwood, P., & Nathans, J. (2011). Expression of the Norrie disease gene (Ndp) in developing and adult mouse eye, ear, and brain. *Gene Expression Patterns, 11*(1-2), 151–155. doi:10.1016/j.gep.2010.10.007 PMID:21055480

Young, S., Moss, D., Sedgwick, O., Fridman, M., & Hodgkins, P. (2015). A meta-analysis of the prevalence of attention deficit hyperactivity disorder in incarcerated populations. *Psychological Medicine, 45*(2), 247–258. doi:10.1017/S0033291714000762 PMID:25066071

Zamir, T. (2006). The moral basis of animal-assisted therapy. *Society & Animals, 14*(2), 179–199. doi:10.1163/156853006776778770 PMID:16862727

Zeisel, S. H. (2008). Is maternal diet supplementation beneficial? Optimal development of infant depends on mother's diet. *The American Journal of Clinical Nutrition, 89*(2), 685S–687S. doi:10.3945/ajcn.2008.26811F PMID:19116319

Zeisel, S. H. (2009). Importance of methyl donors during reproduction. *The American Journal of Clinical Nutrition, 89*(2), 673S–677S. doi:10.3945/ajcn.2008.26811D PMID:19116320

Zemblys, R. (2016). Eye-movement event detection meets machine learning. *Biomedical Engineering, 20*(1).

Zemblys, R., Niehorster, D. C., Komogortsev, O., & Holmqvist, K. (2018). Using machine learning to detect events in eye-tracking data. *Behavior Research Methods, 50*(1), 160–181. doi:10.375813428-017-0860-3 PMID:28233250

Zenker, M., Mayerle, J., Lerch, M. M., Tagariello, A., Zerres, K., Durie, P. R., ... Reis, A. (2005). Deficiency of UBR1, a ubiquitin ligase of the N-end rule pathway, causes pancreatic dysfunction, malformations and mental retardation (Johanson-Blizzard syndrome). *Nature Genetics, 37*(12), 1345–1350. doi:10.1038/ng1681 PMID:16311597

Ziereisen, F., De Munter, C., & Perlmutter, N. (1993). The Keutel syndrome. Report of a case and review of the literature. *Pediatric Radiology, 23*(4), 314–315. doi:10.1007/BF02010925 PMID:8414764

Zijlstra, A., Mancini, M., Chiari, L., & Zijlstra, W. (2010). Biofeedback for training balance and mobility in older populations: A systematic review. *Journal of Neuroengineering and Rehabilitation, 7*(1), 58. doi:10.1186/1743-0003-7-58 PMID:21143921

Zilbovicius, M., Boddaert, N., Belin, P., Poline, J. B., Remy, P., Mangin, J. F., & Samson, Y. (2000). Temporal lobe dysfunction in childhood autism: A PET study. *The American Journal of Psychiatry, 157*(12), 1988–1993. doi:10.1176/appi.ajp.157.12.1988 PMID:11097965

Zimmermann, M. B. (2011). The role of iodine in human growth and development. *Seminars in Cell & Developmental Biology*, *22*(6), 645–652. doi:10.1016/j.semcdb.2011.07.009 PMID:21802524

Zwaigenbaum, L., Thurm, A., Stone, W., Baranek, G., Bryson, S., Iverson, J., ... Rogers, S. (2007). Studying the emergence of autism spectrum disorders in high-risk infants: Methodological and practical issues. *Journal of Autism and Developmental Disorders*, *37*(3), 466–480. doi:10.100710803-006-0179-x PMID:16897376

Zwirner, P., & Wilichowski, E. (2001). Progressive sensorineural hearing loss in children with mitochondrial encephalomyopathies. *The Laryngoscope*, *111*(3), 515–521. doi:10.1097/00005537-200103000-00024 PMID:11224785

About the Contributors

Sanjeev Kumar Gupta is currently working as a Clinical Psychologist (Clinician and Researcher) at All India Institute of Speech and Hearing, India. He has completed MPhil in Medical and Social Psychology from the Central Institute of Psychiatry, Ranchi, PhD in Psychology from the University of Mysore and has more than 10 years of experience in the field of Clinical Psychology. His areas of interest include child and adolescent mental health, executive function training, cognitive behavior therapy, mindfulness meditation, telerehabilitation, stuttering, neurodevelopmental disorders, and cognitive electrophysiology. He has edited one book, contributed two chapters in books and published 15 articles in various national and international peer-reviewed journals. He has chaired scientific sessions and presented several research papers both at national and international conferences. He has also conducted several workshops/symposiums and training programs for professionals, parents and caregivers of children with neurodevelopmental disorders.

Srinivasan Venkatesan is Professor and Head, Department of Clinical Psychology, AIISH, Mysore, Karnataka. He has earlier served at NIMH, Secunderabad-Hyderabad. He has authored 26 books, contributed 24 chapters in books, another 35 varieties of technical literature, and published 135 research papers, served as resource person for workshops for different target groups. He has completed projects through collaboration with national/international agencies, guided students for Ph.D., been on editorial board for journals and peer-reviewed research articles, presented papers in conferences and served as an examiner for adjudication of doctoral theses. Consistently a first class and university rank holder from school to pre-doctoral courses at NIMHANS, Bangalore, 1987; he was awarded the doctorate in 1993. A Fellow of the Society for Advanced Studies in Medical Sciences, New Delhi, in psychiatry, he was decorated with Gold Medal by the former President of India, Sri Giani Zail Singh in 1994; NN Sen Memorial Award for 'Best Research Paper' by Indian Association of Clinical Psychologists in 2002; 'Psycho Oration Award' in January 2009, and Prof. Anima Sen Memorial Award in 2012.

S. P. Goswami holds PhD in Speech and Hearing and also PGDHRM and MBA in Health Care Management. He is the first Speech and Hearing professional to receive the prestigious CV Raman fellowship from UGC, Government of India as Visiting Scholar at College of Applied Health Sciences, Department of Speech & Hearing Science, University of Illinois at Urbana-Champaign under CV Raman fellowship, UGC, GOI, New Delhi (August, 2013 to July, 2014). Presently he is working as Professor and Head Department of Speech-Language Pathology and Academic coordinator and formerly worked as Head Department of Clinical Services, Speech-Language Pathology at AIISH, Mysore. He has more than 18 years of academic, clinical, research and administrative experience. He works in the area of

Aphasia, ageing and neuro-cognitive communication disorders in adults and elderly. He has published more than 31 research articles in national and international journals, 20 in-house publication and 19 Books/chapters/tools/tests with ISBN numbers. Two candidates have been awarded PhD and four are presently pursuing their doctorate program under his guidance.

Rajeev Kumar, Doctoral Researcher at Indian Institute of Technology Kharagpur, availed prestigious Senior Research Fellowship of University Grant Commission, New Delhi. Hold MSW from Tata Institute of Social Sciences, Mumbai, and M.Phil from Central Institute of Psychiatry, Ranchi. Major areas of interest are psychotherapeutic interventions, substance use, mental health and community-epidemiological aspect of HIV/AIDS, children mental health and protection issues and community health issues. Having publications in national and international journals including Taylor and Francis publication group. Mr. Kumar is a member of reviewer board in journals of Sage Publication and Elsevier publication. Mr. Kumar delivered several invited lectures in various state level training programs, and have taught at the undergraduate and postgraduate level at Indian Institute of Technology Kharagpur. Currently teaching as adjunct faculty at Department of Rural Development and Management, Ramakrishna Mission Vivekanand Universtiy, Ranchi. As a national level master trainer, Mr. Kumar conducted nine week-long training in Jharkhand, West Bengal, and Sikkim states for ongoing multi collaborative National Drug Use Survey sponsored by Ministry of Social Justice and Empowerment, New Delhi. Mr. Kumar has presented several research papers at national and international fora, including International Congress of Psychology, Yokohama, Japan.

* * *

Mahesh B. V. M. is a Lecturer in Speech Pathology in the Department of Speech-Language Pathology at the All India Institute of Speech and Hearing (AIISH), Mysore. He previously held a faculty position at the Jawarharlal Institute of Post Graduate Medical Education and Research (JIPMER), Puducherry, India. He has completed his Bachelor's in speech and hearing and Master's in Speech-Language Pathology, AIISH, Mysore. His research interests are language production, bilingualism, language motor interaction, fluency disorders and kinematic analysis of speech in typical and disordered speech motor control.

Kulbhushan Chand received the B.Tech. degree in Electronics and Communication Engineering from the Guru Nanak Dev University, India, in 2010, and the M.Tech. degree in Electronics and Communication Engineering from the Lovely Professional University, India, in 2013. He is currently working towards the PhD degree in Electronics and Communication Engineering with Dr Arun Khosla at the Dr B R Ambedkar National Institute of Technology Jalandhar, India. His research interests include biofeedback, embedded systems, wearable physiological sensors and computing, healthcare and gamification.

Yashodhara Kumar G. Y. is a Clinical Psychologist Gr-II in the Department of Clinical psychology at All India Institute of Speech and Hearing, Mysore. He received M.Sc (Clinical Psychology), M. Phil. in Psychology, PG Diploma in Guidance and Counselling degrees and currently perusing Ph. D. in the University of Mysore. Some of his research interests are disability studies, developmental psychology, psychometrics, Personality studies, Emotional problems, Neuropsychology, Forensic Psychology. He is a member of professional bodies such as National Academy of Psychology and Indian Science Congress. With more than ten years of professional experience, he has contributed to the psychology literature as an author and co-author through more than 17 research articles published in national and international journals. He also served as a resource person in various national level workshops in the field of clinical psychology. He awarded International travel grant by Indian Council of Medical Research (ICMR) to present his research work on "case reports: Tryout of smartphone applications for neuro-psychological rehabilitation in traumatic brain injury" at International Congress of Psychology (ICP) 2016 held at Yokohama, Japan. Also, he presented eight research articles in various national level conferences.

Venkataraman Hariharan is Lecturer in Clinical Psychology, All India Institute of Speech and Hearing, Mysore, Karnataka. He was earlier a Clinical Psychologist at PES Institute of Medical Sciences and Research (PESIMSR), Kuppam, Andhra Pradesh. Hariharan has the publications in the area related to Suicide, Psycho-Dermatology, Anxiety, Depression, Psycho-Ophthalmology and Intelligence.

Saransh Jain is working as a lecturer in audiology at the JSS Institute of speech and hearing, Mysuru from last 7 years. He has secured gold medal from the University of Mysore for his post-graduation in speech and hearing; from University of Rajasthan for post-graduation in clinical psychology and for under-graduation in speech and hearing. He has also received outstanding clinician award from READS society for hearing impaired children, Jaipur. His research interest includes understanding the perception of speech in normal and differently able individuals, psychoacoustic processing in human auditory system, auditory processing disorders, cognitive processing abilities and its association with audition. His research experience includes two book chapters in research handbooks, 17 international paper publications in peer-reviewed journals, 05 national paper publications and 32 paper presentations in national and international conferences. He had also guided 16 master's level dissertation students and presently guiding 4 more students for the academic year 2017-18. He is also pursuing his PhD in understanding the temporal processing abilities by hearing-impaired individuals.

Deepti Kakkar was born in 1982, in Jalandhar, Punjab, India. She did her Bachelor of Technology in Electronics and Communication Engineering from Himachal Pradesh University, India in 2003 and Masters of Engineering in Electronics Product Design and Technology from Punjab University, Chandigarh. She did her PhD in the area of Cognitive Radios from Dr B.R. Ambedkar National Institute of Technology, Jalandhar, India. She has a total academic experience of 11 years and at present; she is Assistant Professor in the Department of Electronics and Communication, Dr B. R. Ambedkar National Institute of Technology, Jalandhar, India. Earlier, she had worked as lecturer in the Department of Electronics and Communication, DAV Institute of Engineering and Technology, Jalandhar, Punjab. She has guided 20 postgraduate engineering dissertations and several projects. She is currently guiding 2 PhD theses. She has 20 papers in the proceedings of various International Journals and Conferences. Her recent research interests include cognitive Neuroscience, Neuro-developmental Disorder, Dynamic Spectrum Allocation, Spectrum Sensing, and Cognitive Radios.

Arun Khosla was a renowned professor in the Department of Electronics and Communication Engineering in Dr B R Ambedkar National Institute of Technology, Jalandhar, Punjab. He pursued his Doctor of Philosophy from School of Information Technology (Guru Gobind Singh Indraprastha University, Delhi). His research interests include Soft Computing, Artificial Intelligence and Machine Learning, Assisted Technologies. He has many International and National Journals on his name in the fields like image processing, neurological disorders, etc.

Sushma Kotnala has done her Masters in Applied Psychology and M. Phil (Clinical Psychology). She is working as a Full-time Clinical Psychologist in New Delhi. She was awarded two gold medals in her Masters as well as in her Post Graduation. She has published 2 research papers. Her area of Interest is taking lectures in Psychiatry, Neuro-psychological rehabilitation, childhood developmental disorders and research methodology.

Swapna N. is a Reader in Speech Pathology, Department of Speech-Language Pathology, All India Institute of Speech and Hearing, Mysuru. She is specialized in the area of speech and its disorders, specifically fluency and motor speech disorders. She has various publications to her credit. She has over 20 years of clinical experience in working with individuals with communication disorders. She completed her PhD on fine-grained auditory discrimination in children with learning disability at the University of Mysore in 2005. She has also publications related feeding and swallowing in typically and atypically developing children. She also contributes to teaching undergraduate and postgraduate students.

Vijaya Kumar Narne worked as Reader in audiology at the JSS Institute of speech and hearing, Mysuru from last 1 year. He has secured his post-graduation and PhD in audiology from University of Mysore. His research interest includes understanding the perception of speech in normal and differently able individuals, psychoacoustic and electrophysiology in human auditory system. He has secured 8 grants from All India Institute of Speech and Hearing and 1 extramural grant from Cognitive Science Initiative, Department of Science and Technology. Further, he collaborates nationally and internationally with eminent professors in the field of Audiology. To his credit, he has 24 publications in highly ranked international peer-reviewed journals. He had also guided 20 master's level dissertation students. He is currently pursuing his Post-Doc at Department of Clinical Research, South Denmark University.

G. S. V. Padmakar completed his masters from Dr B R Ambedkar National Institute of Technology, Jalandhar, Punjab. His main research was based on neurological disorders which made him realise the problems faced by the children having different learning disabilities. Later he designed an application for the dyslexics which made them understand the proper writing of letters and various sound-symbol association.

Nicola Pellew, MHSc, is a PhD Health Sciences student in the Department of Interprofessional Health Sciences and Health Administration at Seton Hall University. Nicola joined the School of Health and Medical Science's PhD program in 2017 and plans to defend her dissertation in March 2021. Nicola holds a Master's degree in Health Science Leadership from Saint Francis University, a Postgraduate BSc Honours degree in Biochemistry, and a Bachelor's degree in Biochemistry and Microbiology, both from the College of Agriculture, Engineering, and Science at the University of KwaZulu Natal Pietermaritzburg. Combining her personal experience with autism and her background in Biomedical and Health Sciences, Nicola's research interests involve the use of Complementary and Alternative Therapies, specifically, Animal-assisted therapy, as a cost-effective strategy in healthcare as well as the use of strategy approaches (e.g., leadership) in research and learning.

Prashanth Prabhu received his Masters in Audiology from the University of Mysuru in 2010. In 2010, he was hired as a clinical audiologist at the Department of Audiology, AIISH, Mysuru and is currently working as Lecturer in Audiology at AIISH, Mysuru. His major interest is in auditory neuropathy spectrum disorder. He has published several research articles and has had conference presentations in the area. He is currently working on developing hearing aid modification strategies to help individuals with auditory neuropathy spectrum disorder.

Brajesh Priyadarshi is a Reader in Linguistics at All India Institute of Speech and Hearing, Mysore and has been working in this Institute for the last eleven years. He previously held a teaching position at Ali Yavar Jung National Institute for Hearing Handicapped (AYJNIHH), New Delhi. He completed M.Phil in linguistics in 2002 from the Jawaharlal Nehru University, New Delhi, and was awarded PhD in Linguistics from the same University in 2014. He presently also holds the position of Head, Department of Material Development at All India Institute of Speech and Hearing, Mysore. His areas of interest are research in clinical linguistics and psycho-linguistics. He has completed three research projects as the principal investigator and two projects as the co-investigator. He also has three ongoing projects. He has over 20 publications to his credit, including journal articles, a book and book chapter.

Sunil Kumar Ravi is working as Associate Professor & Principal at Shravana Institute of Speech & Hearing, Ballari, India. He is also the Faculty Consultant for Bachelors of Health Sciences (Majors in Speech & Hearing) at Gulf Medical University, Ajman, United Arab Emirates. He did his M.Sc (Speech-Language Pathology) & PhD (SLP) at AIISH, Mysore. His areas of interest include but are not limited to aphasia, electrophysiology, bilingualism, dementia and child language disorders. He has written a book chapter on 'Fast mapping of novel words in multilingual context' in the book "Handbook of South & Southeast Asian Psycholinguistics", Cambridge University Press, New York. He has published several research papers in national & international journals (Asia Pacific Journal of SLH, International Journal of Multilingualism). He has presented research papers at both International and national level conferences. He has also delivered guest lectures at various conferences and seminars in India. He has been the chair, co-chair and reviewer for scientific sessions on language for various conferences.

Azeez Rizwana has been directly involved in the education of children of varied social backgrounds and intellectual capacities since the past 15 years. Her career spanning roughly two decades has seen her working in the capacity of a school principal, a student counsellor, a researcher and an assistant professor. She may well be regarded as a woman with strong repute and authority in the said discipline. Apart from juggling a family, she gained a B.Sc. and B.Ed. between 1985 and 2004 following which she pursued M.Phil. in Learning disabilities from the University of Mysore in 2010. The zeal to contribute as an educator led to a PhD from the same university in 2016, where she has pioneered a psycholinguistic study using an eye tracker with Urdu as a language of investigation. Apart from garnering accolades at numerous conferences and workshops, she has also been certified by the Maharashtra Dyslexia Association for using DALI, a screening tool prepared by NBRC, Delhi, to screen children with dyslexia. Dr. Azeez now resides in Mysuru with her family and is in the process of conducting a project with DST to screen children from impoverished backgrounds for cognitive impairments. A vision for a school directed at identifying and nurturing children with specific learning disabilities is a near hope.

Srushti S. is a speech-language pathologist who earlier served as a Research Officer in the Department of Speech-Language Pathology and is presently working as an Assistant Professor (Speech-Language Pathology), Shravana Institute of Speech and Hearing, Ballari, Karnataka. She has some publications in the area of feeding in children with communication disorders.

Arun Pratap Singh is currently working as Assistant Professor and Yoga Trainer at Department of Psychology, Mahatma Gandhi Antarrashtriya Hindi Vishwavidyalaya, Wardha (Maharashtra), where he teaches, assesses and coordinates teaching-learning of mainstream psychological and yogic courses in different programmes including B.Ed, M.Ed, B.A., M.A., & M.Phil. After earning PhD in Yoga and Health Psychology from University of Delhi in 2011, he has taught in reputed colleges and private universities i.e. Zakir Husain College, Indraprastha College of Women, Ambedkar College, Galgotias University, Amity University. His areas of interest include mental health, yogic care and life style, spiritual perspectives and psychological perspectives of health. He contributed five chapters in books published by national and international publications and published 25 articles in various national and international peer-reviewed and indexed journals. He has presented 22 research papers both at National and International conferences and also conducted several workshops/symposiums and training programs for professionals and students on yoga therapy. Recently, he has been awarded "Best Yoga Publication of the Year" by School of Ayush Studies and Research under the aegis of Ministry of Ayush, Government of India.

Lalit Kumar Singh is currently working in Lucknow University, in the Department of Psychology. He is a certified mental health professional recognized and certified by Rehabilitation Council of India. His education of psychology is from Delhi University where he has done his M.A., M.Phil in Clinical Psychology from Institute of Human Behaviour and Allied Sciences. He is a Doctorate from Magadh University. He has a rich experience of working at different places including Institute of Human Behaviour and Allied Sciences Delhi, Institute of Mental Health and Hospital Agra, Gautam Buddha University Greater Noida, Dayalbagh University Agra, and Lok Seva Ayog, Allahabad on the post of Superintendent in Social Welfare Department. His interest areas lie in Psychodynamic Psychotherapy, Psychopathology and Sexual Deviance, Spirituality, Neuro-theology and State of mind, Psychoanalysis, libidinal deviance and development of psychopathology. He has conducted many workshops in the area of psychotherapy, dream work, healthy parental training. He has written articles in many national newspapers. He has presented no. of the symposium in national and international conferences, has been invited to chair the scientific session in conferences both in national and international events, and has presented no. of papers in various seminar and conferences.

Kiran Srivastava is presently working as an Assistant Professor in Amity University, Lucknow and completed her Bachelor's degree in Psychology from Calcutta Univesity (2005-2008) after which she did Masters in Clinical Psychology from Barkutallah University, Bhopal. (2008-2010). Then she did M.Phil (RCI Recognised) in Clinical Psychology from Pandit Ravi Shankar Shukla University, Raipur. She started her career in this field as a Lecturer in Noida International University as well as started practicing independently in Amrapali Hospital, Greater Noida (U.P). In 2013, she was appointed as Assistant Professor in the Department Of Clinical Psychology, at the Institute of Mental Health and Hospital, (IMHH) Agra (U.P). Following in the year 2016, she joined Amity University Lucknow as Assistant professor in the Department of Clinical Psychology. Her key interest areas are Psychotherapy (Psychoanalysis, Cognitive Behavior Therapy, and Behavior Modification), Neuropsychology, Rorschach Inkblot Test, IQ assessments. She has published articles in National and International journals, has chaired the session, attended the conference and presented symposium. She has conducted numerous workshops for enriching students' knowledge in this area thus making them more confident in the Professional field.

Komal Srivastava is working as a Senior Dietician in Apollo Gleneagles Hospitals, Kolkata. She has an experience of 11 years and her key area of interest is in Pediatrics Nutrition. She did her Masters in Foods and Nutrition from RVS College of Arts and Science. She enrolled herself in a 6 months PG Diploma Course in Diabetes Educator (recognized by International Diabetes Federation) in 2009 and after clearing her exams she was selected as one of the Master Trainer to teach students the same course. In 2010 she cleared her Registered Dietician Examination and was certified as a Registered Dietician. In 2012 she has enrolled in PhD program and her study topic is on paediatrics nutrition. She has published articles in national and international journals too. As her area of interest is on paediatrics she wants to educate the mothers regarding the nutritional requirements of their kids and steps to be taken to solve their eating problems because according to her healthy child means healthy nation.

Gaurav Thapliyal has done Masters in Psychology, M. Phil (Clinical Psychology) and Post Graduate Diploma in Psychological Counseling. He has done his Post Graduate Diploma in Human Resource Management. He worked as a clinical psychologist in New Delhi from 2015-2016. He is working as an Assistant Professor and clinical psychologist in Secunderabad, Hyderabad from 2016 till now. His areas of Interest are Neuro-developmental disorders, Behavioral medicine, Cognitive rehabilitation and Psychiatry.

Tanu Wadhera has received the B.Tech degree in Electronics and Communication from Guru Nanak Engineering College, Ludhiana, India and M.Tech degree in Electronics & Communication from Punjabi University, Patiala, India. Currently, she is a Research Scholar in National Institute of Technology, Jalandhar, India. Her research interests are cognitive neuroscience, behavioral understanding, technology in autism spectrum disorder, biomedical signal processing, signal classification and prediction of neurodevelopmental disorders.

Index

E

F

G

H

I

T

V

Y

Z

www.ingramcontent.com/pod-product-compliance
Lightning Source LLC
LaVergne TN
LVHW060403300926
849162LV00006B/1336